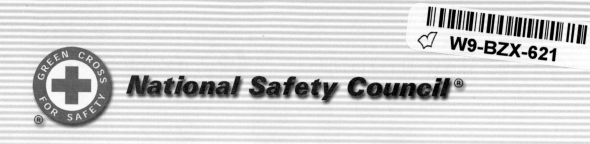

National Safety Council®

First Aid and CPR

Fourth Edition

Alton Thygerson, Ed.D.
Consultant/Medical Writer
National Safety Council

JONES AND BARTLETT PUBLISHERS

Sudbury, Massachusetts

BOSTON   TORONTO   LONDON   SINGAPORE

JONES AND BARTLETT PUBLISHERS

40 Tall Pine Drive, Sudbury, MA 01776
978-443-5000
nsc@jbpub.com
www.nsc.jbpub.com

Jones and Bartlett Publishers Canada
2406 Nikanna Road
Mississauga, ON L5C 2W6
CANADA

Jones and Bartlett Publishers International
Barb House, Barb Mews
London W6 7PA
UK

National Safety Council®

First Aid Institute
1121 Spring Lake Drive
Itasca, IL 60143-3201
(630) 285-1121
(800) 621-7619
www.nsc.org

General Manager of Public Safety Group:
Donna Siegfried

Production Credits

Chief Executive Officer: Clayton E. Jones
Chief Operating Officer: Donald W. Jones, Jr.
Executive V.P. and Publisher: Tom Manning
V.P. and Managing Editor: Judith H. Hauck
V.P., Sales and Marketing: Paul Shepardson
V.P., Production and Design: Anne Spencer
V.P., Manufacturing and
  Inventory Control: Therese Bräuer
Publisher, EMS & Aquatics: Lawrence D. Newell
Emergency Care Senior
  Acquisitions Editor: Tracy Foss
Director of Marketing, EMS
  and Health Sciences: Kimberly Brophy
Emergency Care Associate Editor: Jennifer Reed

Production Editor: Linda S. DeBruyn
Interactive Technology Director: W. Scott Smith
Text Design: Studio Montage
Typesetting and Editorial: Nesbitt Graphics
Illustrations: Rolin Graphics
Interior Photos: Richard Nye
Cover Design: Studio Montage
Cover Photographs (clockwise from top left):
  © Brian Pieters, Masterfile;
  © Wedgworth, Custom Medical Stock Photo;
  Steve Ferry, P&F Communications;
  Richard Nye
Printing and Binding: Courier Company

Library of Congress Cataloging-in-Publication Data

First Aid and CPR/National Safety Council.—4th ed.
    p. cm.
Previous editions entered under title.
Includes index.
ISBN 0-7637-1319-8 (alk. paper)
1. First aid in illness and injury. 2. CPR (First aid) I. National Safety Council. II. Title.
RC86.7.T466 2000
616.02'52–dc21   00-049739

Additional illustrations and photo credits appear on page 448, which constitutes a continuation of the copyright page.

Printed in the United States of America
05 04 03 02 01   10 9 8 7 6 5 4 3 2 1

What's New

When an emergency strikes, knowing what to do is critical. That is why the National Safety Council's First Aid and CPR course is invaluable.

The foundation of the course is *First Aid and CPR*, Fourth Edition. This book is the cornerstone of an integrated training program that combines comprehensive first aid and CPR content with exciting new features, design, and technology to better support instructors and to prepare students for any emergency.

First Aid and CPR, Fourth Edition contains:

 The latest Cardiopulmonary Resuscitation and Emergency Cardiac Care Guidelines

 Expanded Coverage of Automated External Defibrillators

 Interactive Web Activities

 Exciting new features including Newsbytes and First Aid Tips

 Newly designed and easy-to-follow Action Guides and Skill Scans

Resource Preview

This textbook is the core of the First Aid and CPR program with features that will reinforce and expand on the essential information.

Features include:

Action Guides
Accompanying every first aid skill, there is a flowchart to reinforce the decision-making process and appropriate first aid procedures.

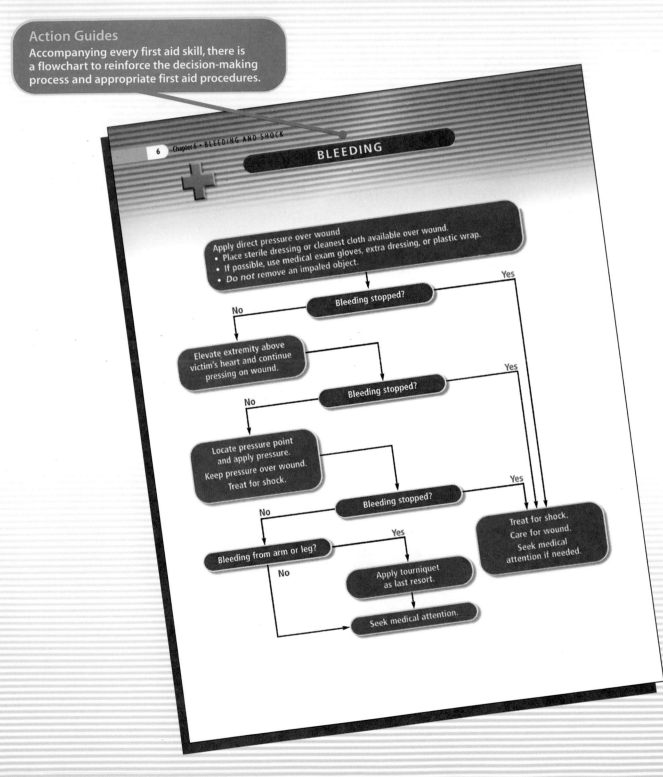

Resource Preview

Skill Scans

Skill Scans provide short, step-by-step visual reviews of first aid procedures discussed in detail within the chapter.

Skill Scan

One-Person Moves

1. *Human crutch* (one person helps victim to walk). If one leg is injured, help the victim to walk on the good leg while you support the injured side.

2. *Cradle carry.* Use for children and lightweight adults who cannot walk.

3. *Firefighter's carry.* If the victim's injuries permit, you can travel longer distances if you carry the victim over your shoulder.

4. *Pack-strap carry.* When injuries make the fireman's carry unsafe, this method is better for longer distances.

5. *Piggyback carry.* Use this method when the victim cannot walk but can use the arms to hang onto the rescuer.

Resource Preview

Caution
Learning what *not* to do in an emergency is critical when seconds count.

First Aid Tips
These tips provide instant experience from masters of the trade.

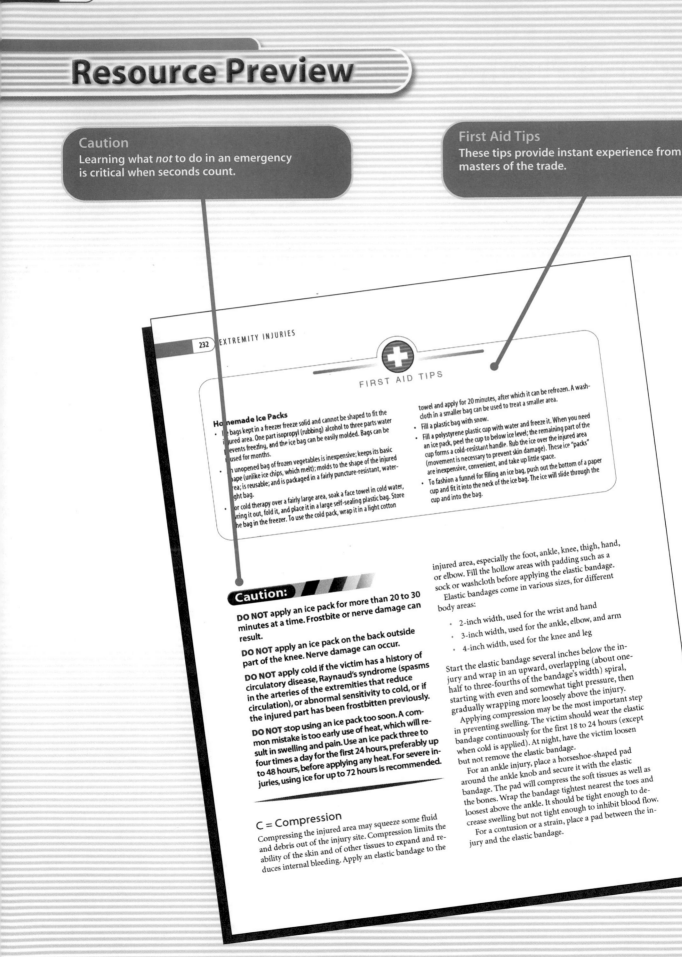

232   EXTREMITY INJURIES

FIRST AID TIPS

Homemade Ice Packs
- Ice bags kept in a freezer freeze solid and cannot be shaped to fit the injured area. One part isopropyl (rubbing) alcohol to three parts water prevents freezing, and the ice bag can be easily molded. Bags can be used for months.
- An unopened bag of frozen vegetables is inexpensive; keeps its basic shape (unlike ice chips, which melt); molds to the shape of the injured area; is reusable; and is packaged in a fairly puncture-resistant, water-tight bag.
- For cold therapy over a fairly large area, soak a face towel in cold water, wring it out, fold it, and place it in a large self-sealing plastic bag. Store the bag in the freezer. To use the cold pack, wrap it in a light cotton

- towel and apply for 20 minutes, after which it can be refrozen. A washcloth in a smaller bag can be used to treat a smaller area.
- Fill a plastic bag with snow.
- Fill a polystyrene plastic cup with water and freeze it. When you need an ice pack, peel the cup to below ice level; the remaining part of the cup forms a cold-resistant handle. Rub the ice over the injured area (movement is necessary to prevent skin damage). These ice "packs" are inexpensive, convenient, and take up little space.
- To fashion a funnel for filling an ice bag, push out the bottom of a paper cup and fit it into the neck of the ice bag. The ice will slide through the cup and into the bag.

Caution:

DO NOT apply an ice pack for more than 20 to 30 minutes at a time. Frostbite or nerve damage can result.

DO NOT apply an ice pack on the back outside part of the knee. Nerve damage can occur.

DO NOT apply cold if the victim has a history of circulatory disease, Raynaud's syndrome (spasms in the arteries of the extremities that reduce circulation), or abnormal sensitivity to cold, or if the injured part has been frostbitten previously.

DO NOT stop using an ice pack too soon. A common mistake is too early use of heat, which will result in swelling and pain. Use an ice pack three to four times a day for the first 24 hours, preferably up to 48 hours, before applying any heat. For severe injuries, using ice for up to 72 hours is recommended.

C = Compression
Compressing the injured area may squeeze some fluid and debris out of the injury site. Compression limits the ability of the skin and of other tissues to expand and reduces internal bleeding. Apply an elastic bandage to the injured area, especially the foot, ankle, knee, thigh, hand, or elbow. Fill the hollow areas with padding such as a sock or washcloth before applying the elastic bandage.

Elastic bandages come in various sizes, for different body areas:

- 2-inch width, used for the wrist and hand
- 3-inch width, used for the ankle, elbow, and arm
- 4-inch width, used for the knee and leg

Start the elastic bandage several inches below the injury and wrap in an upward, overlapping (about one-half to three-fourths of the bandage's width) spiral, starting with even and somewhat tight pressure, then gradually wrapping more loosely above the injury.

Applying compression may be the most important step in preventing swelling. The victim should wear the elastic bandage continuously for the first 18 to 24 hours (except when cold is applied). At night, have the victim loosen but not remove the elastic bandage.

For an ankle injury, place a horseshoe-shaped pad around the ankle knob and secure it with the elastic bandage. The pad will compress the soft tissues as well as the bones. Wrap the bandage tightest nearest the toes and loosest above the ankle. It should be tight enough to decrease swelling but not tight enough to inhibit blood flow.

For a contusion or a strain, place a pad between the injury and the elastic bandage.

Resource Preview

Newsbytes
Newsbytes illustrate first aid issues in the real world.

FYI
FYI delves deeper into topics of interest and provides a better understanding of first aid and CPR.

Balloons: Serious Choking Hazard for Children

Ordinary balloons can be deadly if they are inhaled while inflated, partially inflated, or after bursting into fragments, according to a study of 449 children who died from choking on foreign objects. Balloons were responsible for more deaths than any other non-food object. Balls and marbles were next on the hazard list. Balloons pose a greater threat than solid objects that are swallowed because balloons conform to the shape of the breathing passage and thus block it more completely.

Source: F. L. Rimell, et al., "Characteristics of Objects that Cause Choking in Children," *Journal of the American Medical Association* 274:1763, December 13, 1995.

If the breaths do not go in, retilt the victim's head and try breaths again. If breaths still do not go in, the airway is likely obstructed. See the section on unresponsive choking management on page 87.

If the breaths go in and the infant has a pulse, continue giving rescue breathing. Because infants breathe faster than adults, breathe into an infant once every three seconds. Between breaths, remove your mouth from the victim's to allow air to flow out of the victim's lungs. As you remove your mouth, you should turn your head to the side to see if the victim's chest fell after each breath. For rescue breathing, breathe into the infant for the first second, count "one—one thousand," then take a breath yourself for the third second.

Gastric Distention

Rescue breaths tend to cause stomach or gastric distention more often in infants than in adults. Minimize this problem by limiting the breaths to the amount needed to make the chest rise. Avoid overinflating the lungs. Gastric distention can cause regurgitation and aspiration of stomach contents.

Check for Signs of Circulation

After the two breaths have been given, check for signs of circulation.

If signs of circulation exists but breathing is absent, continue rescue breathing. Give a rescue breath once every three seconds. After 20 breaths, you should activate EMS.

Chest Compressions

An infant without signs of circulation requires both rescue breathing and chest compressions. The proper chest compression point in an infant is midsternum, between the infant's nipples. Place three fingers (index, middle, and ring) on the chest, with the index finger next to the imaginary nipple line on the infant's feet side. Lift the index finger off the chest.

Use the two remaining fingers to apply the chest compressions. Press the infant's midsternum (area between the nipples) ½ to 1 inch into the chest with the middle and ring finger. Either place your other hand under the infant's shoulder to provide support or keep it on the infant's forehead to keep the head tilted. If the infant is carried during CPR, the length of the body is on the rescuer's forearm with the head kept level with the trunk.

The infant compression rate is 100 per minute. External chest compressions must always be combined with rescue breathing. The ratio of compressions to breaths is five to one. Each series of five compressions is performed while the rescuer says aloud "One, two, three, four, five." After

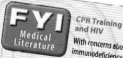

CPR Training and HIV

With concerns about the human immunodeficiency virus (HIV) and other infectious agents, many people are wondering whether disinfection procedures used on CPR-training manikins are adequate to prevent the transmission of diseases. Routine disinfection with 70% isopropyl alcohol is enough to prevent the spread of the virus that causes AIDS.

Although there have been no cases to date of HIV transmitted by CPR manikins, the virus is found in saliva and can survive for a time on plastic material. While the risk is minimal, it is important to ease fears about disease transmission since CPR training is widespread.

The preferred method of disinfecting equipment is to use bleach solution, with isopropyl alcohol available as an option. When isopropyl alcohol is used, it is supposed to be applied to the manikin for 60 seconds.

Source: I. B. Corless, et al., "Decontamination of an HIV-infected CPR Manikin," *American Journal of Public Health* 82:1542–43, 1992.

Resource Preview

Web Activities
The Web Activities further reinforce and expand on information discussed in the chapters through interactive exercises.

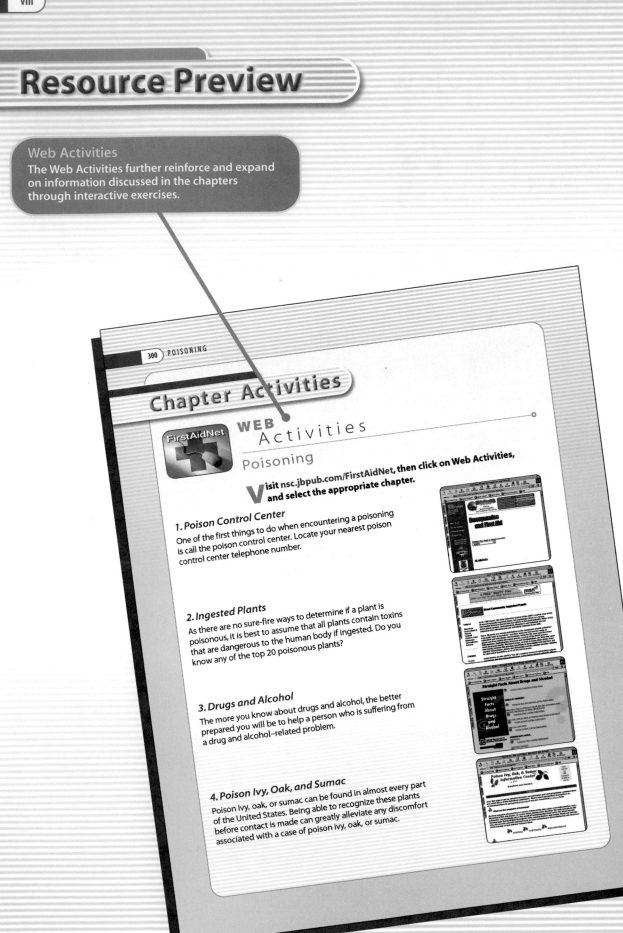

Chapter Activities

WEB Activities

Poisoning

FirstAidNet

Visit nsc.jbpub.com/FirstAidNet, then click on Web Activities, and select the appropriate chapter.

1. Poison Control Center
One of the first things to do when encountering a poisoning is call the poison control center. Locate your nearest poison control center telephone number.

2. Ingested Plants
As there are no sure-fire ways to determine if a plant is poisonous, it is best to assume that all plants contain toxins that are dangerous to the human body if ingested. Do you know any of the top 20 poisonous plants?

3. Drugs and Alcohol
The more you know about drugs and alcohol, the better prepared you will be to help a person who is suffering from a drug and alcohol–related problem.

4. Poison Ivy, Oak, and Sumac
Poison ivy, oak, or sumac can be found in almost every part of the United States. Being able to recognize these plants before contact is made can greatly alleviate any discomfort associated with a case of poison ivy, oak, or sumac.

Resource Preview

Study Questions
Study Questions provide an opportunity to test your knowledge of the first aid skills presented in each chapter. It allows you to discover where your knowledge is strong and where it needs improving.

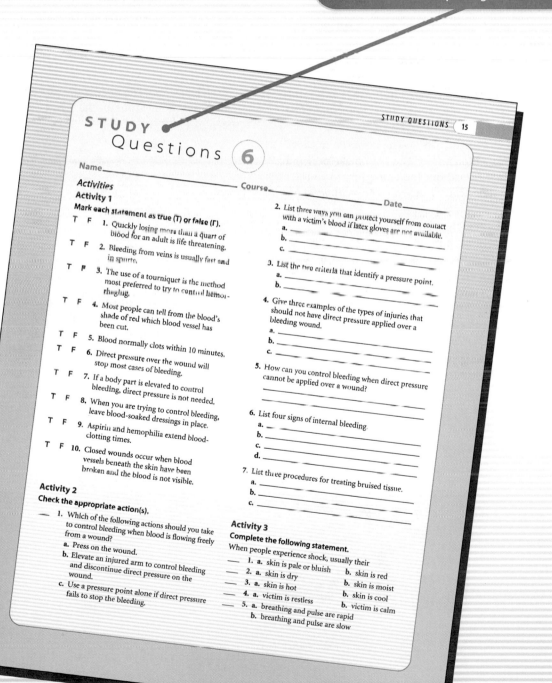

STUDY QUESTIONS 15

STUDY Questions 6

Name_____

Course_____

Date_____

Activities

Activity 1

Mark each statement as true (T) or false (F).

T F 1. Quickly losing more than a quart of blood for an adult is life threatening.

T F 2. Bleeding from veins is usually fast and in spurts.

T F 3. The use of a tourniquet is the method most preferred to try to control hemorrhaging.

T F 4. Most people can tell from the blood's shade of red which blood vessel has been cut.

T F 5. Blood normally clots within 10 minutes.

T F 6. Direct pressure over the wound will stop most cases of bleeding.

T F 7. If a body part is elevated to control bleeding, direct pressure is not needed.

T F 8. When you are trying to control bleeding, leave blood-soaked dressings in place.

T F 9. Aspirin and hemophilia extend blood-clotting times.

T F 10. Closed wounds occur when blood vessels beneath the skin have been broken and the blood is not visible.

Activity 2

Check the appropriate action(s).

_____ 1. Which of the following actions should you take to control bleeding when blood is flowing freely from a wound?

a. Press on the wound.

b. Elevate an injured arm to control bleeding and discontinue direct pressure on the wound.

c. Use a pressure point alone if direct pressure fails to stop the bleeding.

2. List three ways you can protect yourself from contact with a victim's blood if latex gloves are not available.

a. _____

b. _____

c. _____

3. List the two criteria that identify a pressure point.

a. _____

b. _____

4. Give three examples of the types of injuries that should not have direct pressure applied over a bleeding wound.

a. _____

b. _____

c. _____

5. How can you control bleeding when direct pressure cannot be applied over a wound?

_____

_____

6. List four signs of internal bleeding.

a. _____

b. _____

c. _____

d. _____

7. List three procedures for treating bruised tissue.

a. _____

b. _____

c. _____

Activity 3

Complete the following statement.

When people experience shock, usually their

_____ 1. a. skin is pale or bluish   b. skin is red

_____ 2. a. skin is dry   b. skin is moist

_____ 3. a. skin is hot   b. skin is cool

_____ 4. a. victim is restless   b. victim is calm

_____ 5. a. breathing and pulse are rapid

b. breathing and pulse are slow

Instructor Resources

Instructor's ToolKit CD-ROM

Teaching your First Aid and CPR course has never been easier! Putting technology to work for you, the Instructor's ToolKit CD-ROM gives you more options and flexibility than you ever had before, and saves you time! For each chapter in the textbook, you'll find:

Lecture Outlines—This is a complete, ready-to-use lesson plan from the Instructor's Manual that outlines all of the topics covered in the text. It is provided in an electronic format that can be modified and customized to fit your course.

PowerPoint Presentations—The PowerPoint slides provide you with a powerful way to make presentations that are educational and engaging to your students. The slides can be modified and edited to fit your individual presentation.

Lecture Success—This feature makes available images from the textbook, both photographs and illustrations. With Lecture Success, you can incorporate more graphics into your PowerPoint presentations, make handouts, or enlarge a specific image for further classroom discussion.

TestBank—Provides over 1,000 questions that correspond to the chapters in the text.

Video Clips—These clips allow you to illustrate the most important skills students need to learn in a First Aid and CPR course.

ISBN: 0-7637-1618-9

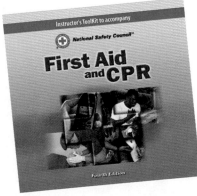

Instructor's Resource Manual

The Instructor's Resource Manual is designed to be your reference guide and includes:

- detailed lesson plans with sample lectures, teaching strategies, supplemental information, and suggested readings
- teaching tips and ideas to enhance your presentation
- proficiency tests and answers to all end-of-chapter study questions found in the text

ISBN: 0-7637-1622-7

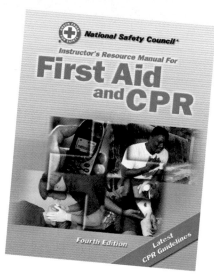

Instructor Resources

First Aid Video

The First Aid Video combines real-life situations with an instructional classroom format to teach the essential skills of first aid.
(approx. 42 minutes)
ISBN: 0-7637-1624-3

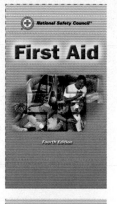

CPR Video

The CPR Video combines real-life situations with an instructional classroom format to teach the essential skills of CPR. This video provides information that is consistent with the 2000 International CPR and ECC guidelines.
(approx. 29 minutes)
ISBN: 0-7637-1625-1

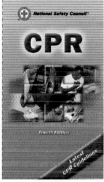

Instructor's Slide Set

80 informative slides emphasize key points and stimulate classroom discussion with realistic examples of first aid and CPR training.
ISBN: 0-7637-1623-5

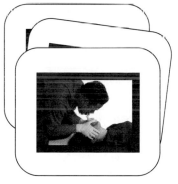

Trauma Slide Set

Bring the real world to your classroom discussion with approximately 80 real-life trauma slides, depicting actual injuries.
ISBN: 0-7637-1700-2

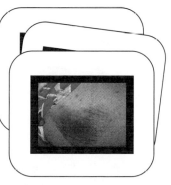

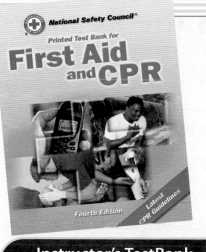

Instructor's TestBank (printed)

Over 1,100 test questions that correspond to the chapters in the text. An electronic version of the TestBank is included on the Instructor's ToolKit CD-ROM.
ISBN: 0-7637-1621-9

Teaching Packages

The Teaching Package combines:
- Instructor's ToolKit CD-ROM
- Instructor's Resource Manual
- First Aid and CPR Videos
- Instructor's Slide Set
- and textbook

all in one convenient box.
ISBN: 0-7637-1672-3

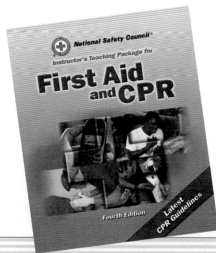

Online Resources | www.nsc.jbpub.com

A key component in our program, innovative and interactive activities help students become first aiders.

Features include:

Chapter Activities
Provide information that expands on the subjects presented in each chapter and interactive exercises to increase understanding.

Anatomy Review
Tests student's knowledge of human anatomy through figure-labeling exercises.

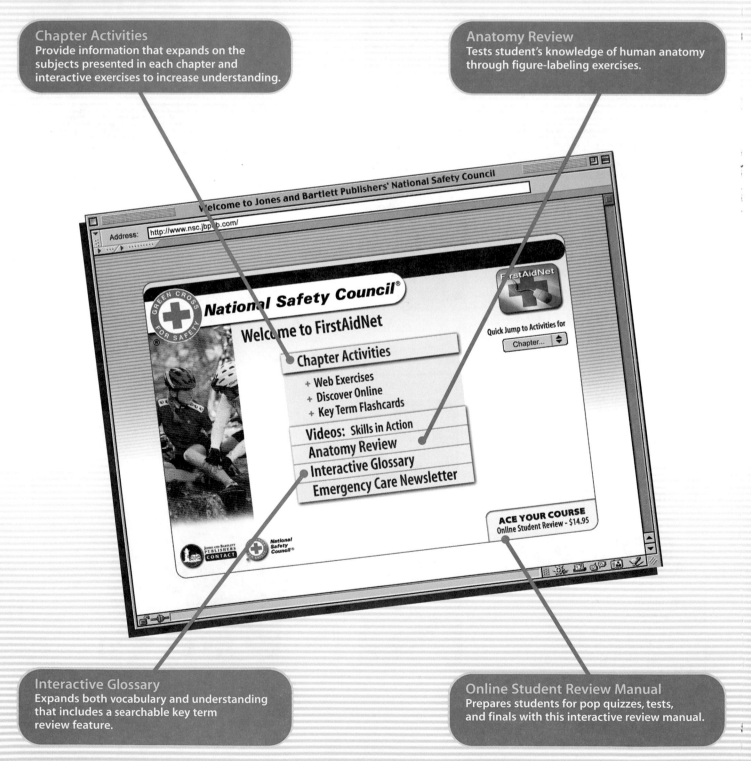

Interactive Glossary
Expands both vocabulary and understanding that includes a searchable key term review feature.

Online Student Review Manual
Prepares students for pop quizzes, tests, and finals with this interactive review manual.

Online Resources | www.nsc.jbpub.com

Make full use of today's teaching and learning technologies.
Instructor Resources include:

Benefits of National Safety Council Educational Training Centers
Provides an administrative overview of the National Safety Council

Becoming a National Safety Council Educational Training Center
Includes online submission of:
• Educational Training Center Department Application Form
• Online Instructor Examination

Address: http://www.nsc.jbpub.com/

Welcome to Jones and Bartlett Publishers' National Safety Council

National Safety Council®

SUBCRIBE to the Emergency Care Newsletter

Benefits of National Safety Council Educational Training Centers

Becoming a National Safety Council Educational Training Center

Obtaining Course Completion Cards

News – Including the Emergency Care Newsletter

National Safety Council Partner Organizations

Becoming a National Safety Council Educational Training Center

Becoming a National Safety Council Educational Training Center is Easy! Academic Instructors, click here to enter.

Attention Academic Instructors!
Challenge your knowledge of first aid and CPR through our on-line testing system.
Click here to enter.

HOME

Online Instructor Resources

National Safety Council Programs

FirstAidNet

JONES AND BARTLETT PUBLISHERS CONTACT

National Safety Council®

Direct Communications Link with the National Safety Council and Jones and Bartlett Publishers
News includes:
• Emergency Care Newsletter, a free resource with the latest trends in emergency care, medical journal reviews, teaching strategies, information on upcoming conferences and conventions, and much more
• Emergency Care Newsletter Archives
• Bulletin Board where instructors share resources and ideas

Obtaining Course Completion Cards Provides
• Terms of Course Completion Cards
• Online Course Completion Card Request Form

Student Resources

Interactive First Aid and CPR CD-ROM

This interactive CD-ROM covers all key first aid and CPR material. It offers students a chance to test their knowledge of key topics and procedures through scenario-based learning and full motion video clips.

ISBN: 0-7637-1617-0

Online Student Review Manual

The Online Student Review Manual is designed to evaluate mastery of material learned in class and covered in *First Aid and CPR,* Fourth Edition. Each chapter in the book is supplemented with:

- an exam consisting of 20 to 40 multiple-choice questions to test students' knowledge of key concepts and procedures
- a special grading feature for immediate results and answers to all of the questions
- a chapter correlation of the question/answer to the *Fourth Edition*

ISBN: 0-7637-1716-9

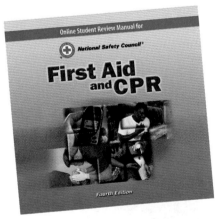

CyberClass Edition of First Aid and CPR, Fourth Edition

CyberClass is a customizable, web-based course management resource that offers distance learning tools for you and your students. It requires no special resources and very little technological expertise on your part. Your set-up time is minimal; post assignments, administer tests, maintain an online grade book, and much more. . .all online.

CyberClass tools include:

Syllabus—Customize the pre-loaded syllabus or load your own and update it during class.

Hot Links—Add your own links to those that come pre-loaded from FirstAidNet.

Assignments—Submit course assignments electronically.

Flashcards and CyberChallenges—Provide an excellent practice and a fun way to learn.

Testing—Create a web-based exam from the pre-loaded question bank that is automatically graded, or create your own custom exam. Students can complete exams online and grades can automatically be added to your online grade book.

Bulletin Board—Post assignments, PowerPoint presentations, discussion topics, and other messages in a central location.

Messaging—Internal e-mail capabilities allow you to communicate with your students.

Chat Sessions—Hold chat sessions for online office hours, mini-lectures, group work, and discussion groups. Respond to students in real time!

Course Administration—Set preferences, modify the student roster, and keep an online grade book.

ISBN: 0-7637-1616-2

About the National Safety Council Program

Congratulations on selecting the National Safety Council's First Aid and CPR program! You join good company, as the National Safety Council has successfully trained over 6 million people worldwide in first aid and cardiopulmonary resuscitation (CPR). The National Safety Council's training network of nearly 10,000 instructors at over 4,000 sites worldwide has established the National Safety Council programs as the standard by which all others are judged.

In setting the standards, the National Safety Council has worked in close cooperation with hundreds of national and international organizations, thousands of corporations, thousands of leading educators, dozens of leading medical organizations, and hundreds of state and local governmental agencies. Their collective input has helped create programs that stand alone in quality. Consider just a few of the National Safety Council's current collaborations:

World's Leading Medical Organizations

The National Safety Council is currently working with both the American Academy of Orthopedic Surgeons (AAOS), Wilderness Medical Society (WMS), and the American Heart Association to help bring innovative, new training programs to the marketplace. The National Safety Council and the AAOS are developing a new First Responder program and the National Safety Council and the WMS are developing the first of its kind wilderness first aid program.

Spanning the Globe

Across the globe, from Boston to Bangkok, from Miami to Milan, from Seattle to Stockholm, people are trained with National Safety Council programs. National Safety Council first aid and CPR programs are already used in your area.

World's Leading Corporations

Thousands of corporations including Westinghouse, Exxon, General Motors, Ameritech, and U.S. West have selected many of the National Safety Council emergency care programs to train employees.

World's Leading Colleges and Universities

Hundreds of leading colleges and universities are working closely with the National Safety Council to fully develop and implement the Internet Initiative that will establish the National Safety Council as the leading online provider of emergency care programs.

Most importantly, in selecting the National Safety Council programs, you can feel confident that the programs are of the highest quality. You can rely on the National Safety Council. Founded in 1913, the National Safety Council is dedicated to protecting life, promoting health, and reducing accidental death. For nearly 90 years, the National Safety Council has been the world's leading authority on safety/injury education.

National Safety Council ®

Benefits Offered Exclusively by the National Safety Council and Jones and Bartlett Publishers

Ease of administration

Academic departments with certified first aid and CPR instructors are able to offer any National Safety Council program by completing a simple application authorized by the department chair or course coordinator.

Academic freedom to structure your course so it meets your needs, and the needs of your students: National Safety Council programs are designed specifically for the academic classroom. Our flexible academic programs allow you to determine the most appropriate course:

- Content
- Length
- Structure
- Testing
- Proficiency Standards

Cutting-edge multimedia teaching and learning tools

Our CD-ROMs, videos, and web-enhanced programs integrate the classroom with technology for an interactive learning experience.

Just for you, we have an Instructor's ToolKit CD-ROM complete with adaptable PowerPoint presentations and a customizable TestBank. You'll also receive a free monthly electronic Emergency Care Newsletter to keep you up-to-date with industry trends.

FREE Course Completion Cards

Once approved as an Educational Training Center, you will be able to obtain nationally recognized and accepted course completion cards for your students with just a quick phone call, e-mail, or online submission.

There are no hoops to jump through or additional fees to you or your students for the course completion cards your students have earned.

One-stop shopping

From first aid to bloodborne pathogens, the National Safety Council can fulfill your training needs with completely integrated teaching and learning systems.

No hidden costs for academic institutions

This includes FREE instructor's support materials to qualified adopters. All Educational Training Centers are eligible to receive free Instructor's Manuals. Qualified Educational Training Centers are also eligible for free Instructor's Teaching Packages, based on the total number of textbooks ordered annually.

A wide variety of teaching support materials are available with every program to make teaching easy, comprehensive, and authoritative. These materials include Instructor's ToolKit CD-ROMs, Instructor's Manuals, Printed and Computerized TestBanks, Instructor's Slide Sets, and Videos.

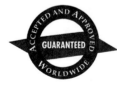

Worldwide acceptance, approval, and guarantee of all programs: Unconditional Guarantee

If for some reason, somewhere, someone does not approve or accept the National Safety Council course completion cards, we will pay all course fees for that student to take a comparable course that is accepted. Simple as that! Now you can be 100% confident in making the switch to the user-friendly National Safety Council programs.

Clayton E. Jones
Chief Executive Officer
Jones and Bartlett Publishers

Reviewers

The National Safety Council acknowledges the following individuals for assistance on reviewing this text and/or previous editions:

Donna Siegfried
National Safety Council

Sharon Adams
Spokane Community College

Frank Amato
Indian River Community College

Michael Ballard
Morehead State University

Lori Carter
University of North Florida

Franklin Carver
Ohio University

Frank Chapman
University of North Carolina - Wilmington

Les Chatelain
University of Utah

Harvey Clearwater
University of Maryland, College Park

Vonnie Clovin
University of Kentucky

Kate Cunningham
Valencia State Community College

Caprice Dodson
Houston Community College

Greg Goebel
Southeast Community College

Robin Gurgainus
James Sprint Community College

John Healey
Lane Community College

Bert Hood
Arizona Chapter, National Safety Council

Kathy Hudson
Hudson County Public Schools

Tim Kayhill
Eastern Kentucky University

Jogoon Kim
Michigan State University

Marian King
North Atlanta High School

Laura Kitzmiller
Texas A&M

Frank Lagotic
Santa Fe Community College

Harold Leibowitz
Brooklyn College

Paula Linder
University of Maine, Orno

Brent Mangus
University of Nevada, Las Vegas

Dwaine J. Marten
University of Idaho

Debbie Moffett
Miami Dade Community College - Kendall Campus

Debra Murray
University of North Carolina, Chapel Hill

Jerry Nauman
Winona State University

Bruce Norris
West Chester University

Sharon Ogle
Brevard Community College

Glen Payton
Texas Christian University

Allan Peterson
Gordon College

Ron Pfeiffer
Boise State University

Scott Richter
University of Montana

Scott Roberts
SUNY College at Buffalo

Sherm Sowby
California State University, Fresno

David Spiro, EMT-P
Hartsdale, NY

Larry Starr
SOS Technologies

Jessie Stoner
Florida Community College at Jacksonville

Jeannie Stream
Danville Area Community College

Lance Tatum
Gordon College

Maggie Tucker
University of Florida, Gainsville

Harry Tyson
Bowling Green University

Andrew Weinberg, MD
Miami University

Deitra Wengert
Towson State University

C. Newton Wilkes
Northwestern State University

John Wingfield
Ball State University

Acknowledgments

The National Safety Council acknowledges the following organizations for assistance reviewing this text and/or previous editions:

American Academy of Ophthalmology

American Academy of Orthopaedic Surgeons

American Academy of Safety Education

American Alliance for Health, Physical Education, Recreation, and Dance

American Burn Association

American Camping Association

American Civil Defense Association

American College of Surgeons

American Dental Association

American Diabetes Association

American Equine Association

American Heart Association

American Medical Association

American Medical Equestrian Association

American Trauma Association

Aquatic Exercise Association

Association for the Advancement of Automotive Medicine

Basic Trauma Life Support

Boy Scouts of America

Canadian Association of Fire Chiefs

Emergency Nurses Association

Emergency Response Institute

Epilepsy Foundation

Girl Scouts, USA

Jeff Ellis & Associates

International Association of Fire Fighters

International Society of Fire Service Instructors

Medic Alert Foundation

Mine Safety and Health Administration

National Academy of Emergency Medical Dispatch

National Association of EMS Physicians

National Athletic Trainers Association

National Center on Child Abuse and Neglect

National Emergency Number Association

National Highway Traffic Safety Administration

National Institute of Burn Medicine

National Oceanic and Atmospheric Association

National Recreation and Park Administration

National Registry of Emergency Medical Technicians

National Rescue Consultants

National Safety Council

National Ski Patrol

Occupational Safety and Health Administration

Prevent Blindness, America

U.S. Airforce

U.S. Army

U.S. Centers for Disease Control and Prevention

U.S. Coast Guard

U.S. Consumer Product Safety Commission

U.S. Department of Health and Human Services

U.S. Public Health Service

Wilderness Medical Society

Young Men's Christian Association

Brief Contents

Table of Contents
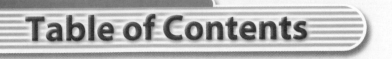

PART 1 INTRODUCTION

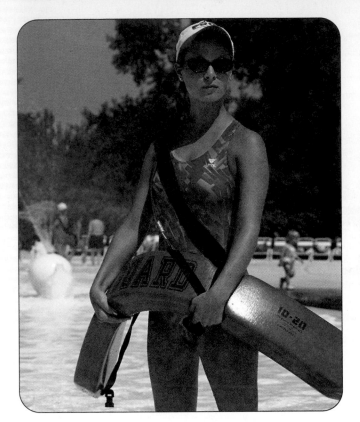

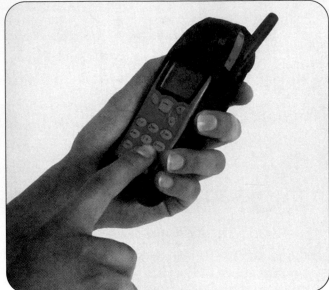

PART 2 VICTIM ASSESSMENT

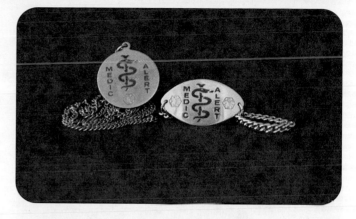

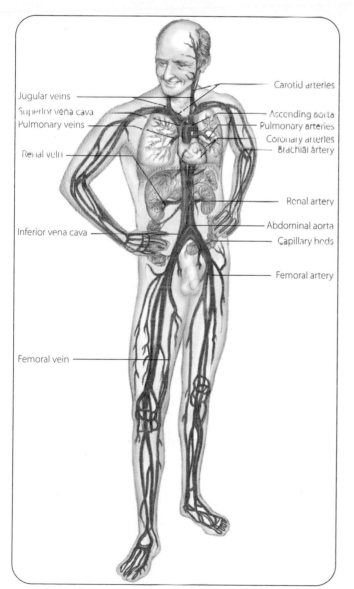

Jugular veins

Superior vena cava

Pulmonary veins

Renal vein

Inferior vena cava

Femoral vein

Carotid arteries

Ascending aorta

Pulmonary arteries

Coronary arteries

Brachial artery

Renal artery

Abdominal aorta

Capillary beds

Femoral artery

PART 3 LIFE-THREATENING EMERGENCIES

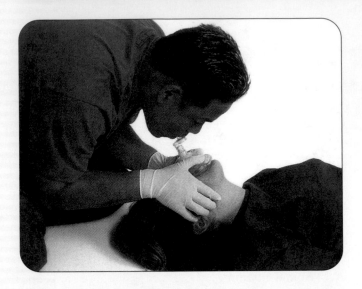

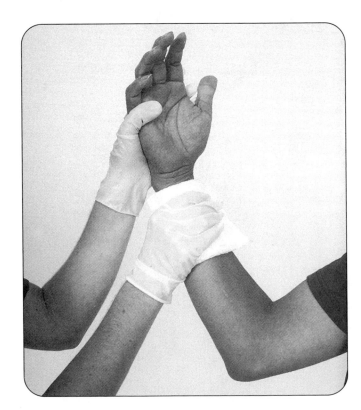

PART 4 INJURIES

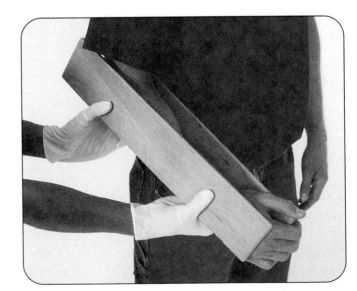

PART 5 MEDICAL EMERGENCIES

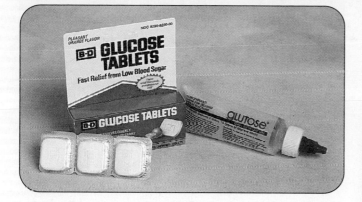

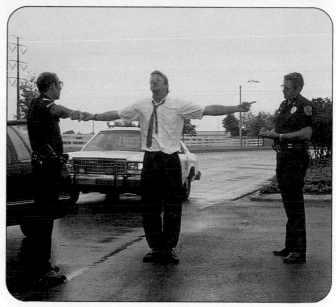

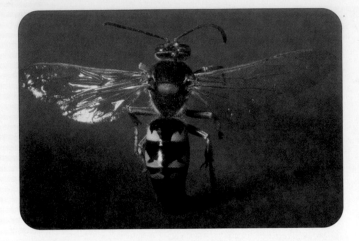

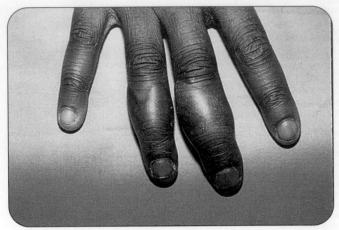

PART 6 SPECIAL SITUATIONS

Your First Aid & CPR IQ

Test your current knowledge. Read each question and place your answer in the "Pre-check" column. After reading this manual and completing your course, read the questions again and place your answers in the "Post-check" column. Compare your answers and see what you have learned.

Question	Pre-check			Post-check		
1. Most communities use 9-1-1 as their emergency telephone number.	T	F	Uncertain	T	F	Uncertain
2. Most injured victims require a complete physical exam.	T	F	Uncertain	T	F	Uncertain
3. Someone coughing forcefully may be choking, and abdominal thrusts should be given.	T	F	Uncertain	T	F	Uncertain
4. Unresponsive breathing victims should be placed on their side.	T	F	Uncertain	T	F	Uncertain
5. Adult CPR requires the rescuer to give 5 chest compressions and 1 rescue breath.	T	F	Uncertain	T	F	Uncertain
6. Rescue breathing should be given to any unresponsive, non-breathing victim.	T	F	Uncertain	T	F	Uncertain
7. Open a victim's airway by tilting the head back and lifting the chin.	T	F	Uncertain	T	F	Uncertain
8. Direct pressure and elevation can control most injuries involving bleeding.	T	F	Uncertain	T	F	Uncertain
9. Heat should be applied quickly to any muscle, bone or joint injuries to reduce swelling.	T	F	Uncertain	T	F	Uncertain
10. Applying butter is an effective treatment for first degree burns.	T	F	Uncertain	T	F	Uncertain
11. An object impaled (stuck) in the body should removed so that bleeding can be controlled.	T	F	Uncertain	T	F	Uncertain
12. A splint is something used to stabilize (reduce movement) a broken bone.	T	F	Uncertain	T	F	Uncertain
13. Chest pain is one of the most frequent signals of a heart attack.	T	F	Uncertain	T	F	Uncertain
14. Sugar should be given to a victim suspected of suffering a diabetic emergency.	T	F	Uncertain	T	F	Uncertain
15. Syrup of ipecac should be given to a person who has ingested a corrosive poisonous substance.	T	F	Uncertain	T	F	Uncertain
16. Ice should be applied to a snakebite wound.	T	F	Uncertain	T	F	Uncertain
17. Rub or massage a frostbitten part to quickly rewarm it.	T	F	Uncertain	T	F	Uncertain
18. Salt tablets should be given to victims of heat emergencies.	T	F	Uncertain	T	F	Uncertain
19. Hypothermia occurs only in subfreezing temperatures.	T	F	Uncertain	T	F	Uncertain
20. Extremely hot skin indicates heat exhaustion.	T	F	Uncertain	T	F	Uncertain

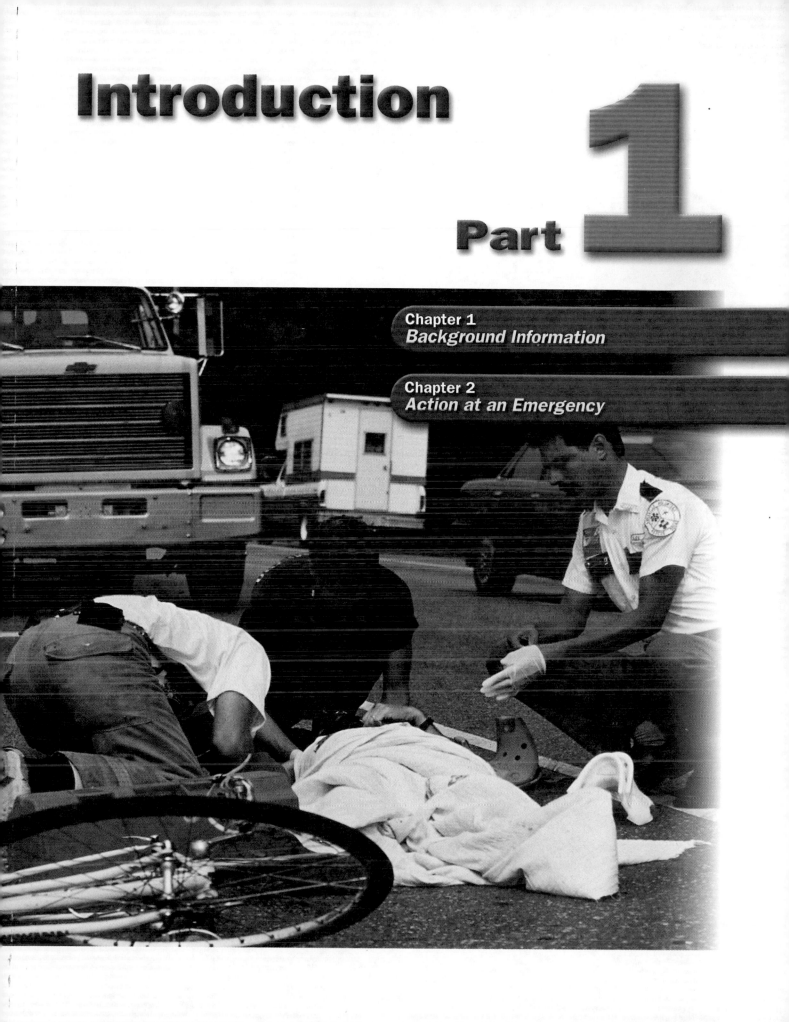

Introduction

Part 1

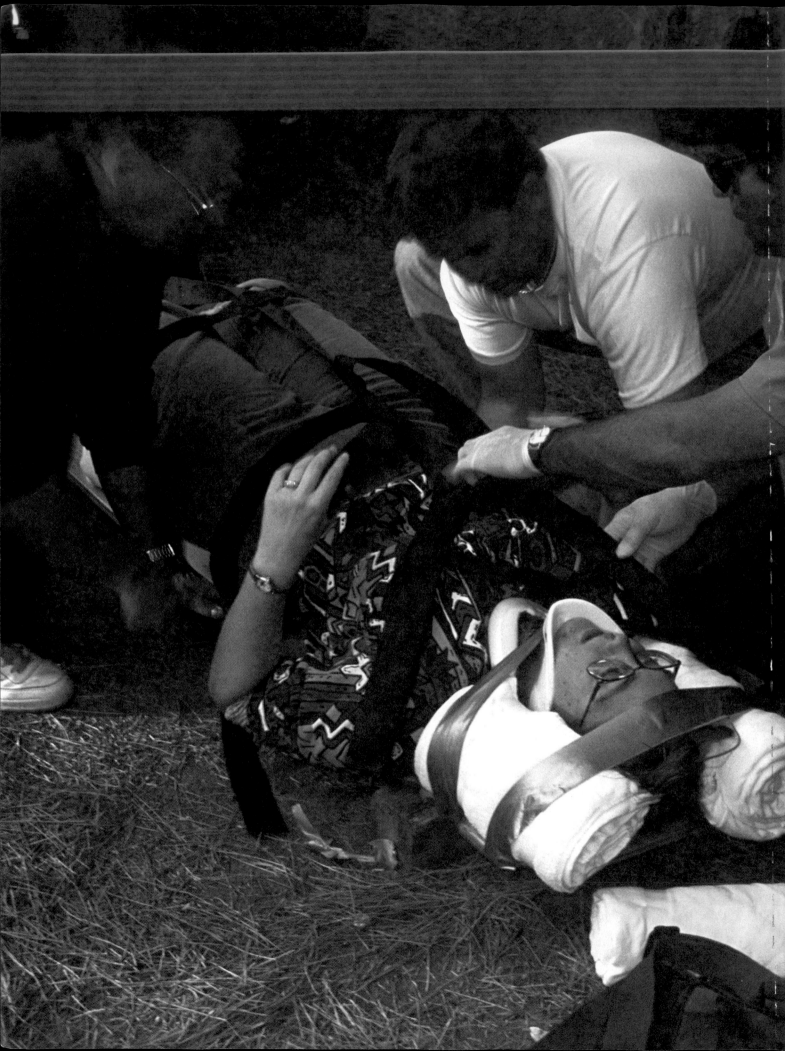

Chapter 1

Background Information

Need for First Aid Training

A large truck swings around a corner, crashes into an automobile, and pushes it over an embankment. Bystanders rush to the rescue. They remove the driver of the car, stop a passing car, lift the injured man to his feet, and send him in a sitting position to a nearby hospital. Because of this unskilled and ignorant handling, the man's spinal cord is injured by the sharp edge of a broken vertebra so that he will remain paralyzed for the rest of his life. But this tragic outcome could have been avoided if someone had known what to do in an emergency.

A backcountry hiker is bitten by a rattlesnake. Her frantic companion "cuts and sucks" the bitten area, not realizing that this is an obsolete and harmful procedure. A trained first aider would have known the proper procedures for taking care of the victim.

A swimmer is pulled unconscious from the water. No one helps because no one knows cardiopulmonary resuscitation (CPR). The emergency medical service (EMS) ambulance arrives too late to revive the swimmer. CPR would have served as an interim action and preserved life for the few minutes needed until the ambulance arrived.

Late at night, a man who had earlier smashed a fingernail in a car door can no longer stand the excruciating pain caused by the pressure of blood accumulating underneath the fingernail. He drives himself to a hospital emergency department where the blood clot is relieved. He later receives a bill for over $100. If he had known the proper first aid procedure, he could have relieved the pain sooner and saved money.

These cases clearly point out the need for first aid training. *It's better to know it and not need it than to need it and not know it.* Everyone should be able to perform first aid because most people will eventually find themselves in a situation requiring it, either for another person or for themselves.

A delay of as little as four minutes when a person's heart stops can mean death. Therefore, what a bystander does can mean the difference between life and death.

However, most injuries do not require life-saving efforts. During their entire lifetime, most people will see only one or two situations involving life-threatening conditions. Saving lives is important, but knowing what to do for less severe injuries demands greater attention and more first aid training.

Throughout the world, injuries are the leading cause of death during the first half of the human life span. Each year, one in four people suffers a nonfatal injury serious enough to need medical attention or to restrict activity for at least a day. Few escape the tragedy of a fatal or permanently disabling injury to a relative or a friend. Then there are those who require care for less severe injuries and sudden illness at home, work, or play. (▶**Table 1-1**), (▶**Table 1-2**), and (▶**Table 1-3**) describe just how often minor injuries happen in a single year.

Despite increased attention and progress in recent years, many people still lack an acceptable level of knowledge and proficiency in first aid. These skills are greatly needed.

> *"Whatever can go wrong, will."*
>
> Murphy's Law

> *"Whatever can happen to one man can happen to every man."*
>
> Lucius Annaeus Seneca (4 B.C.?–A.D. 65)

Value to Self

Although many people learn first aid in order to help others, the training primarily helps oneself. It enables a person to give proper immediate care to one's own injuries and sudden illness. If victims are too seriously injured to help themselves, they may be able to direct others toward proper care.

First aid training also helps develop safety awareness. Discussing injuries promotes injury prevention by showing how injuries occur.

Value to Others

Those with first aid training are more likely to deliver proper assistance to injured family members. Although the main beneficiaries are the trained individual and family, the benefits of knowing appropriate first aid techniques extend further, usually to co-workers, acquaintances, and strangers.

Value in Remote Locations

Should injuries or sudden illness require medical care, time, distance, and availability are major considerations. EMS can reach most victims who are severely injured or suddenly ill within 10 to 20 minutes. However, some victims are long distances from medical care. Although most people associate wilderness settings involving outdoor recreational activities (eg, hiking, camping, hunting, snowmobiling) with long distances and lack of medical care, other settings also demand that people be prepared to give first aid over an extended time:

- urban areas after a natural or manmade disaster that destroys or overwhelms the EMS
- remote occupations (eg, farming, ranching, commercial fishing, forestry)
- remote communities
- developing countries

First aid needed in remote locations is similar to that needed in urban settings, but extra skills are sometimes required. See Chapter 22 for information on delivering first aid in remote locations.

What Is First Aid?

First aid is the immediate care given to an injured or suddenly ill person. First aid does *not* take the place of proper medical treatment. It consists only of furnishing temporary assistance until competent medical care, if needed, is obtained or until the chance for recovery without medical care is assured. Most injuries and illnesses do not require medical care.

Properly applied, first aid may mean the difference between life and death, between rapid recovery and a long hospitalization, or between a temporary disability and permanent injury. First aid involves more than doing things for others; it also includes treatment that people can do for themselves.

Being able to recognize a serious medical emergency and knowing how to get help may make a crucial difference in saving a life. The problem is that people may not recognize an emergency because neither the victim nor bystanders know basic symptoms (eg, a heart attack victim may wait hours after the onset of symptoms before seeking help). Moreover, most people do not know first aid; even if they do, they may panic in an emergency.

Legal Considerations

Legal and ethical issues concern all first aid providers. For example, is a first aider required to stop and give care at an automobile crash? Can a child with a broken arm be treated even when the parents cannot be contacted for their consent? These and many other legal and ethical questions confront first aiders.

Table 1-1: Number and Percent Distribution of Emergency Department Visits by Cause of Injury, United States, 1996

Cause of Injury	Number of Visits (000)	%
All Injury-Related Visits	**34,941**	**100.0%**
Unintentional Injuries	**30,040**	**86.0%**
Accidental Falls	7,210	20.6%
Total Motor Vehicle Accidents	4,546	13.0%
Motor vehicle traffic	4,318	12.4%
Motor vehicle nontraffic	228	0.7%
Striking Against or Struck Accidentally by Objects or Persons	3,533	10.1%
Accidents Caused by Cutting or Piercing Instruments	2,661	7.6%
Overexertion	1,444	4.1%
Accidents Due to Natural and Environmental Factors	1,242	3.6%
Accidental Poisoning by Drugs, Medicinal Substances, Biologicals, Other Solid and Liquid Substances, Gases and Vapors	709	2.0%
Accidents Caused by Fire and Flames, Hot Substances or Object, Caustic or Corrosive Material, and Steam	604	1.7%
Pedalcycle, Nontraffic and Other	510	1.5%
Machinery	484	1.4%
Other Transportation	145	0.4%
Other Mechanism	2,175	6.2%
Mechanism Unspecified	4,654	13.3%
Intentional Injuries	**2,322**	**6.6%**
Self-inflicted Injury	253	0.7%
Poisoning by Solid or Liquid Substances, Gases or Vapors	166	0.5%
Assault	2,019	5.8%
Unarmed Fight or Brawl and Striking by Blunt or Thrown Object	1,038	3.0%
Assault by Cutting and Piercing Instrument	169	0.5%
Assault by Other and Unspecified Mechanism	769	2.2%
Adverse Effects of Medical Treatment	**1,124**	**3.2%**
Other and Unknown	**1,393**	**4.0%**

Source: Adapted from McCaig, L.F., Strussman, B.J. (1997). National Hospital Ambulatory Medical Care Survey: 1996 Emergency Department Summary (Advanced data, Number 295, December 19, 1997).

Consent

A first aider must have the victim's consent before giving first aid. Touching another person without his or her permission or consent is unlawful (known as battery) and could be grounds for a lawsuit. Likewise, giving first aid without the victim's consent is unlawful.

Expressed Consent

Consent must be obtained from every conscious, mentally competent (able to make a rational decision) adult of legal age. Tell the victim your name and that you have first aid training and explain what you will be doing. The victim may give permission either verbally or with a nod of the head.

Table 1-2: Injuries Associated with Consumer Products

Description	Injanies[a]	Description	Injanies[a]
Home Workshop Equipment		Sofas, couches, davenports, divans, etc.	107,812
Saws (hand or power)	79,854	Rugs and carpets	98,693
Hammers	41,518	Toilets	44,335
Drills	16,584	Mirrors or mirror glass	22,623
Welding & soldering equipment	15,803	Electric lighting equipment	22,067
Pliers, wire cutters, or wrenches	14,780	Sinks	20,420
Power grinder, buffers, polishers	14,729		
Hoists, lifts, jacks, or jack stands	14,254	**Home Structures and Construction Materials**	
Screwdrivers	10,090	Stairs or steps	914,887
Batteries (all types)	7,993	Floors or flooring materials	841,022
		Other doors	326,148
Packaging and Containers, Household		Ceilings and walls	238,066
Household containers and packaging	184,097	Household cabinets, racks, and shelves	222,621
Bottles and jars	81,116	Nails, screws, tacks, or bolts	165,623
Bags	21,060	Windows	131,333
Aerosol and pressurized containers	4,456	Porches, balconies, open-side floors	114,287
		Fences or fence posts	110,731
Housewares		Handrails, railings, or banisters	34,421
Knives	435,276	Glass doors	33,952
Tableware and flatware (excluding knives)	107,963	Garage doors (including automatic garage doors)	19,449
Scissors	30,290	Fireplaces	16,331
Waste containers, trash baskets, etc.	26,686		
Slicers and choppers	13,493	**General Household Appliances**	
		Refrigerators	25,133
Home Furnishings, Fixtures, and Accessories		Irons	15,149
Beds	394,939	Vacuum cleaners	14,005
Tables, n.e.c.	287,933	Washing machines	11,402
Chairs	260,055	Ovens	10,203
Bathtubs and showers	164,749	Ranges	2,158
Ladders	143,297		

Implied Consent

Implied consent involves an unresponsive victim in a life-threatening condition. It is assumed or implied that an unresponsive victim would consent to lifesaving interventions. A conscious victim who does not resist the administrations of a first aider is also assumed to have given consent.

Children and Mentally Incompetent Adults

Consent must be obtained from the parent or guardian of a child victim, as legally defined by the state. The same is true for an adult who is mentally incompetent. When life-threatening situations exist and the parent or legal guardian is not available for consent, first aid should be given based on implied consent. Do not withhold first aid from a minor just to obtain parental or guardian permission.

Psychiatric emergencies present difficult problems of consent. Under most conditions, a police officer is the only person with the authority to restrain and transport a person against that person's will. A first aider should not intervene unless directed to do so by a police officer

Table 1-2: continued

Description	Injuries[a]	Description	Injuries[a]
Heating, Cooling, and Ventilating Equipment		Chainsaws	29,684
Pipes (excluding smoking pipes)	26,926	Greenhouse or gardening supplies	12,654
Fans	16,073	Hatchets or axes	11,875
Radiators (excluding vehicle radiators)	13,212	Tractors	9,167
Air conditioners	11,479	Manual snow or ice removal tools	7,337
Furnaces	7,077		
Coal or wood-burning stoves	4,925	**Sports and Recreation Equipment**	
		Trampolines	82,722
Home Communication and Entertainment Equipment		Swings or swing sets	73,923
Televisions	37,401	Monkey bars or other playground climbing equipment	71,828
Sound recording and reproducing equipment	22,086	Swimming pool	62,812
Telephones or telephone accessories	14,432	All terrain vehicles	55,400
Computers (equipment and electronic games)	6,701	Skateboards	48,186
		Slides or sliding boards	45,767
Personal Use Items		Sleds	26,067
Footwear	75,804	Mopeds or power-assisted cycles	7,853
Jewelry	54,720		
Razors and shavers	40,773	**Miscellaneous Products**	
Hair grooming equipment and accessories	24,974	Toys, n.e.c.	68,777
Coins	24,755	Baby walkers or jumpers	16,487
Luggage	13,510	Fireworks	8,299
		Car seats (for infants and children)	7,954
Yard and Garden Equipment			
Lawn mowers	60,804		
Pruning, trimming, and edging equipment	32,217		

Source: U.S. Consumer Product Safety Commission, National Electronic Injury Surveillance System, *Product Summary Report, All Products, CY1997*. Not all product categories are shown. Products were selected for either high injury frequency or apparent interest in the product.

[a]Estimated number of product-related injuries in the United States and territories that were treated in hospital emergency departments.

n.e.c. = not elsewhere classified.

or unless it is obvious that the victim is about to do life-threatening harm to himself or herself or to others.

Refusing Help

Although it seldom happens, a person may refuse assistance for countless reasons, such as religious grounds, avoidance of possible pain, or the desire to be examined by a physician rather than by a first aider. Whatever the reason for refusing medical care, or even if no reason is given, the conscious and mentally competent adult can reject help.

Generally, the wisest approach is to inform the victim of his or her medical condition, what you propose to do, and why the help is necessary. If the victim understands the consequences and still refuses treatment, there is little else you can do. Call the EMS and, while awaiting their arrival:

- Try again to persuade the victim to accept care and encourage others at the scene to persuade the victim. A victim may have a change of mind after a short period of time.

Table 1-3: Sports Injuries

Sport	Participants	Injuries
Archery	4,800,000	3,213
Baseball and softball	30,400,000	326,714
Basketball	33,300,000	644,921
Bicycle riding[b]	45,100,000	544,561
Billiards, pool	36,000,000	3,685
Bowling	44,800,000	23,317
Boxing	(a)	7,257
Exercising with equipment[c]	47,900,000	86,024
Fishing	44,700,000	72,598
Football[d]	20,100,000	334,420
Golf	26,200,000	39,473[e]
Gymnastics	(a)	33,373[f]
Handball	(a)	2,517
Horseback riding	(a)	58,709
Ice hockey	1,900,000	77,491[g]
Ice skating	7,900,000	25,379[h]
Racquetball[i]	4,500,000	10,438
Roller skating	37,500,000	153,023[h,j]
Skateboarding	6,300,000	48,186
Snowboarding	2,800,000	37,638
Snowmobiling	(a)	12,676
Soccer	13,700,000	148,913
Swimming	59,500,000	83,772
Tennis	11,100,000	22,294
Volleyball	17,800,000	67,340
Water skiing	6,500,000	10,657
Wrestling	(a)	39,829

Source: Participants—National Sporting Goods Association (NSGA); figures include those seven years of age or older who participated more than once per year except for bicycle riding and swimming, which include those who participated six or more times per year. Injuries—Consumer Product Safety Commission (CPSC); figures include only injuries treated in hospital emergency departments.

[a]Data not available.

[b]Excludes mountain biking.

[c]Includes weight lifting.

[d]Includes touch and tackle football.

[e]Excludes golf carts (8,304 injuries).

[f]Excludes trampolines (82,722 injuries).

[g]There were 4,444 injuries in street hockey, 5,584 in roller hockey, 4,830 in field hockey, and 45,306 in hockey, unspecified.

[h]There were 22,748 injuries in skating, unspecified.

[i]Includes squash and paddle ball.

[j]Includes 2×2 (54,609 injuries) and in-line (98,414 injuries).

- Make certain you have witnesses. All too often a victim will refuse consent and then deny having done so.
- Consider calling for law enforcement assistance. In most locations, the police can place a person in protective custody and require him or her to go to a hospital.

Abandonment

Abandonment means terminating the care of a victim without ensuring continued care at the same level or higher. Once you have responded to an emergency, you must not leave a victim who needs continuing first aid until another competent and trained person takes responsibility for the victim. This may seem obvious, but there have been cases in which critically ill or injured victims were left unattended and then died. Thus, a first aider must stay with the victim until another equally or better trained person takes over.

Negligence

Negligence means not following the accepted standards of care, resulting in further injury to the victim. Negligence involves:

1. Having a duty to act
2. Breaching that duty (substandard care)
3. Causing injury and damages

Duty to Act

No one is required to render first aid unless a legal duty to act exists. For example, a physician could ignore a stranger suffering a heart attack or a fractured bone. While moral obligations may exist, they are not always the same as a legal obligation to help. Duty to act may apply in the following situations:

- *When employment requires it.* If your employer designates you as the individual responsible for rendering first aid to meet OSHA (Occupational Safety and Health Administration) requirements and you are called to an injury scene, you have a duty to act. Other examples of occupations that involve a legal obligation to give first aid include law enforcement officers, park rangers, athletic trainers, lifeguards, and teachers.
- *When a pre-existing responsibility exists.* You may have a pre-existing relationship with other persons that makes you responsible for them, which means that you must give first aid should they need it. For example, a parent has a pre-existing responsibility for a child or a driver for a passenger.

Duty to act means following guidelines for standards of care. Standards of care ensure quality care and protection for injured or suddenly ill victims. The elements that make up standards of care include the following:

- *The type of rescuer.* A first aider should provide the level and type of care expected of a reasonable person with the same amount of training and in similar circumstances. Different standards of care apply to physicians, nurses, emergency medical technicians (EMTs), and first aiders.

- *Published recommendations.* Emergency care–related organizations and societies publish recommended first aid procedures. For example, the American Heart Association publishes guidelines for giving CPR, and the Wilderness Medical Society publishes guidelines for assisting victims who are more than one hour from medical care.

Breach of Duty

Generally, a first aider breaches ("breaks") his or her duty to a victim by failing to provide the type of care that would be provided by a person having the same or similar training. There are two ways to breach one's duty: acts of omission and acts of commission. An *act of omission* is the failure to do what a reasonably prudent person with the same or similar training would do in the same or similar circumstances. An *act of commission* is doing something that a reasonably prudent person would *not* do under the same or similar circumstances. Forgetting to put on a dressing is an act of omission; cutting a snake-bite site is an act of commission.

Injury and Damages Inflicted

In addition to physical damage, injury and damage can include physical pain and suffering, mental anguish, medical expenses, and sometimes loss of earnings and earning capacity.

Confidentiality

First aiders may become privy to information that would be embarrassing to the victim or the victim's family if it were publicly revealed. It is important that you be extremely cautious about revealing information you learn while caring for someone. The law recognizes that people have the right to privacy.

Do not discuss what you know with anyone other than those who have a medical need to know. Some state laws do, however, require the reporting of certain incidents, such as rape, abuse, and gunshot wounds.

Good Samaritan Laws

Starting in the early 1960s, a number of states (beginning with California in 1959) enacted laws designed to protect physicians and other medical personnel from legal actions that might arise from emergency treatment they provided while not in the line of duty. These laws, known as Good Samaritan laws, encourage people to assist others in distress by granting them immunity against lawsuits. While the laws vary from state to state, Good Samaritan immunity generally applies only when the rescuer is (1) acting during an emergency, (2) acting in good faith, which means he or she has good intentions, (3) acting without compensation, and (4) not guilty of any malicious misconduct or gross negligence toward the victim (deviating from rational first aid guidelines).

Although Good Samaritan laws primarily cover medical personnel, several states have expanded them to include laypersons serving as first aiders. In fact, some states have several Good Samaritan laws that cover different types of people in various situations (eg, California has fifteen, New York has eight, and Florida has four different Good Samaritan laws).

Many legal experts believe Good Samaritan laws have given first aiders a false sense of security. These laws will not protect first aiders from lawsuits regardless of their actions. Good Samaritan laws are not a substitute for competent first aid or for keeping within the scope of your training.

Fear of lawsuits has made some people wary of getting involved in emergency situations. First aiders, however, are rarely sued; those who are usually obtain a favorable ruling from the courts.

STUDY
Questions (1)

Name_____ **Course**_____ **Date**_____

Activities

Activity 1

Mark each statement as true (T) or false (F).

T F 1. Every year one in four Americans is injured seriously enough to require medical attention or activity restriction for at least one day.

T F 2. Correct application of first aid can mean the difference between life or death.

T F 3. Proper first aid includes seeking medical care for all injuries and sudden illness.

T F 4. First aiders often face lawsuits.

T F 5. A layperson is under no legal obligation to render assistance to an injured person.

T F 6. The primary purpose of Good Samaritan laws is for first aider protection.

T F 7. Many people lack proficiency in first aid.

T F 8. Some people are required to give first aid as part of their job descriptions.

T F 9. A physician is required by law to treat all persons.

T F 10. An athletic trainer has a "duty to act" toward his or her school's injured athletes.

T F 11. If you are involved in a traffic accident, you are legally required to render assistance to injured victims.

T F 12. If you observe a traffic accident while driving in a remote location, you are legally required to stop and give assistance to injured victims.

T F 13. After giving first aid, you must remain with the victim until someone equally or more qualified takes over.

T F 14. Before providing first aid to children, you should first attempt to contact the parents or guardian unless the injury is life threatening.

15. What are the two key words or phrases in the definition of "first aid"?
   a. _____
   b. _____

16. With what two conditions does first aid care concern itself?
   a. _____
   b. _____

17. Is a physician needed in all first aid cases? Explain your answer.

   _____

   _____

Activity 2

Pretest of first aid information. **Mark each statement as true (T) or false (F). The information is not covered in the first chapter, but previews some of the book's content. Let's see what you already know.**

T F 1. If someone is bitten by a rattlesnake, immediately cut through the fang marks and suck out the venom.

T F 2. When an adult is choking, slap him or her on the back to dislodge the obstruction.

T F 3. A victim who has swallowed poison should be placed on his or her left side.

T F 4. Antibiotic ointments can be placed on shallow wounds.

T F 5. To kill bacteria in a wound, apply an antiseptic such as Merthiolate or hydrogen peroxide.

T F 6. Rub or massage frostbitten toes, and then thaw them slowly in cold water.

T F 7. Inducing vomiting is necessary in most cases of swallowed poisoning.

T F 8. Put butter on a burn.

T F 9. First aiders never have an occasion to cut the skin.

T F 10. Remove an embedded tick by applying a heavy oil to smother it or touch it with a heated object to cause it to back out.

STUDY
Questions (1)

Activity 3
Values clarification: What do you think?

____ 1. If a friend of yours were giving improper first aid, what would you do?
   a. Report him to the National Safety Council or other certifying organization.
   b. Ignore it.
   c. Ask him to stop.
   d. Show how to give the proper first aid.

____ 2. If a stranger were giving improper first aid, what would you do?
   a. Report her to the National Safety Council or other certifying organization.
   b. Ignore it.
   c. Ask her to stop.
   d. Show how to give the proper first aid.

____ 3. What motivated you to take a first aid course?
   a. The chance to expand my knowledge.
   b. My job requires it.
   c. Curiosity about snakebites, hypothermia, and other situations requiring first aid.
   d. I want to be prepared to render aid to others.
   e. Other.

   _____

   _____

   _____

____ 4. Which of these facts would discourage you from giving first aid?
   a. You could possibly be sued for negligence.
   b. First aid equipment and supplies are unavailable.
   c. The victim has a known, highly contagious disease.
   d. Another first aider is helping the victim.
   e. The victim is a stranger.

____ 5. What is your attitude about first aid training?
   a. Everyone should be skilled in giving first aid.
   b. Only those designated as a first aider on the job need training.
   c. At least one member of every household should have first aid training.
   d. Training received as a youth is sufficient.

6. First aid training should be a required course for those attending (put yes or no for each item):
   a. elementary schools   _____
   b. high schools   _____
   c. colleges/universities   _____
   d. worksite training   _____
   e. should never be required _____

Chapter Activities

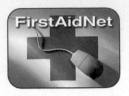

WEB Activities

Background Information

Visit nsc.jbpub.com/FirstAidNet, then click on Web Activities, and select the appropriate chapter.

National Center for Injury Prevention and Control

The National Center for Injury Prevention and Control monitors trends in unintentional injuries in the United States in an effort to reduce injury, disability, death, and costs associated with injuries outside the workplace.

Good Samaritan Laws

The question of Good Samaritan Law protection for a person helping at an emergency scene always arises during a first aid class. It is important to know the background of the "Good Sam" laws, as well as knowing how your state supports the law.

The National Safety Council

The National Safety Council is dedicated to the protection of life, promotion of health, and reduction of accidental death. For more than 80 years, the National Safety Council has been the world's leading authority on safety and injury education.

Law Guide

Do you have some law-related questions? Need some advice, a lawyer, or just need to better understand law concepts? If so, get free help to simple, useful knowledge about the law in all 50 states, and every county, including personal injury and medical malpractice law.

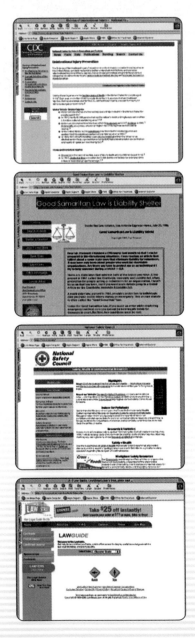

Chapter 2

Action at an Emergency

Bystander Intervention

The bystander is a vital link between the emergency medical service (EMS) and the victim. Typically it is a bystander who recognizes a situation as an emergency and acts to help the victim. A bystander must perform the following actions quickly and reliably:

1. recognize the emergency
2. decide to help
3. contact EMS, if needed
4. assess the victim
5. provide first aid

Compared with health care professionals, ordinary bystanders are significantly less likely to offer help in emergencies that occur in public places. Some reasons for this fact include:

- ignorance
- confusion about what is an emergency
- characteristics of the emergency (eg, unpleasant physical characteristics of the victim, the presence of other bystanders)

Ignorance and Helping Behavior

The average layperson is ignorant of many aspects of emergency care and has difficulty recognizing common medical emergencies and deciding to call an ambulance.

Also, a person who does not feel competent to deal with an emergency is not likely to offer even minimal help. The person who does not feel competent may escape this uncomfortable feeling by failing to acknowledge the situation as an emergency. The implication is that bystanders who are uncertain of their ability to deal with a seriously injured victim may be more likely to assume that the victims are not seriously injured.

Confusion about What Is an Emergency

Sometimes, laypersons have a great deal of difficulty deciding when an emergency exists. For example, motor vehicle crashes may be easier to recognize as emergencies than heart attacks. This can lead to delays in contacting the EMS and to inappropriate decisions, such as transporting victims with life-threatening problems by private vehicles rather than contacting EMS.

Other Factors That Influence Whether a Bystander Helps

In addition to ignorance and confusion, bystanders encounter other barriers that can slow or prevent action in an emergency. Many people are put off by unpleasant physical characteristics such as blood, vomit, or alcohol on the breath. Reluctance to help may reflect an unwillingness to approach or touch a bloody victim. The current public attention on human immunodeficiency virus (HIV) and acquired immunodeficiency syndrome (AIDS) may make this problem more difficult.

Another factor involved in helping behavior is the bystander's time of arrival. A bystander who sees the emergency happen is more likely to help than a bystander who arrives after the event.

Quality of Help Provided by Bystanders

Some evidence suggests that much first aid treatment by bystanders is inadequate or potentially dangerous. Failure to keep an open airway and the decision to transport the victim in a private vehicle rather than EMS are two examples. One study concluded that 9% of the emergency victims who died would have had a greater chance for survival if they had received better care from laypersons and professionals. An Australian study examined 13 deaths from head and spinal injuries. For several of those deaths, inadequate first aid rendered by a layperson and the decision to transport the victim in a private vehicle were cited as potential contributing factors for the deaths.

What Should Be Done?

As stated at the beginning of this chapter, victims would benefit if bystanders could quickly and reliably do the following:

1. recognize the emergency
2. decide to help
3. contact EMS, if needed
4. assess the victim
5. provide first aid

Recognize the Emergency

To help in an emergency, the bystander first has to notice that something is wrong. Noticing that something is wrong is related to four factors:

- *Severity.* Severe, catastrophic emergencies such as a traffic collision involving an overturned car or several vehicles attract attention.
- *Physical distance.* The closer a bystander is to an emergency situation, the more likely he or she will notice it.
- *Relationship.* Knowing the victim increases the likelihood of noticing an emergency. For example, you would notice your child's injuries before you might notice a total stranger with the same injuries.
- *Time exposed.* Evidence indicates that the longer a bystander is aware of the situation, the more likely he or she will notice it as an emergency.

Decide to Help

At some time, everyone will have to decide whether to help another person. Unless the decision to act in an emergency is considered well in advance of an actual emergency, the many obstacles that make it difficult or unpleasant for a bystander to help a stranger are almost certain to impede action. One important strategy that people use to avoid action is to refuse (consciously or unconsciously) to acknowledge the emergency. Many emergencies do not look like the ones portrayed on television, and the uncertainty of the real event can make it easier for the bystander to avoid acknowledging the emergency.

> *"I shall pass through this life but once.*
> *Any good, therefore, that I can do*
> *Or any kindness I can show to any fellow creature*
> *Let me do it now.*
> *Let me not defer or neglect it,*
> *For I shall not pass this way again."*
>
> Etienne de Grellet

Making a quick decision to get involved at the time of an emergency is unlikely to occur unless the bystander has considered, in advance, the possibility of helping. Thus, the most important time to make the decision to help is *before* you ever encounter an emergency.

Deciding to help is an attitude about emergencies and about one's ability to deal with emergencies. It is an attitude that takes time to develop and is affected by a number of factors.

> *"A hero is no braver than an ordinary man, but he is brave five minutes longer."*
>
> Emerson

Developing such an attitude means that you must:

- appreciate the importance of bystander help to an injured or suddenly ill person

- feel confident enough about helping someone who is seriously injured or suddenly ill to offer help even if someone else is present
- be willing to take the time to help
- be able to put the potential risks of helping in perspective
- feel comfortable about taking charge at an emergency scene
- feel comfortable about seeing or touching a victim who may be bleeding or vomiting or who may appear dead

Deciding Not to Help

A bystander can always find excuses for not helping in emergency situations. The following excuses are possible reasons for why people fail to aid others.

- It could be harmful. Bystanders have lost their lives or been severely injured while attempting to rescue others. One example is Oklahoma teacher Ronnie Darden, who lost his left leg and part of his right foot when he tripped over a power line as he tried to help passengers in a crashed car. Another example is Joe Delancy, a star halfback for the Kansas City Chiefs, who died while trying to rescue three drowning boys in Louisiana. The fear of being sued or contracting a disease such as HIV or tuberculosis can also act as a deterrent. And some would-be rescuers have been attacked by dogs protecting their disabled owners.
- "Helping doesn't matter." Some bystanders may feel that the victim is getting what he or she deserves. Others may be repulsed by a negative image of the victim (eg, if the victim is drunk or homeless). Rewards, if any, are not high for rescuers, possibly consisting of a newspaper write-up or a small cash prize. Often the rescuer gets nothing more than a hurried "Thanks," and in some cases rescuers are never known.
- Obstacles may prevent helping. Many bystanders do not know how to help. They cannot swim, do not know how to control bleeding or perform cardiopulmonary resuscitation (CPR), or do not have other necessary rescue and first aid skills. Ironically, the more bystanders there are, the less likely it is that one of them will respond.

Some would-be rescuers are adversely affected by the sight of blood, vomit, and other appalling conditions sometimes found at emergency scenes.

Contact EMS, If Needed

Laypeople often make inappropriate decisions concerning EMS. They delay contacting EMS until they are

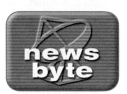

Won't Help at Car Crash

Nearly half of Americans say they might not stop to help the victims of a roadside accident if they were the only ones available to help, according to a survey conducted by the National Highway Traffic Safety Administration (NHTSA). When asked for their reasons for not stopping, respondents mentioned concern about not knowing how to help, fear for personal safety, and worry about being sued. NHTSA reported that the number of potential "Good Samaritans" among the American population declined when compared with the results of a similar survey conducted in 1994.

Source: National Highway Traffic Safety Administration, 1996 Motor Vehicle Occupant Safety Survey, April 1998. *Annals of Emergency Medicine,* 1998; 31(4):518-520.

absolutely sure that an emergency exists, or they elect to bypass EMS and transport the victim to medical care in a private vehicle. Such actions present significant dangers to victims.

Assess the Victim

The bystander must decide if life-threatening conditions exist and what kind of help a victim needs immediately.

Provide First Aid

Often the most critical life-support measures are effective only if started immediately by the nearest available person. That person usually will be a layperson— a bystander.

Rescuer Reactions

The sight of blood and the cries of victims can be very upsetting to people attempting to rescue and assist the injured. Seeing a grotesque amputation, being splattered with vomitus or blood, or smelling disagreeable odors

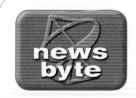

Actual vs. Perceived EMS Response Time

Patient's perceptions of ambulance response times are inaccurate. They tend to overestimate response time while underestimating scene time and time to medical care.

Source: Allison H. Harvey, W.C. Gerard, George F. Rice, and Holmes Finch, Actual vs. Perceived EMS Response Time, *Prehospital Emergency Care,* January/March 1999 Vol. 3 #1, pp. 11-14.

from urine and feces can be quite unnerving. More than one rescuer has felt nauseated and weak, vomited, or fainted when helping injured victims. Even the toughest of physicians and EMTs have difficult moments when exposed to certain situations.

It is essential that rescuers stay conscious and working at an injury scene. A rescuer who collapses while aiding the injured detracts attention from the original victim, whose condition is usually more serious. All the knowledge and skills a rescuer has are useless if he or she collapses or has to leave the scene because of weakness or fainting.

Some emergency care workers seem to have "ice in their veins." They always appear calm and unaffected by even the worst injuries. These people may seem callous, but the proper psychological term is *desensitized*. A specialty within psychology deals with desensitization and suggests ways of overcoming anxieties caused by unpleasant sights and sounds. Desensitization is a deconditioning or a counterconditioning process that can be effective in eliminating fears and anxieties. The idea is to weaken an undesirable response such as fainting by strengthening an incompatible response. When responses are incompatible (calmness versus anxiety), the occurrence of either one prevents the occurrence of the other. By desensitizing, you learn to associate relaxation with situations that elicit anxiety so that eventually you do not experience anxiety. But you first need to learn how to invoke relaxation before gradually exposing yourself to anxiety-producing situations such as the sight of blood.

There are some simple ways to desensitize (calm) yourself while helping another person:

- Close your eyes for a moment and take several long, deep breaths. Let your mind go blank and just say the number "one" as you breathe out. Do not count—just repeat the number "one" at the end of each exhalation.

- Change your thought patterns from the unpleasant to the pleasant by singing a favorite song to yourself (not out loud, of course, for the obvious reason of how you might appear to the victim or observers).

After you have learned a relaxation response technique, you can begin a process of gradual exposure to unpleasant scenes by viewing videos, slides, or pictures of injuries in medical journals. Another step in the process of conditioning yourself might be to volunteer at a hospital emergency department.

In a number of cases, a rescuer who fainted had failed to eat breakfast. It is strongly recommended that everyone maintain an adequate blood sugar level through proper eating habits.

Post-Care Reactions

After giving first aid for severe injuries, rescuers often feel an emotional "letdown," which is frequently overlooked. Discussing your feelings, fears, and reactions within 24 to 72 hours of helping at a traumatic injury scene helps prevent later emotional problems. You could discuss your feelings with a trusted friend, a mental health professional, or a member of the clergy. Bringing out your feelings quickly helps to relieve personal anxieties and stress.

Scene Survey

If you are at the scene of an emergency situation, do a 10-second survey (▼Figure 2-1) that includes looking for three things: (1) hazards that could be dangerous to you, the victim(s), or bystanders; (2) the mechanism or cause of the injury or injuries; and (3) the number of victims.

As you approach an emergency scene, scan the area for immediate dangers to yourself or to the victim. For example, if a vehicle involved in an automobile accident is in the roadway obstructing traffic, you have to consider whether you can safely go to that vehicle to help the victim. Or you might notice that gasoline is dripping from the gas tank and that the battery has shorted out and is sparking. In these circumstances, you should withdraw

(**Figure 2-1**) Scene survey

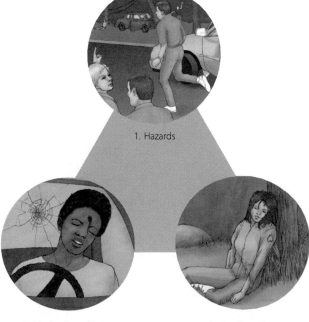

Do a 10-second scene survey by looking for three things:

1. Hazards

2. Mechanism of injury or nature of a victim's sudden illness

3. Number of victims

and get help before proceeding. You are not being cowardly, merely realistic. Never attempt a rescue that you have not been specifically trained to do. You cannot help another if you also become a victim. Always ask yourself: Is the scene safe to enter? (For details about hazards at an emergency scene, refer to Chapter 23.)

The second thing to do in the first 10 seconds is to try to determine the cause of the injury (mechanism of injury). For example, if the emergency department physician knows that a victim was thrown against a steering wheel, he or she will check for liver, spleen, and cardiac injuries. Be sure to tell the EMS personnel about your conclusions, so that they can fully recognize the extent of the injuries.

Finally, determine how many people are injured. There may be more than one victim, so look around and ask about others involved.

Seeking Medical Attention

Knowing the difference between a minor injury and a life-threatening one is important. For example, upper abdominal pain can be indigestion, ulcers, or an early sign of a heart attack. An unresponsive person may have tripped and received a concussion or be having an allergic reaction to an insect sting.

Not every cut needs stitches, nor does every burn require medical attention. It is, however, always best to err on the side of caution.

According to the American College of Emergency Physicians (ACEP), if the answer to any of the following questions is yes, or if you are unsure, call 9-1-1 or the local emergency number for help.

- Is the victim's condition life-threatening?
- Could the condition get worse and become life-threatening on the way to the hospital?
- Does the victim need the skills or equipment of emergency medical technicians (EMTs) or paramedics?
- Would distance or traffic conditions cause a delay in getting to the hospital?

ACEP also recommends that the following conditions are warning signs that require an immediate trip to the hospital emergency department either by ambulance or by private vehicle:

- fainting
- chest or abdominal pain or pressure
- sudden dizziness, weakness, or change in vision
- difficulty breathing, shortness of breath
- severe or persistent vomiting

- sudden severe pain anywhere in the body
- suicidal or homicidal feelings
- bleeding that does not stop after 10 to 15 minutes of pressure
- a gaping wound with edges that do not come together
- problems with movement or sensation following an injury
- cuts on the hand or face
- puncture wounds
- the possibility that foreign bodies such as glass or metal may have entered a wound
- most animal bites and all human bites
- hallucinations and clouding of thoughts
- a stiff neck in association with a fever or a headache
- a bulging or abnormally depressed fontanel (soft spot) in infants
- stupor or dazed behavior accompanying a high fever that is not alleviated by acetaminophen or aspirin
- unequal pupil size, loss of consciousness, blindness, staggering, or repeated vomiting after a head injury
- spinal injuries
- severe burns
- poisoning
- drug overdose

When a serious situation occurs, call EMS (9-1-1 in most communities) *first*. Do *not* call your doctor, the hospital, a friend, relatives, or neighbors for help before you call EMS. Calling anyone else first only wastes time.

Calling EMS has several advantages over driving to the hospital emergency department:

- Many victims should not be moved except by trained personnel.
- The EMTs who arrive with the ambulance know what to do. In addition, they are in radio contact with hospital physicians.
- Care provided by EMTs at the scene and on the way to the hospital can increase a victim's chances of survival and rate of recovery. The condition could get worse and become life-threatening on the way.
- An EMS ambulance usually can get a victim to the hospital quicker.

If the situation is not an emergency, call your doctor. However, if you are in *any* doubt as to whether the situation is an emergency, call EMS.

How to Call the EMS

In most communities, to receive emergency assistance of every kind you simply phone 9-1-1 (▶Figure 2-2). Check to see if this is true in your community. Emergency telephone numbers are usually listed on the inside front cover of telephone directories. Keep these numbers near or on every telephone. Dial "0" (the operator) if you do not know the emergency number. A community 9-1-1 number has several benefits:

- There is only one number to remember.
- Calls are received by specially trained personnel.
- Response time is reduced.

When you call EMS, be ready to give the dispatcher the following information. Speak slowly and clearly.

1. The victim's location. Give the address, names of intersecting roads, and other landmarks, if possible. This information is the most important you can give. Also, tell the specific location of the victim (eg, "in the basement"). When calling from a cellular phone, give the address immediately, because if you are cut off, the dispatcher cannot track a cellular phone call.

2. Your phone number and name. This prevents false calls and allows a dispatch center without the enhanced 9-1-1 system to call back for additional information if needed.

3. What happened. State the nature of the emergency (eg, "My husband fell off a ladder and is not moving").

4. Number of persons needing help and any special conditions (eg, "car crash, two cars, three people trapped").

5. Victim's condition (eg, "My husband's head is bleeding") and any first aid you have tried (such as pressing on the site of the bleeding).

Do *not* hang up the phone unless the dispatcher instructs you to do so. Enhanced 9-1-1 systems can track a call, but some communities lack this technology or are still using a seven-digit emergency number. Also, the EMS dispatcher may tell you how to best care for the victim. If you send someone else to call, have the person report back to you so you can be sure the call was made. Other tips include:

- Teach children what 9-1-1 is for and how and when to call. Refer to "nine-one-one," not "nine-eleven," because children may expect to find an 11 on the dial or on the push buttons.

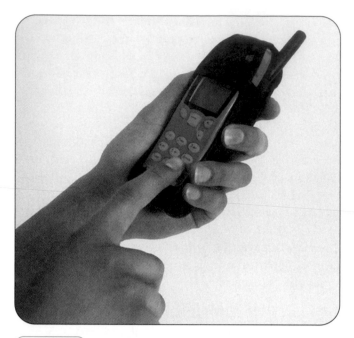

Figure 2-2 For help, phone 9-1-1 or the local emergency number.

- Do not hang up without explanation if you call 9-1-1 by mistake, or the dispatcher will have to call back to see if you need help.

- If your area does not have a 9-1-1 system, add EMS, fire, and police numbers to a list by your phones. During an emergency, you may not have the time or presence of mind to find a directory listing.

Disease Precautions

First aiders must understand the risks from infectious diseases, which can range in severity from mild to life-threatening. First aiders should know how to reduce

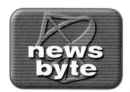

Lights and Sirens

Using lights and siren during victim transport puts both emergency personnel and the general public at a significant risk from automobile crashes. The authors found that nearly 40% of victims were transported with lights and siren despite being defined as stable. Other studies have evaluated the effect of lights and siren on time and found that using them saves only slightly more than 30 seconds.

Source: M.E. Lacher and J.C. Baushel; Lights and Siren Use in Pediatric 9-1-1 Ambulance Transportation: Are They Being Misused? *Annals of Emergency Medicine*, 1997; 29:223-227.

the risk of contamination to themselves and to others. Precautionary measures help protect against infection from viruses and bacteria.

Bloodborne Disease

Some diseases are caused by microorganisms that are "borne" (carried) in a person's bloodstream. Contact with blood infected with such microorganisms may cause infection. Of the many bloodborne pathogens, three pose significant health threats to first aiders: hepatitis B virus (HBV), hepatitis C virus (HCV), and HIV.

Hepatitis B

Hepatitis B, the most common form of hepatitis, is a viral infection of the liver. Types A, B, and C are each caused by a different virus.

A vaccine for hepatitis B is available and is recommended for all infants and for adults who may have contact with carriers of the disease or with blood. Medical and laboratory workers, police, intravenous drug users, people with multiple sexual partners, and those living with someone who has a lifelong infection are at high risk of hepatitis B (and hepatitis C as well). Vaccination is the best defense against HBV. There is no chance of developing hepatitis B from the vaccine. Federal laws require employers to offer a series of three vaccine injections free to all employees who may be at risk of exposure.

Without vaccination shots, exposure to hepatitis B may produce symptoms within two weeks to six months following exposure. People with hepatitis B infection may be symptom free, but that does *not* mean they are not contagious. These people may infect others through exposure to their blood. Symptoms of hepatitis B resemble those of the flu and include fatigue, nausea, loss of appetite, stomach pain, and perhaps a yellowing of the skin.

Hepatitis B starts as an inflammation of the liver and usually lasts one to two months. In a few people, the infection is very serious, and in some, mild infection continues for life. The virus may stay in the liver and can lead to severe damage (cirrhosis) and liver cancer. Medical treatment that begins immediately after exposure may prevent infection from developing.

Hepatitis C

Hepatitis C, first identified in the 1980s, is caused by a different virus than HBV, but both diseases have much in common. Like hepatitis B, hepatitis C affects the liver and can lead to long-term liver disease and liver cancer. Hepatitis C varies in severity and there may not be any

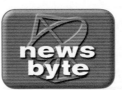

What Is the Risk of HIV Transmission from Contacting Blood?

In professional football, there are almost four bleeding injuries per game, yet researchers estimate the risk of HIV transmission in an NFL game to be less than one in one million.

Source: L. S. Brown et al: Bleeding Injuries in Professional Football: Estimating the Risk for HIV Transmission. *Annals of Internal Medicine* 122:271–74 (1995).

symptoms at the time of infection. Currently, there is no vaccine or effective treatment for hepatitis C.

HIV

Estimates are that over 1.5 million people in the United States are infected with HIV but have no symptoms. A person infected with HIV can infect others, and those infected with HIV almost always develop AIDS, which interferes with the body's ability to fight off other diseases. No vaccine is available to prevent HIV infection, which eventually proves fatal. The best defense against AIDS is to avoid becoming infected.

How Bloodborne Pathogens Are Transmitted

HIV and HBV are usually transmitted (passed on) when disease organisms in body fluids enter the body through mucous membranes or through breaks in the skin. The most common forms of transmission are:

- blood to blood contact
- sexual contact with an infected person
- from an infected mother to her unborn child
- sharing needles with infected intravenous drug users

A first aider may be exposed to HIV and HBV in two ways. An open sore or wound may come in contact with a victim's infectious blood or other body fluids that contain blood. Or the first aider might not be wearing the proper personal protective equipment (PPE) (▶Figure 2-3) to protect against contact with infectious material.

Protection

In most cases, you can control the risk of exposure to bloodborne pathogens by wearing the proper PPE and by following some simple procedures.

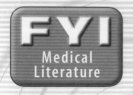

Facts about the Human Immunodeficiency Virus and Its Transmission

Research has revealed a great deal of valuable information about the human immunodeficiency virus (HIV) and acquired immunodeficiency syndrome (AIDS). The ways in which HIV can be transmitted have been clearly identified.

HIV is spread by sexual contact with an infected person, by needle-sharing among injecting drug users, or, less commonly (and now very rarely in countries where blood is screened for HIV antibodies), through transfusions of infected blood or blood clotting factors. Babies born to HIV-infected women may become infected before or during birth, or through breastfeeding after birth.

In the health-care setting, workers have been infected with HIV after being stuck with needles containing HIV-infected blood or, less frequently, after infected blood gets into the worker's bloodstream through an open cut or splashes into a mucous membrane (eg, eyes or inside of the nose).

Some people fear that HIV might be transmitted in other ways; however, no scientific evidence to support any of these fears has been found. The Centers for Disease Control and Prevention (CDC) reports:

1. Because HIV does not survive well outside its living host, it does not spread or remain infectious outside its host.

2. Although HIV has been transmitted between family members in a household setting, this type of transmission is very rare. These transmissions are believed to have resulted from contact between skin or mucous membranes and infected blood or body fluids.

3. Closed-mouth or "social" kissing is not a risk for HIV transmission. Because of the theoretical potential for contact with blood during "French" or open-mouthed kissing, the CDC recommends against engaging in this activity with an infected person. However, no case of AIDS reported to the CDC can be attributed to transmission through any kind of kissing.

4. HIV has been found in saliva and tears in only minute quantities from some AIDS patients. HIV has not been recovered from the sweat of HIV-infected persons. Contact with saliva, tears, or sweat has never been shown to result in HIV transmission.

5. There is no evidence of HIV transmission through biting or blood-sucking insects, even in areas where there are many cases of AIDS and large populations of mosquitoes. When an insect bites a person, it does not inject its own or a previous victim's blood into the new victim. Rather, it injects saliva (yellow fever and malaria are transmitted through the saliva of certain mosquito species).

6. No transmission has occurred involving rescue breathing during CPR manikin practice or actual resuscitation attempts.

CDC National AIDS Hotline: 1-800-342-AIDS (2437)

Spanish: 1-800-344-7432

Deaf: 1-800-243-7889

Source: Adapted from the Centers for Disease Control and Prevention

Personal Protective Equipment (PPE)

This equipment blocks entry of an organism into the body. The most common type of protection is gloves. The Food and Drug Administration (FDA), the Centers for Disease Control and Prevention (CDC), and the Occupational Safety and Health Administration (OSHA) have stated that vinyl and latex gloves are equally protective. Research indicates that latex has fewer micropores (very small holes) and thus offers the most protection. However, latex tends to break down faster over time (several years) while they sit in a first aid kit, waiting to be used. All first aid kits should have several pairs of gloves. Because some rescuers have allergic reactions to latex, non-latex gloves (vinyl or nitrile) should also be available (▶Figure 2-4).

Protective eyewear and a standard surgical mask may be necessary at some emergencies; first aiders ordinarily will not have or need such equipment.

Mouth-to-barrier devices are recommended for rescue breathing and CPR. There is no documented case of disease transmission to a rescuer as a result of performing unprotected CPR on an infected victim. Nevertheless, a mouth-to-barrier device should be used whenever possible (▶Figure 2-5).

(**Figure 2-3**) Whenever possible, use gloves as a barrier.

Figure 2-4 A–D Glove removal

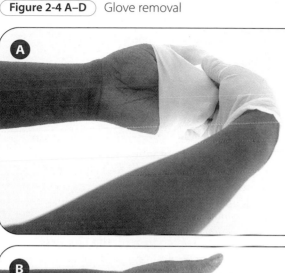

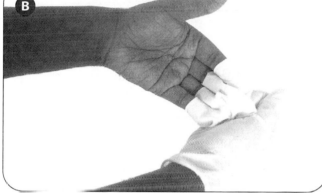

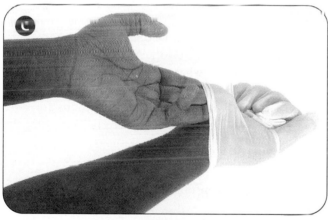

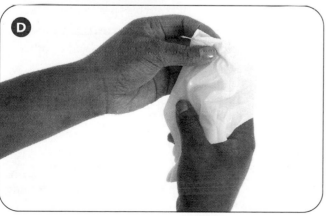

How to Remove Gloves

Take them off without touching their outside surface following these steps.

A. Pull the top towards the fingers, turning the glove inside out

B. As the glove comes off, hold it in the palm of your other hand.

C. Slide your fingers under the top of the other glove. Do not touch the outside of the glove.

D. First glove is inside the second. Dispose of properly.

Figure 2-5 Pocket face mask, one-way valve

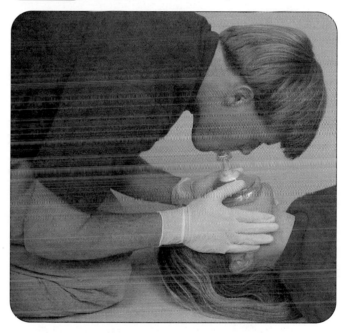

Universal Precautions or Body Substance Isolation?

Individuals infected with HBV or HIV may not show symptoms and may not even know they are infectious. For that reason, all human blood and body fluids should be considered potentially infectious, and precautions should be taken to avoid contact. *Body substance isolation* (BSI) procedures assume that *all* body fluids are a possible risk. EMS personnel routinely follow BSI procedures, even if blood or body fluids are not visible.

OSHA requires any company with employees who are expected to give first aid in an emergency to follow *universal precautions*, which assume that *all* blood and *certain* body fluids pose a risk for transmission

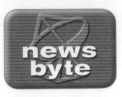

Latex Allergies: A Growing Risk

Allergies to latex, or natural rubber, can be disabling and even life-threatening, producing reactions ranging from mild dermatitis to wheezing, urticaria (skin eruptions with intense itching), and anaphylaxis (life-threatening anaphylactic shock). With the emphasis on protection against HIV and other bloodborne pathogens, latex products are becoming very common, increasing the opportunities for and likelihood of exposure to latex. Alternatives to latex examination gloves are products made of nitrile, neoprene, or vinyl. Latex allergy may be a serious barrier to pursuing a career in health care. For those in the health-care field who are severely allergic and react even to latex particles in the air, the only option may be to abandon the field of health care.

Source: Joby Kolsun; Latex Allergies: A Growing Risk, *Emergency Medicine*, Vol. 30, #10, pp. 66, 71; October 1998.

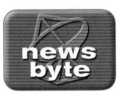

Do Gloves Really Protect?

A study tested the effectiveness of vinyl and latex gloves as barriers to hand contamination. Gloves were checked according to the American Society for Testing and Materials and leaks occurred with 43% of vinyl gloves and 9% of latex gloves. The researchers concluded that latex gloves, and to a lesser extent vinyl gloves, provide substantial protection during hand contact with moist body substances, functioning as a barrier even when leaks are present. Since leaks are not always detected by the wearer, hand washing should routinely follow the use of disposable gloves.

Source: R. J. Olsen et al; Examination Gloves as Barriers to Hand Contamination in Clinical Practice. *Journal of the American Medical Association,* 270:350–353; July 21, 1993.

of HBV and HIV. OSHA applies the "Good Samaritan" definition to an employee who assists another with a nosebleed or a cut. Such acts, however, are not considered occupational exposure unless the employee who provides the assistance is a member of a first aid team or is designated or expected to render first aid as part of his or her job. In essence, OSHA's requirement excludes unassigned employees who perform unanticipated first aid.

Whenever there is a chance that you could be exposed to bloodborne pathogens, your employer must provide

Handwashing

Wearing Personal Protective Equipment (PPE) and washing your hands are the best ways to protect against disease. If you have been exposed to blood or body fluids, follow these steps:

1. Remove your gloves and immediately wash your hands and contaminated body area with soap and water. Rub your hands together vigorously for at least 10 to 15 seconds (work up a lather), then rinse your hands and dry them with a paper towel.

2. Use a paper towel to turn off the faucet so you do not recontaminate yourself or others.

3. If you cannot wash immediately with soap and water, use antiseptic towelettes and wash with soap and water as soon as possible.

4. Flush your eyes, nose, and other mucous membranes with water if they have been exposed.

appropriate PPE, which might include eye protection, gloves, gowns, and masks. The PPE must be accessible, and your employer must provide training to help you choose the right PPE for your work.

While EMS personnel follow BSI procedures and OSHA requires designated worksite first aiders to follow universal precautions, what should a typical first aider do? It makes sense for first aiders to follow BSI procedures and assume that *all* blood and body fluids are infectious and follow appropriate protective measures.

Coping with Emergencies

When an injury occurs, first aiders can protect themselves and others against bloodborne pathogens by following these steps:

1. Wear appropriate PPE, such as gloves.

2. If you have been trained in the correct procedures, use absorbent barriers to soak up blood or other infectious materials.

3. Clean the spill area with an appropriate disinfecting solution, such as diluted bleach.

4. Discard contaminated materials in an appropriate waste disposal container.

If you have been exposed to blood or body fluids:

1. Use soap and water to wash the parts of your body that have been contaminated.

2. If the exposure happened at work, report the incident to your supervisor. Otherwise, contact your personal physician. Early action can prevent the development of hepatitis B and enable affected workers to track potential HIV infection.

The best protection against bloodborne disease is using the safeguards described here. By following these guidelines, first aiders can decrease their chances of contracting bloodborne illnesses.

Airborne Disease

Infective organisms such as bacteria or viruses introduced into the air by coughing or sneezing are said to be "airborne." Droplets of mucus that carry those bacteria or viruses can be inhaled by other individuals. The rate of tuberculosis (TB) has increased recently and is receiving much attention. TB, caused by bacteria, sometimes settles in the lungs and can be fatal. In most cases, a first aider will not know that a victim has TB. Assume that any person with a cough, especially one who is in a nursing home or a shelter, may have TB. Other symptoms include fatigue, weight loss, chest pain, and coughing up blood. If a surgical mask is available, wear it or wrap a handkerchief over your nose and mouth.

Death

There are few incidents that involve more emotional stress than the life-and-death situations that you might face. Death and dying are the unfortunate parts of providing emergency care.

The Dying Victim

A dying person presents a difficult situation. To assist such a victim:

- Avoid negative statements about the victim's condition. Even a semiconscious person can hear what is being said.
- Assure the victim that you will locate and inform his or her family of what has happened. Attempt to have family members present—they can provide great comfort to the victim.
- Allow some hope. Don't tell the victim that he or she is dying. Instead, say something like, "I don't know for sure. I won't give up on you, so don't give up on yourself. Keep trying."
- Do not volunteer information about the victim or others who may also be injured. However, if the victim asks a question about a family member, tell the truth. Provide simple, honest, clear information if it is requested and repeat it as often as necessary.
- Use a gentle tone of voice.
- Use a reassuring touch, if appropriate.
- Let the person know that everything that can be done to help will be done.

The Stages of Grieving

Both the dying and the surviving go through a grieving process that has been described as having the following five stages:

1. Denial ("Not me"). This is an attempt to create a buffer against the shock of dying and dealing with the illness or injury.
2. Anger ("Why me?"). Bystanders may be the target of the anger. Do not take the anger or insults personally. Be tolerant, use good listening skills, and be empathetic.
3. Bargaining ("OK, but first let me . . ."). In the victim's mind, an agreement will postpone the death for a short time.
4. Depression ("OK, but I haven't . . ."). This stage is characterized by sadness and despair. The person is usually silent and retreats into his or her own world.
5. Acceptance ("OK, I am not afraid"). This does not mean the person is happy about dying. The family often requires more support during this stage than the victim does.

Dealing with Survivors

Deal with the family members of a dead or dying victim as follows:

- Do not pronounce death; leave the confirmation of death to a physician.
- Allow survivors to grieve in whatever way seems right to them (anger, rage, crying).
- Provide simple, honest, clear information as it is requested, and repeat it as often as necessary. The survivors should not be told everything at once.
- Offer as much support and comfort as possible, by your presence as well as by your words. Do not leave an individual survivor alone, but do respect that person's right to privacy.
- Use a gentle tone of voice.
- Use a reassuring touch, if appropriate.

STUDY Questions ②

Name_____ Course_____ Date_____

Activities

Activity 1

Mark each statement as true (T) or false (F).

T   F   1. Every community in the United States uses the 9-1-1 telephone number.

T   F   2. Wearing medical exam gloves relieves first aiders of handwashing after caring for a wounded victim.

T   F   3. Bystanders are more likely to help with people around.

T   F   4. At some time, everyone will have to make the decision whether to help another person.

T   F   5. Deciding to help others should be done before encountering an emergency.

T   F   6. Fear of being injured stops some bystanders from helping another person.

T   F   7. A victim's negative image or appearance repulses some bystanders from helping.

T   F   8. Being negatively affected by the sight of blood is impossible to overcome.

T   F   9. Cases of HIV and HBV transmission have resulted from giving rescue breathing.

Activity 2

Choose the best answer.

____ 1. Bloodborne pathogens include
   a. HIV and HBV
   b. tuberculosis and meningitis
   c. hepatitis and tuberculosis

____ 2. Which is the most prevalent?
   a. HIV
   b. HBV
   c. HCV

____ 3. A vaccine is available for
   a. HIV
   b. HBV
   c. HCV

____ 4. Body Substance Isolation (BSI)
   a. assumes blood and all body fluids are infectious
   b. assumes blood and only certain body fluids are infectious
   c. is the same thing as "universal precautions"

____ 5. Latex gloves
   a. are not affected by chemicals
   b. are less porous than vinyl gloves
   c. may not be washed and reused

____ 6. Transmission of HIV
   a. is not possible through the mucous membranes
   b. can occur through nonintact skin
   c. is prevented by vaccination

____ 7. If you are exposed to blood,
   a. use soap and water to wash the exposed parts of your body
   b. contact your personal physician
   c. if on the job, report it to your supervisor
   d. all of the above

Activity 3

1. What five actions should a bystander perform at an emergency?

   a. _____

   b. _____

   c. _____

   d. _____

   e. _____

STUDY
Questions (2)

2. What three things should a first aider look for during a scene survey?

    a. _____

    b. _____

    c. _____

3. When calling for emergency assistance, you should be ready to give the EMS dispatcher the following information:

    a. _____

    b. _____

    c. _____

    d. _____

    e. _____

4. List two reasons why the caller should be the last to hang up the phone when talking to an EMS dispatcher.

    a. _____

    b. _____

5. How can first aiders protect themselves against bloodborne pathogens?

    a. _____

    b. _____

    c. _____

    d. _____

6. What can you do if you have been exposed to blood or body fluids?

    a. _____

    b. _____

7. How can you assist a family member of a deceased person?

    a. _____

    b. _____

    c. _____

8. What are the five stages of grieving?

    a. _____

    b. _____

    c. _____

    d. _____

    e. _____

9. List ways of desensitizing (calming) yourself while helping an injured victim at a scene involving blood, vomitus, etc.

    a. _____

    b. _____

    c. _____

Chapter Activities
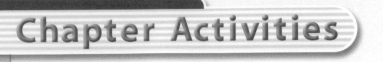

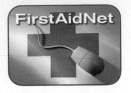

WEB
Activities

Action at an Emergency

Visit nsc.jbpub.com/FirstAidNet, then click on Web Activities, and select the appropriate chapter.

Post-Traumatic Stress Disorders

Many times, those helping an injured victim may experience Post-Traumatic Stress Disorder, which involves feeling terrified, powerless, and/or horrified. While not everyone will experience all of these feeling, some cases will be more severe than others.

Emergency Telephone Numbers

In most communities, you only need to know 9-1-1 during an emergency. However, keeping a list of emergency telephone numbers near the phone will save crucial minutes when you need to call for help.

CDC and Hepatitis

Hepatitis is a serious disease caused by a virus that attacks the liver. The virus can cause lifelong infection and damage including cirrhosis (scarring) of the liver, liver cancer, liver failure, and death. Hepatitis B vaccine is available for all age groups to prevent hepatitis B virus infection. Prevention guidelines are available for all forms of hepatitis.

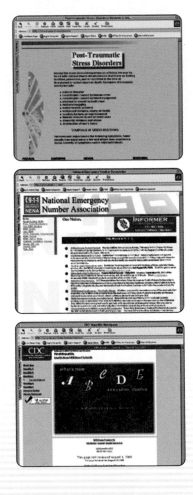

Victim Assessment

Part 2

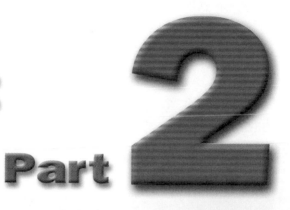

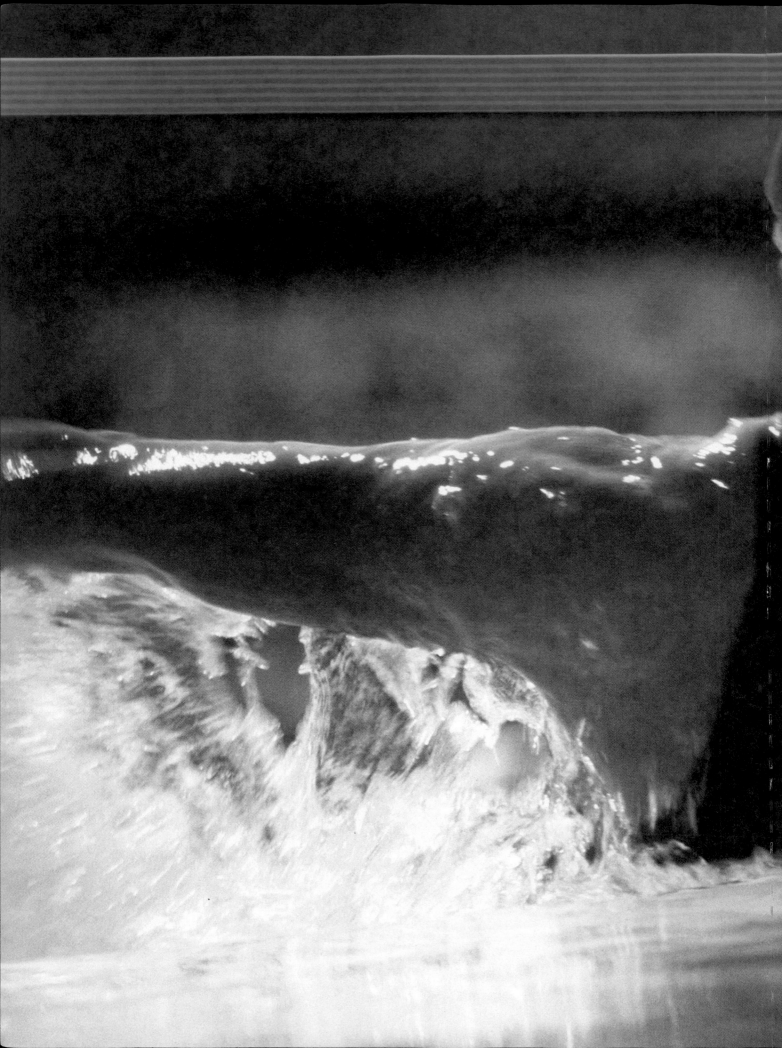

Chapter 3

The Human Body

To adequately assess a victim's condition and to give effective first aid, a first aider must be familiar with the anatomy and physiology of the human body. This knowledge provides a solid cornerstone for building the essentials of quality victim assessment and emergency first aid.

In injuries and illnesses, most life-threatening conditions affect the respiratory, circulatory, and nervous systems. These three body systems include the most important and sensitive organs: the lungs, the heart, the brain, and the spinal cord.

The other body systems are also important, and a good victim assessment can locate injury and/or sudden illnesses affecting them as well. The major body systems described in this chapter are the respiratory, circulatory, nervous, skeletal, and muscular systems, and the skin. The other body systems—the endocrine, gastrointestinal, and genitourinary systems—are not discussed.

The Respiratory System

The body can store food to last several weeks and water to last several days, but it can store enough oxygen for only a few minutes. Ordinarily this does not matter because we have only to inhale air to get the oxygen we need. If the body's oxygen supply is cut off, as in drowning, choking, or smothering, death will result in about four to six minutes unless the oxygen intake is restored. Oxygen from air is made available to the blood through the respiratory system and then to the body cells by the circulatory system.

Nose

Air normally enters the body during inhalation through the nostrils. It is warmed, moistened, and filtered as it flows over the damp, sticky lining (mucous membrane) of the nose. When a person breathes through the mouth instead of the nose, there is less filtration and warming. After passing through the nasal passages, air enters the nasal portion of the pharynx (throat).

Pharynx and Trachea

From the back of the nose or the mouth, the air enters the throat or **pharynx** (▼Figure 3-1). The pharynx is a common passageway for food and air. At its lower end, the pharynx divides into two passageways, one for food and the other for air. Muscular control in the back of the throat routes food to the food tube (**esophagus**), which leads to the stomach; air is routed from the pharynx to the windpipe (**trachea**), which leads to the lungs. The trachea and the esophagus are separated by a small flap of tissue (**epiglottis**), which acts as a valve to close the trachea when food is being swallowed. At all other times, the trachea remains open to permit breathing. Usually this diversion works automatically to keep food out of the trachea and to prevent air from entering the esophagus. If the epiglottis fails to close, food or liquid can enter the trachea instead of the esophagus.

However, normal swallowing controls do not operate if a person is unconscious. *That is why a first aider should never pour liquid into the mouth of an unconscious person in an attempt to revive him or her. The liquid may flow down into the windpipe and suffocate the victim.* Foreign objects, such as false teeth or a piece of food, may also lodge in the throat or windpipe and cut off the passage of air.

In the upper two inches of the trachea, just below the epiglottis, is the voice box (**larynx**), which contains the vocal cords. The larynx can be felt in the front of the throat (Adam's apple).

(**Figure 3-1**) Respiratory system

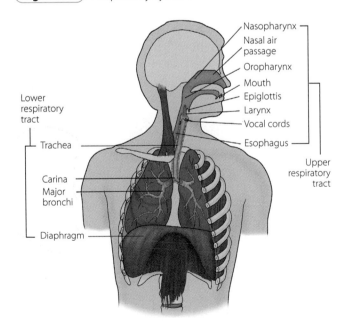

- Lower respiratory tract
  - Trachea
  - Carina
  - Major bronchi
  - Diaphragm

- Nasopharynx
- Nasal air passage
- Oropharynx
- Mouth
- Epiglottis
- Larynx
- Vocal cords
- Esophagus

Upper respiratory tract

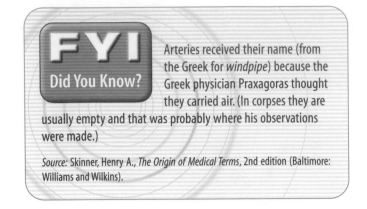

FYI
Did You Know?

Arteries received their name (from the Greek for *windpipe*) because the Greek physician Praxagoras thought they carried air. (In corpses they are usually empty and that was probably where his observations were made.)

Source: Skinner, Henry A., *The Origin of Medical Terms*, 2nd edition (Baltimore: Williams and Wilkins).

Lungs

The trachea branches into two main tubes (bronchial tubes or bronchi), one for each lung. Each bronchus divides and subdivides somewhat like the branches of a tree. The smallest bronchi end in thousands of tiny pouches (alveoli or air sacs), just as the twigs of a tree end in leaves. Each air sac is enclosed in a network of capillaries. The walls that separate the air sacs and the capillaries are very thin. Through those walls, oxygen combines with hemoglobin in red blood cells to form oxyhemoglobin, which is carried to all parts of the body. Carbon dioxide and certain other waste gases in the blood move across the capillary walls into the air sacs and are exhaled from the body. The lungs occupy most of the chest cavity.

Mechanics of Breathing

The passage of air into and out of the lungs is called **respiration.** Breathing in is called **inhalation**; breathing out is **exhalation.**

Respiration is a mechanical process brought about by alternately increasing and decreasing the size of the chest cavity. When the diaphragm (the dome-shaped muscle dividing the chest from the abdomen) contracts, the chest expands, drawing air into the lungs (inhalation). An exchange of oxygen and carbon dioxide takes place in the lungs. When the diaphragm expands, it exerts pressure on the lungs, causing air to flow out (exhalation).

Infants and children differ from adults. Their respiratory structures are smaller and more easily obstructed than those of adults. Infants' and children's tongues take up proportionally more space in the mouth than do adults'. The trachea is more flexible in infants and children. The primary cause of cardiac arrest in infants and children is an uncorrected respiratory problem.

The average rate of breathing in an adult at rest is 12 to 20 complete respirations per minute (▶Table 3-1).

Table 3-1: Normal Respiration Rate Ranges

Breaths per Minute*	
Adults	12 to 20
Children	15 to 30
Infants	25 to 50

*To obtain the breathing rate in a person, count the number of breaths in a 30-second period and multiply by 2. Avoid letting the person know you are counting to prevent influencing the rate.

Normal rates for children are from 15 to 30 times per minute; infant rates will be between 25 and 50 times per minute. Normally the rate slows when a person is lying down, and speeds up during vigorous exercise. The rate of breathing is controlled by a nerve center in the brain (the respiratory center).

Signs of inadequate breathing include a rate of breathing outside normal ranges, cool or clammy skin with a pale or cyanotic (blue-gray) color, and nasal flaring, especially in children.

When a person performs hard muscular work, the lungs cannot get rid of carbon dioxide or take in oxygen fast enough at the normal rate. As carbon dioxide increases in the blood and tissues, the respiratory center sends impulses along its nerves to cause deeper and more rapid respirations. At the same time, the heart rate increases. This increases the supply of oxygen available to the body, as the heart pumps more blood through the lungs.

The Circulatory System

The circulatory system (▶Figure 3-2) is made up of the blood, the heart, and the blood vessels. Blood is the great delivery system for cells throughout the body. It carries nutrients and other products from the digestive tract in its plasma, and oxygen from the lungs in its hemoglobin. It also transports wastes produced by the cells to the lungs, kidneys, and other excretory organs for removal from the body.

Heart

The human circulatory system is a completely closed circuit of tubelike vessels through which blood flows. The heart (▶Figure 3-3), by contracting and relaxing, pumps blood through the vessels. It is a powerful,

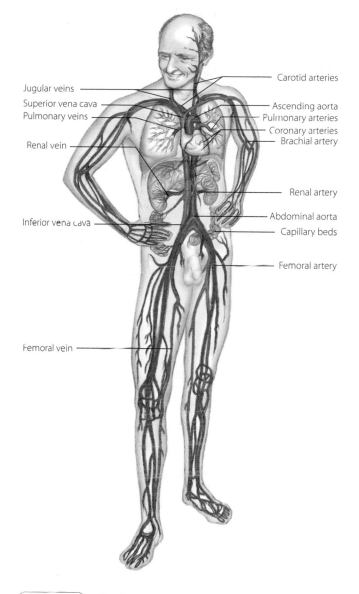

Jugular veins
Superior vena cava
Pulmonary veins
Renal vein
Inferior vena cava
Femoral vein

Carotid arteries
Ascending aorta
Pulmonary arteries
Coronary arteries
Brachial artery
Renal artery
Abdominal aorta
Capillary beds
Femoral artery

(Figure 3-2) Circulatory system

hollow, muscular organ about as big as a man's clenched fist, shaped like a pear, and located in the left center of the chest, behind the sternum (breast bone). The heart is divided by a wall in the middle. Right and left compartments are divided into two chambers, atrium above, ventricle below. Check valves are located between each atrium and its corresponding ventricle and at the exit of the major arteries leading out of each ventricle. The opening and shutting of these valves at just the right time in the heartbeat keeps the blood from backing up.

At each beat, or contraction, the heart pumps blood rich in carbon dioxide and low in oxygen from the right ventricle to the lungs and returns oxygen-rich blood to

A

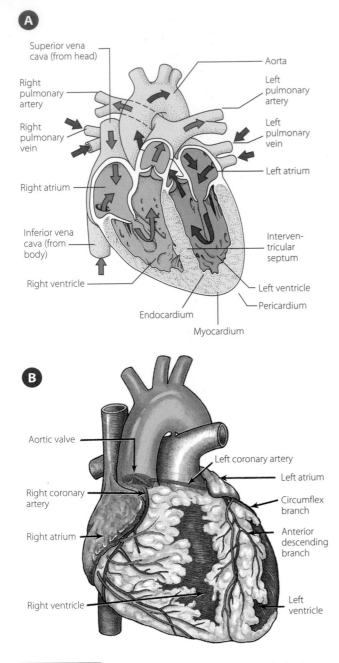

Superior vena cava (from head)

Aorta

Right pulmonary artery

Left pulmonary artery

Right pulmonary vein

Left pulmonary vein

Left atrium

Right atrium

Inferior vena cava (from body)

Interventricular septum

Right ventricle

Left ventricle

Pericardium

Endocardium

Myocardium

B

Aortic valve

Left coronary artery

Left atrium

Right coronary artery

Circumflex branch

Anterior descending branch

Right atrium

Right ventricle

Left ventricle

(**Figure 3-3, A–B**) **A.** Heart—circulation (internal view) **B.** Heart—coronary arteries (external view)

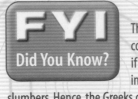
tubes: the pulmonary artery, which carries blood to the lungs for the carbon dioxide–oxygen exchange, and the aorta, which carries blood to all the other parts of the body. The aorta divides and subdivides until it ends in networks of extremely fine vessels (**capillaries**) smaller than hairs. Through the thin walls of the capillaries, oxygen and food pass out of the bloodstream into the stationary cells of the body, while the body cells discharge their waste products into the bloodstream. In the capillaries of the lungs, carbon dioxide is released and oxygen is absorbed. Capillaries, having reached their limit of subdivision, begin to join together again into **veins.** The veins become larger and larger and finally form major trunks that empty blood returning from the body into the right atrium and blood from the lungs into the left atrium.

It is impossible to prick normal skin anywhere without puncturing capillaries. Because the flow of blood through the capillaries is relatively slow and under little pressure, blood merely oozes from a punctured capillary and usually has time to clot, promptly plugging the leak.

Each time the heart contracts, the surge of blood can be felt as a pulse at any point where an artery lies close to the surface of the body, near the skin surface and

the left atrium of the heart. The left ventricle pushes blood rich in oxygen freshly obtained to the rest of the body and returns oxygen-poor blood to the right atrium. At each relaxation of the heart, blood flows into the left atrium from the lungs and into the right atrium from the rest of the body (▶**Table 3-2**).

Blood Vessels

The **arteries** are elastic, muscular tubes that carry blood away from the heart. They begin at the heart as two large

Table 3-2: Normal Heart Rates	
Beats per Minute*	
Adults	60 to 100
Children	80 to 100
Toddlers	100 to 120
Newborns	120 to 140

*To obtain a heart rate in most people, count the number of beats over a 30-second period and multiply by 2.

over a bone. When an artery is cut, blood spurts out. There is no pulse in a vein because the pulse is lost by the time the blood has passed through the capillaries. Hence, blood from a cut vein flows out in a steady stream. It has much less pressure behind it than blood from a cut artery.

Major locations for feeling pulses include the following:

- **Carotid:** the major artery of the neck, which supplies the head with blood. Pulsations can be palpated (felt) on either side of the neck (do not try to feel both at the same time). Use the carotid to check an unconscious person's pulse.

- **Femoral:** the major artery of the thigh supplying the lower extremities with blood. Pulsations can be palpated in the groin area (the crease between the abdomen and thigh).

- **Radial:** the major artery of the lower arm. Pulsations can be palpated at the palm side of the wrist on the thumb side. Use the radial to check a conscious person's pulse.

- **Brachial:** an artery of the upper arm. Pulsations can be palpated on the inside of the arm between the elbow and the armpit. Use the brachial to determine a pulse in an infant.

- **Posterior tibial:** located behind the inside ankle knob. Pulsations can be palpated on the posterior surface of the medial malleolus.

- **Dorsalis pedis:** Pulsations can be palpated on the top surface of the foot (▶**Figure 3-4**) (20% of the population have no pulsations).

Blood Pressure

Blood pressure is a measure of the pressure exerted by the blood on the walls of the flexible arteries. Blood pressure may be high or low according to the resistance offered by the walls to the passage of blood. This difference in resistance may be due to several causes. For example, if blood does not fill the system, as following hemorrhage, the pressure will be low (**hypotension**). High blood pressure (**hypertension**) may be present when the arterial walls have become hard and cannot expand readily.

Blood

Blood has liquid and solid portions. The liquid portion is called *plasma*. The solid portion, which is transported by the plasma, includes disk-like red blood cells; slightly larger, irregularly shaped white blood cells; and an immense number of smaller bodies called platelets.

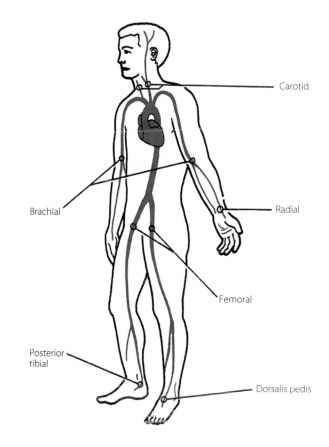

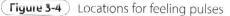
(**Figure 3-4**) Locations for feeling pulses

Plasma, the liquid part of the blood, is about 90% water, in which minerals, sugar, and other materials are dissolved. Plasma carries food materials picked up from the digestive tract and transports them to the body cells. It also carries waste materials produced by cells to the kidneys, digestive tract, sweat glands, and lungs for elimination (excretion) in urine, feces, sweat, and expired breath.

The red blood cells, which give blood its color, carry oxygen to the organs. The white blood cells are part of the body's defense against bacteria. These cells can go wherever they are needed in the body to fight infection, for example, a wound in the skin or other tissue that is diseased or injured. Pus, a sign of wound infection, gets its yellowish-white color from the innumerable white blood cells that are fighting the invading bacteria.

Platelets are essential for the formation of blood clots. If blood plasma did not clot at the site of a wound, the slightest cut or abrasion would produce death from bleeding. Clots plug the openings through which blood escapes from punctured blood vessels. Bleeding from a large blood vessel may be too rapid to permit the formation of a clot. **Hemorrhage** is the term for profuse bleeding.

Perfusion refers to the circulation of blood through an organ or a structure. **Hypoperfusion** is the inadequate circulation of blood through an organ or a structure. The average-size adult male has about six quarts (12 pints) of blood.

Inadequate circulation is known as **shock** (hypoperfusion). Shock is a state of profound depression of the vital processes of the body, characterized by the following signs and symptoms: pale, cyanotic (bluish), cool, clammy skin; rapid pulse; rapid breathing; restlessness, anxiety, or mental dullness; nausea and vomiting; reduction in total blood volume; low or decreasing blood pressure; and subnormal temperature.

The Nervous System

The nervous system is a complex collection of nerve cells (neurons) that coordinate the work of all parts of the human body and keep the individual in touch with the outside world. Neurons receive stimuli from the environment and transmit impulses to nerve centers in the brain and spinal cord. Then, by a complicated process of thinking (reasoning) plus reflex and automatic reactions, they produce nerve impulses that regulate and coordinate all bodily movements and functions and govern behavior and consciousness.

Once nerve cells have been destroyed, the body cannot regenerate them. Some limited nerve repair is possible, however, as long as the vital cell body is intact. If a nerve fiber is cut or injured, the section attached to the cell body remains alive, but the part beyond the injury withers away.

The nervous system can be classified in different ways. From a structural standpoint, there is (1) the central nervous system, which includes the brain and the spinal cord, and (2) the peripheral nervous system, a network of nerve cells that originates in the brain and spinal cord and extends to all parts of the body, including the muscles, the surface of the skin, and the special sense organs, such as the eyes and the ears. The peripheral nervous system is further subdivided into the voluntary and the autonomic (involuntary) nervous systems.

Central Nervous System

The central nervous system (CNS) consists of the brain (▶Figure 3-5), which is enclosed within the skull, and the spinal cord, which is housed in a semi-flexible bony column of vertebrae. The CNS serves as the controlling organ of the body. The brain enables us to think, judge, and act. The spinal cord is a major communication pathway between the brain and the rest of the body.

Brain

The brain, which is the headquarters of the human nervous system, is probably the most highly specialized organ in the body. It weighs about three pounds in the average adult, is richly supplied with blood vessels, and requires considerable oxygen to perform effectively.

The brain has three main subdivisions: the cerebrum (large brain), which occupies nearly all (75%) of the cranial cavity; the cerebellum (small brain), and the brain stem. The cerebrum is divided into two hemispheres by a deep cleft. The outer surface of the cerebrum, the cerebral cortex, is about one-eighth of an inch thick, composed mainly of cell bodies of nerve cells and often referred to as "gray matter."

Certain sections of the cerebrum are localized to control specific body functions such as sensation, thought, and associative memory, which allows us to store, recall, and make use of past experiences. The sight center of the brain is located at the back of the cerebrum, and is called the occipital lobe. The temporal lobes, at the sides of the head, deal with smell and hearing.

The cerebellum is located at the back of the cranium (skull) and below the cerebrum. Its main function is to coordinate muscular activity.

The third major area of the brain is the brain stem, which extends from the base of the cerebrum to the foramen magnum (a large opening at the base of the skull).

Small cavities in the brain contain the **cerebrospinal fluid** (CSF), a clear, watery solution similar to blood plasma. Circulating throughout the brain and the spinal cord, CSF serves as a protective cushion and exchanges food and waste materials. The total quantity of CSF in the brain-spinal cord system is 100 to 150 ml, although up to several liters may be produced daily. It is constantly being produced and reabsorbed.

(**Figure 3-5**) Brain

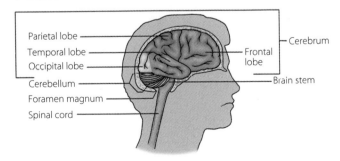

Parietal lobe
Temporal lobe
Occipital lobe
Cerebellum
Foramen magnum
Spinal cord
Cerebrum
Frontal lobe
Brain stem

Their knowledge of nerve structure and function enables physicians to locate diseased brain sections. Because nerves from one side of the body eventually connect with the opposite side of the brain, a person whose left arm is paralyzed after a stroke will have suffered damage to the right side of the brain.

Spinal Cord

The spinal cord (▼Figure 3-6) is a soft column of nerve tissue continuous with the lower part of the brain that is enclosed in the bony vertebral column. The spinal cord exits the brain through the foramen magnum. Thirty-one pairs of spinal nerves branch from the spinal cord. These nerves are large trunks that are similar to telephone cables because they house many nerve fibers. Some fibers carry impulses into the spinal cord; others carry impulses away from it. Spinal nerves at different levels of the cord regulate activities of various parts of the body.

Because the spinal cord lies close to the bony walls of the vertebra, especially in the cervical (neck) and thoracic (chest) regions, it is particularly vulnerable to injury. Damage to the cord is almost always irreversible. An injury to the lumbar (lower back) spine causes paralysis and loss of sensation in the legs; an injury to the cervical cord causes paralysis and loss of sensation in the arms as well as in the legs.

(Figure 3-6) Spinal cord

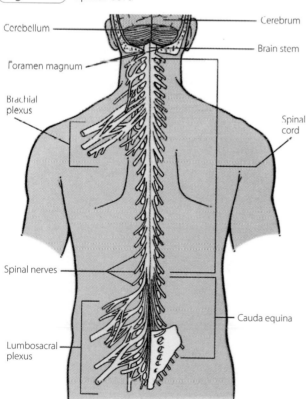

- Cerebellum
- Foramen magnum
- Brachial plexus
- Spinal nerves
- Lumbosacral plexus
- Cerebrum
- Brain stem
- Spinal cord
- Cauda equina

Peripheral Nervous System

At each vertebral level and on each side of the spinal cord, a spinal nerve exits the spinal cord through an opening in the bony canal. These nerves make up the peripheral nervous system.

The peripheral nervous system consists of the sensory and motor nerves. The sensory nerves carry sensations such as smell, touch, heat, and sound from the body to the brain and the spinal cord. The motor nerves carry information from the brain and the spinal cord to the body.

Autonomic Nervous System

The autonomic nervous system consists of a group of nerves that control heart rate, digestion, sweating, and other automatic body processes. These processes are not controlled by the conscious mind, but they can be influenced by the CNS to a limited extent.

If a nerve is cut or seriously damaged, disrupting the connection between the brain and the body, the body part will not be able to work. For example, if the motor nerve going to the right leg is cut, the leg will be unable to move. This may be a permanent loss. Injuries to the nerves in the spinal cord can be very serious.

Fortunately, the CNS is well protected against injury. The brain is enclosed in the cranial cavity of the skull. The spinal cord is contained in the hollow space of the vertebrae. The brain and the spinal cord are also protected by three layers of tissue known as the meninges. The space between the layers of the meninges is filled with CSF, which also helps protects the brain and spinal cord from injury.

The Skeletal System

The human body is shaped by its bony framework. Without its bones, the body would collapse. The adult skeleton (▶Figure 3-7) has 206 bones. Bones are composed of living cells surrounded by hard deposits of calcium. The bone cells are well supplied by blood vessels and nerves. The calcium deposits give bones their strength and rigidity. Broken bones are repaired by bone-building cells lying in the bone and its covering sheath, the periosteum. New bone is formed at the site of the break, much as two pieces of steel are welded together.

Skull

The skull rests at the top of the spinal column. It contains the brain, certain special-purpose glands (such as the pituitary and the pineal), and the centers of special senses—sight, hearing, taste, and smell. The skull has two parts, the brain case (cranium) and the face (▶Figure 3-8).

Figure 3-7 Skeletal system

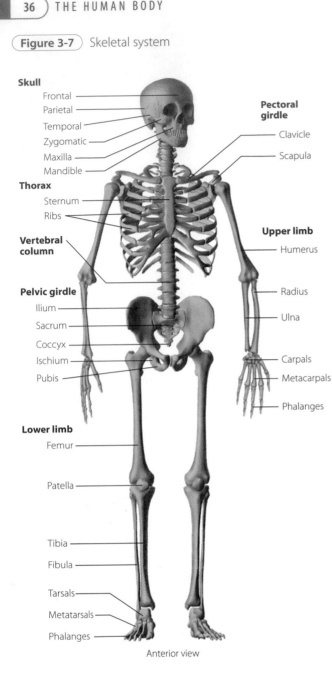

Skull
- Frontal
- Parietal
- Temporal
- Zygomatic
- Maxilla
- Mandible

Thorax
- Sternum
- Ribs

Vertebral column

Pelvic girdle
- Ilium
- Sacrum
- Coccyx
- Ischium
- Pubis

Lower limb
- Femur
- Patella
- Tibia
- Fibula
- Tarsals
- Metatarsals
- Phalanges

Pectoral girdle
- Clavicle
- Scapula

Upper limb
- Humerus
- Radius
- Ulna
- Carpals
- Metacarpals
- Phalanges

Anterior view

Figure 3-8 Skull

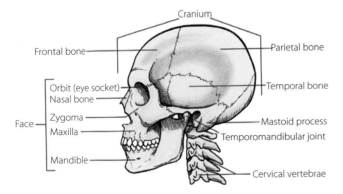

- Cranium
- Frontal bone
- Orbit (eye socket)
- Nasal bone
- Face
  - Zygoma
  - Maxilla
- Mandible
- Parietal bone
- Temporal bone
- Mastoid process
- Temporomandibular joint
- Cervical vertebrae

Blood vessels and nerve trunks pass to and from the brain through openings in the skull, mostly at the base. The largest opening is the foramen magnum, where the spinal cord joins the brain. The brain, which fits snugly in the cranium, is covered by the meninges membranes. The very narrow spaces between the membranes are filled with CSF.

Although the skull is very tough, a blow may fracture it. Even if there is no fracture, a sudden impact may tear or bruise the brain and cause it to swell, as any soft tissue will swell following an injury or bruise. Because the skull does not "give," injury to the brain is magnified by the contained pressure. Unconsciousness or even death may result from swelling (**edema**), a tearing wound (**laceration**), bleeding, or other damage to the brain.

The face extends from the eyebrows to the chin and forms the eyes, nose, cheeks, mouth, and lower jaw (mandible).

Spinal Column

The spinal column (▼**Figure 3-9**) is made up of irregularly shaped bones called **vertebrae** (singular is *vertebra*). Lying one on top of the other to form a strong flexible column, the vertebrae are bound firmly together by strong ligaments. Between each two vertebrae is an intervertebral disk, a pad of tough elastic cartilage that acts as a shock absorber.

The spinal column can be damaged by disease or by injury. A crushed or displaced vertebra can squeeze, stretch, tear, or sever the spinal cord. Moving the disabled part by the injured person or careless handling by well-

Figure 3-9 Spinal column (spine)

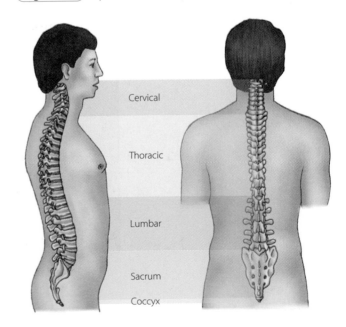

- Cervical
- Thoracic
- Lumbar
- Sacrum
- Coccyx

meaning but uninformed persons can further displace sections of the spinal column, resulting in additional injury to the cord and possibly permanent paralysis. For that reason, a person with a back or neck injury must be handled with extreme care.

Thorax

The thorax (rib cage) is made up of ribs and the sternum (breastbone). The sternum is a flat, narrow bone in the middle of the front wall of the chest. The collar bones and certain ribs are attached to the sternum.

The 24 ribs are semiflexible arches of bone. There are 12 on each side of the chest. The back ends of the 12 pairs of ribs are attached to the 12 thoracic vertebrae. Strong ligaments bind the back ends of the ribs to the backbone but allow slight gliding or tilting movements. The front ends of the top 10 pairs of ribs are attached to the sternum by cartilage. The front ends of the last two pairs (pairs 11 and 12) hang free, giving them the name "floating ribs."

Fractures of the sternum or the ribs usually result from crushing or squeezing the chest. A fall, blow, or penetration of the chest wall by an object may have the same effect. The chief danger from such injuries is that the lungs or heart may be punctured by the sharp ends of the broken bones.

The lowest portion of the sternum is the **xiphoid process**, which is used as the landmark for determining the hand position for chest compressions given in CPR.

Pelvis

The two hipbones and the sacrum form the pelvic girdle (pelvis). Muscles help attach the pelvic bones, the trunk, the thighs, and the legs. The pelvis forms the floor of the abdominal cavity. The lower part of the cavity, sometimes called the pelvic cavity, holds the bladder, rectum, and internal parts of the reproductive organs. The floor of the pelvic cavity helps to support the intestines.

Leg Bones

Upper Leg (Thigh)

At the outer side of each hipbone is a deep socket into which the round head of the thighbone (**femur**) fits, forming a ball-and-socket joint. The lower end of the femur is flat and has two knobs. These knobs articulate with the shinbone (**tibia**) at the knee joint. Although the femur is the longest and strongest bone in the skeleton, it is a common fracture site. A fractured femur is always serious because it is difficult to align the broken or splintered ends to create a strong union. Because of the force required to break the femur, laceration of the surrounding tissues, pain, and blood loss may be extensive.

Knee

The knee joint is the largest joint in the body and is a strong hinge joint. The joint is protected and stabilized in the front by the kneecap (**patella**). The patella is a small triangular-shaped bone in front of and between the femur and the tibia and within the tendon of the large muscle of the front of the thigh. Because the patella usually receives the force of falls or blows to the knee, it is frequently bruised or dislocated and sometimes fractured.

Lower Leg

The lower leg refers to that portion of the lower extremity between the knee and the ankle. Its two bones are the **tibia** and the **fibula** (▼Figure 3-10). The tibia (shin bone) is at

Figure 3-10   Lower extremity bones

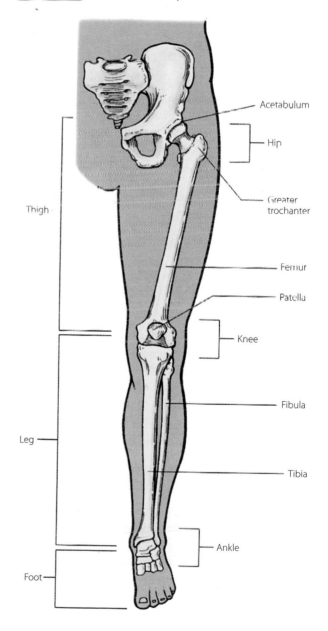

the front and inner side of the leg. It is palpable throughout its length. Its broad upper surface receives the end of the femur to form the knee joint. The lower end, much smaller than the upper end, forms the inner rounded knob of the ankle (medial malleolus). The fibula, which is not a part of the true knee joint, is attached at the top to the tibia. Its lower end forms the outside ankle knob (lateral malleolus). The fibula is more often fractured alone than is the tibia.

Ankle, Feet, and Toes

The ends of the tibia and fibula form the socket of the ankle joint. Both ankle knobs are easily palpated. The seven ankle bones (**tarsals**) are bound firmly together by tough ligaments. The heel bone (calcaneus) transmits the weight of the body to the ground and forms a base for the muscles of the calf of the leg when walking (▼**Figure 3-11**).

The sole and the instep of the foot are formed by the five long **metatarsals**. These articulate with the tarsals and with the front row of toe bones (phalanges).

Shoulder

The collar bone (**clavicle**) and the shoulder blade (**scapula**) form the shoulder girdle. Each clavicle—a long, slightly double-curved bone—is attached to the sternum at its inner end and to the scapula at its outer end. Each clavicle can be palpated (felt) throughout its length. Fractures are common because the clavicle lies close to the surface and must absorb blows.

Each scapula—a large, flat, triangular bone—is located over the upper ribs at the back of the thorax.

Arm Bones

Upper Arm

The bone of the upper arm, the **humerus,** is the arm's largest bone. Its upper end (the head) is round; its lower

end is flat. The round head fits into a shallow cup in the shoulder blade, forming a ball-and-socket joint. This is the most freely movable joint in the body and is easily dislocated. Dislocations may tear the capsule of the joint (synovial membrane) and cause damage. Improper manipulation during attempts to reduce or "set" the dislocation may add to the damage. Therefore, it is important to treat dislocations of the shoulder with gentle care.

Forearm

The two bones of the forearm (**radius** and **ulna**) lie side by side. The larger of the two, the ulna, is on the little finger side, and part of it forms the elbow. The flat, curved lower end of the humerus fits into a big notch at the upper end of the ulna to form the elbow joint. This hinge joint permits movement in one direction only. The radius, shorter and smaller than the ulna, is on the thumb side of the forearm (▼**Figure 3-12**).

Wrist, Hand, and Fingers

The wrist is composed of eight small, irregularly shaped bones (**carpals**) united by ligaments. Tendons extending from the muscles of the forearm to the bones of the hand and fingers pass down the front and the back of the wrist close to the surface. Wrist lacerations may sever these tendons, resulting in total or partial immobility of the fingers.

(**Figure 3-12**) Arm bones

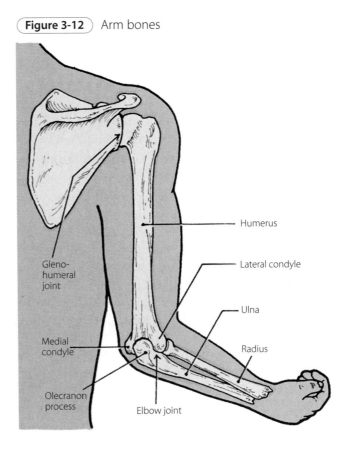

(**Figure 3-11**) Ankle, foot bones

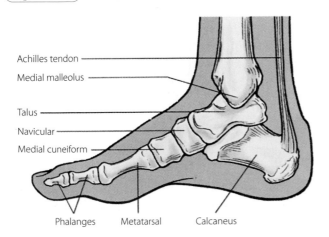

The palm of the hand has five long bones (**meta-carpals**). The 14 bones of the fingers (phalanges) give the hand its great flexibility. The thumb is the most important digit. A good thumb and one or two fingers make a far more useful hand than four fingers minus the thumb (▼Figure 3-13).

Joints

A joint is where two or more bones meet or join. Some joints, such as those in the cranium, allow little, if any, movement of the bones. Other joints, such as the hip and the shoulder, allow a wide range of motion. In a typical joint, a layer of cartilage (gristle), which is softer than bone, acts as a pad or buffer. The bones of such a joint are held in place by firmly attached ligaments, which are bands of very dense, tough, but flexible connective tissue. Joints are enclosed in a capsule, a layer of thin tough material, strengthened by the ligaments. The inner side of the capsule (synovial membrane) secretes a thick fluid (**synovial fluid**) that lubricates and protects the joint.

Muscular System

Body movement is due to work performed by muscles (▶Figure 3-14) Examples are walking, breathing, the

(Figure 3-13) Wrist, hand, finger bones

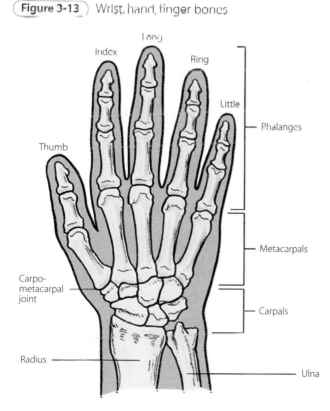

beating of the heart, and the movements of the stomach and the intestines. What enables muscle tissue to perform work is its ability to contract—that is, to become shorter and thicker— when stimulated by a nerve impulse. The cells of a muscle, usually long and threadlike, are called *fibers*. Each muscle has countless bundles of closely packed, overlapping fibers bound together by connective tissue. The three different kinds of muscles are skeletal muscle (voluntary), smooth muscle (involuntary), and cardiac muscle (heart). They differ both in appearance and in the specific jobs they do.

Skeletal Muscles

The skeletal muscles, which are under the control of a person's will, make possible all deliberate acts: walking, chewing, swallowing, smiling, frowning, talking, moving the eyeballs. Most voluntary muscles are attached by one or both ends to the skeleton by tendons. However, some muscles are attached to skin, cartilage, and special organs, such as the eyeball, or to other muscles, such as the tongue.

Muscles help to shape the body and to form its walls. Most skeletal muscles end in tough, whitish cords (**tendons**) that attach them to the bones they move. Tendons continue into the fascia, which covers the skeletal muscles. The fascia is much like the skin of a sausage in that it surrounds the muscle tissue. At either end of the muscle, the fascia extends beyond the muscle to attach to a bone. That area is lined with a synovial membrane, which secretes a lubricating substance, the synovial fluid. This makes it easier for the tendon to move when the muscle contracts or relaxes. Muscular contraction pulls the bone in the direction permitted by a joint.

When they are not working, muscles become comparatively slack. But they never completely relax; some fibers are contracting all the time. They always have some tension (muscle tone).

Muscles can be injured in many ways. Overexerting a muscle can break fibers. Muscles can be bruised, crushed, cut, torn, or otherwise injured, with or without breaking the skin. Muscles injured in any of those ways are likely to become swollen, tender, painful, or weak.

Smooth Muscles

A person has little or no control over the smooth muscles and usually is not conscious of them. Smooth muscles line the walls of tubelike structures such as the gastrointestinal tract, the urinary system, the blood vessels, and the bronchi of the lungs.

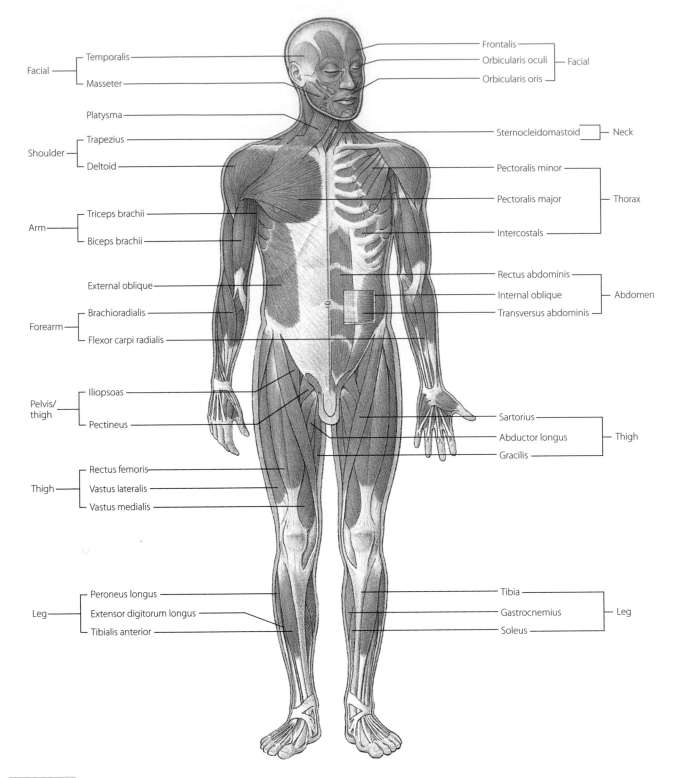

Facial
— Temporalis
— Masseter

Platysma

Shoulder
— Trapezius
— Deltoid

Arm
— Triceps brachii
— Biceps brachii

External oblique

Forearm
— Brachioradialis
— Flexor carpi radialis

Pelvis/thigh
— Iliopsoas
— Pectineus

Thigh
— Rectus femoris
— Vastus lateralis
— Vastus medialis

Leg
— Peroneus longus
— Extensor digitorum longus
— Tibialis anterior

Frontalis
Orbicularis oculi — Facial
Orbicularis oris

Sternocleidomastoid — Neck

Pectoralis minor
Pectoralis major — Thorax
Intercostals

Rectus abdominis
Internal oblique — Abdomen
Transversus abdominis

Sartorius
Abductor longus — Thigh
Gracilis

Tibia
Gastrocnemius — Leg
Soleus

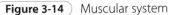

Figure 3-14 Muscular system

Cardiac Muscle

Cardiac muscle is a specialized form of muscle found only in the heart. A continuous supply of oxygen and glucose is needed for cardiac muscle to work properly.

Skin

The skin covers the entire body, protecting the deep tissues from being injured, drying out, or being invaded by bacteria and other foreign bodies. The skin helps to regulate body temperature, by aiding in the elimination of water and various salts. The skin senses heat, cold, touch, pressure, and pain and transmits that information to the brain and the spinal cord.

The skin (▼Figure 3-15) consists of two layers: the outer layer (**epidermis**) and the inner layer (**dermis**). The epidermis varies in thickness in different parts of the body (the palms and the soles of the feet are thickest), and its dead cells are constantly worn off. The dermis has a rich supply of blood vessels and nerve endings. Hair grows from the dermis through openings called hair folli-

cles. Sweat glands and oil glands in the dermis empty onto the surface of the epidermis through pores in the skin. Beneath the dermis is the subcutaneous ("under the skin") layer, which is well supplied with fat cells and blood vessels.

Sweat (perspiration) glands occur in nearly all parts of the skin. Sweat contains essentially the same minerals as blood plasma and urine, but it is more dilute. Normally, only traces of the waste products excreted in urine are in sweat. But when sweating is profuse or when the kidneys are diseased, the amounts of such wastes excreted in the sweat may be considerable. Several mineral salts are removed from the body in sweat. Chief among those in quantity is sodium chloride (the same mineral as common table salt).

A general knowledge of the human body, similar to that outlined in this chapter, should help in understanding the other chapters in this book. Even though you will not be making a medical diagnosis, you will be able to suspect what is wrong with a victim and provide proper first aid. You will also be able to communicate correct information to medical personnel with the least possible confusion.

(Figure 3-15) Skin

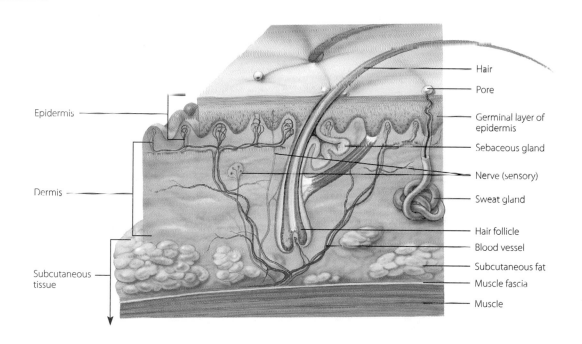

STUDY
Questions ③

Name_____ Course_____ Date_____

Activities

Activity 1

Mark each statement as true (T) or false (F).

T F **1.** Conditions involving the respiratory, nervous, and skeletal systems can threaten life.

T F **2.** Cerebrospinal fluid (CSF) is blood found on the surfaces of the brain and spinal cord.

T F **3.** The brain can swell and press against the skull.

T F **4.** Floating ribs are the bottom two pairs of ribs hanging free.

T F **5.** The longest and strongest bone in the body is the sternum.

T F **6.** Normal swallowing controls do not work in an unconscious person.

T F **7.** The malleolus in the ankle are the lower ends of the tibia and fibula bones.

T F **8.** Of the two bones in the forearm, the ulna is on the thumb side.

T F **9.** The epiglottis closes when food is being swallowed.

T F **10.** The Adam's apple is a common term for the front of the larynx.

T F **11.** The heart is about the size of a clenched fist and shaped like a pear.

T F **12.** A pulse happens where a vein passes near the skin's surface and over a bone.

T F **13.** Hemorrhage is the term for profuse bleeding.

Activity 2

Choose the best answer.

____ **1.** How many quarts of blood are in the body of an average sized adult?
  a. 4 quarts
  b. 6 quarts
  c. 8 quarts
  d. 10 quarts

____ **2.** The bone between the shoulder and elbow is the
  a. femur
  b. humerus
  c. scapula
  d. radius
  e. tibia

____ **3.** The _____ is the pulse point used in unconscious victims.
  a. carotid
  b. aorta
  c. brachial
  d. femoral

____ **4.** The collarbone is known as the
  a. ulna
  b. metacarpal
  c. tarsal
  d. clavicle

____ **5.** The major artery that leaves the left side of the heart and carries freshly oxygenated blood to the body is referred to as the
  a. vena cava
  b. carotid artery
  c. aorta
  d. pulmonary vein

Match the following:

____ **6.** prevents food and liquid from entering the lungs

____ **7.** part of the larynx that can be felt in front of the throat

____ **8.** outer layer of skin

____ **9.** attaches muscle to bone

____ **10.** kneecap

  a. tendon
  b. patella
  c. epiglottis
  d. Adam's apple
  e. epidermis

____ **11.** The trachea is the
  a. passageway leading to the stomach
  b. passageway leading to the lungs
  c. opening from the stomach to the small intestines
  d. opening between the esophagus and stomach

STUDY
Questions (3)

Which structure(s) are located in the upper arm?

___ **12.** scapula

___ **13.** humerus

___ **14.** sciatic nerve

___ **15.** radial pulse

___ **16.** The bones of the upper extremity include which of the following?

    a. occipital

    b. femur

    c. ulna

    d. patella

What is the average rate of breathing for

17. _____ adults

18. _____ children

19. _____ infants

What is the average pulse rate for

20. _____ adults

21. _____ children

22. _____ toddlers

23. _____ newborns

Name the major locations for feeling each of the following pulses.

    Name   Location

24. Carotid   _____

25. Radial   _____

26. Brachial   _____

27. Posterior tibial   _____

28. Dorsalis pedis   _____

Which of the following statements are true?

___ **29.** The heart receives its nutrients and oxygen via the coronary veins.

___ **30.** The heart is cone-shaped and about the size of a golf ball.

___ **31.** The right ventricle pumps blood to the body.

___ **32.** The heart has four chambers.

Match the following elements of blood with their corresponding definition(s).

    a. red blood cells

    b. white blood cells

    c. plasma

    d. platelets

___ **33.** tiny, disk-shaped elements that, when ruptured, release chemical factors needed to form blood clots

___ **34.** carry oxygen to and carbon dioxide away from the tissues

___ **35.** involved in destroying germs and producing antibodies that help the body resist infection

___ **36.** watery, salty fluid that makes up more than half the blood's volume

37. List the three types of blood vessels:

    a. _____

    b. _____

    c. _____

38. List the three most important body systems sustaining life:

    a. _____

    b. _____

    c. _____

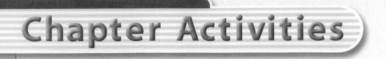

Chapter Activities

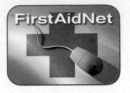

WEB Activities

The Human Body

Visit **nsc.jbpub.com/FirstAidNet, then click on Web Activities, and select the appropriate chapter.**

The Skeletal System

This web site offers extensive visuals for a review of the body's skeletal system. Keeping up on the basics of the human anatomy can help a first aider recognize and treat an injury or illness.

The Inner Body

Most first aiders can still provide effective care without extensive knowledge of the human body. But there are advantages to knowing the basics of human anatomy.

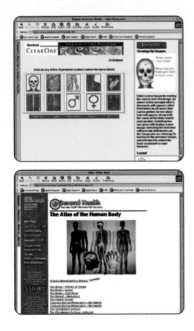

Chapter 4

Finding Out What's Wrong

Victim Assessment

Victim assessment is an important first aid skill. It requires an understanding of each assessment step as well as decision-making skills.

Every time you encounter a victim, first check out the scene. The scene survey determines the safety of the scene, the victim's cause of injury or nature of illness, and the number of victims. Without a scene survey, a potentially dangerous situation could result in further injury to the victim or to you and others.

The scene survey is followed by the initial victim assessment. During the initial victim assessment, the first aider identifies and corrects immediate life-threatening conditions involving problems with the victim's airway, breathing, and circulation (the ABCs). Victims with immediate life-threatening conditions can die within minutes unless their problems are quickly recognized and corrected. Determining the type of injury or illness is also part of the initial assessment.

A physical examination and medical history follow the initial assessment. These steps can reveal information that will help identify the injury or illness, its severity, and appropriate first aid. Detailed information is gained about the victim's injury (eg, painful ankle, bleeding nose) or chief complaint (eg, chest pain, itchy skin).

If two or more people are injured, attend to the quiet one first. A quiet victim might not be breathing or have a heartbeat. A victim who is talking, crying, or otherwise alert is obviously breathing.

Initial Assessment

The goal of the initial assessment is to determine whether there are life-threatening problems that require quick care ▶Skill Scan . This assessment involves evaluating the victim's responsiveness, airway (A), breathing (B), and circulation (C) ▶Figure 4-1 . The following step-by-step initial assessment should not be changed. It takes less than a minute to complete, unless first aid is required at any point. By the end of the initial assessment, the victim's

Skill Scan | Initial Assessment

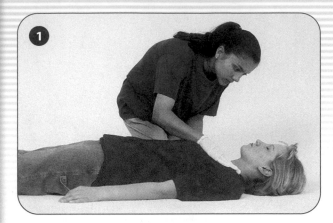

1. Responsive? Tap and shout.

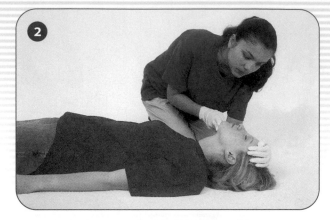

2. A = Airway open? Head-tilt/chin-lift.

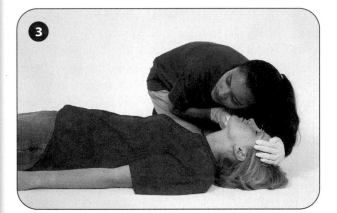

3. B = Breathing? Look, listen, and feel.

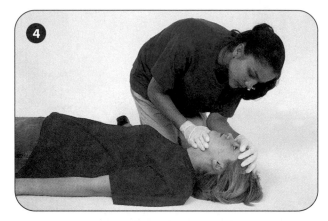

4. C = Circulation? Check for signs of circulation.

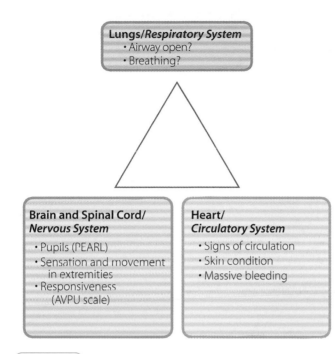

Lungs/Respiratory System
• Airway open?
• Breathing?

Brain and Spinal Cord/ Nervous System
• Pupils (PEARL)
• Sensation and movement in extremities
• Responsiveness (AVPU scale)

Heart/ Circulatory System
• Signs of circulation
• Skin condition
• Massive bleeding

Figure 4-1 How to assess the three most important body systems

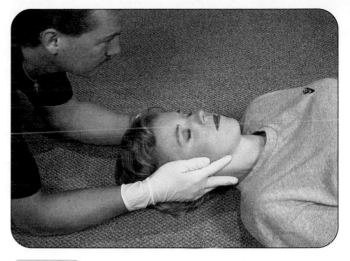

Figure 4-2 Immobilizing the head with the hands

Table 4-1: The AVPU Scale

A = Alert and aware
V – Responds to verbal stimulus
P = Responds to painful stimulus
U = Unresponsive

A: Alert. The victim's eyes are open, and he or she can answer questions clearly. A victim who knows the date (time), where he or she is (place), and his or her own name (person) is said to be alert.

V: Responsive to verbal stimulus. The victim might not be oriented to time, place, and person but does respond in some meaningful way when spoken to.

P: Responsive only to painful stimulus. The eyes do not open, and the victim does not respond to questions. The victim does respond when the muscle between the neck and shoulder is pinched.

U: Unresponsive to any stimulus. The eyes do not open, and the victim does not respond to pinching of the muscle between the neck and shoulder.

problem will most likely be identified as being an injury or an illness.

Begin the initial assessment with a check for responsiveness. If there is a possibility of a spinal injury, have another person hold the victim's head to minimize movement and avoid causing further damage (►Figure 4-2).

Check for responsiveness by speaking to the victim. If the person can talk, breathing and heartbeat are present. If the victim does not respond, tap his or her shoulder and ask, "Are you okay?" If there is no response, consider the victim as being unresponsive.

The level of responsiveness, from alert to unresponsive, is one of the most important indicators of the victim's overall condition. The AVPU scale is used to describe the level of responsiveness (►Table 4-1).

Immediate Threats to Life

A: Airway

The airway must be open for breathing. If the victim is speaking or crying, the airway is open. If a responsive victim cannot talk, cry, or cough forcefully, the airway is probably obstructed and must be checked and cleared. In this case, abdominal thrusts (Heimlich maneuver) can be given to clear an obstructed airway in a responsive adult victim. Refer to Chapter 5 where the Heimlich maneuver is described in detail.

In an unresponsive victim lying face up, the most common airway obstruction is the tongue. Snoring is evidence of this. If there is no suspected spinal injury, use the head tilt–chin lift method to open the airway. If a spinal injury is likely, use the jaw-thrust method to prevent further injury. Chapter 5 outlines these maneuvers in full detail.

Once the victim's airway is clear of obstruction, the initial assessment can continue.

VICTIM ASSESSMENT

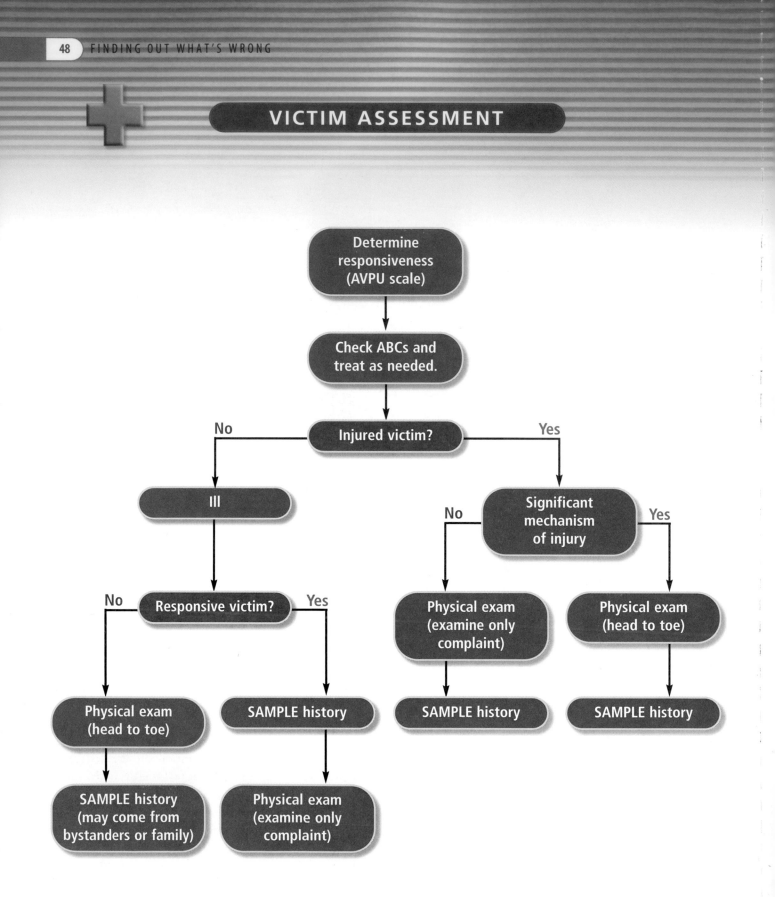

Victim Assessment Checklist

1. **Scene Survey**
   Hazards?
   Number of victims?
   Mechanism (cause) of injury?
2. **Initial Assessment**
   A = Airway open?
   B = Breathing?
   C = Circulation
   - breathing? coughing? movement?
   - hemorrhage?
   - skin condition (temperature, moisture, color)
3. **Physical Exam**
   Head: D-O-T-S, CSF
   Eyes: PEARL
   Neck: D-O-T-S
   Chest: D-O-T-S (squeeze)
   Abdomen: D-O-T-S (push)
   Pelvis: D-O-T-S (squeeze and push)
   Extremities: D-O-T-S, CSM
4. **Victim's History** (for sudden illness, may be completed before physical exam)
   SAMPLE
   Medical-alert tag?

Victim Assessment Sequence

- Determine responsiveness (AVPU scale)
- Perform the initial assessment (ABCs)

Injured Victim

1. Significant Mechanism of Injury:
   a. Physical exam (head to toe)
   b. SAMPLE history
2. No Significant Mechanism of Injury:
   a. Physical exam (examine only complaint)
   b. SAMPLE history

Ill Victim

1. Responsive:
   a. SAMPLE history
   b. Physical exam (examine only complaint)
2. Unresponsive:
   a. Physical exam (head to toe)
   b. SAMPLE history (from bystanders)

B: Breathing

A breathing rate between 12 and 20 times per minute is normal for adults. Victims who are having difficulty moving air and who are breathing less than eight times per minute or more than 24 times per minute need care. Note any breathing difficulties or unusual breathing sounds such as wheezing, crowing, gurgling, or snoring. This step primarily focuses upon whether or not the victim is breathing and obvious breathing difficulties rather than the breathing rate.

Check for breathing in an unresponsive victim after opening the airway. Watch for the victim's chest to rise and fall as you place your ear next to the victim's mouth. "Look, listen, and feel" for about ten seconds to check for breathing. If the victim is not breathing, keep the airway open and breathe two slow breaths into the victim. Refer to Chapter 5 for details. Whenever possible, use a mouth-to-barrier device (mask or face shield).

C: Circulation

After checking and correcting any airway and breathing problems, check the victim's circulation. Note victim's signs of circulation —breathing, coughing, movement, the skin color and temperature, and search for severe bleeding.

Signs of circulation. Check the victim for normal breathing, coughing, or movement in response to the rescue breaths.

Severe Bleeding Check for severe bleeding by looking over the victim's entire body for blood (blood-soaked clothing or blood pooling on the floor or the ground). Controlling bleeding requires the application of direct pressure or a pressure bandage. Avoid contact with the victim's blood, if possible, by using medical exam gloves or extra layers of dressings or cloth. Control any bleeding with pressure as described in Chapter 6.

Skin Condition A quick check of the victim's skin can also provide information about circulatory status. Check skin temperature, color, and condition (eg, moist, dry). Skin color, especially in light-skinned people, reflects the circulation under the skin as well as oxygen status. In darkly pigmented people, changes might not be readily apparent but can be assessed by the appearance of the nail beds, the inside of the mouth, and the inner eyelids. When the skin's blood vessels constrict or the pulse slows, the skin becomes cool and pale or cyanotic (blue-gray color). When the skin's blood vessels dilate or blood flow increases, the skin becomes warm.

You can get a rough idea of temperature by putting the back of your hand or wrist on the victim's forehead. If the

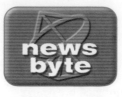

Detecting a Pulse

Researchers performed a study of 449 lay people to evaluate their skills in checking the carotid pulse. The majority of the participants had just completed a 16-hour or 8-hour first aid course. A small group were evaluated before attending a course. All volunteers were asked to check the carotid pulse in a young, healthy, nonobese person by counting aloud the detected pulse rate. The average time was 9.46 seconds. Only 47.7% of the participants could detect a carotid pulse within five seconds, and 73.3% within 10 seconds. It took more than 35 seconds for 95% of the volunteers to detect the pulse correctly. Checking for a pulse by lay persons has been discontinued.

Source: Bahr, J., et al., Skills of Lay People in Checking the Carotid Pulse. *Resuscitation*, 1997; 35:23–26.

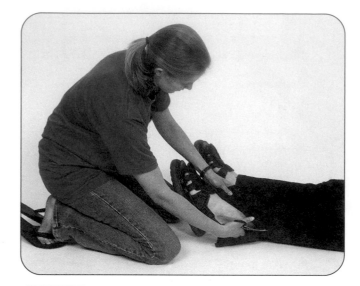

Figure 4-3 Expose the injury. Remove as much clothing as necessary, while trying to maintain privacy.

victim has a fever, you should be able to feel it. Abnormal skin temperature will feel hot, cool, cold, or clammy (cool and moist).

What is the purpose of a physical examination?

The goal of doing a "hands-on" physical exam is to identify immediately any potentially life-threatening illness or injury. It also helps to provide an objective database on which to establish emergency care. A good physical exam plus a well-taken medical history are the essential elements in discovering what is wrong. If you don't know what's wrong, you can't treat it.

Expose the Injury

Clothing may have to be removed to check for an injury and to give proper first aid. If you need to remove clothing, explain what you intend to do and why. Remove as much as necessary, try to maintain privacy, and prevent exposure to cold. Damage clothing only if necessary—cut along the seams ▶**Figure 4-3**.

Physical Exam and SAMPLE History

The initial assessment is followed by a physical examination and the SAMPLE history ▶**Skill Scan**. Up to this point, the initial assessment has been the same for both ill and injured victims. Likewise, whether the victim has an injury or an illness, the steps in the physical exam and SAMPLE history are similar.

Injured Victim

The physical exam and SAMPLE history of the injured victim take place immediately after the initial assessment. Start by reconsidering the mechanism (cause) of injury that you identified previously, during the scene survey. This allows you to determine which procedures to use in checking an injured victim.

Injured Victim with a Significant Mechanism of Injury ▶**Table 4-2**. For an injured victim with a significant mechanism of injury, take the following steps in this order: stabilize the head to keep it from moving, monitor the ABCDs, perform a physical examination, and obtain a SAMPLE history.

In addition to the significant mechanisms of injury, assume that a victim with a head injury may also have a spinal injury until proven otherwise. About 15% to 20% of head injury victims also have a spinal injury.

Assess a responsive victim for a spine injury by asking:

- Can you feel me squeezing your fingers and toes?
- Can you wiggle your fingers and toes?
- Can you squeeze my hand and push your foot against my hand?

Skill Scan · Physical Exam: Injury

Briefly Inspect by Looking and Feeling for D-O-T-S Throughout the Body

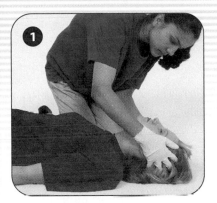

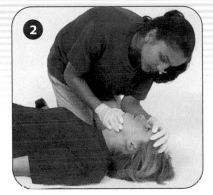

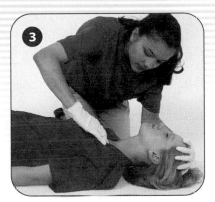

1. Head: Check the skull and scalp. Look and feel for D-O-T-S. Check for clear fluid in ears (cerebrospinal fluid).

2. Eyes: Gently open both eyes and compare the pupils—they should be the same size. Check to see if they react to light.

3. Neck: Look and gently feel for D-O-T-S. Check for a medical-alert necklace.

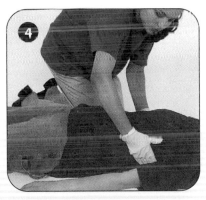

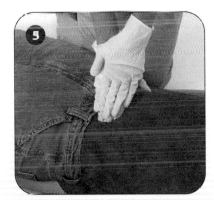

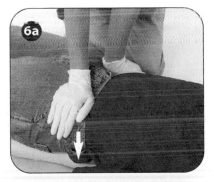

4. Chest: Check for D-O-T-S. Gently squeeze the chest for rib pain.

5. Abdomen: Check for D-O-T-S. Gently press the four abdominal quadrants.

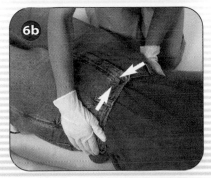

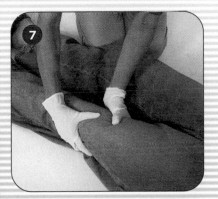

7. Extremities: Check the full length of both arms and legs for D-O-T-S. Check for CSM—circulation (pulse), sensation, movement.

6. Pelvis: Check for D-O-T-S:
   a. Gently press downward on the tops of the hips for pain.
   b. Gently press towards each other for pain.

Table 4-2: Significant Mechanisms (Causes) of Injury

- Falls of more than 15 feet for adults, more than 10 feet for children, or more than three times the victim's height
- Vehicle collisions involving ejection, a rollover, high speeds, a pedestrian, a motorcycle, or a bicycle
- Unresponsive or altered mental status
- Penetrations of the head, chest, or abdomen (eg, stab or gunshot wounds) of the muscle between the neck and shoulder.

For an unresponsive victim, test the integrity of the spinal cord by stroking the bottom of the foot firmly toward the big toe with a key or similar sharp object. This is known as the Babinski reflex test. The normal response is an involuntary reflex that makes the big toe go down (except in infants where it goes in the opposite direction). If the spinal cord or brain is injured, the toe will flex upward for both adults and children.

If you suspect a spinal injury, do not move the victim's head or neck. Stabilize the victim against any movement, and be sure to tell him or her not to move.

Physical Examination A good physical exam is very important for the injured victim who is unresponsive or has a significant mechanism of injury.

Check the victim's head, neck, chest, abdomen, pelvis, and extremities. To evaluate these areas, look and feel for the following signs of injury: deformities, open injuries, tenderness, and swelling. The mnemonic "D-O-T-S" is helpful in remembering the signs of injury (▶Skill Scan):

- **D**eformities occur when bones are broken, causing an abnormal shape.
- **O**pen wounds break the skin.
- **T**enderness is sensitivity to touch.
- **S**welling is the body's response to injury that makes the area look larger than usual.

Head Have someone stabilize the victim's head and neck to keep it from moving. Look and feel for D-O-T-S over the entire head. Look for leakage of blood or fluid (cerebrospinal fluid) from the nose or ears.

Eyes Check the pupils of the eyes for equality and reactivity to light. (PEARL: **P**upils **E**qual **A**nd **R**eact to **L**ight.) The pupils are normally equal in size. Unequal pupils occur normally in 2% to 4% of the population, but in others, the pupils should be of equal size when the brain

is not injured (▼Figure 4-4). To check for reactivity to light, use a flashlight or cover and then uncover the victim's eyes with your hand. Pupils normally quickly constrict in response to light.

Neck Look and feel for D-O-T-S.

Caution:

WHEN DOING A PHYSICAL EXAM

DO NOT aggravate injuries or contaminate wounds.

DO NOT move a victim with a possible spinal injury.

Chest Look and feel the entire chest for D-O-T-S. Squeeze or compress the sides together for rib pain.

Abdomen Look and feel for D-O-T-S. Gently press all four abdominal quadrants for rigidity and tenderness, using the pads of your fingers (▶Figure 4-5). If the victim complains of pain in a particular area, ask the victim to point to it; press that area last.

Pelvis Look and feel for D-O-T-S. Gently squeeze the hips inward together and gently press the hips downward.

(**Figure 4-4**) Changes in pupil size can have medical significance.

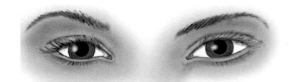

Dilated pupils

Constricted pupils

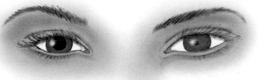

Unequal pupils

Extremities Look and feel the entire length and girth of each extremity (arms and legs) for D-O-T-S. Check the **C**irculation, **S**ensation, and **M**ovement (use the mnemonic "CSM" as a way of remembering) of each extremity. Check for circulation in the arms by feeling for the radial pulse on the victim's thumb side of the wrist and check the circulation of the legs by feeling for the posterior tibial pulse between the inside of the ankle bone and the Achilles tendon. To check for sensation, ask the victim whether he or she can feel you pinching his or her fingers and toes. To check for movement, ask the victim to wiggle his or her fingers and toes, to squeeze your hand with his or her hands, and to push his or her feet against your hand. Compare the responses of one extremity against the responses of the other for any differences.

SAMPLE History The information in a SAMPLE history can affect the first aid you give. It is called a SAMPLE history because the letters in the word "SAMPLE" stand for the elements of the history (▶Table 4-3).

If the victim is unresponsive, you may be able to obtain the SAMPLE history information from family, friends, or bystanders.

Injured Victim with No Significant Mechanism of Injury Focus the physical examination of a victim without a significant mechanism of injury on areas that

Table 4-3: SAMPLE History	
Description	**Sample Questions**
S = Symptoms	"What's wrong?" (known as the chief complaint)
A = Allergies	"Are you allergic to anything?"
M = Medications	"Are you taking any medications? What are they for?"
P = Past medical history	"Have you had this problem before? Do you have other medical problems?"
L = Last oral intake	"When did you last eat or drink anything? What was it?"
E = Events leading up to the illness or injury	Injury: "How did you get hurt?" Illness: "What led to this problem?"

the victim complains about and areas that you think might be injured, based on the mechanism of injury. If the victim has no significant mechanism of injury and no immediately life-threatening injuries, the steps of the physical exam and the SAMPLE history are simplified.

Determine the chief complaint— the problem as the victim describes it. For example, one victim might complain of a cut finger while another tells you about pain from twisting an ankle. Begin the physical examination at the site of the injury or the chief complaint, using the mnemonic "D-O-T-S." Your assessment focuses on just the areas that the victim tells you are painful or that you suspect may be injured. After the physical exam, conduct a SAMPLE history.

Suddenly Ill Victim

With a responsive ill victim, first obtain the victim's SAMPLE history then conduct a physical examination focused on the victim's chief complaint (symptoms). With an unresponsive ill victim, perform a rapid physical examination first, followed by the victim's SAMPLE history.

Responsive Ill Victim A responsive ill victim's SAMPLE history is obtained before the physical examination. The victim should be the main source of information; additional sources could include family, friends, and bystanders.

The main reason for talking to the victim is to find out his or her chief complaint—the one thing that seems

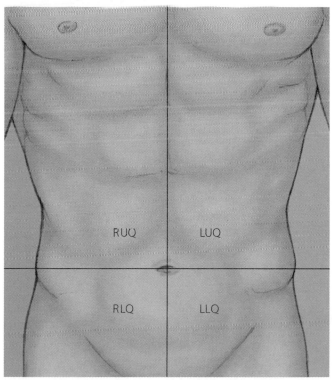

(**Figure 4-5**) Gently press the four quadrants for firmness and softness.

RUQ LUQ

RLQ LLQ

Skill Scan D-O-T-S

Examine an Area by Looking and Feeling for Deformity, Open Wounds, Tenderness, and Swelling (D-O-T-S)

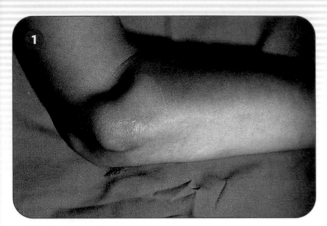

1. D = Deformity.

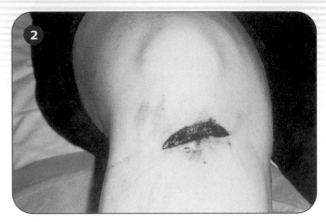

2. O = Open wounds.

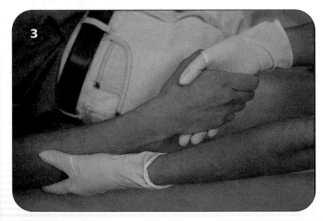

3. T = Tenderness.

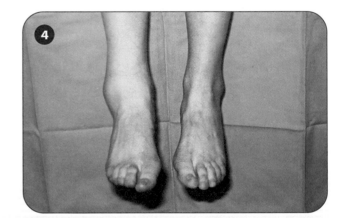

4. S = Swelling.

most seriously wrong with him or her. After finding out what is wrong, get the rest of the SAMPLE history. This information can affect the first aid you give.

After obtaining the SAMPLE history, perform a physical examination. Focus the physical examination on the victim's chief complaint. For example, if the victim's complaint is chest pain, the physical exam focuses on that area. After the physical examination, provide first aid based on what you found.

Unresponsive Ill Victim For an unresponsive ill victim, the assessment sequence is different. Because you cannot obtain a SAMPLE history from the victim, you begin with the physical exam. After this, gather as much of the SAMPLE history as you can from any family, friends, or bystanders.

Another difference between what you do for responsive and unresponsive ill victims is the type of physical exam that you perform. For a responsive victim, you can focus the physical exam on the victim's main complaint.

Because an unresponsive ill victim can't tell you where the problem is, you will need to do a rapid physical examination of the entire body.

The physical exam of an unresponsive ill victim will be almost the same as the physical exam of an injured victim. You rapidly check the victim's head, neck, chest, abdomen, pelvis, and extremities. As you check each area, look for deformities, an open wound, tenderness, and swelling (D-O-T-S). For the specific physical examination steps, see the earlier section "Injured Victim with a Significant Mechanism of Injury." Medic Alert® identification tags also provide important information (▶**Figure 4-6**). Because an unresponsive ill victim cannot talk, interview bystanders as a possible source of SAMPLE history.

Medical Identification Tags

Look for medical identification tags, which may be beneficial in identifying allergies, medications, or medical

Signs/Symptoms

+ Signs = victim's conditions you can see, feel, hear, or smell

+ Symptoms = things the victim feels and is able to describe; known as the "chief complaint"

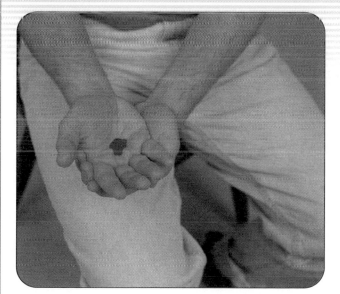

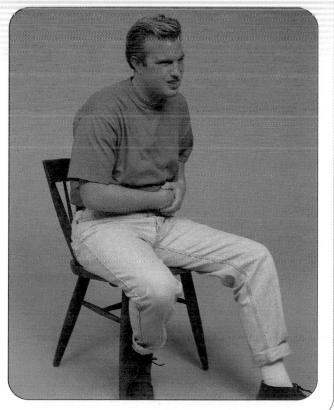

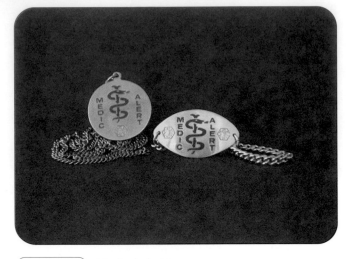

Figure 4-6 Medical-alert tag

history. A medical-alert tag, worn as a necklace or as a bracelet, contains the wearer's medical problem(s) and a 24-hour telephone number that offers, in case of an emergency, access to the victim's medical history plus names of doctors and close relatives. Necklaces and bracelets are durable, instantly recognizable, and less likely than cards to be separated from the victim in an emergency.

What to do Until EMS Arrives

The initial assessment, physical examination, and SAMPLE history are done quickly so that injuries and illnesses can be identified and given first aid and, if necessary, transportation can be arranged. After the most serious problems have been cared for, regularly recheck the victim.

Check the victim's responsiveness, airway, breathing, circulation, and the effectiveness of first aid. Do this at least every 15 minutes for an alert victim, who has no serious injury or illness, and at least every five minutes for a victim who is unresponsive; has difficulties with airway, breathing, or circulation, including major blood loss; or has a significant mechanism of injury. When in doubt, repeat the ongoing assessment every five minutes or as frequently as possible.

Advantages of the Left-Side Position

Left-side positioning is referred to by several terms: recovery position, left lateral recumbent position, left lateral decubitus position, and stable-side position. Positioning a person on his or her left side has several advantages:

+ It keeps the airway open in an unresponsive breathing victim without a spinal injury.

+ It delays vomiting by placing the esophagus above the stomach.

+ It delays a poison's effects by retaining the poison in the stomach (the pyloric sphincter is kept straight up). A poison can be better dealt with in the stomach than in the small intestines.

+ It relieves pressure on a pregnant woman's vena cava (the body's largest vein). Many pregnant women will pass out or at least feel dizzy if they lie supine (on their backs), because of the reduced blood flow.

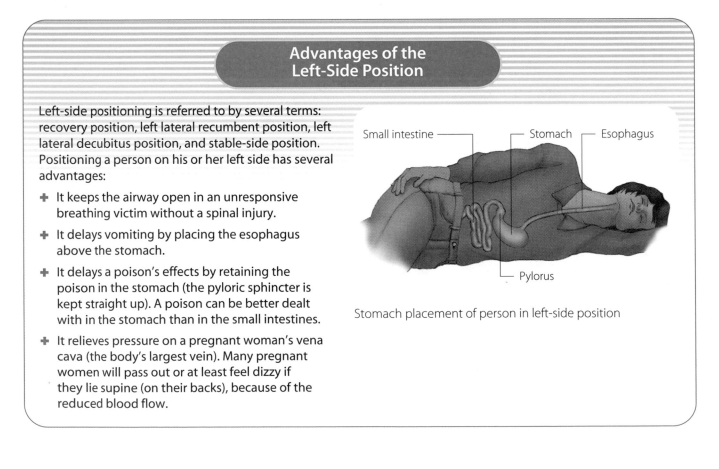

Small intestine — Stomach — Esophagus

— Pylorus

Stomach placement of person in left-side position

When EMS personnel arrive, provide the following information:

1. victim's chief complaint
2. responsiveness (AVPU scale)
3. ABCD (airway, breathing, circulation, disability) status
4. physical exam findings
5. SAMPLE history
6. any first aid that has been provided

First-in-the-United States 9-1-1

Haleyville, Alabama was the first 9-1-1 emergency telephone service in the United States. The first ceremonial 9-1-1 call in the town of 4,500 rang on February 16, 1968. On February 22, 1968, Nome, Alaska implemented 9-1-1 service.

But the concept of a national number had been around for three decades before that. Britain created the first—using 999—in 1937. In the United States, the first catalyst for a nationwide emergency telephone number was in 1957, when the National Association of Fire Chiefs recommended use of a single number for reporting fires. The U.S. Congress recommended a national number in 1958 and, a decade later, the Federal Communications Commission (FCC) and AT&T designated 9-1-1 as the emergency number throughout the United States. It was chosen because it is brief, easily remembered, quickly dialed, and was not used in any telephone exchange at the time.

Today, 9-1-1 covers about 93 percent of the United States population. 95 percent of that coverage is Enhanced 9-1-1 that gives a caller's address. Approximately 96% of the geographic U.S. is covered by some type of 9-1-1.

Examples of some other countries' national emergency numbers: Australia, 000; Canada, 911; Denmark, 112; Irish Republic, 999; Italy, 113; Kenya, 999; Switzerland, 112; Venezuela, 171.

Source: Adapted from the National Emergency Number Association, *The Development of 9-1-1*; www.nena 9-1-1.org

STUDY Questions ④

Name_____ Course_____ Date_____

Activities

Activity 1

Mark each statement as true (T) or false (F).

T   F   1. Laypersons should check for a pulse.

T   F   2. The mnemonic D-O-T-S helps in remembering what to look for during a physical exam.

T   F   3. For an unresponsive victim, use the signs of circulation.

T   F   4. Unequal pupils of the eyes are an indication of a brain injury or a stroke.

T   F   5. The absence of the signs of circulation may indicate that the victim has suffered a heart attack.

T   F   6. Limited use of one side of the body is a sign of stroke.

T   F   7. If the victim is unresponsive, look for a medical-alert tag.

T   F   8. If you find hemorrhaging during a victim assessment, continue the assessment and come back to the bleeding later.

T   F   9. Most victims require a complete physical exam.

T   F   10. Medical-alert identification can help in collecting a victim's SAMPLE history.

____ 11. In the case of multiple victims, which victim should you go to first?
   a. one who is quiet
   b. one who is talking
   c. one who is crying
   d. one who is yelling

Designate the following as signs (A) or symptoms (B).

____ 12. Sherry states that she feels dizzy.

____ 13. After a fall, Matt has a deformed lower leg.

____ 14. Steve's skin is red and blistered.

____ 15. Scott's pulse rate is 88 beats per minute.

____ 16. Justin's skin feels hot when touched.

____ 17. Mike begins to vomit.

____ 18. Jim says he has no feeling in his left arm.

____ 19. Whitney is wheezing.

Activity 2

1. Name the steps in a victim assessment.
   a. _____
   b. _____
   c. _____

2. Identify what you should check during the primary, or initial, survey.
   A = _____
   B = _____
   C = _____

3. Describe each level of the AVPU scale.
   A = _____
   V = _____
   P = _____
   U = _____

4. List some unusual breathing sounds that might indicate breathing difficulties.
   a. _____
   b. _____
   c. _____
   d. _____

5. What does the mnemonic D-O-T-S remind a first aider to look for?
   D = _____
   O = _____
   T = _____
   S = _____

6. Explain what the acronym PEARL represents.
   P = _____
   E = _____
   A = _____
   R = _____
   L = _____

STUDY
Questions 4

_____ 7. Where can CSF appear?

  a. nose

  b. ear

  c. eye

  d. both a and b

_____ 8. How would you check a victim's chest for tenderness?

  a. Squeeze it inward between your hands.

  b. Thump it with your finger.

  c. Look at it closely.

  d. Gently press the four quadrants.

_____ 9. How would you check a victim's abdomen for tenderness?

  a. Squeeze it inward between your hands.

  b. Thump it with your finger.

  c. Rub it with your hands.

  d. Gently press the four quadrants.

_____ 10. How would you check a victim's pelvis for tenderness?

  a. Squeeze it inward between your hands.

  b. Thump it with your finger.

  c. Gently press downward.

  d. Both a and c.

_____ 11. How would you check a victim's extremity for tenderness?

  a. Squeeze it inward between your hands.

  b. Thump it with your finger.

  c. Rub it with your hand.

12. One method of checking the extremities is to use the acronym CSM, which represents:

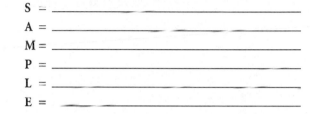

  C = _____

  S = _____

  M = _____

13. If time permits, collect the victim's SAMPLE history. SAMPLE helps identify:

  S = _____

  A = _____

  M = _____

  P = _____

  L = _____

  E = _____

14. What three major body systems are assessed during the initial assessment?

  a. _____

  b. _____

  c. _____

_____ 15. When examining a victim's eyes, you should look for:

  a. color of the iris

  b. reaction of pupils to light

  c. equal or unequal size of the pupils

  d. both b and c

_____ 16. What is a sign?

  a. what the victim tells you is wrong

  b. what the victim tells you about pain

  c. what you see, hear, or feel when assessing a victim

  d. an indication that death is imminent

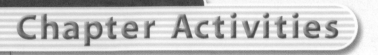

Chapter Activities

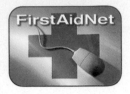

WEB Activities

Finding Out What's Wrong

Visit **nsc.jbpub.com/FirstAidNet**, then click on **Web Activities**, and select the appropriate chapter.

Medical Identification

People with special medical conditions who are around close friends or family members may be relatively safe if they need sudden medical attention. But if they need emergency care in a public place or when surrounded by strangers, they may not be able to quickly and accurately convey their medical histories to a first aider.

Examination of an Unresponsive/Unconscious Victim

Remember, unresponsive/unconscious victims require special attention. Usually an EMS ambulance with trained personnel will arrive within minutes, but sometimes the wait is much longer.

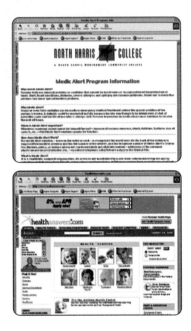

Life-Threatening Emergencies

Part 3

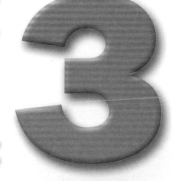

Chapter 5
Basic Life Support

Chapter 6
Bleeding and Shock

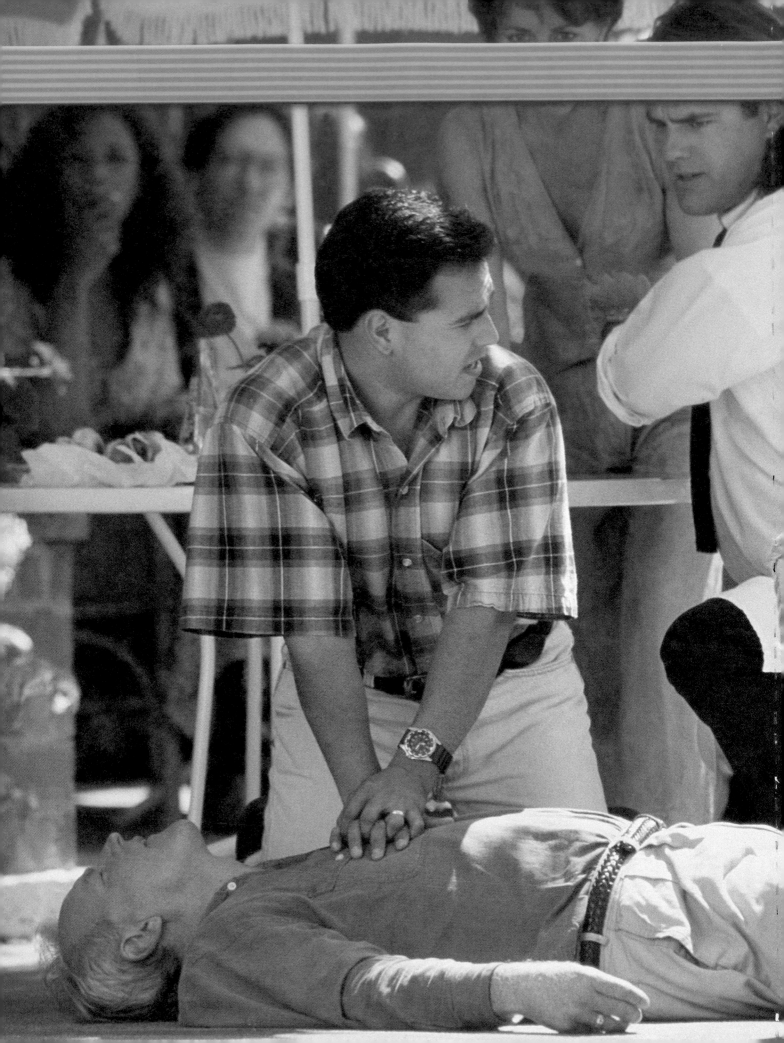

Basic Life Support

The American Heart Association reports that, in the United States, nearly 250,000 deaths each year are due to heart attacks. Heart attacks are the most prominent medical emergency in North America. In addition, drownings, suffocations, electrocutions, and drug intoxication cause cardiac arrest. Many deaths could be prevented if the victims got prompt help—if someone trained in CPR provided the proper life-saving measures until trained EMS professionals could take over.

Adult and Child Basic Life Support

If a victim is not breathing, rescue breathing must be started immediately. This is one of the most important procedures that you as a first aider can perform. For best results, you must understand the process so well that you can proceed automatically. Every second you spend trying to recall the proper procedure is a precious second lost in resuscitating a victim.

Essentially, there are eight steps for performing basic life support:

1. Check the victim's responsiveness.
2. Call 9-1-1.
3. Open airway.
4. Check breathing.
5. Check circulation.
6. Perform CPR.
7. Recheck circulation.
8. Perform rescue procedures based on findings.

Check Responsiveness

The first step is to recognize that a person is unresponsive. The simplest method to determine unresponsiveness is to tap the victim's shoulder and shout, "Are you okay?". Do not forcefully shake the victim, because he or she may have a spinal injury. Start resuscitation efforts at once. Brain damage occurs without oxygen.

Activate EMS

If the victim is unresponsive, activate the EMS *immediately*, to avoid losing any time unnecessarily in acquiring advanced cardiac life support. Direct a bystander to activate the EMS (usually by telephoning 9-1-1). If no bystanders are present, activate the EMS yourself ▼**Figure 5-1** .

Position the Unresponsive Victim

If you are able to tell that the unresponsive victim is breathing, place the victim in the recovery position (if no suspected spinal injury). If you are uncertain if the victim is breathing, roll the victim over, keep the head, neck, and shoulders aligned to avoid any twisting of the body. The victim must be on a firm, flat surface.

Open the Airway

The most important maneuver in performing rescue breathing is opening the victim's airway. The most common cause of airway obstruction in an unresponsive person is blockage by the tongue. When a victim's airway is opened, the lower jaw moves forward, bringing the base of the tongue (which is attached to the lower jaw) forward also and away from the back of the throat. The easiest way to open an injured person's airway is by tilting the head and lifting the chin.

To perform the head-tilt/chin-lift maneuver, place one hand, palm down, on the victim's forehead and push downward so the head tilts back. Then place the index and middle fingers of your other hand under the lower edge of the chin to lift the jaw. Simply opening the victim's airway can sometimes restore breathing.

Remove any visible object or vomit from mouth. Another technique to use with a victim who has a possible

Figure 5-1 Start resuscitation efforts at once. Brain damage occurs without oxygen.

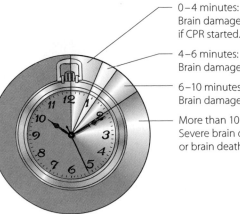

0–4 minutes:
Brain damage unlikely if CPR started.

4–6 minutes:
Brain damage possible.

6–10 minutes:
Brain damage probable.

More than 10 minutes:
Severe brain damage or brain death certain.

Advantages of the Left-Side Position

Left-side positioning is referred to by several terms: recovery position, left lateral recumbent position, left lateral decubitus position, and stable-side position. Positioning a person on his or her left side has several advantages:

✦ It keeps the airway open in an unresponsive breathing victim without a spinal cord injury.

✦ It protects the lungs from aspiration should vomiting occur.

✦ It delays vomiting by placing the esophagus above the stomach.

✦ It delays a poison's effects by retaining the poison in the stomach (the pyloric sphincter is kept straight up). A poison can be better dealt with in the stomach than in the small intestines.

✦ It relieves pressure on a pregnant woman's vena cava (the body's largest vein). Many pregnant women will pass out or at least feel dizzy if they lie supine (on their backs), because of the reduced blood flow.

spinal injury is a jaw thrust without a head tilt. Stabilize the victim's head, place your fingers behind the angles of the victim's lower jaw on each side of the head, and move the lower jaw forward without tilting the head backward.

Check for Breathing

After determining unresponsiveness and opening the airway, the next step is to look, listen, and feel for breathing. *Look* to see whether there is any visible movement of the victim's chest, *listen* for air by placing your ear next to the victim's mouth and nose, and *feel* for air by placing your cheek next to the victim's mouth and nose. If breathing is present, you will see the victim's chest rise and fall, hear air coming from the victim's mouth and nose, and feel air against your cheek. This process should take about ten seconds.

Signs of Poor Circulation

✦ No breathing or coughing

✦ No movement after receiving breaths

✦ Abnormal skin condition (low temperature, color)

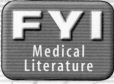

FYI
Medical Literature

Chain of Survival

The Chain of Survival includes four links: (1) early access; (2) early cardiopulmonary resuscitation (CPR); (3) early defibrillation; and (4) early advanced care. A missing link decreases the chance of survival.

1. **Early access.** Early access of the emergency medical service (EMS) means that defibrillation-trained and equipped personnel will arrive at the victim's side more rapidly and enables trained emergency dispatchers to coach bystanders in providing CPR until help arrives. The bystander must recognize the emergency, be willing to help, and be able to notify the local EMS.

2. **Early CPR.** Early CPR, which combines rescue breathing and chest compressions, serves as a holding action providing blood and oxygen to vital organs for a few extra minutes until defibrillation and advanced care can be mobilized. It takes more than CPR to save a life when the heart stops.

CPR, as we do it today, was first described in 1960. Since then, the technique has changed very little. The earlier it is used, the better. Bystander CPR improves a victim's likelihood of survival. However, CPR alone has a minimal effect without early defibrillation, and experts claim that poorly performed CPR may be no more effective than no CPR at all.

3. **Early defibrillation.** In most cases of adult cardiac arrest, the heart is in an abnormal rhythm called ventricular fibrillation that can only be reversed by delivering an electrical shock with a machine known as a defibrillator. Each minute delayed for attempted defibrillation reduces the likelihood of survival.

4. **Early advanced care.** Early advanced care includes the three above links plus special care (eg, intravenous medications) to help stabilize the victim and prevent recurrence of cardiac arrest.

Perform Rescue Breathing

If a victim is not breathing, perform rescue breathing by using one of the following methods: mouth-to-mouth, mouth-to-nose, mouth-to-barrier device, or mouth-to-stoma.

Mouth-to-Mouth Method

The mouth-to-mouth method of rescue breathing is the simplest, quickest, and most effective method for providing oxygen to a victim.

Effective mouth-to-mouth rescue breathing causes the chest to rise and fall with each breath. Exhaled air is about 16% oxygen which is enough to sustain life in comparison to room air, which is 21% oxygen.

Mouth-to-mouth breathing is preferred over mouth-to-nose breathing, especially if there is nasal bleeding, injury, or blockage. To perform mouth-to-mouth rescue breathing, follow these steps:

1. Make sure the victim's head is positioned with the neck extended and the head tilted backward to open the airway.

2. Pinch the victim's nose closed to prevent air from escaping, using the same hand that is on the victim's forehead to keep the neck extended.

3. Take a deep breath.

4. Make a tight seal with your mouth around the victim's mouth.

5. Slowly blow air into the victim's mouth until you see the chest rise.

6. Remove your mouth to allow the air to come out and turn your head away as you take another breath.

7. Repeat one more breath.

If the first two breaths do not go in, retilt the victim's head and try breaths again. If the breaths do not go in, use the procedure to aid an unresponsive choking victim described later in this chapter (page 77).

Definitions

+ **Cardiopulmonary resuscitation (CPR)** combines rescue breathing (also known as mouth-to-mouth breathing) and external chest compressions. *Cardio* refers to the heart, and *pulmonary* refers to the lungs. *Resuscitation* means "to revive." Proper and prompt CPR serves as a holding action by providing oxygen to the brain and heart until advanced cardiac life support can be provided.

+ **Basic life support (BLS)** refers to lifesaving procedures that focus on the victim's airway, breathing, and circulation. BLS includes rescue breathing, CPR, and obstructed airway management.

Skill Scan Turning a Victim Face Up

No Suspected Spinal Injury:

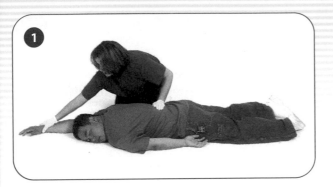

1. Raise arm nearest you over the head.

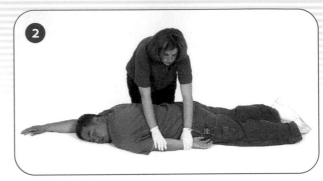

2. Tuck the other arm against the victim's side.

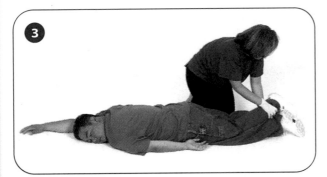

3. Adjust victim's legs so they are straight.

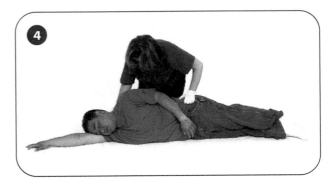

4. Support the head and neck with one hand. Firmly grip the clothing or edge of the hip with your other hand. Roll the victim over.

Skill Scan

Moving the Victim into Recovery Position

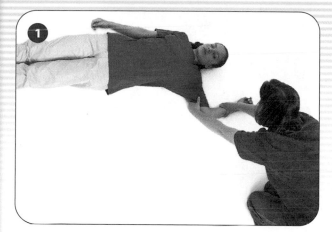

1. Place one arm away from body.

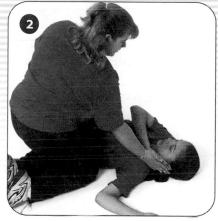

2. Place the other arm with back of hand over the left cheek.

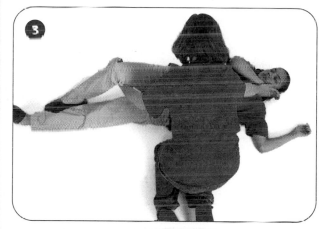

3. Bend and grab the far knee.

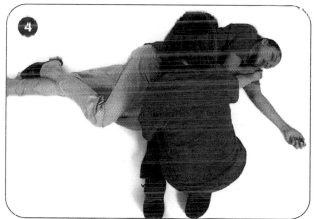

4. Roll the victim towards you by pulling the far knee towards you and to the ground. Protect the head during the roll.

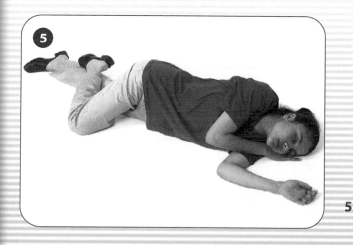

5. Recovery position. The hand supports the head. Chin tilted. Bent knee and arm gives stability.

Do not remove a victim's dentures unless they interfere with rescue breathing. Even loose dentures give form and shape to the victim's mouth.

Mouth-to-Nose Method

Although mouth-to-mouth breathing is successful in the majority of cases, certain complications may necessitate that you use mouth-to-nose rescue breathing. For example, the victim's mouth cannot be opened, a good seal cannot be made around the victim's mouth, the victim's mouth is severely injured, or the victim's mouth is too large or has no teeth.

The mouth-to-nose technique is performed like mouth-to-mouth breathing, except that you force your exhaled breath through the victim's nose while holding his or her mouth closed with one hand by pushing up on the chin. Then hold the victim's mouth open so any nasal obstruction does not impede exhalation of air from the victim's lungs.

Mouth-to-Stoma Method

Cancer and other diseases of the vocal cords often make surgical removal of the larynx necessary. This operation is called a *laryngectomy*, and an individual who has had the larynx removed is called a *laryngectomee*. Laryngectomees do not have a connection between the upper airway and the lungs. They breathe through a small permanent opening called a *stoma*, which is surgically made in the lower part of the neck and joined to the trachea. Some laryngectomees have a tracheostomy tube temporarily inserted inside their surgically created airway until the surrounding tissues mature. A person with a tracheostomy tube can be recognized by the tube that projects out of the front of the neck.

In mouth-to-stoma rescue breathing, the victim's mouth and nose must be closed during the delivery of breaths because the air can flow upward into the upper airway through the larynx as well as downward into the lungs. You can close the victim's mouth and nose with one hand. Determine breathing by looking at, listening to, and feeling at the stoma. Keep the victim's head and neck level.

Mouth-to-Barrier Device

A mouth-to-barrier device (▶**Figure 5-3, A–B**) is an apparatus that is placed over a victim's face as a disease prevention for the rescuer during rescue breathing. There are two types of mouth-to-barrier devices:

- *Masks.* Resuscitation masks cover the victim's mouth and nose. Most have a one-way valve so exhaled air from the victim does not enter the rescuer's mouth.

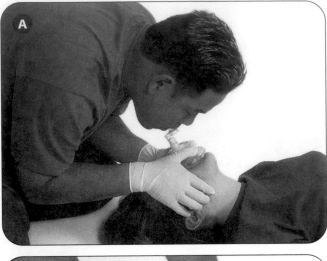

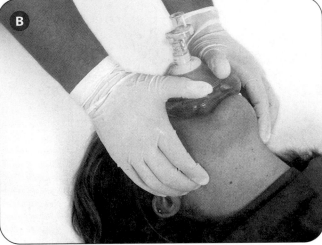

(**Figure 5-3, A–B**) Mouth-to-barrier device. Thumbs hold mask, fingers lift the jaw, and tilt the head.

- *Face shields.* These clear plastic devices have a mouthpiece through which the rescuer breathes, but lack a one-way valve. Some models have a short airway that is inserted into the victim's mouth over the tongue. They are smaller and less expensive than masks, but air can leak around the shield. Also, they cover only the victim's mouth, so the nose must be pinched (▶**Figure 5-4**).

Use of a barrier device requires the victim's airway to be opened. After the mask is in place, the rescuer breathes through the device. The technique is performed like mouth-to-mouth breathing.

Check for Signs of Circulation

After you have given the first two breaths, check the victim for signs of circulation to see if the heart is beating.

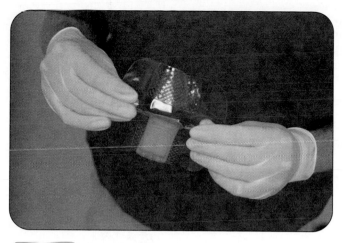

Figure 5-4 Face shield

If the victim has no signs of circulation, CPR must be started immediately.

If the victim has signs of circulation but is not breathing, continue rescue breathing at a rate of one breath every five seconds, or 12 times per minute (adult). Give a child one breath every three seconds. Between breaths, remove your mouth to take a breath and to permit air to flow out of the victim's lungs. As you remove your mouth, turn your head toward the victim's feet to see whether the victim's chest falls after each breath.

Perform External Chest Compressions

External chest compressions are required when the signs of circulation are absent.

Chest compressions and rescue breathing are combined in a procedure known as **cardiopulmonary resuscitation (CPR).** Chest compressions require a smooth application of pressure over the lower half of the sternum (breastbone). External pressure applied to the sternum increases pressure in the chest (intrathoracic pressure), and moves blood to the brain. Compressions must not be sharp or jabbing or applied over the tip of the sternum (xiphoid process). Proper hand position and placement on the victim's chest are necessary to avoid internal injury such as bruising of the heart, laceration of the liver, or rupture of the spleen.

Blood flow in the carotid arteries as a result of external chest compressions is only one-fourth to one-third the normal flow, but it is adequate until advanced life support can be given. Because the blood circulates oxygen, chest compressions must be accompanied by rescue breathing. Follow these steps for effective chest compressions:

1. Place the victim on his or her back on a firm, flat surface.

2. Locate the lower part of the victim's sternum by placing your hands between the nipples on the center of the chest. Another method is to slide your middle and index fingers along the margin of the victim's rib cage until you locate the notch in the center of the lower chest where the ribs and the sternum meet. Keep the middle finger on the center of the notch and place your index finger on the lower end of the victim's sternum, next to your middle finger. Place the heel of your hand next to your index finger nearer the victim's head.

3. Place the heel of the other hand on the back of the first hand. Your fingers should be pointing away from you. Interlace or extend your fingers but keep them off the victim's chest wall to avoid rib fractures and other internal injuries. The heel of the hand that is in direct contact with the sternum must remain in contact with the chest during both the compression and the release to prevent bouncing or jerking movements. If you have arthritic hands or wrists, grasp the wrist of the hand touching the sternum, instead of placing one hand on top of the other.

4. Lean forward so your shoulders are directly over your hands. Keeping your arms straight, press straight downward on the sternum $1^{1}/_{2}$ to 2 inches, using the weight of the upper part of your body, then relax pressure on the sternum completely. The pressure and relaxation phases of each chest compression should be of equal duration; do not pause between each phase. Be sure to push straight downward on each compression. Pushing at an angle is less effective and creates pressure over the ends of the ribs where they attach to the sternum, resulting in injury to the victim.

5. Give 15 chest compressions at a rate of about 100 per minute. The compression rate refers to the speed of compressions and not the actual number given in one minute.

6. After 15 compressions, immediately give two slow breaths (take a breath between them). After the two breaths, quickly reassess your hand location and position, then begin another cycle of 15 compressions and two breaths.

7. After you have completed four cycles (which should take about one minute), check the victim for signs of circulation for 10 seconds. If there are no signs of circulation, continue CPR starting with 15 compressions. Check the signs of circulation every few minutes.

Recognizing Immediate Threats to Life and Basic LIfe Support

If you see a motionless person ...

1

Are you okay?

Check responsiveness.
- Tap victim and shout, "Are you okay?"
- Shout for help.
- If unresponsive, go to step #2.

2

9-1-1

Call 9-1-1 or emergency telephone number.
- If the victim is 8 years of age or older and an AED is available, get it.

3

Open airway.
- Tilt the head back and lift the chin.
- Remove any obvious obstructions.
- If you suspect a spinal injury, use jaw-thrust method without head-tilt.

Recognizing Immediate Threats to Life and Basic LIfe Support

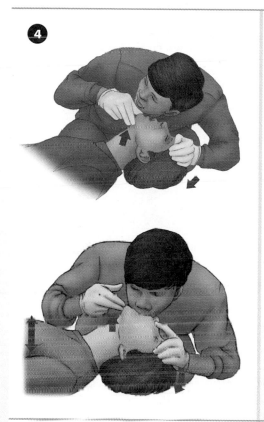

④

Check breathing (10 seconds).

• Look, listen and feel for breathing.

• If breathing, place victim in recovery position.

• If not breathing, give 2 slow rescue breaths (2 seconds each).

• If breaths do not cause the chest to rise, the airway may be blocked. Reposition the head and try breaths again. If chest does not rise, begin CPR (see step 8). When you open the airway to give a breath, look for an object in the throat and if seen, remove it.

• If two breaths cause the chest to rise, continue to step #5.

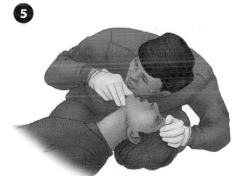

⑤

Check circulation (10 seconds).

Signs of circulation include—

• Breathing

• Coughing

• Movement

• Normal skin condition (temperature and color)

• Improved level of responsiveness

• Pulse

If signs of circulation exist but no breathing, give one breath about every five seconds. Recheck signs of circulation every minute.

If no signs of circulation, begin CPR (step #6).

Recognizing Immediate Threats to Life and Basic LIfe Support

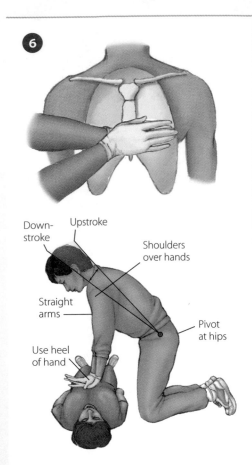

6

Down-stroke · Upstroke

Shoulders over hands

Straight arms

Pivot at hips

Use heel of hand

Perform CPR.

- Place heel of one hand on the center of the chest between the nipples (lower half of the sternum).

- Using two hands, depress chest downward 1$\frac{1}{2}$ to 2 inches.

- Give 15 chest compressions at a rate of about 100 per minute.

- Open airway and give two slow breaths (two seconds each).

- Continue cycles of 15 chest compressions and two rescue breaths until an AED is available (see AED information below).

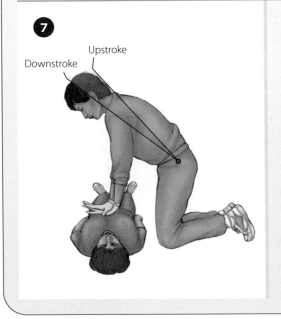

7

Downstroke · Upstroke

Recheck circulation.

After four cycles of compressions and breaths (about one minute), recheck for signs of circulation.

- If not breathing and no other signs of circulation exist, resume CPR.

Recognizing Immediate Threats to Life and Basic LIfe Support

7

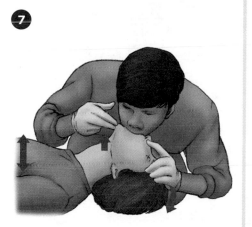

- If breathing, place victim in recovery position.
- If not breathing, but other signs of circulation exist, provide one rescue breath about every five seconds.
- Recheck for signs of circulation every few minutes.

8

Early defibrillation

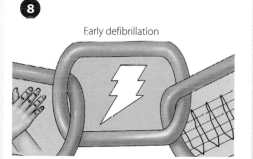

If you are trained to use an AED, follow this sequence:
- Perform CPR until an AED is available.
- Turn on the AED.
- Attach AED pads.
- "Analyze" the heart rhythm.
- Shock (up to three times if advised by AED).

After three shocks or after any AED prompt of "no shock indicated:"
- Check for signs of circulation (including carotid pulse).
- If no signs of circulation, perform CPR for one minute.

Check for signs of circulation. If absent:
- "Analyze" and follow the AED's prompts.
- Shock, if prompted.
- Repeat analyze, shock, and CPR as needed.

BASIC LIFE SUPPORT

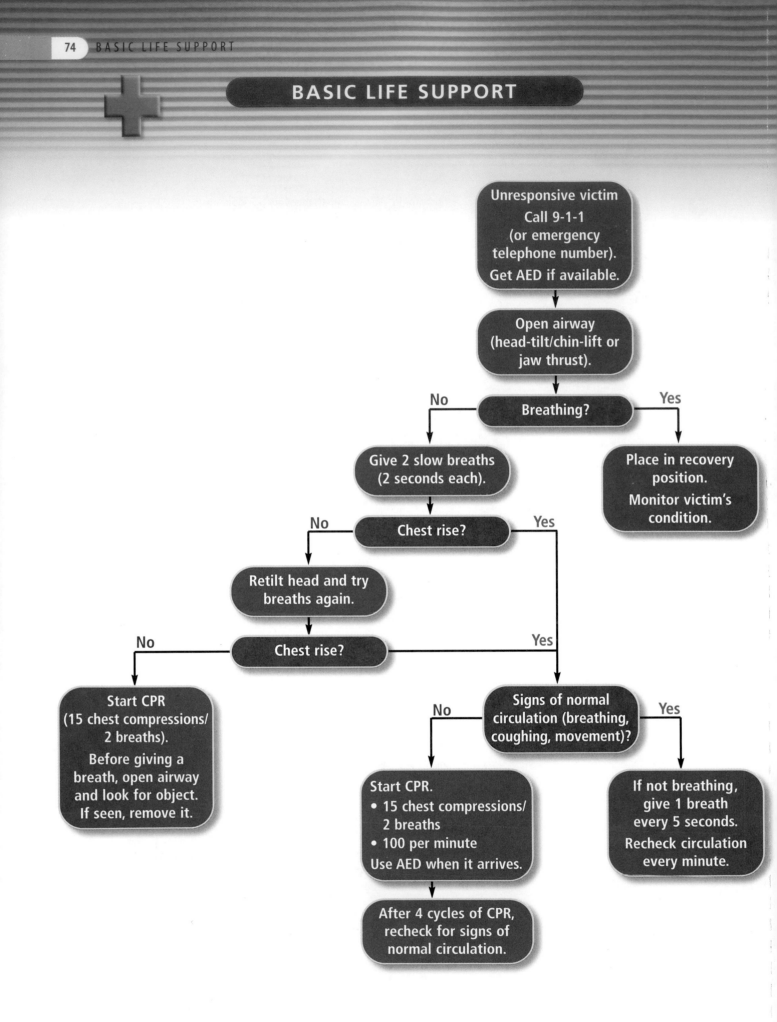

Unresponsive victim
Call 9-1-1
(or emergency telephone number).
Get AED if available.

Open airway
(head-tilt/chin-lift or jaw thrust).

No — Breathing? — **Yes**

Give 2 slow breaths (2 seconds each).

Place in recovery position.
Monitor victim's condition.

No — Chest rise? — **Yes**

Retilt head and try breaths again.

No — Chest rise? — **Yes**

Start CPR (15 chest compressions/ 2 breaths).
Before giving a breath, open airway and look for object. If seen, remove it.

No — Signs of normal circulation (breathing, coughing, movement)? — **Yes**

Start CPR.
• 15 chest compressions/ 2 breaths
• 100 per minute
Use AED when it arrives.

If not breathing, give 1 breath every 5 seconds.
Recheck circulation every minute.

After 4 cycles of CPR, recheck for signs of normal circulation.

Airway Obstruction (Choking)— Adult and Child

Recognizing Choking

Choking victims vary as to whether the victim (1) is responsive and has a partial airway obstruction, (2) is responsive and has a complete airway obstruction, (3) becomes unresponsive as a result of a complete airway obstruction, or (4) is found unresponsive with a complete airway obstruction.

A foreign body lodged in the airway may cause a partial or complete airway obstruction. When a foreign body partially blocks the airway, either good or poor air exchange may result. When good air exchange is present, the victim is able to make forceful coughing efforts in an attempt to relieve the obstruction. The victim should be permitted and encouraged to cough. Sometimes, a good air exchange may progress to a poor air exchange.

A choking victim who has poor air exchange has weak and ineffective coughs, and breathing becomes more difficult. The skin, the fingernail beds, and the inside of the mouth may appear bluish-gray in color (indicating cyanosis). Each attempt to inhale is usually accompanied by a high-pitched noise. A partial airway obstruction with poor air exchange should be treated as if it were a complete airway blockage.

Complete airway obstruction in a responsive victim commonly occurs when the victim has been eating. The victim is unable to speak, breathe, or cough. When asked, "Can you speak?" the victim is unable to respond verbally. Choking victims with complete foreign body obstruction of the airway may instinctively reach up and clutch their necks to communicate that they are choking. This motion is known as the universal distress signal for choking

Types of Upper Airway Obstruction

+ **Tongue.** Unconsciousness relaxes soft tissues, and the tongue can fall into the airway. "Swallowing one's tongue" is impossible, but the widespread belief that this can happen is explained by slippage of the relaxed tongue into the airway. The tongue is the most common cause of airway obstruction.

+ **Foreign body.** The National Safety Council reports that 3,000 deaths occur in the United States each year because of foreign body airway obstruction. People, especially children, inhale all kinds of objects. Foods such as hot dogs, candy, peanuts, and grapes are major offenders because of their shapes and consistencies. Meat is the main cause of choking in adults. Balloons are the top cause of nonfood choking deaths in children, followed by balls, marbles, toys, and coins. The airways of unconscious victims can also be obstructed by a foreign body (eg, vomit, teeth).

+ **Swelling.** Severe allergic reactions (anaphylaxis) and irritants (eg, smoke, chemicals) can cause swelling. Even a nonallergic person who is stung inside the throat by a bee, yellow jacket, or flying insect can experience swelling in the airway.

+ **Spasm.** Water that is suddenly inhaled can cause a spasm in the throat. This happens in about 10% of all drownings. When such a spasm does not allow the lungs to fill with water, it is known as a "dry drowning."

+ **Vomit.** Most people vomit when they are at or near death. Therefore, always expect vomit during CPR.

▶Figure 5-5). The victim becomes panicked and desperate and may appear pale in color. Because a complete obstruction prevents air from entering the lungs, oxygen deprivation occurs within a few minutes.

Abdominal Thrusts (Heimlich Maneuver)

Giving abdominal thrusts to a choking victim older than one year can dislodge the foreign body from the airway. To give abdominal thrusts to a choking victim who is sitting or standing, position yourself behind the victim.

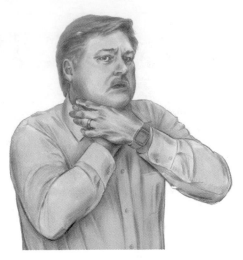

Figure 5-5 Universal sign of choking distress.

Place your arms around the victim's waist and form a fist with one hand. Place the thumb side of the fist with the knuckles up against the victim's abdomen slightly above the navel. With your other hand, grasp and hold your fist, then give quick upward and inward thrusts to the victim's abdomen. If the victim is sitting in a chair, you probably will have to turn the victim, because reaching around the victim and the back of the chair usually is not practical.

Causes of Choking

There are many reasons why people choke on objects, including:

✛ They try to swallow large pieces of food.

✛ Loose dentures (false teeth) inhibit the proper chewing of food.

✛ Eating too fast.

✛ Eating while talking or laughing.

✛ Walking, running, or playing with objects in the mouth.

✛ Drunkenness contributes to choking for several reasons:
  • Alcohol can deaden sensations in the mouth and interfere with swallowing.
  • An excessive amount of alcohol can affect one's judgment as to proper chewing and swallowing of food.
  • Before-dinner drinking delays the start of eating, so the hungry eater may attempt to swallow large chunks of food without proper chewing.

Basic Life Support Steps for Adult Victims

RAP ABC

R: Responsiveness of victim?

A: Activate EMS (usually call 9-1-1).

P: Position victim on back.

A: Airway open. Use head-tilt/chin-lift or jaw thrust.

B: Breathing check. Look, listen, and feel for 10 seconds.

✛ If victim is breathing and spinal injury is not suspected, place victim in recovery position.

✛ If victim is not breathing, give 2 slow breaths; watch chest rise.
  • If 2 breaths go in, proceed to step C.
  • If breaths do not go in, retilt head and try again.
  • If breaths still do not go in, give CPR. Before giving breaths, look for object in throat and if seen, remove it.

C: Circulation check for signs of circulation (10 seconds)

✛ If there are signs of circulation but no breathing, give rescue breathing (1 breath every 5 seconds).

✛ If there are no signs of circulation, give CPR (cycles of 15 chest compressions followed by 2 breaths).

After 1 minute (4 cycles of CPR or 10 to 12 rescue breaths), check for signs of circulation.

✛ If no signs of circulation, give CPR (cycles of 15 compressions and 2 breaths) starting with chest compressions.

✛ If there are signs of circulation but no breathing, give 1 breath every 5 seconds.

Continue the thrusts until the object is expelled or the victim becomes unresponsive. Should that happen, call 9-1-1 and start CPR.

A responsive choking victim who is alone can self-administer abdominal thrusts. The victim places the thumb side of a closed fist in the same position described above, covers the first with the other hand, then gives inward, upward thrusts. Also, if a firm object such as a chair or table is available, the victim can lean over the back of the chair or a corner of the table, pressing the abdomen upward and inward.

Resonsive Adult and Child Airway Obstruction (Choking)

If person is responsive and cannot speak, breathe, or cough...

1

Check victim for choking.

• Ask "Are you choking? Can you speak?"

• A choking victim cannot speak, breathe or cough and may clutch the neck with the hand.

2

Give abdominal thrusts (Heimlich maneuver).

• Place a fist against the victim's abdomen just above the navel.

• Grasp the fist with your other hand and press into victim's abdomen with quick inward and upward thrusts.

• Continue thrusts until object is removed or victim becomes unresponsive.

• Give chest thrusts instead of abdominal thrusts for women in late stages of pregnancy or large victims.

3

If the victim becomes unresponsive.

• Call 9-1-1 or emergency telephone number to activate the EMS system (or send someone to do it).

• Assess the victim and give CPR if needed.

• Each time you open the airway to give a breath, look for an object in the throat and if seen, remove it.

Adult Basic Life Support Proficiency Checklist

S = self check / P = partner check / I = instructor check

Adult Rescue Breathing

	S	P	I
1. Check responsiveness.	○	○	○
2. Activate EMS.	○	○	○
3. Airway open.	○	○	○
4. Breathing check.	○	○	○
5. 2 slow breaths.	○	○	○
6. Check circulation.	○	○	○
7. Rescue breathing (1 every 5 seconds).	○	○	○
8. Recheck circulation and breathing after first minute, then every few minutes.	○	○	○

Adult CPR

	S	P	I
1. Check responsiveness.	○	○	○
2. Activate EMS.	○	○	○
3. Airway open.	○	○	○
4. Breathing check.	○	○	○

	S	P	I
5. 2 slow breaths.	○	○	○
6. Check circulation.	○	○	○
7. Position hands.	○	○	○
8. 15 compressions.	○	○	○
9. 2 slow breaths.	○	○	○
10. Continue CPR (3 more cycles, for total of 4).	○	○	○
11. Recheck circulation.	○	○	○
12. Continue CPR (start with compressions).	○	○	○
13. Recheck circulation every few minutes.	○	○	○

Adult Choking

	S	P	I
1. Position hands.	○	○	○
2. Give abdominal thrusts until object removed or victim unresponsive.	○	○	○
3. Assess the victim and begin CPR if needed.	○	○	○

Differences between Adult and Child (1 – 8 years) Basic Life Support

IF child ...	THEN ...
Is unresponsive and rescuer is alone	**Activate the EMS system after one minute of resuscitation** (in adults, activate EMS immediately after determining unresponsiveness).
Is **not** breathing but other signs of circulation exist	• Give **1 to 1$^1/_2$ second breaths** (in adults give 1$^1/_2$ to 2 second breaths). • Give **one breath every 3 seconds** (in adults give one breath about every 5 seconds).
Does **not** have any signs of circulation	• Give **chest compressions with one hand** (hand nearest feet) while keeping other hand on child's forehead (adult requires two hands on victim's chest for compressions). • Give **one breath after every 5 chest compressions** (adult one-rescuer CPR requires two breaths after every 15 compressions). • Compress sternum 1 to $^1/_2$ inches (adults require 1$^1/_2$ to 2 inches). • Do not use an AED on children (AEDs may be used on persons over the age of eight years).

Child Basic Life Support Proficiency Checklist

S = self check / P = partner check / I = instructor check

Child Rescue Breathing

	S	P	I
1. Check responsiveness.	○	○	○
2. Send a bystander, if available, to call EMS.	○	○	○
3. **A**irway open.	○	○	○
4. **B**reathing check.	○	○	○
5. 2 slow breaths.	○	○	○
6. **C**heck circulation.	○	○	○
7. Rescue breathing (1 every 3 seconds).	○	○	○
8. If alone, call EMS after 1 minute.	○	○	○
9. Recheck circulation and breathing after first minute, then every few minutes.	○	○	○

Child CPR

	S	P	I
1. Check responsiveness.	○	○	○
2. Send a bystander, if available, to call EMS.	○	○	○
3. Airway open.	○	○	○
4. Breathing check.	○	○	○
5. 2 slow breaths.	○	○	○
6. Check circulation.	○	○	○
7. Position hand.	○	○	○
8. 5 compressions with only 1 hand.	○	○	○
9. 1 slow breath.	○	○	○
10. Continue CPR for 1 minute (19 more cycles, for total of 20).	○	○	○
11. If alone, call EMS after 1 minute.	○	○	○
12. Recheck circulation.	○	○	○
13. Continue CPR	○	○	○
14. Recheck circulation every few minutes.	○	○	○

Child Choking

	S	P	I
1. Postion hands.	○	○	○
2. Give abdominal thrusts until object removed or victim unresponsive.	○	○	○
3. If unresponsive, access the victim and give CPR if needed.	○	○	○

If the choking victim is obese or in late stages of pregnancy, give chest thrusts. Position yourself behind the victim and place the thumb side of a fist on the middle of the victim's sternum. Then thrust straight back until the object is expelled or the victim becomes unresponsive. If the pregnant or large victim is lying down, kneel at the victim's side and give CPR.

Responsive Choking Victims

First determine if the victim has good or poor air exchange. A victim with good air exchange is able to speak, cough forcefully, and make effective breathing efforts. Encourage such a victim to cough; do not interfere with the victim's efforts to expel the object.

Treat a responsive victim with a partial airway obstruction and poor air exchange as you would for a complete obstruction. Poor air exchange is marked by ineffective, weak coughing, high-pitched noise, breathing difficulty, possible cyanosis, and inability to speak. To assist these victims:

1. Ask, "Can you speak?"
2. If the victim is unable to speak, give abdominal thrusts.
3. Repeat thrusts until the airway is clear or the victim becomes unresponsive.

Unresponsive Choking Victims

To help an unresponsive choking victim:

1. Determine the victim's responsiveness.
2. Call for help—either send someone or call yourself.
3. Open the victim's airway using the head-tilt/chin-lift method.
4. Determine if the victim is breathing by looking at the chest and listening for air coming out of the mouth and nose.
5. Give two slow breaths. If the breaths do not go in, retilt the victim's head and try breaths again. *The breaths not causing the chest to rise indicates choking.*
6. If unsuccessful, begin CPR. Each time you open the airway to give a breath, look for an object in the throat and if seen, remove it.

Infant Basic Life Support

Basic life support techniques for an infant differ from those for an adult or child. Initially occurring cardiac arrest in infants is rare. Usually, infants have a respiratory arrest with cardiac arrest developing later because the heart muscle did not receive sufficient oxygen.

Infant Rescue Breathing and CPR

Check Responsiveness

Check responsiveness by tapping the infant and speaking loudly. If alone, give resuscitation for one minute before activating EMS. If a bystander is nearly, have him or her call 9-1-1.

Positioning an Unresponsive Infant

Properly position the victim so that if any resuscitation efforts are needed, they can be performed. If the victim is found lying facedown, roll the infant onto his or her back. The victim's head and neck should always be supported with one of your hands so that they remain aligned with the rest of the body and do not twist.

Opening the Airway

After unresponsiveness has been determined and the infant has been properly positioned, open the infant's airway using the head-tilt/chin-lift method. You will usually only need to tilt the infant's head a small amount to open the airway. Do not overtilt the head backward because the pliability of the infant's tissues can block the airway. To lift the chin, place the finger(s) of your other hand under the bony part of the jaw. Then lift your fingers to bring the chin up. The fingers should not press on the soft tissue under the victim's chin because this can interfere with the opening of the airway. As you lift the chin, your other hand on the forehead maintains the head-tilt position of the victim. Sometimes, opening the airway may be all that is necessary for the infant to breathe.

For a suspected spinal-injured victim use a jaw thrust without a head tilt. While stabilizing the head, place the fingers of each hand behind the angles of the victim's lower jaw on each side of the head and move the lower jaw forward without tilting the head backward.

Check for Breathing

After unresponsiveness has been determined and the airway has been opened, you should look, listen, and feel for breathing. You should (1) look to see whether there is any visible movement of the infant's chest, (2) listen for air by placing your ear next to the infant's mouth and nose, and (3) feel for air by placing your cheek next

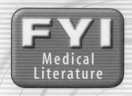

Reduce the Risk of Sudden Infant Death Syndrome (SIDS)

Sudden Infant Death Syndrome (SIDS) is the sudden and unexplained death of an infant under one year of age. SIDS, sometimes known as crib death, strikes nearly 5,000 babies in the United States every year. More boys than girls are victims and most deaths occur during the fall, winter, and early spring months Doctors and nurses don't know what causes SIDS, but they have found some things that can be done to make babies safer.

One of the most important things to do to help reduce the risk of SIDS is to put a healthy baby on his or her back to sleep. Do this when the baby is being put down for a nap or to bed for the night.

Other Things that Can be Done to Help Reduce the Risk of SIDS

1. **Bedding.** Make sure a baby sleeps on a firm mattress or other firm surface. Don't use fluffy blankets or comforters under the baby. Don't let the baby sleep on a waterbed, sheepskin, pillow, or other soft materials. When the baby is very young, don't place soft stuffed toys or pillows in the crib with him or her.

2. **Temperature.** Babies should be kept warm, but they should not be allowed to get too warm. Keep the temperature in the baby's room so that it feels comfortable to you.

3. **Smoke-free.** Create a smoke-free zone around babies. Babies and young children exposed to smoke have more colds and other diseases, as well as an increased risk of SIDS.

4. **Prenatal care.** Early and regular prenatal care can also help reduce the risk of SIDS. The risk of SIDS is higher for babies whose mothers smoke during pregnancy.

5. **Doctor or clinic visits.** If your baby seems sick, call your pediatrician right away. Make sure your baby receives his or her shots on schedule.

6. **Breastfeeding.** If possible, consider breastfeeding your baby.

SIDS: "Back to Sleep" Campaign

The American Academy of Pediatrics recommendations on sleep position:

1. A supine position, where an infant is completely on his or her back, carries the lowest risk of SIDS. Side sleeping also lowers the risk of potentially life-threatening breathing problems, and is a "reasonable alternative" to stomach-down sleeping.

2. Infants should not have soft surfaces or pillows while sleeping, which have the potential to trap air.

3. The sleeping position recommendation is for healthy infants. Some pediatricians may recommend that babies with certain medical problems or birth defects need to sleep in the prone, or face-down, position.

4. The recommendation is intended for sleeping infants. Indeed, a certain amount of time spent in the stomach-down position is recommended for infants who are awake and being watched.

These recommendations are considered to be primarily important during the first six months of age, when a baby's risk of SIDS is greatest. Parents should discuss these recommendations with their baby's doctor.

Source: National Institute of Child Health and Human Development.

---

to the infant's mouth and nose. If breathing is present, you will see the infant's chest rise and fall, hear air coming from the infant's mouth and nose, and feel air against your own cheek.

Rescue Breathing

To give rescue breaths to an infant, place your mouth over the infant's nose and mouth or over only the nose, forming an airtight seal. Give two slow breaths, taking time to quickly breathe between them.

If both breaths go into the infant, check for signs of circulation. If the breaths do not cause the chest to rise, retilt the infant's head and try again.

Breaths should be limited to the amount needed to raise the infant's chest.

To perform rescue breathing for an infant, follow these steps:

1. Make sure the infant's airway is open.

2. Form an airtight seal over the victim's nose and mouth, or over only the mouth, or only the nose.

3. Give two slow breaths.

4. Watch to see if the infant's chest rises.

5. Remove your mouth to allow the air to come out and move your head away as you take another breath.

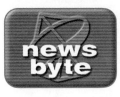

Balloons: Serious Choking Hazard for Children

Ordinary balloons can be deadly if they are inhaled while inflated, partially inflated, or after bursting into fragments, according to a study of 449 children who died from choking on foreign objects. Balloons were responsible for more deaths than any other non-food object. Balls and marbles were next on the hazard list. Balloons pose a greater threat than solid objects that are swallowed because balloons conform to the shape of the breathing passage and thus block it more completely.

Source: F. L. Rimell, et al., "Characteristics of Objects that Cause Choking in Children," *Journal of the American Medical Association* 274:1763, December 13, 1995.

If the breaths do not go in, retilt the victim's head and try breaths again. If breaths still do not go in, the airway is likely obstructed. See the section on unresponsive choking management on page 87.

If the breaths go in and the infant has a pulse, continue giving rescue breathing. Because infants breathe faster than adults, breathe into an infant once every three seconds. Between breaths, remove your mouth from the victim's to allow air to flow out of the victim's lungs. As you remove your mouth, you should turn your head to the side to see if the victim's chest fell after each breath. For rescue breathing, breathe into the infant for the first second, count "one—one thousand," then take a breath yourself for the third second.

Gastric Distention

Rescue breaths tend to cause stomach or gastric distention more often in infants than in adults. Minimize this problem by limiting the breaths to the amount needed to make the chest rise. Avoid overinflating the lungs. Gastric distention can cause regurgitation and aspiration of stomach contents.

Check for Signs of Circulation

After the two breaths have been given, check for signs of circulation.

If signs of circulation exists but breathing is absent, continue rescue breathing. Give a rescue breath once every three seconds. After 20 breaths, you should activate EMS.

Chest Compressions

An infant without signs of circulation requires both rescue breathing and chest compressions. The proper chest compression point in an infant is midsternum, between the infant's nipples. Place three fingers (index, middle, and ring) on the chest, with the index finger next to the imaginary nipple line on the infant's feet side. Lift the index finger off the chest.

Use the two remaining fingers to apply the chest compressions. Press the infant's midsternum (area between the nipples) ½ to 1 inch into the chest with the middle and ring finger. Either place your other hand under the infant's shoulder to provide support or keep it on the infant's forehead to keep the head tilted. If the infant is carried during CPR, the length of the body is on the rescuer's forearm with the head kept level with the trunk.

The infant compression rate is 100 per minute. External chest compressions must always be combined with rescue breathing. The ratio of compressions to breaths is five to one. Each series of five compressions is performed while the rescuer says aloud "One, two, three, four, five." After

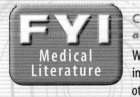

CPR Training and HIV

With concerns about the human immunodeficiency virus (HIV) and other infectious agents, many people are wondering whether disinfection procedures used on CPR-training manikins are adequate to prevent the transmission of diseases. Routine disinfection with 70% isopropyl alcohol is enough to prevent the spread of the virus that causes AIDS.

Although there have been no cases to date of HIV transmitted by CPR manikins, the virus is found in saliva and can survive for a time on plastic material. While the risk is minimal, it is important to ease fears about disease transmission since CPR training is widespread.

The preferred method of disinfecting equipment is to use bleach solution, with isopropyl alcohol available as an option. When isopropyl alcohol is used, it is supposed to be applied to the manikin for 60 seconds.

Source: I. B. Corless, et al., "Decontamination of an HIV-infected CPR Manikin," *American Journal of Public Health* 82:1542–43, 1992.

Infant (under 1 year)
Rescue Breathing and CPR

If you see a motionless infant ...

1

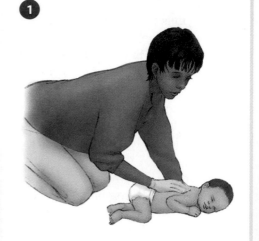

Check responsiveness.

- Tap the victim and shout, "Are you okay?"

2

Activate EMS.

- Ask a bystander to call the local emergency telephone number, usually 9-1-1.

- If you are alone, call EMS after one minute of resuscitation, unless a bystander can be sent.

Infant (under 1 year) Rescue Breathing and CPR

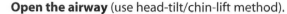

③

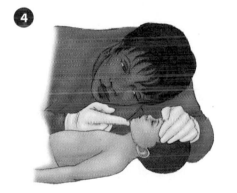

Open the airway (use head-tilt/chin-lift method).

- Place your hand that is nearest victim's head on victim's forehead and tilt head back slightly.

- Place the fingers of your other hand under the chin and lift gently. Avoid pressing on the soft tissues under the jaw.

④

Check for breathing (10 seconds).

- Place your ear over the victim's mouth and nose while keeping the airway open.

- *Look* at the victim's chest to check for rise and fall; *listen* and *feel* for breathing.

⑤

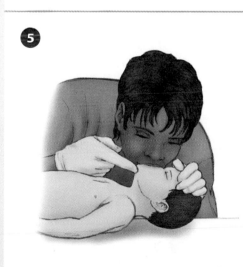

If not breathing, give 2 slow breaths.

- Keep the airway open.

- Take a breath and place your mouth over the victim's mouth and nose, or nose only.

- Give 2 slow breaths.

- Watch chest rise to see if your breaths go in.

- Allow for chest deflation after each breath.

If breaths do not go in

- Retilt the head and try again.

- If unsuccessful; give CPR.

Infant (under 1 year)
Rescue Breathing and CPR

6

Check for signs of circulation (10 seconds).

Signs of circulation include—

- Breathing
- Coughing
- Movement
- Normal skin condition (temperature and color)
- Improved level of responsiveness
- Pulse

7

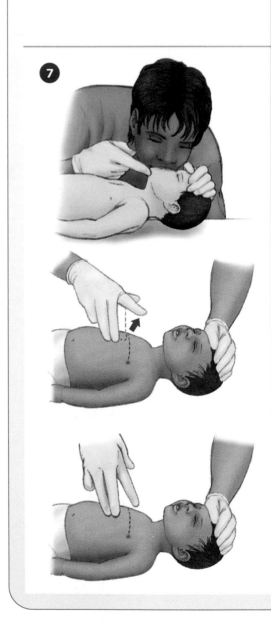

If no breathing, but other signs of circulation.

- Give 1 breath every 3 seconds.
- Recheck signs of circulation every minute.

If there are no signs of circulation.

- Begin CPR.

    1. Place 2-3 fingers in the center of the chest.

    2. Compress the chest 5 times.

    3. Push sternum straight down ½ to 1 inch.

    4. Do smooth compressions, counting "One, two, three, four, five."

- Give 1 slow breath.
- Continue cycles of 5 compressions and one breath for one minute, then check for signs of circulation. If absent, restart CPR with chest compressions. Recheck the signs of circulation every few minutes. If there are signs of circualtion but no breathing, give rescue breathing.
- Give CPR until:
- Infant revives.

OR

- Trained help, such as emergency medical technicians (EMTs), arrives and relieves you.

OR

- You are completely exhausted.

the fifth compression, the rescuer opens the victim's airway and gives one breath.

After the first minute of CPR, and if a second rescuer is not available, activate the EMS. Every few minutes feel the pulse.

The procedures for performing rescue breathing and external chest compressions on an infant are as follows:

1. Determine responsiveness by tapping the infant; if the infant is lying facedown, turn him or her onto their back. Place on a firm, flat surface.

2. Open the airway using the head-tilt/chin-lift method.

3. Check for breathing.

4. If breathing is absent, form an airtight seal over the victim's nose and mouth or nose only, and give two slow breaths; watch to see if the infants's chest rises. Remove your mouth to allow the air to come out and move your head away as you take another breath. If the breaths did not go in, retilt the victim's head and try breaths again. If breaths do not go in, give CPR checking for objects before breaths.

5. Check for signs of circulation. If the breaths caused the chest to rise and the victim has signs of circulation, continue giving rescue breathing. Breathe into an infant once every three seconds. Between breaths, remove your mouth from the victim's to allow air to flow out of the victim's lungs. As you remove your mouth, turn your head to the side to see if the victim's chest fell after each breath. For rescue breathing, breathe into the infant for the first second, count "one—one thousand" for the second, then take a breath yourself for the third second.

6. If the signs of circulation are absent, begin CPR.

7. After one minute of CPR, activate the EMS if another rescuer has not already.

Airway Obstruction—Infant

People, especially children and infants, choke on all kinds of objects (▶Figure 5-6). Foods such as hot dogs, candy, peanuts, and grapes are major offenders because of their shape and consistencies. Non-food choking deaths are caused by balloons, balls and marbles, toys, and coins. Balloons are the top cause of non-food choking deaths in children.

As discussed before, the airway may be partially or completely blocked. With a partial airway obstruction, an infant is able to make persistent coughing efforts

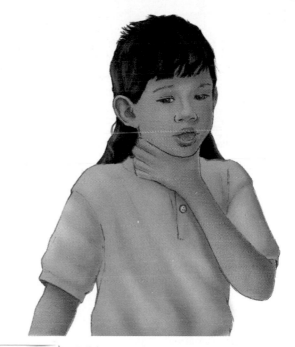

(Figure 5-6) Children can choke on all kinds of objects.

that should not be hampered. If good air exchange becomes poor exchange or if there is initially poor air exchange, the victim should be managed as having a complete airway obstruction. Poor air exchanges are indicated by ineffective coughing, high-pitched noises, breathing difficulty, and blueness of the lips and fingernail beds.

Back Blows and Chest Thrusts

To perform back blows on an infant, straddle the infant facedown over your forearm. The infant's head should be lower than the trunk. Your hand should be around the jaw and neck of the infant to support the infant's head. For more support, rest your forearm on your thigh. Using the heel of the other hand, you are ready to give five rapid back blows between the infant's shoulder blades.

To give chest thrusts, turn the infant onto his or her back. After delivering the five back blows, immediately place your free hand on the back of the infant's head and neck and keep the other hand in place. Using both hands and forearms to sandwich the infant—one supporting the jaw, neck, and chest, and the other the back—turn the infant over. After you have turned the infant onto his or her back, the infant should be resting on your thigh. The infant's head should be lower than the trunk.

With the infant in this position, give five chest thrusts in rapid succession. The thrusts are given to the sternum (between the nipples), using two fingers. The technique used to locate and perform chest thrusts is the same as that used to perform external chest compressions for CPR.

Unresponsive Choking Infant

To help an unresponsive choking infant, you should give CPR. Before giving breaths, open the airway, look for an object and is seen, remove it.

Responsive Victim

Help for a responsive infant also combines back blows and chest thrusts. They should be given when an infant has complete airway obstruction as evidenced by the inability to breathe, cough, or cry. Back blows and chest thrusts should be used until the object is removed or the infant becomes unresponsive.

Responsive Choking Infant

If infant is conscious and cannot speak, breathe, or cough…

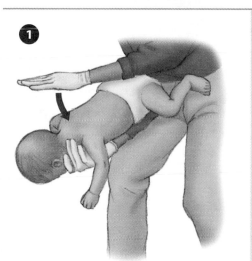

1

Give up to 5 back blows.

- Hold the infant's head and neck with one hand by firmly supporting the infant's jaw between your thumb and fingers.

- Lay the infant face down over your forearm with head lower than his or her chest. Brace your forearm and the infant against your thigh.

- Give up to 5 distinct and separate back blows between the infant's shoulder blades with the heel of your hand.

2

Give up to 5 chest thrusts.

- While supporting the back of the infant's head, roll the infant face up.

- Place 3 fingers on the infant's sternum with your ring finger next to and below the imaginary nipple line toward the infant's feet.

- Lift your ring finger off the chest.

- Give up to 5 separate and distinct thrusts with your index and middle fingers on the infant's sternum in a manner similar to CPR chest compressions, but at a slower rate.

3

Repeat:

- Until the infant becomes unresponsive. Call 9-1-1, assess the victim, and begin CPR if needed. Each time you open the airway to give a breath, look for an object in the throat and if seen, remove it.

OR

- Object is expelled and infant begins to breathe or cough forcefully.

Infant Basic Life Support Proficiency Checklist

S = self check / P = partner check / I = instructor check

Infant Rescue Breathing

	S	P	I
1. Check responsiveness.	○	○	○
2. Send a bystander, if available, to call EMS.	○	○	○
3. Airway open.	○	○	○
4. Breathing check.	○	○	○
5. 2 slow breaths.	○	○	○
6. Check circulation.	○	○	○
7. Rescue breathing (1 every 3 seconds).	○	○	○
8. If alone, call EMS after 1 minute.	○	○	○
9. Recheck circulation and breathing after first minute, then every few minutes.	○	○	○

Infant CPR

	S	P	I
1. Check responsiveness.	○	○	○
2. Send a bystander, if available, to call EMS.	○	○	○
3. Airway open.	○	○	○
4. Breathing check.	○	○	○
5. 2 slow breaths.	○	○	○
6. Check circulation.	○	○	○
7. Position fingers.	○	○	○
8. 5 chest compressions.	○	○	○
9. 1 slow breath.	○	○	○
10. Continue CPR for 1 minute (19 more cycles, for total of 20).	○	○	○
11. If alone, call EMS after 1 minute.	○	○	○
12. Recheck circulation.	○	○	○
13. Continue CPR.	○	○	○
14. Recheck circulation every few minutes.	○	○	○

Infant Choking

	S	P	I
1. Position infant.	○	○	○
2. Give up to 5 back blows.	○	○	○
3. Give up to 5 chest thrusts .	○	○	○
4. Repeat Steps 2 and 3 until object removed or victim unresponsive.	○	○	○
5. If unresponsive, assess the victim and begin CPR if needed.	○	○	○

Basic Life Support Review

These techniques are the same for all victims regardless of age:

- Check responsiveness—tap and shout.
- Open airway—head-tilt/chin-lift; for suspected spinal injury use jaw-thrust without head-tilt.
- Check breathing—look at chest to rise and fall and listen and feel for breathing.
- If breathing, place in recovery position.
- If not breathing, give 2 slow breaths (#1 in table).
- If breaths do not cause chest to rise, retilt head and give breaths again.
- If breaths still unsuccessful, give CPR (#2 in table).
- Check for signs of circulation (breathing, coughing, movement, normal skin condition).
- If not breathing but other signs of circulation exist, give rescue breaths (#3 in table).
- If not breathing and no other signs of circulation exist, perform CPR (#4 in table).

Action	Adult (>8 years)	Child (1-8 years)	Infant (<1 year)
1. Breathing methods	Mouth-to-barrier device Mouth-to-mouth Mouth-to-nose Mouth-to-stoma	Mouth-to-barrier device Mouth-to-mouth Mouth-to-nose	Mouth-to-barrier device Mouth-to-mouth and nose Mouth-to-nose
2. Foreign-body airway obstruction in unresponsive victim	CPR cycles of 15 compressions to 2 breaths. Before giving a breath, look for an object in throat and if seen, remove it.	CPR cycles of 5 compressions to 1 breath. Before giving a breath, look for an object in throat and if seen, remove it.	5 back blows, 5 chest thrusts
3. Rescue breathing but other signs of circulation exist	1 breath every 5 seconds. Should cause chest to rise.	1 breath every 3 seconds. Should cause chest to rise.	1 breath every 3 seconds. Should cause chest to rise.
4. Compressions:			
• Locating hand positions	• Lower half of sternum, between nipples	• Lower half of sternum, between nipples	• 1 finger width below nipple line
• Method	• Heel of 1 hand, other hand on top	• Heel of 1 hand	• 2 fingers
• Depth	• $1\frac{1}{2}$ inch to 2 inches	• 1 to $1\frac{1}{2}$ inches	• $\frac{1}{2}$ to 1 inch
• Rate	• 100 per minute	• 100 per minute	• 100+ per minute
• Ratio of chest compressions to breaths	• 15:2	• 5:1	• 5:1
5. When to activate EMS when alone	Immediately after establishing unresponsiveness	After 1 minute of resuscitation, unless bystander available who can call	After 1 minute of resuscitation, unless bystander available who can call
6. Automated external defibrillation (AED)	Yes	No	No

STUDY
Questions (5)

Name_____ Course_____ Date_____

Activities

Activity 1

Choose the best answer.

____ 1. Are chest compressions likely to work if the victim is on a soft surface?
a. Yes, a soft surface is okay.
b. No, the surface should be hard.

____ 2. When you tilt the head with the chin lift, where do you place your fingertips?
a. Under the soft part of the throat near the chin
b. Under the bony part of the jaw near the chin

____ 3. Which is the safer way to open the airway of a person who may have a spinal injury?
a. Push the jaw forward from the corners.
b. Stabilize head and lift the jaw.
c. Use either method.

____ 4. How should you check for stopped breathing?
a. Look at the chest; listen and feel for air coming out of the mouth.
b. Look at the pupils of the eyes.
c. Check the pulse.

____ 5. When you give breaths to any victim, the breaths should be:
a. Slow
b. Fast

____ 6. Before deciding whether to give CPR, check the victim's signs of circulation for:
a. three seconds
b. five seconds
c. 10 seconds
d. 20 seconds

____ 7. To find where to push on the chest for adult chest compressions, you should measure up:
a. Two hand-widths from the navel
b. One finger-width from the middle finger on the sternum's tip

____ 8. Give chest compressions:
a. With a quick jerk
b. Smoothly and regularly

____ 9. Push on a victim's chest:
a. At an angle
b. Straight down

____ 10. Compress an adult's chest at least:
a. $1/2$ to 1 inch
b. 1 to $1^1/_2$ inches
c. $1^1/_2$ to 2 inches

____ 11. In one-rescuer CPR, give chest compressions to an adult at the rate, per minute, of:
a. 100
b. 80
c. 60
d. 40

____ 12. What is the pattern of compressions and breaths in one-rescuer CPR for an adult victim?
a. 15 compressions, 2 breaths
b. 15 compressions, 1 breath
c. 5 compressions, 2 breaths
d. 5 compressions, 1 breath

Activity 2

Choose the best answer.

____ 1. An adult victim is coughing forcefully. Should you give back blows and thrusts?
a. Yes
b. No

____ 2. A person is coughing weakly and making wheezing noises. You should:
a. Give abdominal thrusts.
b. Let the person alone and watch closely.

____ 3. A victim who seems to be choking *can* speak. Should you give abdominal thrusts?
a. Yes
b. No

____ 4. A responsive person is coughing forcefully, trying to dislodge an object. Then the person stops coughing and cannot speak. You should:
a. Give abdominal thrusts.
b. Let the person alone and watch closely.

STUDY
Questions (5)

___ **5.** When you give abdominal thrusts to a responsive adult victim, what part of your wrist do you place against the victim?
   a. The palm side
   b. The little finger side
   c. The thumb side

___ **6.** Give abdominal thrusts quickly:
   a. Inward and upward
   b. Straight back

___ **7.** Where do you place your fist on an adult to give abdominal thrusts?
   a. Over the breastbone
   b. Slightly above the navel
   c. Below the navel

___ **8.** To give abdominal thrusts to an adult victim who is lying down, place the heel of one hand:
   a. Slightly above the navel
   b. On the edge of the breastbone
   c. Below the navel

___ **9.** For an adult victim who is obese or in advanced pregnancy, it is better to give:
   a. Abdominal thrusts
   b. Chest thrusts

Activity 3
Choose the best answer.

___ **1.** How should you check for stopped breathing?
   a. Look at the chest; listen and feel for air coming out of the mouth.
   b. Look at the pupils of the eyes.
   c. Check the pulse.

___ **2.** If your amount of breath is enough:
   a. The stomach will form a pouch.
   b. The chest will rise.
   c. Your air backs up against incoming air.

___ **3.** Lay rescuers do not check for an infant's pulse:
   a. True
   b. False

___ **4.** To give a baby chest compressions use:
   a. Two fingers
   b. The heel of one hand

___ **5.** Push on the chest of a child or baby one finger-width:
   a. Above nipple line
   b. Below nipple line
   c. Above xiphoid process

___ **6.** How far should you compress a baby's chest?
   a. $1\frac{1}{2}$ to 2 inches
   b. $\frac{1}{2}$ to 1 inch

___ **7.** Give a baby chest compressions at the rate per minute of:
   a. 100
   b. 80
   c. 60

___ **8.** Give babies and children:
   a. 15 compressions, 2 breaths
   b. 5 compressions, 2 breaths
   c. 15 compressions, 1 breath
   d. 1 compressions, 1 breath

___ **9.** When giving chest compressions to a child, use:
   a. Two or three fingers or heel of one hand
   b. The heel of one hand and the other hand on top

Activity 4
Choose the best answer.

___ **1.** You believe a baby has an object caught in its airway; it cannot cough or cry. What do you do first?
   a. Let it alone and watch closely.
   b. Give abdominal thrusts.
   c. Give chest thrusts.
   d. Give back blows.

___ **2.** Use your finger to remove an object from an unconscious baby or child's mouth:
   a. Whenever back blows and chest thrusts fail
   b. Only if you see the object

STUDY
Questions ⑤

Case Situations

Case 1

You find a 50-year-old male lying in an office building hallway, suffering from cardiac arrest.

1. Describe how to locate the proper hand positioning for giving CPR.

   _____

   _____

   _____

2. Describe:

   ____ **a.** How many hands should you use to compress an adult's chest?

   ____ **b.** Compression depth in inches

   ____ **c.** Compressions per minute

   ____ **d.** Compression to ventilation ratio

3. List four common CPR compression mistakes:

   a. _____

   _____

   b. _____

   _____

   c. _____

   _____

   d. _____

   _____

Case 2

At a family picnic you find an uncle unconscious. You open his airway and unsuccessfully attempt to give one rescue breath.

1. What do you do now?

   a. _____

   _____

   _____

   b. _____

   _____

   _____

2. If that fails, what should you do?

   _____

   _____

   _____

3. If that fails, what should you try next?

   _____

   _____

4. Then what, if you are still unsuccessful?

   _____

   _____

   _____

Case 3

A six-year-old, whose face is cyanotic, appears to be choking and violently gasping for air.

1. What is the immediate emergency care to alleviate the problem? What should be done?

   _____

   _____

   _____

2. Describe the proper procedure for the immediate emergency care necessary in this situation.

   _____

   _____

   _____

Case 4

A frantic mother calls to report that her infant suddenly has stopped breathing. Within seconds, you cross the street to her house and find the mother giving rescue breathing. A check of the infant's pulse reveals no pulse.

1. What is the immediate emergency care in this situation?

   _____

   _____

   _____

STUDY
Questions 5

____ 2. For an infant, how many cardiac compressions per minute should you complete?

    a. 80

    b. 100

    c. 120

____ 3. For a small infant, how many inches down should you compress the chest wall?

    a. $1/4$

    b. $1/4$ to $1/2$

    c. $1/2$ to 1

    d. 1 to $1^1/_2$

____ 4. When checking infant's signs of circulation, use the:

    a. coughing

    b. breathing

    c. both of these

Case 5

While eating at a local fast-food restaurant, you see a young male kneeling against a table bench, grasping his throat with one hand. You find that he is cyanotic about the lips. He is unable to speak. The victim's friends tell you that he is allergic to aspirin.

____ 1. This victim is most likely experiencing:

    a. an acute asthma attack

    b. an airway obstruction

    c. an allergic reaction

    d. a respiratory infection

____ 2. Immediate care of this victim would include:

    a. giving two rescue breaths

    b. hitting him repeatedly between the shoulder blades

    c. trying to dislodge the food with your finger

    d. if he is sitting or standing, applying upward, inward abdominal thrusts with your hands

Chapter Activities

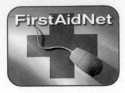

WEB Activities

Basic Life Support

Visit nsc.jbpub.com/FirstAidNet, then click on Web Activities, and select the appropriate chapter.

AIDS and CPR

According to the federal government's Centers for Disease Control and Prevention (CDC), AIDS *cannot* be transmitted via saliva. Nevertheless, to reduce the risk of spreading any disease, face masks with one-way valves are recommended for trained rescuers who perform CPR.

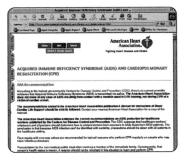

CPR STATS

Though no single agency collects information about how many people get CPR and how many people are trained to perform CPR, many studies have been done examining CPR in specific communities. While they show varying rates of success, all are consistent in showing benefits from early CPR.

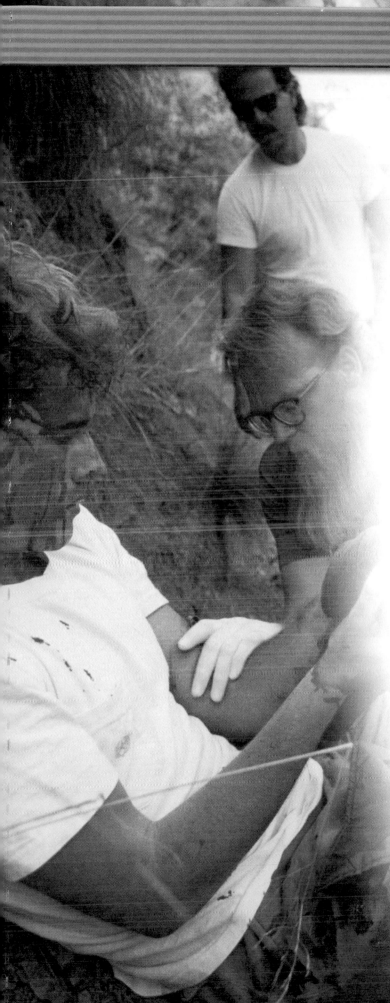

Chapter 6

Bleeding and Shock

Bleeding

The average-size adult has about five to six quarts (10 to 12 pints) of blood and can safely donate a pint during a blood donation. However, rapid blood loss of one quart or more can lead to shock and death. A child who loses one pint of blood is in extreme danger.

External Bleeding

External bleeding occurs when blood can be seen coming from an open wound. The term **hemorrhage** refers to a large amount of bleeding in a short time.

Types of External Bleeding

External bleeding can be classified into three types according to its source. In **arterial bleeding,** blood spurts (up to several feet) from the wound. Arterial bleeding is the most serious type of bleeding because a great deal of blood can be lost in a very short time. Arterial bleeding also is less likely to clot because blood can clot only when it is flowing slowly or not at all. However, unless a very large artery has been cut, it is unlikely that a person will bleed to death before the flow can be controlled. Nevertheless, arterial bleeding is dangerous, and must be controlled.

In **venous bleeding,** blood from a vein flows steadily or gushes. Venous bleeding is easier to control than arterial bleeding. Most veins collapse when cut. Bleeding from deep veins, however, can be as massive and as hard to control as arterial bleeding.

In **capillary bleeding,** blood oozes from capillaries. It is the most common form of bleeding, and usually is not serious, and can be controlled easily. Quite often, this type of bleeding will clot and stop by itself.

Each type of blood vessel—artery, vein, capillary—contains blood of a different shade of red. An inexperienced person may have difficulty detecting the differences. Identifying the type of bleeding by its color is not important.

The body naturally responds to bleeding in the following way:

- *Blood vessel spasm.* Arteries contain small amounts of muscle tissue in their walls. If a blood vessel is completely severed, it draws back into the tissue, constricts its diameter, and slows the bleeding dramatically. If an artery is only partially cut across its diameter, however, constriction is incomplete. The vessel may not contract, and the loss of blood may not slow as dramatically.

- *Clotting.* Special elements (platelets) in blood form a clot. Clotting (▶Figure 6-1) serves as a protective covering for a wound until the tissues underneath can repair themselves. In a healthy individual, initial clot formation normally takes about 10 minutes. Clotting time is longer in people who have lost a great deal of blood over a prolonged period of time, are taking aspirin or anticoagulants, are anemic, are hemophiliacs, or have severe liver disease.

Caution:

DO NOT contact blood with your bare hands. Protect yourself with medical exam gloves, extra gauze pads, or clean cloths, or have the victim apply the direct pressure. If you must use your bare hands, do so only as a last resort. After the bleeding has stopped and the wound has been cared for, vigorously wash your hands with soap and water.

DO NOT use direct pressure on an eye injury, a wound with an embedded object, or a skull fracture.

DO NOT remove a blood-soaked dressing. Apply another dressing on top and keep pressing.

What to Do

Regardless of the type of bleeding or the type of wound, the first aid is the same. First, and most important, you must control the bleeding (▶Skill Scan):

1. Protect yourself against disease by wearing medical exam gloves. If medical exam gloves are not available, use several layers of gauze pads, clean cloths, plastic wrap, a plastic bag, or waterproof material. You can even have the victim apply pressure on the wound with his or her own hand. After bleeding has stopped and the wound has been cared for, vigorously wash your hands with soap and water.

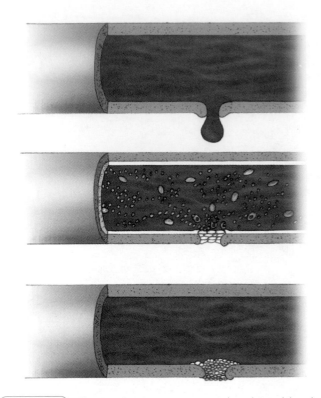

Figure 6-1 Clotting begins as soon as a break in a blood vessel wall occurs (top). Platelets (the oval disks in the middle drawing) stick to the vessel wall and release adenosine diphosphate (ADP) (the smaller round objects), which recruits more platelets. Finally, the temporary platelet plug is replaced by a tough fibrin clot (bottom).

2. Expose the wound by removing or cutting the victim's clothing to find the source of the bleeding.

3. Place a sterile gauze pad or a clean cloth such as a handkerchief, washcloth, or towel over the entire wound and apply direct pressure with your fingers or the palm of your hand. The gauze or cloth allows you to apply even pressure. Direct pressure stops most bleeding. Applying direct pressure to the wound compresses the sides of the torn vessel and helps the body's natural clotting mechanisms to work. Be sure the pressure remains constant, is not too light, and is applied to the bleeding source. Do not remove blood-soaked dressings; simply add new dressings over the old ones.

4. If the bleeding is from an arm or leg, elevate the injured area above heart level to reduce blood flow as you continue to apply pressure. Elevation allows gravity to make it difficult for the body to pump blood to the affected extremity. Elevation alone, however, will not stop bleeding and must be used in combination with direct pressure over the wound.

Skill Scan) Bleeding Control

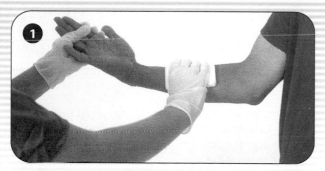

1. Direct pressure stops most bleeding. Wear medical exam gloves, and place a sterile gauze pad or a clean cloth over wound.

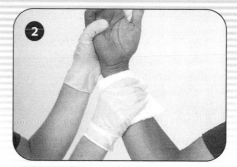

2. If bleeding continues, use elevation to help reduce blood flow. Combine with direct pressure over the wound.

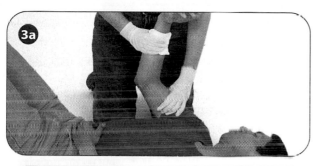

3a

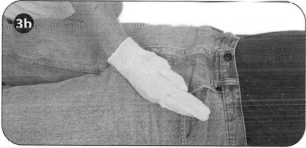

3b

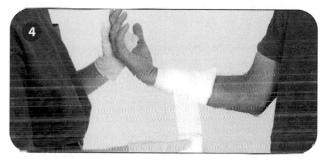

4. A pressure bandage can free you to attend to other injuries or victims.

3. If bleeding continues, apply pressure at a pressure point to slow blood flow. Locations are: (a) brachial or (b) femoral. Combine with direct pressure over the wound.

5. To free you to attend to other injuries or victims, use a pressure bandage to hold the dressing on the wound. Wrap a roller gauze bandage tightly over the dressing and above and below the wound site.

"Blood is a very special juice."

Goethe (1749–1832)

6. If the bleeding continues, apply pressure at a pressure point as you continue putting direct pressure over the wound to slow the flow of blood (▼ **Figure 6-2**). A pressure point is where an artery near the skin's surface passes close to a bone, against which it can be compressed. The most accessible pressure points on both sides of the body are the brachial point in the upper inside arm and the femoral point in the groin. Using pressure points requires skill, because unless the exact location of the pulse point is used, the pressure-point technique is useless. Many first aiders have difficulty finding the precise pressure-point location. Direct pressure, however, stops most bleeding.

7. When direct pressure cannot be applied such as in the case of a protruding bone, skull fracture, or embedded object, use a doughnut-shaped (ring) pad to control bleeding (▶ **Figure 6-3**). To make a ring pad, wrap one end of a narrow bandage (roller or cravat) several times around your four fingers to form a loop. Pass the other end of the bandage through the loop and wrap it around and around until the entire bandage is used and a ring has been made.

8. When bleeding stops, use procedures in Chapter 7 for wound care.

Some people panic when they see even the smallest amount of blood. The sight of more than a couple of tablespoonfuls of blood generally is enough to scare victims and bystanders. Take time to reassure the victim that everything possible is being done. Don't belittle the victim's concerns.

Caution:

DO NOT apply a pressure bandage so tightly that it cuts off circulation. Check the radial pulse if the bandage is on an arm; for a leg, check the pulse between the inside ankle bone knob and the Achilles tendon (posterior tibial).

DO NOT use a tourniquet. They are rarely needed and can damage nerves and blood vessels. A tourniquet may cause the loss of an arm or leg. If you do use one, apply wide, flat materials—never rope or wire—and do not loosen it. Remember: Using a tourniquet usually means the extremity will have to be amputated.

Internal Bleeding

Internal bleeding occurs when the skin is not broken and blood is not seen. It can be difficult to detect but can be life threatening. Internal bleeding comes from injuries that do not break the skin or from nontraumatic disorders such as ulcers.

What to Look for

The signs of internal bleeding may take days to appear:

- bruises or contusions of the skin
- painful, tender, rigid, bruised abdomen
- vomiting or coughing up blood
- stools that are black or contain bright red blood

(**Figure 6-2**) Proper hand positions for applying pressure on brachial and femoral arteries.

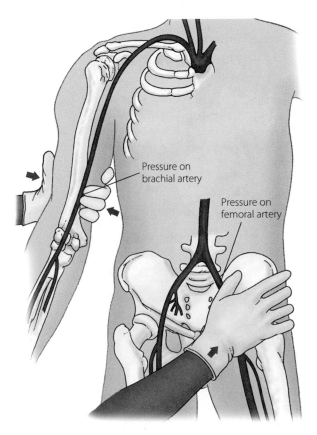

Pressure on brachial artery

Pressure on femoral artery

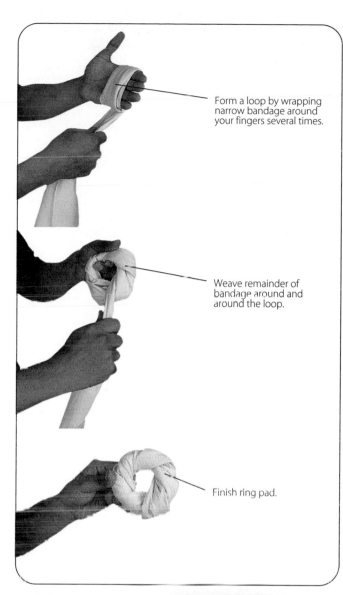

Form a loop by wrapping narrow bandage around your fingers several times.

Weave remainder of bandage around and around the loop.

Finish ring pad.

What to Do

For severe internal bleeding, follow these steps:

1. Monitor ABC.

2. Expect vomiting. If vomiting occurs, keep the victim lying on his or her left side to allow drainage and to prevent both inhalation of vomitus (aspiration) and expulsion of vomit from the stomach.

3. Treat for shock by raising the victim's legs 8 to 12 inches and cover the victim with a coat or blanket to keep warm. See page 106 for when to use other body positions.

4. Seek immediate medical attention.

Caution:

DO NOT give a victim anything to eat or drink. It could cause nausea and vomiting, which could result in aspiration. It could cause complications if surgery is needed.

Bruises are a form of internal bleeding but are not life threatening. To treat bruises:

1. Apply an ice pack directly on the skin for 20 minutes.

2. If the bruise is on an arm or leg, raise the limb if it is not broken.

3. If an arm or a leg is involved, apply an elastic bandage for compression.

Shock (Hypoperfusion)

Shock refers to circulatory system failure, which happens when oxygenated blood is not provided in sufficient amounts for every body part. Because every injury affects the circulatory system to some degree, first aiders should automatically treat injured victims for shock. Shock is one of the most common causes of death in an injured victim (▶Table 6-1).

The damage caused by shock depends on which body part is deprived of oxygen and for how long. For example, without oxygen, the brain will be irreparably damaged in 4 to 6 minutes, the abdominal organs in 45 to 90 minutes, and the skin and muscle cells in 3 to 6 hours.

To understand shock, think of the circulatory system as having three components: a working pump (the heart), a network of pipes (the blood vessels), and an adequate amount of fluid (the blood) pumped through the pipes.

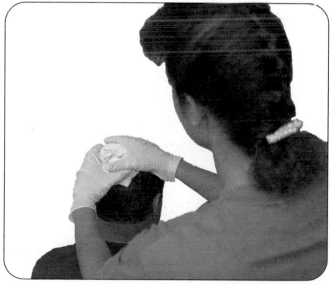

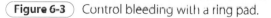

Figure 6-3 Control bleeding with a ring pad.

BLEEDING

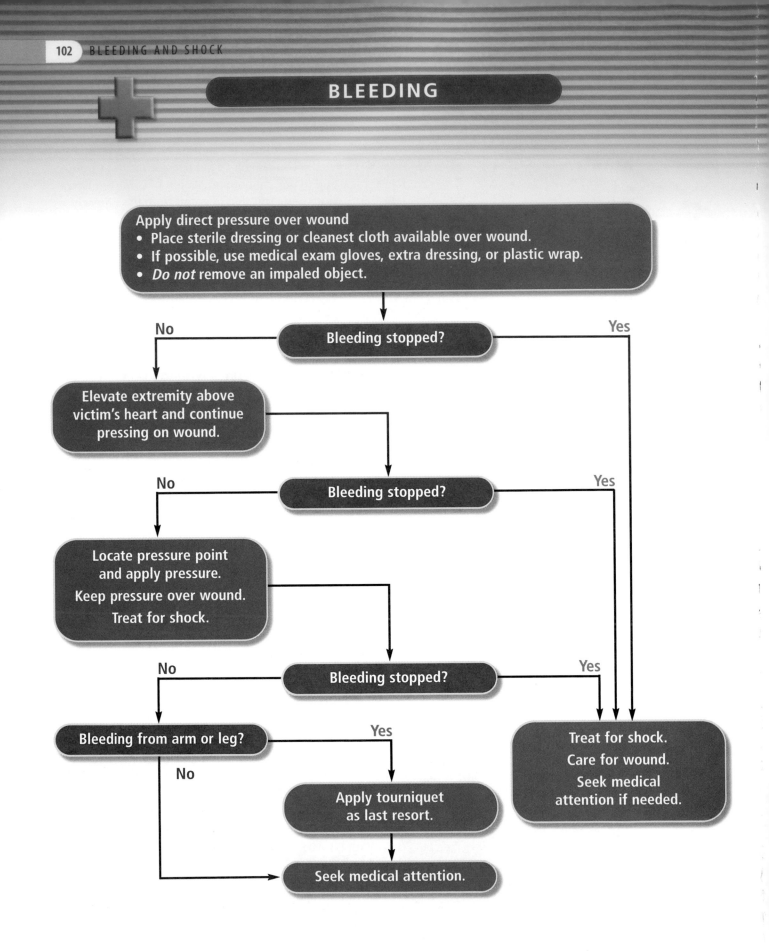

Apply direct pressure over wound
- Place sterile dressing or cleanest cloth available over wound.
- If possible, use medical exam gloves, extra dressing, or plastic wrap.
- *Do not* remove an impaled object.

Bleeding stopped?
No → Yes →

Elevate extremity above victim's heart and continue pressing on wound.

Bleeding stopped?
No → Yes →

Locate pressure point and apply pressure.
Keep pressure over wound.
Treat for shock.

Bleeding stopped?
No → Yes →

Bleeding from arm or leg?
Yes → No

Apply tourniquet as last resort.

Treat for shock.
Care for wound.
Seek medical attention if needed.

Seek medical attention.

Table 6-1: Signs of Shock

Signs (in order of appearance)	Reason
1. Altered mental status: • anxiety • restlessness • combativeness	Brain not receiving enough oxygen.
2. Skin: • pale • cold • clammy	Body attempts to correct problem by diverting blood from nonvital to vital organs (i.e., from skin to heart and brain).
3. Nausea and vomiting	Blood diverted from digestive system, which causes nausea and occasional vomiting.

4. Changes in vital signs	As body tries to pump more blood:
	• pulse increases—
	  60 to 100 = normal;
	  >120 = serious.
	• respirations increase—
	  12 to 20 = normal;
	  >24 = serious.

5. Other signs: • thirst • dilated pupils • sometimes cyanosis (blue color), especially of lips and nail beds	

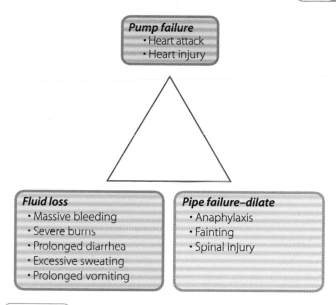

Figure 6-4 Causes of shock.

- *Pipe failure.* When the nervous system is damaged such as in injury to the spinal cord or an overdose of certain drugs, **neurogenic shock** may result. In neurogenic shock, the blood vessels (pipes) enlarge and the blood supply is insufficient to fill them. **Septic shock** develops in some victims with bacterial infection when damaged blood vessels lose their ability to contract. First aiders seldom see cases of septic shock because victims usually are already hospitalized for a serious illness, injury, or operation.

Shock resulting from blood or fluid loss is the most common type.

Damage to any of those components can deprive tissues of blood and produce the condition known as shock ▶**Figure 6-4**).

Shock can be classified as one of three types according to which component has failed.

- *Pump failure.* **Cardiogenic shock** results from a failure of the heart to pump sufficient blood. For example, a major heart attack can damage the heart muscle so the heart cannot squeeze and therefore cannot push blood through the blood vessels.

- *Fluid loss.* **Hypovolemic shock** happens with the loss of a significant amount of fluid from the system. If the lost fluid is blood, this type of shock is best known as **hemorrhagic shock**. People experiencing dehydration due to vomiting, diarrhea, diabetes, insufficient fluid intake, or misuse of diuretics can lose large amounts of fluid. Profuse sweating can also result in a sizable amount of fluid loss.

Caution:

DO NOT raise the legs of victims with head injuries or strokes. Slightly raise the victim's head if no spinal injury is suspected.

DO NOT place victims with breathing difficulties, chest injuries, penetrating eye injuries, or heart attack on their backs. Place them in a half-sitting position to help breathing.

DO NOT place victims rated as V, P, or U (see page 47) or vomiting victims on their backs. Use the recovery position (see page 67). If a spinal injury is suspected, do not move the victim.

DO NOT place an advanced (third trimester) pregnant woman on her back—instead, place her on her left side to avoid pressing the vena cava.

What to Look for

- altered mental status: anxiety and restlessness
- pale, cold, and clammy skin, lips, and nail beds
- nausea and vomiting
- rapid breathing and pulse
- unresponsiveness when shock is severe

What to Do

Even if an injured victim does not have signs or symptoms of shock, first aiders should care for shock ▶Skill Scan. You can prevent shock from getting worse; you cannot reverse it.

1. Treat life-threatening injuries and other severe injuries.
2. Lay the victim on his or her back.
3. Raise the victim's legs 8 to 12 inches. Raising the legs allows the blood to drain from the legs back to the heart ▼Figure 6-5.
4. Prevent body heat loss by putting blankets and coats under and over the victim.

"If the face is red,

Raise the head.

If the face is pale,

Raise the tail."

Old first aid axiom

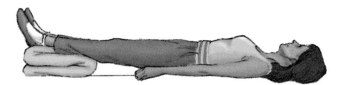
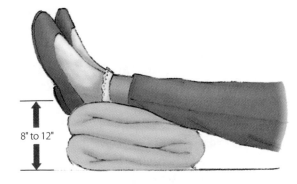

Figure 6-5 Elevate the legs to circulate blood to the vital organs.

8" to 12"

Caution:

DO NOT raise the legs more than 12 inches because that will affect the victim's breathing by pushing the abdominal organs up against the diaphragm.

DO NOT lift the foot of a bed or stretcher—breathing will be affected, and the blood flow from the brain may be retarded and lead to brain swelling.

DO NOT raise the legs of a victim with head injuries, stroke, chest injuries, breathing difficulty, or unconsciousness. Place the victim in the proper position, as described above.

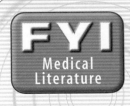

Emergency Blankets

At rest, 75% of the body's heat production is lost by radiation and convection from the body surface. Such heat loss can be detrimental to an injured victim. An inexpensive—but controversial—"emergency" blanket now has scientific backing. These aluminized covers or blankets reduce body heat loss by protecting the body surface from exposure to cool temperatures and air currents and by blocking the escape of radiant body heat to the atmosphere.

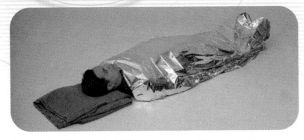

Sources: R. S. Erickson, et al: "Effect of Aluminized Covers on Body Temperature." *Heart and Lung* 20(3):255–264 (May 1991); K. B. Hindsholm, et al: "Reflective Blankets Used for Reduction of Heat Loss." *British Journal of Anaesthesia* 68:531–533 (1992)

Caution:

DO NOT overheat the victim.

DO NOT give the victim anything to eat or drink. It could cause nausea and vomiting, which could result in aspiration. It could also cause complications if surgery is needed.

SHOCK

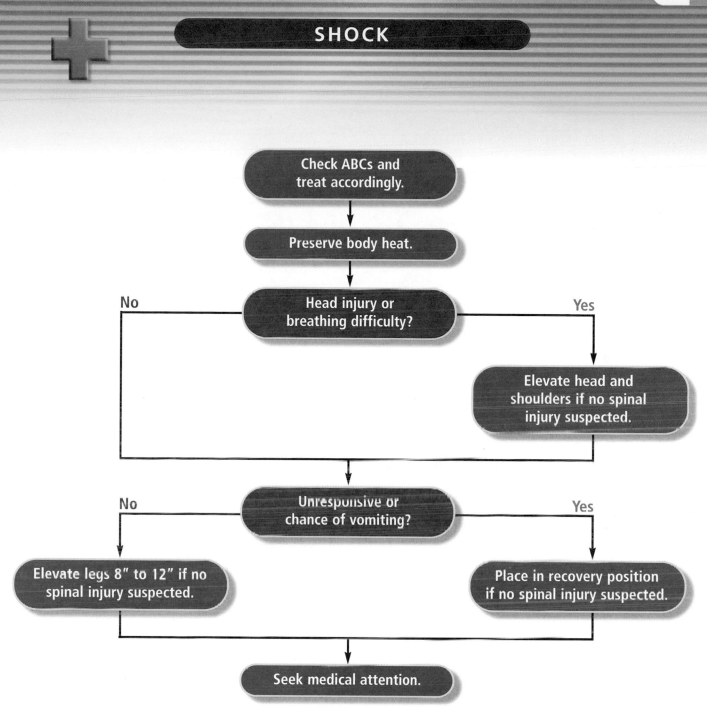

Check ABCs and treat accordingly.

↓

Preserve body heat.

↓

Head injury or breathing difficulty?

No →   ← Yes

Elevate head and shoulders if no spinal injury suspected.

↓

Unresponsive or chance of vomiting?

No →   ← Yes

Elevate legs 8" to 12" if no spinal injury suspected.

Place in recovery position if no spinal injury suspected.

↓

Seek medical attention.

Skill Scan

Positioning the Shock Victim

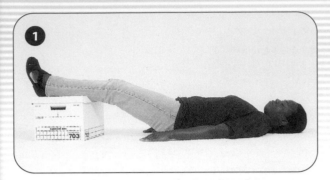

1. Usual shock position. Elevate the legs 8 to 12 inches (if spinal injury is not suspected).

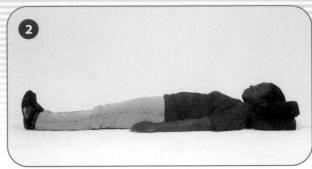

2. Elevate the head for head injury (if spinal injury is not suspected).

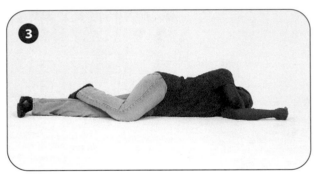

3. Position an unresponsive or stroke victim in the recovery position.

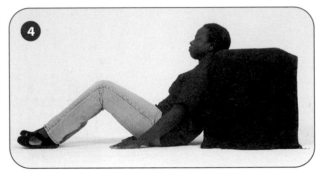

4. Use a half-sitting position for those with breathing difficulties, chest injuries, or a heart attack.

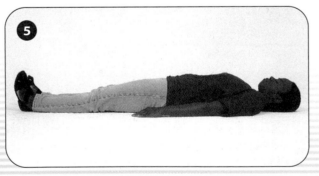

5. Keep victim flat if a spinal injury is suspected or victim has leg fractures.

Anaphylaxis

Allergies are usually thought of as causing rashes, itching, or some other short-term discomfort that disappears when the offending agent is removed from contact with the allergic person. However, a more powerful reaction to substances ordinarily eaten or injected can occur within minutes or even seconds. This reaction, called **anaphylaxis,** can cause death if it is not treated immediately.

Anaphylaxis is a massive allergic reaction by the body's immune system. Normally, the immune system functions to recognize and eliminate foreign materials such as bacteria and viral particles. In the case of anaphylaxis, however, the immune system forms an antibody to a foreign protein upon its first exposure. When the individual is again exposed to the foreign protein (an antigen), the established antibody immediately attempts to neutralize the exposure by binding with the antigen. When the antibody and the antigen combine, they form an antigen-antibody complex. That triggers certain cells in body tissues and in the bloodstream to release a series of chemicals. Those released chemicals are the cause of the severe cardiac, respiratory, skin, and gastrointestinal signs and symptoms that occur in anaphylaxis.

Common Causes of Anaphylaxis

Like less severe allergic reactions, anaphylaxis is an abnormal response to an antigen that doesn't bother most people but causes symptoms in those who have a hypersensitivity to it. Well-known antigens that can cause anaphylaxis include:

- medications (penicillin and related drugs, aspirin, sulfa drugs)
- food and food additives (shellfish, nuts, eggs, monosodium glutamate, nitrates, nitrites)
- insect stings (honeybee, yellow jacket, wasp, hornet, fire ant)
- plant pollen
- radiographic dyes

Since the mid-1900s, penicillin has been by far the most common cause of anaphylaxis. Most allergic reactions to penicillin are local skin reactions such as hives or a rash or systemic reactions (wheezing, swelling, redness).

Insect stings are another major cause of anaphylactic death. Hymenoptera (honeybees, bumblebees, wasps, hornets, yellow jackets, and fire ants) are the offending insects. Although millions of people in the United States are allergic to insect venom, and hundreds of thousands of them have allergic reactions to stings each year, the number of deaths reported from those reactions is estimated at only 50 to 100 per year.

The best way to prevent anaphylaxis is to avoid the instigator (bees, aspirin, certain foods).

What to Look for

Anaphylaxis typically comes on within minutes of exposure to the offending substance, peaks in 15 to 30 minutes, and is over within hours.

The first symptom is usually a sensation of warmth followed by intense itching, especially on the soles of the feet and the palms of the hands. The skin flushes, hives may appear, and the face may swell. Breathing becomes difficult, and the victim may feel faint and anxious. Convulsions, shock, unconsciousness, even death may follow. Other signs and symptoms of anaphylaxis include:

- sneezing, coughing, wheezing
- shortness of breath
- tightness and swelling in the throat
- tightness in the chest
- increased pulse rate
- swelling of the mucous membranes (tongue, mouth, nose)
- blueness around lips and mouth
- dizziness
- nausea and vomiting

About 60% to 80% of anaphylactic deaths are caused by the victims' inability to breathe because swollen airway passages obstruct airflow to the lungs. The second most common cause of anaphylactic deaths—about 24% by one estimate—is shock, caused by insufficient blood circulating through the body's dilated blood vessels.

Caution:

DO NOT mistake anaphylaxis for other reactions such as hyperventilation, anxiety attacks, alcohol intoxication, or low blood sugar.

What to Do

Because the main causes of death resulting from anaphylaxis are the collapse of the circulatory system and respiratory compromise, first aiders must focus on caring for those two body systems. Rapid identification of breathing difficulty and shock will allow the appropriate first aid to be started.

Rescue breathing or CPR may be needed. If a bee sting is involved, remove the stinger by scraping, not squeezing. An ice pack to the sting area may decrease the absorption of more antigen.

Epinephrine

The drug epinephrine can reverse many of the life-threatening processes of anaphylaxis on the circulatory and respiratory systems (vessel dilation and bronchospasm). Epinephrine produces bronchodilation, increases cardiac output, and constricts blood vessels. Injectable epineph-

rine for use by a first aider is available only through a victim's physician-prescribed emergency epinephrine kit. Two such kits are available: AnaKit® and EpiPen®. The advantage of an AnaKit® is that it includes two separate injections in prefilled syringes (▼Figure 6-6). The advantage of the EpiPen® is that the needle of the prefilled syringe is hidden from view (▼Figure 6-7).

The recommended injection site when using an EpiPen® is the front outside part of the thigh (▶Figure 6-8). Do not inject into the buttock or into a vein. To use an EpiPen®, remove the safety cap and place the tip of the autoinjector against the thigh, at a right angle to the leg. Push the autoinjector firmly until it activates, then hold it in place for about 10 seconds. That allows time for the

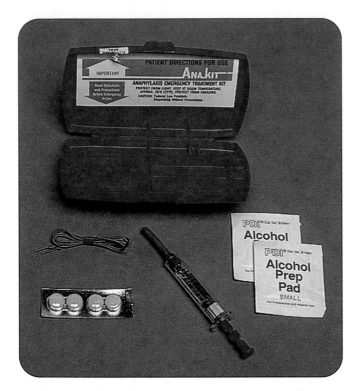

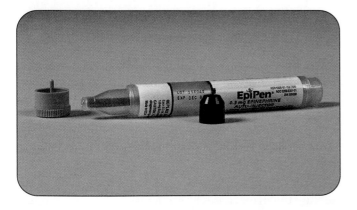

Figure 6-6 Physician-prescribed preloaded epinephrine with 2 shots.

Figure 6-7 Physician-prescribed preloaded epinephrine autoinjector.

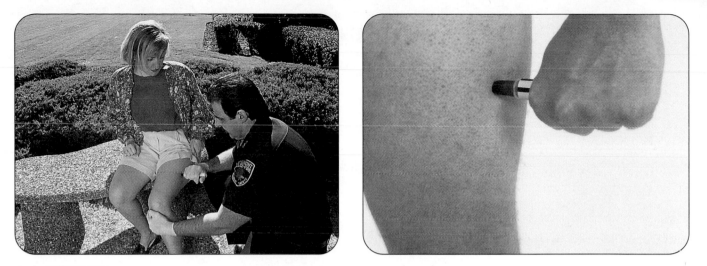

Figure 6-8, A–B Push the autoinjector against the thigh and hold in place until medication is injected (10 seconds).

medication to be injected. Remove the injector and massage the site for several seconds. Some relief of symptoms may appear as soon as one or two minutes after administration.

If you believe that you or a family member is susceptible to anaphylaxis, consult your physician about the need to have an epinephrine kit. If you are in a situation that has all the signals of a severe allergic reaction and the victim's breathing is being affected, ask the victim or anyone else around if the victim has a physician-prescribed epinephrine kit. Although most emergency situations are not life threatening, anaphylaxis is—so be prepared.

Parents, relatives, neighbors, friends, and school personnel must be taught how to recognize and handle an attack. In addition to injectable epinephrine, the allergic victim should wear a medical-alert tag or necklace at all times. If food is the culprit, food labels and restaurant menus must be scrutinized for potential allergens. If flying insects such as bees are the culprit, sensitive individuals must avoid them and not wear perfume, cologne, or bright colors, which attract the insects.

An antihistamine such as Benadryl, though not as life saving a medication as epinephrine, can prevent further reactions. They take about 20 minutes to work.

ANAPHYLAXIS

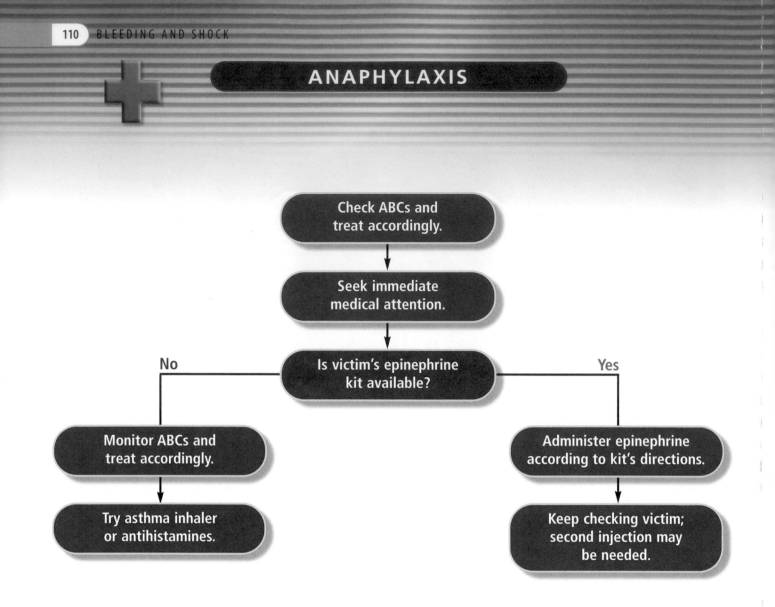

Check ABCs and
treat accordingly.

Seek immediate
medical attention.

No — Is victim's epinephrine
kit available? — Yes

Monitor ABCs and
treat accordingly.

Administer epinephrine
according to kit's directions.

Try asthma inhaler
or antihistamines.

Keep checking victim;
second injection may
be needed.

STUDY
Questions (6)

Name_____ Course_____ Date_____

Activities

Activity 1

Mark each statement as true (T) or false (F).

T F **1.** Quickly losing more than a quart of blood for an adult is life threatening.

T F **2.** Bleeding from veins is usually fast and in spurts.

T F **3.** The use of a tourniquet is the method most preferred to try to control hemorrhaging.

T F **4.** Most people can tell from the blood's shade of red which blood vessel has been cut.

T F **5.** Blood normally clots within 10 minutes.

T F **6.** Direct pressure over the wound will stop most cases of bleeding.

T F **7.** If a body part is elevated to control bleeding, direct pressure is not needed.

T F **8.** When you are trying to control bleeding, leave blood-soaked dressings in place.

T F **9.** Aspirin and hemophilia extend blood-clotting times.

T F **10.** Closed wounds occur when blood vessels beneath the skin have been broken and the blood is not visible.

Activity 2

Choose the best answer.

____ **1.** Which of the following actions should you take to control bleeding when blood is flowing freely from a wound?
   a. Press on the wound.
   b. Elevate an injured arm to control bleeding and discontinue direct pressure on the wound.
   c. Use a pressure point alone if direct pressure fails to stop the bleeding.

2. List three ways you can protect yourself from contact with a victim's blood if medical exam gloves are not available.
   a. _____
   b. _____
   c. _____

3. List the two criteria that identify a pressure point.
   a. _____
   b. _____

4. Give three examples of the types of injuries that should not have direct pressure applied over a bleeding wound.
   a. _____
   b. _____
   c. _____

5. How can you control bleeding when direct pressure cannot be applied over a wound?

   _____

   _____

6. List four signs of internal bleeding.
   a. _____
   b. _____
   c. _____
   d. _____

7. List three procedures for treating bruised tissue.
   a. _____
   b. _____
   c. _____

Activity 3

Complete the following statement.

When people experience shock, usually their

____ **1. a.** skin is pale or bluish   **b.** skin is red

____ **2. a.** skin is dry   **b.** skin is moist

____ **3. a.** skin is hot   **b.** skin is cool

____ **4. a.** victim is restless   **b.** victim is calm

____ **5. a.** breathing and pulse are rapid
         b. breathing and pulse are slow

STUDY
Questions 6

Mark each statement as true (T) or false (F).

T   F   **6.** Shock results when parts of the body do not receive enough blood.

T   F   **7.** Shock is a concern in life-threatening injuries.

T   F   **8.** People's lives can be threatened by shock.

Check the relevant action(s).

9. A victim begins showing signs of shock. Which of the following would you do?

   a. Attempt to warm the victim.

   b. Give fluids to the victim.

   c. Handle the victim gently.

   d. Help a responsive victim walk around to aid blood flow to the extremities.

   e. Place a responsive victim on his or her back and elevate the feet and legs, if injuries will not be aggravated.

   f. Elevate the head of a victim with a head injury.

Match the position with condition/injury.

10. Write A, B, or C to match the best position for a victim with each condition or injury.

Condition or Injury	Best Position
___ crushed chest injury	**A.** on victim's side
___ vomiting	**B.** victim flat on back with legs elevated 8″–12″
___ unresponsive	
___ heart attack	**C.** half sitting and supported
___ head injury	
___ stroke	
___ amputated fingers	

Activity 4

1. Circle the causes of anaphylaxis (allergic reaction) in sensitive people.

   a. hornet sting

   b. eating nuts

   c. taking penicillin

2. Circle the signs and symptoms of anaphylaxis.

   a. blueness around lips and mouth

   b. coughing or wheezing

   c. breathing difficulty

   d. severe itching or hives

   e. nausea and vomiting

   f. bleeding from the nose

   g. extreme thirst

Mark each statement true (T) or false (F) regarding anaphylaxis.

____ **3.** Although the victim appears in distress, these reactions are *not* life threatening.

____ **4.** The only really effective treatment for anaphylaxis is an immediate injection of epinephrine.

____ **5.** Antihistamines can substitute for epinephrine.

____ **6.** Epinephrine can be purchased without a physician's prescription.

____ **7.** Several doses of epinephrine may be needed.

____ **8.** Anaphylaxis is a massive allergic reaction by the body.

Case Situations
Case 1

A person's right hand has been badly mangled by a power saw. You arrive soon afterward to find the victim's hand bleeding profusely.

1. What sequence of first aid procedures would you provide in this situation?

   a. _____

   _____

   b. _____

   _____

   c. _____

   _____

   d. _____

   _____

____ 2. What is probably the most effective method for controlling bleeding in this situation?

   a. direct pressure over the wound

   b. direct pressure and elevation

   c. a tourniquet

   d. running cold water over the bleeding area

STUDY
Questions 6

___ 3. What is the most effective method for controlling most types of bleeding?
   a. direct pressure over the wound
   b. pressure-point technique
   c. a tourniquet
   d. running cold water over the bleeding area

4. Is the use of a tourniquet ever an appropriate method to control bleeding like that described in this case? Why or why not? Check your choice and explain your answer in the space provided.

   ___ a. Yes   ___ b. No

   _____
   _____
   _____

5. What are the major signs and corresponding first aid for the three types of external bleeding? Write your answers in the following chart.

Capillary
Flow: _____
First Aid: _____
   _____

Venous
Flow: _____
First Aid: _____
   _____

Arterial
Flow: _____
First Aid: _____
   _____

Case 2

While chopping firewood for his evening campfire, a middle-aged man deeply lacerates his lower left leg. Fellow campers manage initial control of the profuse bleeding.

___ 1. Upon arrival at the campground, a first aider would probably find this man:
   a. unresponsive
   b. having a severe allergic reaction
   c. in hypovolemic shock
   d. in septic shock

2. This victim may be expected to exhibit which of the following signs and symptoms? Check *all* appropriate answers.
   ___ a. ashen gray skin
   ___ b. high skin temperature
   ___ c. body covered with a clammy sweat
   ___ d. rapid pulse
   ___ e. complaints of thirst

3. The most important action for the first aider to consider in this and most other emergency situations involving shock is to:

   _____
   _____

Case 3

In an orchard, you see a woman lying next to a pickup truck with several bystanders gathered around. A short distance away is a wooden outbuilding that appears to have an active beehive. The victim is in apparent respiratory distress; she is wheezing, and her eyelids appear swollen.

1. This victim is in what type of shock?

   _____

2. Give three causes and examples of this type of shock.
   Causes:
   a. _____
   b. _____
   c. _____

   Examples:
   a. _____
   b. _____
   c. _____

3. The first aid for the type of shock experienced by this victim would include which of the following? Check all appropriate answers.
   ___ a. emergency transport to a medical facility
   ___ b. transport in a prone position to ease respiration
   ___ c. determine if victim has an emergency epinephrine kit
   ___ d. give liquid if the victim requests it

Chapter Activities

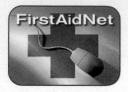

WEB Activities

Action at an Emergency

Visit nsc.jbpub.com/FirstAidNet, then click on Web Activities, and select the appropriate chapter.

MD Care for Cuts

It is important to know if you should consult a doctor about needing stitches or a tetanus shot after an injury.

Shock

Although hemorrhaging is a major cause of shock, other factors can contribute.

Anaphylaxis

Anaphylaxis is the serious and rapid allergic reactions usually involving more than one part of the body that, if severe enough, can kill. Some common causes of anaphylaxis include nuts, shellfish, drugs, latex, and insect stings.

Using an EpiPen®

Emergency treatment for anaphylaxis requires the use of epinephrine. The EpiPen® is a common device used to administer this drug.

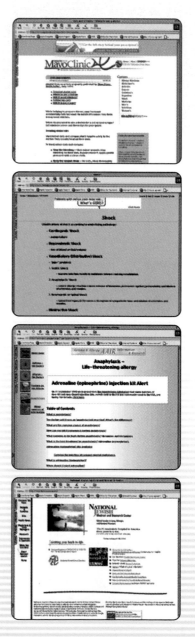

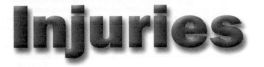

Injuries

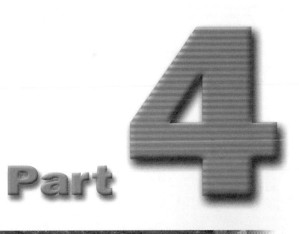

Part 4

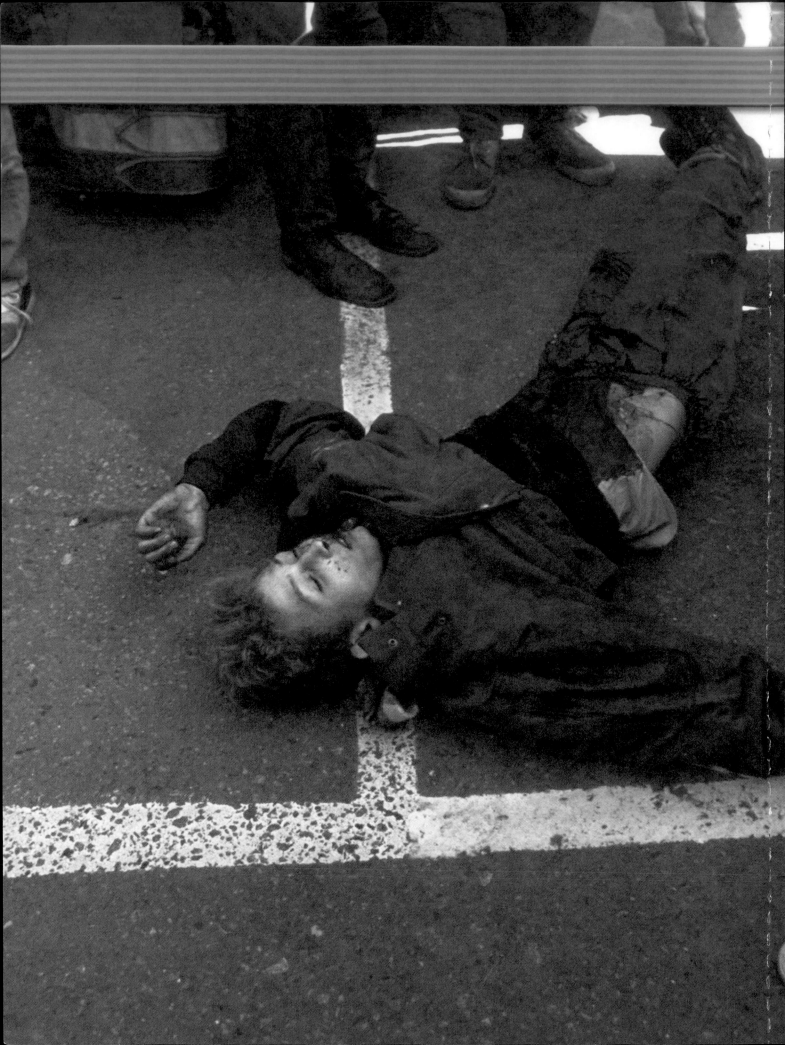

Chapter 7

Wounds

Open Wounds

An open wound is a break in the skin's surface resulting in external bleeding. It may allow bacteria to enter the body, causing an infection. There are several types of open wounds (▶Figure 7-1). Recognizing the type of wound helps to give proper care. With an **abrasion,** the top layer of skin is removed, with little or no blood loss. Abrasions tend to be painful, because the nerve endings often are abraded along with the skin. Ground-in debris may be present. This type of wound can be serious if it covers a large area or becomes embedded with foreign matter. Other names for an abrasion are "scrape," "road rash," and "rug burn."

A **laceration** is cut skin with jagged, irregular edges (▶Figure 7-2). This type of wound is usually caused by a forceful tearing away of skin tissue.

Incisions tend to be smooth-edged, resembling a surgical or paper cut (▶Figure 7-3). The amount of bleeding depends on the depth, the location, and the size of the wound.

Punctures are usually deep, narrow wounds in the skin and underlying organs such as a stab wound from a nail or a knife (▶Figure 7-4). The entrance is usually small, and the risk of infection is high. The object causing the injury may remain impaled in the wound.

With an **avulsion,** a piece of skin is torn loose and is either hanging from the body or completely removed. This type of wound can bleed heavily. If the flap is still attached and folded back, lay it flat and realign it into its normal position. Avulsions most often involve ears, fingers, and hands (▶Figure 7-5).

An **amputation** involves the cutting or tearing off of a body part, such as a finger, toe, hand, foot, arm, or leg.

What to Do

1. Protect yourself against disease by wearing medical exam gloves. If medical exam gloves are not available, use several layers of gauze pads, plastic wrap or bags, or waterproof material. You can even have the victim apply pressure with his or her own hand. Your bare hand should be used only as a last resort.

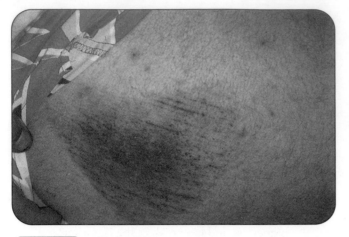

Figure 7-1 Abrasion.

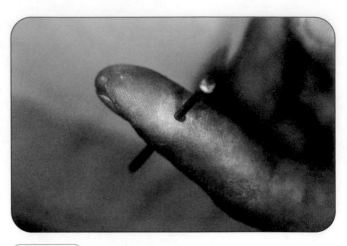

Figure 7-4 Puncture.

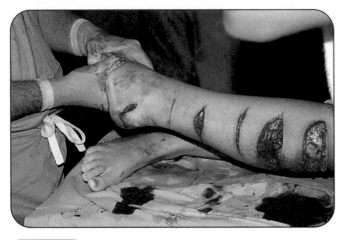

Figure 7-2 Laceration.

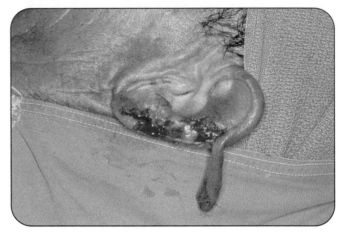

Figure 7-5 Avulsion.

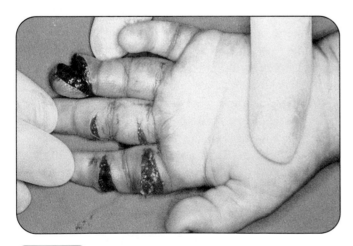

Figure 7-3 Incision.

2. Expose the wound by removing or cutting the clothing to find the source of the bleeding.

3. Control bleeding by using direct pressure and, if needed, the other methods described in the previous chapter.

Caution:

DO NOT clean large, extremely dirty, or life-threatening wounds. Let hospital emergency department personnel do the cleaning.

DO NOT scrub a wound. Scrubbing a wound is debatable, and it can bruise the tissue.

Cleaning a Wound

A victim's wound should be cleaned to help prevent infection. Wound cleaning usually restarts bleeding by disturbing the clot, but it should be done anyway for shallow wounds. For wounds with a high risk factor for infection, leave the pressure bandage in place since medical personnel will clean the wound.

1. Scrub your hands vigorously with soap and water. Put on medical exam gloves, if available.

2. Expose the wound.

3. Clean the wound.

   For a shallow wound:

   - Wash inside the wound with soap and water.

   - Irrigate the wound with water ▼Figure 7-6 (use water that is clean enough to drink). Run water directly into the wound and allow it to run out. Irrigation with water needs pressure (minimum 5 to 8 psi) to adequately cleanse the tissue. Water from a faucet provides sufficient pressure

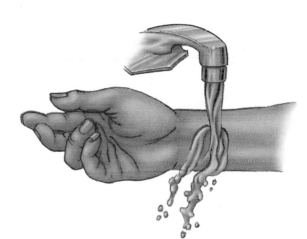
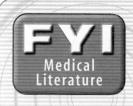
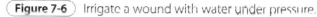

Figure 7-6 Irrigate a wound with water under pressure.

and quantity. Pouring water on the wound or using a bulb syringe will not generate enough force for adequate cleaning.

For a wound with a high risk for infection (eg, an animal bite, a very dirty or ragged wound, a puncture), seek medical attention for wound cleaning. If you are in a remote setting (greater than one hour from medical attention), clean the wound as best you can.

4. Remove small objects not flushed out by irrigation with sterile tweezers. A dirty abrasion or other wound that is not cleaned will leave a "tattoo" on the victim's skin.

5. If bleeding restarts, apply pressure over wound.

FYI
Medical Literature

Wound Irrigation Prevents Wound Infection

Emergency physicians treat an estimated 10 million traumatic wounds annually in the United States. Different methods of wound management have been developed to help minimize wound infection. Use of systemic and topical antibiotics remains controversial. Numerous studies show the benefits of high-pressure irrigation of wounds. One study used 531 patients with traumatic wounds to compare three of the more commonly used wound irrigants in preventing wound infections: normal saline, 1% Betadine, and Shur-Clens™. The researchers concluded that no difference in infection rates among the three irrigants existed and that the mechanical action of high-pressure irrigation, not the solution used, is the most important method of preventing wound infection.

Source: D. J. Dire: "A Comparison of Wound Irrigation Solutions Used in the Emergency Department." *Annals of Emergency Medicine;* 1990, 19(6):704–708.

FYI
Medical Literature

Wound Irrigation

This study compared the effectiveness of tap water or saline solution for irrigating simple skin lacerations to remove bacteria. The results showed no significant difference between bacterial counts in wounds irrigated with normal saline and those irrigated with tap water. The removal of bacteria from a wound depends more on the mechanical effects (speed and pressure) than on the type of solution. Tap water has these advantages over saline—it is more continuous and therefore takes less time, it is less expensive, and it does not require other materials such as sterile syringes or splash guards. Other irrigants with bactericidal properties and detergents have an anticellular effect that impairs wound healing and/or resistance to infection. Irrigation pressures over the 20 to 30 psi range are discouraged because the higher pressure can damage tissue.

Source: R. Moscati, et al., "Comparison of Normal Saline with Tap Water for Wound Irrigation," *American Journal of Emergency Medicine.* July 1998;16:379-381.

High-Risk Wounds

High potential for infection:

+ Bite wounds

+ Very dirty, contaminated wounds

+ Crushing, ragged wounds

+ Wounds over injured bone, joint, or tendon

+ Puncture wounds

Caution:

DO NOT irrigate a wound with full-strength iodine preparations such as Betadine (1%) or isopropyl alcohol (70%). They kill body cells as well as bacteria and are painful. Also, some people are allergic to iodine.

DO NOT use hydrogen peroxide. It does not kill bacteria, it adversely affects capillary blood flow, and it extends wound healing.

DO NOT use antibiotic ointment on wounds that require sutures or on puncture wounds (the ointment may prevent drainage). Use an antibiotic ointment only on abrasions and shallow wounds.

DO NOT soak a wound to clean it. No evidence supports the effectiveness of soaking.

DO NOT close the wound with tape such as butterfly tape. Infection is more likely when bacteria are trapped in the wound. If an unsightly scar later develops, it can be fixed by a plastic surgeon. An extremity (hand, foot) wound can be sutured within six to eight hours of the injury. Suturing of a head or trunk wound can wait up to 24 hours after the injury. Some wounds can be sutured three to five days after the injury.

DO NOT breathe or blow on a wound or the dressing.

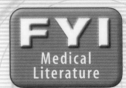

Wound Care: What the Medical Literature Says

- Soaking wounds is not effective.
- Scrubbing wounds is debatable.
- Irrigating wounds requires a minimum of 5 to 8 psi of pressure for tissue cleansing.
- Not closing a wound (eg, with butterfly bandages, Steri-Strips), especially a dirty wound, reduces the risk of infection.
- Applying antiseptic solutions such as Merthiolate™, Mercurochrome™, iodine, isopropyl alcohol, hydrogen peroxide can injure wounded tissues.
- Applying an antibiotic ointment such as Neosporin™ or Polysporin™ reduces the risk of infection.

Source: J. M. Howell, et al: "Outpatient Wound Preparation and Care: A National Survey." *Annals of Emergency Medicine,* 1992, 21: 976–981.

Covering a Wound

For a small wound that does not require sutures:

1. Cover it with a thin layer of antibiotic ointment such as Polysporin™ or Neosporin™. These ointments can kill a great many bacteria and rarely cause allergic reactions. No physician prescription is needed.

2. Cover the wound with a sterile dressing. Do not close the wound with tape or butterfly bandages. Bacteria may remain, leading to a greater chance of infection than if the wound were left open and covered by a sterile dressing. Closing a wound should be left to a physician.

3. If a wound bleeds after a dressing has been applied and the dressing becomes stuck, leave it on as long as the wound is healing. Pulling the scab loose to change the dressing retards healing and increases the chance of infection. If you must remove a dressing that is sticking, soak it in warm water to help soften the scab and make removal easier.

4. If a dressing becomes wet or dirty, change it. Dirt and moisture are both breeding grounds for bacteria.

Dressings and bandages are two different kinds of first aid supplies. A **dressing** is applied over a wound to control bleeding and prevent contamination. A **bandage** holds the dressing in place. Dressings should be sterile or as clean as possible; bandages need not be.

When to Seek Medical Attention

High-risk wounds should receive medical attention. Examples of high-risk wounds include those with embedded foreign material (such as gravel), animal and human bites, puncture wounds, and ragged wounds. Sutures, if needed, are best placed within 6 to 8 hours after the injury. Anyone who has not had a tetanus vaccination within 10 years, 5 years in the case of a dirty wound, should seek medical attention within 72 hours to update his or her tetanus inoculation status.

Wound Infection

Any wound, large or small, can become infected. Once an infection begins, damage can be extensive, so prevention is the best way to avoid the problem. A wound should be cleaned using the procedures described above.

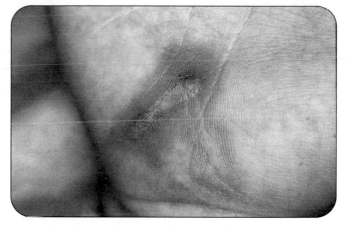

Figure 7-7 Infected wound.

OTC Treatments for Wounds (Days to Heal)

Polysporin™—8.2 days

Neosporin™—9.2 days

Johnson & Johnson First Aid Cream™—9.8 days

Mercurochrome™—13.1 days

No treatment—13.3 days

Bactine™ spray—14.2 days

Merthiolate™—14.2 days

Hydrogen peroxide (3%)—14.3 days

Campho-Phenique™—15.4 days

Tincture of iodine—15.7 days

Source: J. J. Leyden: "Comparison of Topical Antibiotic Ointments, a Wound Protectant, and Antiseptics for the Treatment of Human Blister Wounds Contaminated with *Staphylococcus aureus*." *Journal of Family Practice* 1987, 24(6):601–604.

It is important to know how to recognize and treat an infected wound.

The signs and symptoms of infection include:

- swelling and redness around the wound
- a sensation of warmth
- throbbing pain
- pus discharge
- fever
- swelling of lymph nodes
- one or more red streaks leading from wound toward the heart

The appearance of one or more red streaks leading from the wound toward the heart is a serious sign that the infection is spreading and could cause death. If chills and fever develop, the infection has reached the circulatory system (known as blood poisoning). Seek immediate medical attention ▶**Figure 7-7**.

Factors that increase the likelihood for wound infection include:

- dirty and foreign material left in the wound
- ragged or crushed tissue
- injury to an underlying bone, joint, or tendon
- bite wounds (human or animal)
- hand and foot wounds
- puncture wounds or other wounds that cannot drain

In the early stages of an infection, a physician may allow a wound to be treated at home. Such home treatment would include:

- keeping the area clean
- soaking the wound in warm water or applying warm, wet packs
- elevating the infected part
- applying antibiotic ointment
- changing dressings daily
- seeking medical help if the infection persists or becomes worse

Tetanus

Tetanus is also called "lockjaw" because of its best-known symptom, tightening of the jaw muscles. Tetanus is caused by a toxin produced by a bacterium. The bacterium, which is found throughout the world,

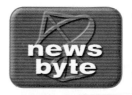

Tetanus Prevalence

Despite the wide availability of immunization against tetanus in the United States, many people are inadequately protected against that uncommon but often lethal disease. Protection was found in only 70% of people studied, with levels of immunity varying widely.

About 50 cases of tetanus occur in the United States each year, principally among the elderly and those who never received a primary series of vaccinations. Adults should have booster shots for tetanus every 10 years.

Source: P. J. Gergen, et al: "A Population-Based Serologic Survey of Immunity to Tetanus in the United States." *New England Journal of Medicine* 1995, 332:761.

forms a spore that can survive in a variety of environments for years. The World Health Organization reports that tetanus causes at least 500,000—perhaps even up to one million—deaths each year.

Millions of adults in the United States have let their tetanus immunizations lapse; a smaller number have never been vaccinated. In addition, antibody levels in immunized children decline over time; one-fifth of youngsters ages 10 to 16 do not have protective levels. Tetanus is not communicable from one person to another.

The bacterium by itself does not cause tetanus. But when it enters a wound such as a puncture wound that contains little oxygen, the bacterium can produce a **toxin,** which is a powerful poison. The toxin travels through the nervous system to the brain and the spinal cord. It then causes certain muscle groups, particularly in the jaw, to contract. There is no known antidote to the toxin once it enters the nervous system.

It is not just stepping on a rusty nail that can bring on the disease. Tetanus bacteria are commonly found in soil, street dust, organic garden fertilizers, and pet feces, and even minor cuts can introduce them into the bloodstream.

A vaccination can completely prevent tetanus. Everyone needs an initial series of vaccinations to prepare the immune system to defend against the toxin. Then a booster shot once every 5 to 10 years is sufficient to maintain immunity.

The guidelines for tetanus immunization boosters are as follows:

- Anyone with a wound who has never been immunized against tetanus should be given a tetanus vaccine and booster immediately.

- A victim who was once immunized but has not received a tetanus booster within the last 10 years should receive a booster.

- A victim with a dirty wound who has not had a booster for within the past five years should receive a booster.

- Tetanus immunization shots must be given within 72 hours of the injury to be effective.

Amputations

In 80% to 90% of cases, an amputated extremity can be successfully replanted (reattached).

Types of Amputations

Amputations usually involve fingers, hands, and arms rather than legs. Amputations are classified according to the type of injury:

- A **guillotine amputation** is a clean-cut, complete detachment. Examples would include a finger cut off with an ax or an arm severed with a saw ▼Figure 7-8A .

- A **crushing amputation** occurs when an extremity separates by being crushed or mashed off, such as when a hand is caught in a roller machine.

- **Degloving** is when the skin is peeled off, much as you would take off a glove ▼Figure 7-8B .

A crushing amputation, the most common type, has a poor chance of reattachment. A guillotine type has a much better chance because it is clean cut. Microsurgical techniques allow amputated parts to be effectively reattached 80% to 90% of the time so they function normally or nearly so.

A complete amputation may not involve heavy blood loss. That is because blood vessels tend to go into spasm, recede into the injured body parts, and shrink in diameter, resulting in a surprisingly small blood loss. More blood is seen in a partial amputation.

Figure 7-8A Amputation.

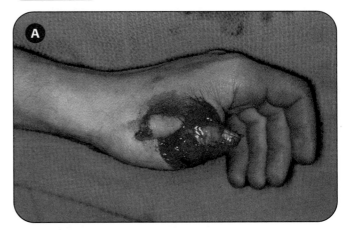

Figure 7-8B Degloving.

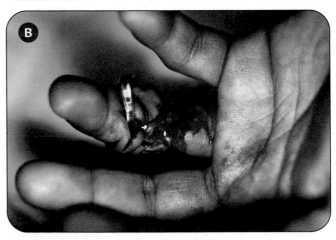

AMPUTATION

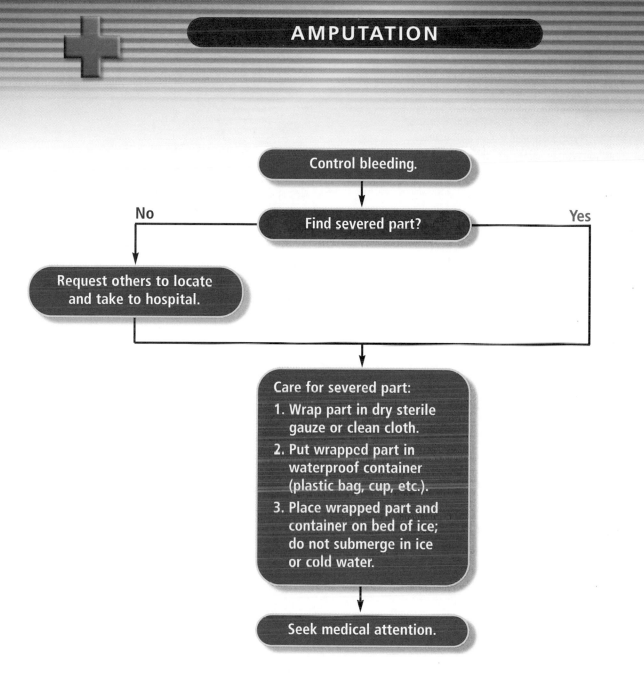

Control bleeding.

Find severed part?

No → Request others to locate and take to hospital.

Yes

Care for severed part:

1. Wrap part in dry sterile gauze or clean cloth.
2. Put wrapped part in waterproof container (plastic bag, cup, etc.).
3. Place wrapped part and container on bed of ice; do not submerge in ice or cold water.

Seek medical attention.

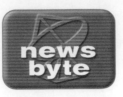

Amputations

Ronald Malt, MD, performed the first successful replantation in 1962 on a young boy's severed arm. In the 1960s, the replantation success rate ranged from 25% to 39%, compared to today's 80% to 90% success rate when appropriate actions are taken.

Apply direct pressure and elevate the damaged extremity. Salvage as much amputated tissue as possible. The tissue should be wrapped in a dry, sterile gauze and placed in a dry, sealed plastic bag or container. Place the container on ice, but avoid freezing it. Don't bury the tissue in ice and don't allow it to get wet. Moisture can cause waterlogging and maceration. The amputated portion does not need to be cleaned.

Source: Emergency, February 1996.

What to Do

1. Control the bleeding with direct pressure and elevate the extremity. Apply a dry dressing or bulky cloths. Be sure to protect yourself against disease. Tourniquets are rarely needed and, if used, will destroy tissue, blood vessels, and nerves necessary for replantation.

2. Treat the victim for shock.

3. Recover the amputated part and, whenever possible, take it with the victim. However, in multicasualty cases, in reduced lighting conditions, or when untrained people transport the victim, someone may be requested to locate and take the severed body part to the hospital after the victim's departure.

4. To care for the amputated body part (▶Figure 7-9):
   • The amputated portion does not need to be cleaned.
   • Wrap the amputated part with a dry, sterile gauze or other clean cloth.
   • Put the wrapped amputated part in a plastic bag or other waterproof container.
   • Place the bag or container with the wrapped part on a bed of ice.

5. Seek medical attention immediately.

Amputated body parts left uncooled for more than six hours have little chance of survival; 18 hours is probably the maximum time allowable for a part that has been cooled properly. Muscles without blood lose

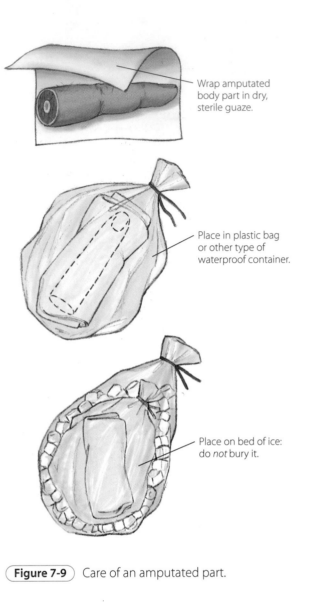

Wrap amputated body part in dry, sterile guaze.

Place in plastic bag or other type of waterproof container.

Place on bed of ice: do *not* bury it.

Figure 7-9 Care of an amputated part.

viability within four to six hours. Fingers with tendons and ligaments can tolerate a longer amputated time period than limbs.

Caution:

DO NOT try to decide whether a body part is salvageable or too small to save—leave the decision to a physician.

DO NOT wrap an amputated part in a wet dressing or cloth. Using a wet wrap on the part can cause waterlogging and tissue softening, which will make reattachment more difficult.

DO NOT bury an amputated part in ice—place it *on* ice. Reattaching frostbitten parts is usually unsuccessful.

DO NOT use dry ice.

DO NOT cut a skin "bridge," a tendon, or other structure that is connecting a partially attached part to the rest of the body. Instead, reposition the part in the normal position, wrap the part in a dry sterile dressing or clean cloth, and place an ice pack on it.

Blisters

A blister is a collection of fluid in a "bubble" under the outer layer of skin. (This section applies only to friction blisters and does not apply to blisters from burns, frostbite, drug reactions, insect or snake bites, or contact with a poisonous plant.)

Repeated rubbing of a small area of the skin will produce a blister. Blisters are so common that many people assume they are a fact of life. But blisters are avoidable, and life for many people could be more comfortable if they knew how to treat and prevent blisters.

Rubbing—as between a sock and a foot—causes stress on the skin's surface because the underlying supporting tissue remains stationary. The stress separates the skin into two layers, and the resulting space fills with fluid. The fluid may collect either under or within the skin's outer layer, the epidermis. Because of differences in skin, blister formation varies considerably from person to person (▼ Figure 7-10).

What to Do

When caring for a friction blister, try to (1) avoid the risk of infection, (2) minimize the victim's pain and discomfort, (3) limit the blister's development, and (4) help a fast recovery.

The best care for a particular blister is determined mainly by its size and location.

If an area on the skin becomes a "hot spot" (painful, red area), tightly apply a piece of tape (adhesive or duct), or apply several layers of moleskin or molefoam cut in a doughnut shape and secured by tape on top of each other.

If a blister on a foot is closed and not very painful, a conservative approach is to tape the blister tightly with duct tape or waterproof adhesive tape. The tape must remain on the blister for several days; removing it may tear off the blister's roof and expose unprotected skin. Unfortunately, the tape may become damp and contaminated and have to be replaced, risking a tear. You could also cut a hole in several pieces of moleskin or molefoam in layered stacks around the blister, make a doughnut-shaped pad, and apply it over the blister. Small blisters, especially on weight-bearing areas, generally respond better if left alone.

If a blister on the foot is open, or a very painful closed blister affects walking or running:

1. Clean the area with soap and water or rubbing alcohol.

(**Figure 7-10**) Friction blister.

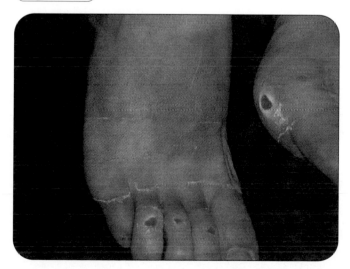

Preventing Blisters

Keeping the skin lubricated and protected will reduce the potential for blister formation. Applying duct or adhesive tape to problem areas, such as around a big toe, can help reduce blister formation by allowing the sock to rub against the tape instead of directly against the skin.

Wearing proper clothing also can prevent blisters. For example, acrylic socks are considered superior to cotton socks in avoiding foot blisters because they are made in layers that are designed to absorb friction. Socks with CoolMax™ construction are highly recommended. Avoid tube socks made of any material because their less precise fit tends to cause more friction than regular, fitted socks. Wear gloves to protect the skin on your hands.

Anything that can be done to keep the skin dry can also reduce blister formation. Moist skin is more susceptible to blisters than either very dry or very wet skin. One method is to wear socks that wick moisture from the skin. Interestingly, the application of antiperspirants to the feet has been shown to reduce the formation of serious blisters.

BLISTERS

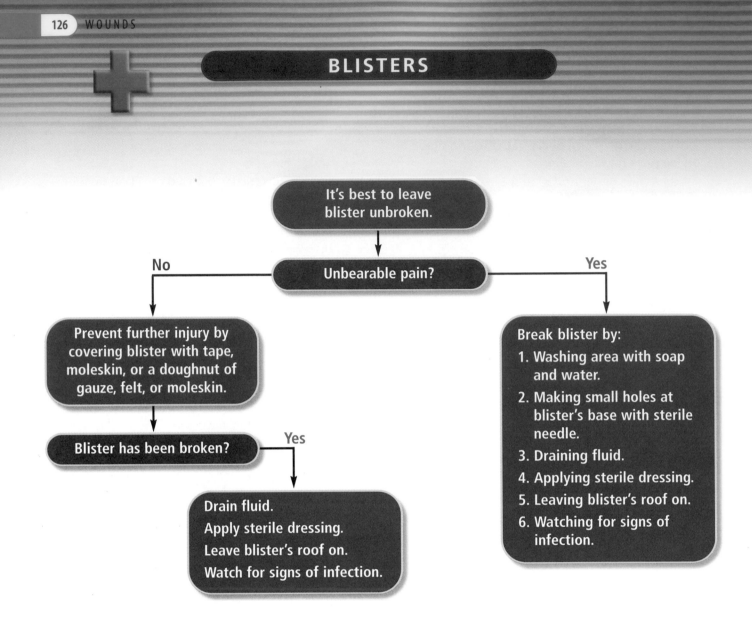

It's best to leave blister unbroken.

Unbearable pain?

No

Prevent further injury by covering blister with tape, moleskin, or a doughnut of gauze, felt, or moleskin.

Blister has been broken? **Yes**

Drain fluid.
Apply sterile dressing.
Leave blister's roof on.
Watch for signs of infection.

Yes

Break blister by:

1. Washing area with soap and water.
2. Making small holes at blister's base with sterile needle.
3. Draining fluid.
4. Applying sterile dressing.
5. Leaving blister's roof on.
6. Watching for signs of infection.

2. Drain all fluid out of the blister by making several small holes at the base of the blister with a sterilized needle. Press the fluid out. Do not remove the blister's roof unless it is torn.

3. Apply several layers of moleskin or molefoam cut in a doughnut shape on top of each other (▼Figure 7-11).

4. Apply antibiotic ointment in the hole and cover it tightly with tape. The pressure dressing ensures that the blister's roof sticks to the underlying skin and that the blister does not refill with fluid after it has been drained.

With few exceptions, the blister's roof, which is the best and most comfortable "dressing," should be removed only when an infection is present. Once a blister has been opened, the area should be washed with soap to prevent further infection. For 10 to 14 days, or until new skin forms, a protective bandage or other cover should be used.

Even with no evidence of infection, you should consider removing the blister's roof when a partially torn blister roof may tear skin adjacent to the blister site, resulting in an even larger open wound. In such cases, use sterilized scissors to remove the loose skin of the blister's roof up to the edge of the normal tissue. Treat the same as for an open blister.

Impaled Objects

Impaled objects come in all shapes and sizes, from pencils and screwdrivers to knives, glass, fence posts, and cactus spines (▼Figure 7-12). Proper first aid requires that the impaled object be stabilized, because there can be significant internal damage.

What to Do

1. Expose the area. Remove or cut away any clothing surrounding the injury. If clothes cover the object, leave them in place; removing them could cause the object to move.

2. Do not remove or move the object. Movement of any kind could produce additional bleeding and tissue damage. Cheeks are the exception because the object or the bleeding could cause an airway obstruction. See the section on impaled object in the cheek for more information.

3. Control any bleeding with pressure around the impaled object. Straddle the object with gauze. Do not press directly on the object or along the wound next to the cutting edge, especially if the object has sharp edges.

4. Stabilize the object. Secure bulky dressings or clean cloths around the object. Some experts suggest

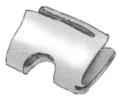

Figure 7-11   Blister care

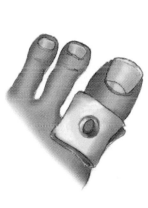

Cut holes in several gauze pads or moleskin.

Place gauze pads or moleskin with hole over blister.

Painful blister can be drained by making small hole with sterilized needle.

Do not remove blister's roof.

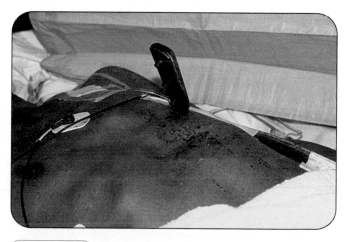

Figure 7-12   Impalement

securing 75% of the object with bulky dressings or cloths to reduce motion.

5. Shorten the object only if necessary. In most cases, do not shorten the object by cutting or breaking it. There are times, however, when cutting or shortening the object allows for easier transportation. Be sure to stabilize the object before shortening it. Remember that the victim will feel any vibrations from the object's being cut and that the injury could be worsened.

Impaled Object in the Cheek

The only time it is safe to remove an impaled object outside a medical setting is when the object is in the victim's cheek.

What to Do

1. Examine the injury inside the mouth. If the object extends through the cheek and you are more than one hour from medical help, consider removing it.

2. Remove the object. Place two fingers next to the object, straddling it. Gently pull it in the direction from which it entered. If it cannot be removed easily, leave it in place and secure it with bulky dressings.

3. Control bleeding. After you have removed the object, place dressings over the wound inside the mouth, between the cheek and the teeth. The dressings will help control bleeding and will not interfere with the victim's airway. Also place a dressing on the outside wound.

Impaled Object in the Eye

If an object is impaled in the eye, it is vital that pressure not be put on the eye. The eyeball consists of two chambers, each filled with fluid. *Do not exert any pressure against the eyeball;* fluid can be forced out of it, worsening the injury.

What to Do

1. Stabilize the object. Use bulky dressings or clean cloths to stabilize a long protruding object. You can place a protective paper cup or cardboard folded into a cone over the affected eye to prevent bumping of the object. For short objects, surround the eye with-

out touching the object with a doughnut-shaped (ring) pad held in place with a roller bandage.

2. Cover the undamaged eye. Most experts suggest that the undamaged eye should be covered to prevent sympathetic eye movement (ie, the injured eye moves when the undamaged eye does, aggravating the injury). Remember that the victim is unable to see when both eyes are covered and may be anxious. Make sure you explain to the victim everything you are doing.

3. Seek medical attention immediately.

Slivers

Small slivers of wood, glass, thorns, or metal can be painful and irritating. They also can cause infection. Because of their size and common location in the fingers, these slivers can usually be easily removed with tweezers. Sometimes, it is necessary to tease one end of the object with a sterile needle to place it in a better position for removal with tweezers. After you have removed the sliver, clean the area with soap and water and apply an adhesive strip (Band-Aid™).

Cactus Spines

Cacti are a part of the desert environment. They also are used as ornamental plants. Infection from cactus-spine punctures is rare. Removing cactus spines is time-consuming because they usually are acquired in bunches, are difficult to see, and are designed by nature to resist removal. Usually spines can easily, yet tediously, be removed with tweezers.

Another method for removing a large number of cactus spines is to coat the area with a thin layer of white woodworking glue or rubber cement and allow it to dry for at least 30 minutes. Slowly roll up the dried glue from the margins. Applying the glue in strips rather than puddles will make the rolling procedure go more smoothly. A single layer of gauze gently pressed onto the still damp glue helps to remove it after it has dried. Using tweezers and glue will remove most of the spines.

Using adhesive tape, duct tape, or Scotch tape, although quick and easy, removes only 30% of the spines, even after multiple attempts. Do not use Super Glue (or other similar product) to remove cactus spines. Not only does it fail to roll up when applied to the skin, it welds the spines to the skin. There is also the risk that the skin will permanently bond to anything it touches.

Fishhooks

Tape an embedded fishhook in place and do *not* try to remove it if injury to a nearby body part such as the eye or an underlying structure such as a blood vessel or nerve is possible or if the victim is uncooperative.

If the point of a fishhook has penetrated the skin but the barb has not, remove the fishhook by backing it out. Then treat the wound like a puncture wound. Seek medical advice for a possible tetanus shot.

If the hook's barb has entered the skin, follow these procedures:

1. If medical care is near, transport the victim and have a physician remove the hook.

2. If you are in a remote area, far from medical care, remove the hook using either the pliers method or the fishline method.

Pliers Method ("Push and Cut")

Use extreme care with the pliers method of fishhook removal because it can produce further severe injury if the hook is pushed into blood vessels, nerves, or tendons (►Figure 7-13). Use pliers with tempered jaws that can cut through a hook. The proper kind of pliers is usually unavailable, or sometimes the barb is buried too deep to be pushed through. Test the pliers by first cutting a similar fishhook.

1. Use cold or hard pressure around the hook to provide temporary numbness.

2. Push the embedded hook further in, in a shallow curve, until the point and the barb come out through the skin.

3. Cut the barb off, then back the hook out the way it came in.

4. After removing the hook, treat the wound and seek medical attention for a possible tetanus shot.

Fishline Method ("Push and Pull")

1. Loop a piece of fishline over the bend or curve of the embedded hook (►Figure 7-14).

2. Stabilize the victim's hooked body area.

3. Use cold or hard pressure around the hook to provide temporary numbness.

4. With one hand, press down on the hook's shank and eye while the other hand sharply jerks the fishline that is over the hook's bend or curve. The jerk movement should be parallel to the skin's surface. The hook will neatly come out of the same hole it entered, causing little pain.

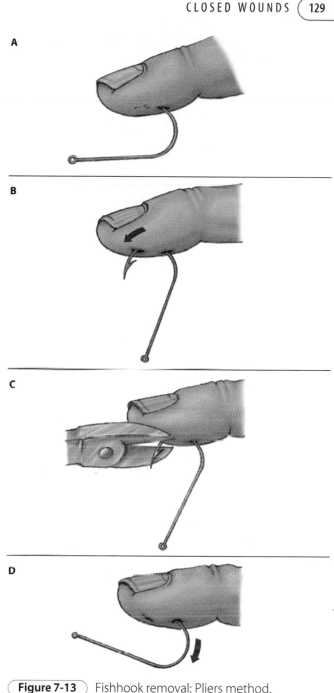

Figure 7-13 Fishhook removal: Pliers method.

5. After removing the hook, care for the wound and seek medical attention for a possible tetanus shot.

Closed Wounds

A closed wound happens when a blunt object strikes the body. The skin is not broken, but tissue and blood vessels beneath the skin's surface are crushed, causing bleeding within a confined area. There are three types of closed wounds:

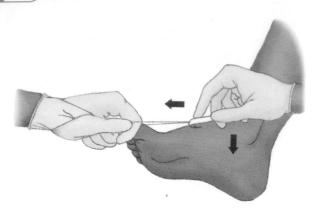

Figure 7-14 Fishhook removal: Fishline method.

- **Bruises and contusions** occur when blood collects under the skin in the injured area. The victim will experience pain and swelling (immediately or within 24 to 48 hours). As blood accumulates, a black-and-blue mark may appear.
- A **hematoma** is a clot of blood under the skin. There may be a lump or bluish discoloration.
- **Crush injuries** are caused by extreme forces, which can injure vital organs and bones without breaking open the skin. Crush injuries may indicate an underlying problem such as a fracture. Signs and symptoms include discoloration, swelling, pain, and loss of use.

What to Do

1. Control bleeding by applying an ice pack directly on the skin for no more than 20 minutes.
2. If the injury involves a limb, apply an elastic bandage for compression.
3. Check for a possible fracture.
4. Elevate an injured extremity above the victim's heart level to decrease pain and swelling.

Wounds That Require Medical Attention

At some point, you will probably have to decide whether medical assistance is needed for a wounded victim. As a guideline, seek medical attention for the following conditions:

- arterial bleeding
- uncontrolled bleeding

- a deep incision, laceration, or avulsion that
  goes into the muscle or bone
  is located on a body part that bends such as the elbow or knee
  tends to gape widely
  is located on the thumb or palm of the hand (nerves may be affected)
- a large or deep puncture wound
- a large embedded object or a deeply embedded object of any size
- foreign matter left in the wound
- human or animal bite
- possibility of a noticeable scar (sutured cuts usually heal with less scarring than unsutured ones)
- a wide, gaping wound
- an eyelid cut (to prevent later drooping)
- a slit lip (easily scarred)
- internal bleeding
- any wound you are not certain how to treat
- victim's immunization against tetanus not up to date

Sutures (Stitches)

If sutures are needed, they should be done by a physician within six to eight hours of the injury. Suturing wounds allows faster healing, reduces infection, and lessens scarring.

Some wounds do not usually require sutures:

- wounds in which the skin's cut edges tend to fall together
- shallow cuts less than one inch long

Rather than close a gaping wound with butterfly bandages or Steri-Strips, cover the wound with sterile gauze. Closing the wound might trap bacteria inside, resulting in an infection. In most cases, a physician can be reached in time for sutures to be made; if not, a wound without sutures will still heal but with scars. Scar tissue can be attended to later by a plastic surgeon.

Gunshot Wounds

Guns are abundant in the United States. It is estimated that about one-half of all American homes have a firearm.

A bullet causes injury in the following ways, depending on its velocity, or speed:

- *Laceration and crushing.* When the bullet penetrates the body, it crushes tissue and forces it apart. That is the main effect of low-velocity bullets. The crushing and laceration caused by the passage of the bullet usually is not serious unless vital organs or major blood vessels are injured. The bullet damages only those tissues that it directly contacts, and the wound is comparable to that caused by weapons such as knives.

- *Shock waves and temporary cavitation.* When a bullet penetrates the body, a shock wave exerts outward pressure from the bullet's path. That pushes tissues away and creates a temporary cavity that can be as much as 30 times the diameter of the bullet. As the cavity forms, a negative pressure develops inside, creating a vacuum. The vacuum then draws debris in with it. Temporary cavitation occurs only with high-velocity bullets and is the main reason for their immensely destructive effect. The cavitation lasts only a millisecond but can damage muscles, nerves, blood vessels, and bone.

In a *penetrating* wound (▼Figure 7-15A), there is a bullet entry point but no exit. In a *perforating* wound (▼Figure 7-15B), there are both entry and exit points.

The exit wound of a high-velocity bullet is larger than the entrance wound; the exit wound from a low-velocity bullet is about the same size as the entry wound. If the bullet was fired at very close range, the entrance wound may be larger than the exit wound because the gases from the gun's muzzle contribute to the surface tissue damage.

Bullets sometimes hit hard tissue such as bones and may bounce around in the body cavities, causing a great deal of damage to tissue and organs. Moreover, bone chips can riccochet to other body areas and cause damage. Because a split or misshapen bullet tumbles and exerts its force over a larger area, it does more damage than a smooth bullet going in a straight line.

What to Do

Regardless of the type of gunshot wound, initial care is roughly the same as for any other wound.

1. Check ABC.
2. Expose the wound(s). Look for entrance and exit wounds.
3. Control bleeding with direct pressure.
4. Apply dry, sterile dressing(s) to the wound(s) and bandage securely in place.

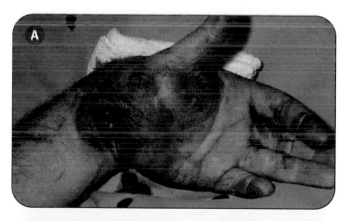

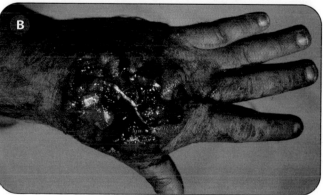

(Figure 7-15A) An entrance wound from a gunshot may have burns around the edges.

(Figure 7-15B) An exit wound is larger and results in greater damage to soft tissues.

5. Treat for shock.
6. Keep the victim calm and quiet.
7. Seek immediate medical care.

Caution:

DO NOT try to remove material from a gunshot wound. The hospital emergency department personnel will clean the wound.

Legal Aspects

Because gunshot wounds will involve contact with law enforcement agencies and possibly testifying in court, carefully observe the scene and the victim. Keep an accurate record of your observations. Preserve possible evidence, such as cartridge casings or shells, for the police. Do not touch or move anything unless absolutely necessary to treat the victim. All gunshot wounds must be reported to the police regardless of whether they are intentional (suicide, assault, murder, self-defense) or unintentional.

STUDY
Questions (7)

Name_____ Course_____ Date_____

Activities
Activity 1
Mark each statement as true (T) or false (F).

T **(F)** 1. Pouring water into a wound provides adequate pressure for irrigating.

T **(F)** 2. Avoid soap and water inside a wound.

T **(F)** 3. Antibiotic ointments can be placed in deep wounds.

(T) F 4. A tetanus immunization booster, if needed, should be given within 72 hours of the injury.

(T) F 5. When washing a wound with soap and water, wash inside a shallow wound.

T **(F)** 6. Hydrogen peroxide kills bacteria (germs) in a wound.

T **(F)** 7. If using rubbing alcohol, apply it on the skin around the wound, not in the wound.

(T) F 8. Topical antibiotic ointments can be placed in shallow wounds.

(T) F 9. If a dressing must be removed and part of the scab sticks to it, soak the dressing in warm water for easier removal.

(T) F 10. Cuts to eyelids and lips should be sutured by a physician.

(T) F 11. Sutures can be placed by a physician hours after the injury occurred.

Choose the best answer regarding types of wounds.

____ 12. A smooth cut made by a sharp object, such as a razor blade, is called
(a.) an incision   b. a laceration
c. an avulsion   d. an abrasion

____ 13. Skinned elbows and knees are examples of:
a. hematomas   b. avulsions
c. lacerations   **(d.)** abrasions

____ 14. Which type of wound has a jagged cut where the tissues are snagged and torn, forming a rough edge around the wound?
a. incision   **(b.)** laceration
c. contusion   d. hematoma

____ 15. The most common form of closed wound is:
a. an abrasion   **(b.)** a contusion
c. a laceration   d. an incision

____ 16. Which type of wound is caused by sharp, pointed objects, such as nails, splinters, and knives?
a. abrasions   b. avulsions
(c.) punctures   d. contusions

____ 17. Which of the following is most likely to lead to the development of tetanus?
a. laceration   b. amputation
c. incision   **(d.)** puncture

____ 18. Which of the following describes a piece of skin torn loose?
a. abrasion   b. amputation
(c.) avulsion   d. laceration

Choose the best answer regarding dressings.

____ 19. The material used to hold sterile material over a wound
a. must be sterile
b. must be adhesive
c. is a dressing
(d.) is a bandage

____ 20. Any material applied directly to a wound in an effort to control bleeding and prevent further contamination
a. is a bandage
b. is a dressing
c. should not be sterile
(d.) should be loosely secured so the wound can be inspected easily

STUDY
Questions ⑦

___ 21. Use of a sterile dressing on an open wound will
   a. reduce further contamination
   b. kill any bacteria present in the wound
   c. be necessary only if the wound is bleeding profusely
   ⓓ prevent shock

___ 22. If, after a dressing has been applied to a wound, bleeding continues, you should
   a. remove the blood-soaked dressing and replace it with a clean, sterile dressing
   ⓑ leave the original dressing in place and place a new dressing over the blood-soaked one

Activity 2
Mark each statement as true (T) or false (F).

Ⓣ F 1. Immediately wash a wound with soap and water.

T Ⓕ 2. Get a tetanus booster shot every year.

Ⓣ F 3. Soaking a wound is not recommended.

T Ⓕ 4. Use Mercurochrome™ or Merthiolate™ instead of soap and water on wounds.

Ⓣ F 5. Use any one of several recommended skin-wound antibiotics.

T Ⓕ 6. Use hydrogen peroxide.

Activity 3
Choose the best answer.

___ 1. After a blister forms, what should you try first?
   a. Drain the blister by making a small hole at the blister's edge.
   b. Use scissors to remove the blister's top.
   ⓒ Cover with gauze or moleskin cut into the shape of a doughnut.

___ 2. When can a blister be broken?
   ⓐ when very painful
   b. at least three days after its appearance
   c. never by a first aider

___ 3. Which is the proper procedure for breaking a blister?
   a. Cut the entire roof of the blister off.
   ⓑ Drain the fluid by making a small hole at the blister's edge.
   c. Use a red-hot paper clip to puncture the skin.
   d. Pinch or squeeze the blister off.
   e. Soak the blister off in hot water.
   f. None of these, since blisters should never be broken.

Case Situations
Case 1

A 39-year-old man has accidentally cut off several of his toes with a lawn mower. You find him sitting on the front steps of his house, firmly holding his foot wrapped in a towel. A minute later, the victim turns pale and slumps onto the grass.

___ 1. This victim is most likely experiencing:
   a. cardiogenic shock
   ⓑ hypovolemic shock
   c. acute blood poisoning
   d. heart attack

___ 2. Care for this victim includes
   ⓐ keeping him flat and elevating his legs
   b. tightening any loose clothing
   c. giving him sugar
   d. performing rescue breathing

___ 3. How should you transport the amputated toes to the hospital?
   ⓐ Wrap them in a dry, sterile gauze dressing, enclose them in something waterproof, and keep them cool.
   b. Place them into a container of warm, clean water.
   c. Place them directly onto several pieces of ice in a plastic cup.
   d. Wrap them in a dry, nonsterile bandage, enclose them in an aluminum wrap, and keep them warm.

STUDY
Questions (7)

T **F** **4.** Amputated parts older than six hours without proper cooling have little chance of survival.

T **F** **5.** Locate any amputated part, regardless of size, and take it with the victim to the nearest hospital emergency department.

T **F** **6.** Cut off a partially attached part.

Case 2

An 8-year-old child steps on a nail while playing in the backyard.

___ **1.** This wound is likely a(n)
  a. puncture wound   **b.** laceration
  c. avulsion   **d.** contusion

___ **2.** If a nail is impaled in your own child's foot, you should pull the nail out.
  a. true
  b. false

___ **3.** Care for the victim includes
  a. cleaning the wound with rubbing alcohol
  b. seeking medical attention
  c. cleaning the wound with hydrogen peroxide
  d. soaking the wound in water

___ **4.** An impaled object may be safely removed from the _____.
  a. chest
  b. abdomen
  c. neck
  d. cheek
  e. foot

Case 3

At the scene of a car accident, you find a victim who is cyanotic and whose right hand has just been completely amputated a little above the wrist.

1. Blood loss in cases of complete amputations is often

_____

_____

_____

2. Explain why.

_____

_____

_____

_____

3. If not adequately cooled, a severed body part has _____ hours for survival; if adequately cooled, the part may survive for _____ hours.

4. Describe the steps for caring for an amputated part.

  a. _____

  _____

  b. _____

  _____

  c. _____

  _____

  d. _____

  _____

Case 4

While on a five-mile hike, a blister appears on your foot. It is painful enough to prevent you from continuing.

1. What could you try first?

  _____

  _____

2. When should you break a blister?

  _____

  _____

3. What are the procedures to break and care for a painful blister?

  a. _____

  _____

  b. _____

  _____

  c. _____

  _____

  d. _____

  _____

  e. _____

  _____

Chapter Activities

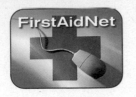

WEB Activities
Wounds

Visit nsc.jbpub.com/FirstAidNet, then click on **Web Activities,** and select the appropriate chapter.

Caring for Stitches

About 1 in 100 wounds become infected. Learning about wound care will help prevent infection and promote healing.

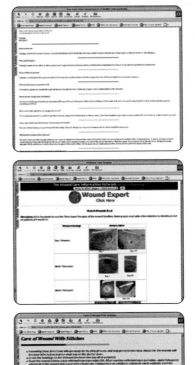

Watch Wounds Heal

Wounds will heal quicker if certain measures are taken. For example, keeping the area clean and protected from bacteria is a big help in the healing process.

Tetanus

Tetanus, a serious disease affecting the nervous system, is caused by a bacterial poison. Symptoms include painful muscle spasms, irritability, drooling, and fever. Tetanus is preventable through safe and effective vaccination.

Chapter 8

Dressings and Bandages

Dressings

A dressing covers an open wound—it touches the wound. Whenever possible, a dressing should be:

- sterile. If a sterile dressing is not available, use a clean cloth, handkerchief, washcloth, or towel
- larger than the wound
- thick, soft, and compressible so pressure is evenly distributed over the wound
- lint free

The purpose of using a dressing is to:

- control bleeding
- prevent infection and contamination
- absorb blood and wound drainage
- protect the wound from further injury

Types of Dressings

Use commercial dressings whenever possible. Dressings used in most first aid situations are commercially prepared, but dressings may need to be improvised.

- *Gauze pads* are used for small wounds. They come in separately wrapped packages of various sizes (eg, 2 inch by 2 inch; 4 inch by 4 inch) and are sterile, unless the package is broken. Some gauze pads have a special coating to keep them from sticking to the wound and are especially helpful for burns or wounds secreting fluids (▶Figure 8-1).
- *Adhesive strips* (eg, Band-Aids™) are used for small cuts and abrasions and are a combination of both a sterile dressing and a bandage (▶Figure 8-2).
- *Trauma dressings* are made of large, thick, absorbent, sterile materials. Individually wrapped sanitary napkins can serve because of their bulk and absorbency, but they usually are not sterile (▶Figure 8-3).

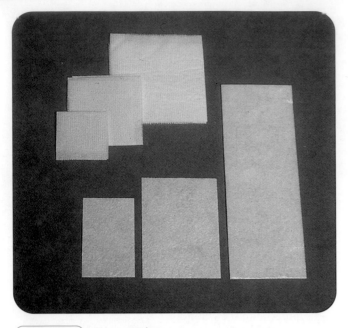

Figure 8-1 Gauze pads

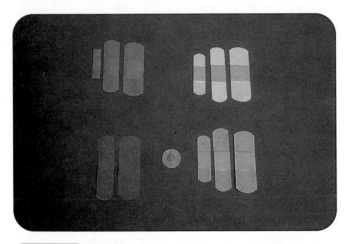

Figure 8-2 Adhesive strips

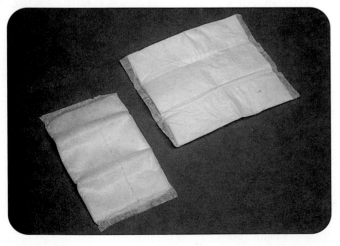

Figure 8-3 Trauma dressings

- When commercial sterile dressings are not available, an *improvised dressing* should be as clean, absorbent, soft, and free of lint as possible (eg, handkerchief, towel). Either use the cleanest cloth available or, in some conditions and if time allows, sterilize a cloth by boiling it and allowing it to dry, by ironing it for several minutes, or by soaking it in rubbing alcohol and allowing it to dry.

Caution:

DO NOT use fluffy cotton or cotton balls as a dressing. Cotton fibers can get in the wound and be difficult to remove.

DO NOT remove a blood-soaked dressing until the bleeding stops. Cover it with a new dressing.

DO NOT pull off a dressing stuck to a wound. If it needs to be removed, soak it off in warm water.

Applying a Sterile Dressing
What to Do

1. If possible, wash your hands and wear medical exam gloves.
2. Use a dressing large enough to extend beyond the edges of the wound. Hold the dressing by a corner. Place the dressing directly over the wound. Do not slide it on.
3. Cover the dressing with one of the types of bandages described below.

Caution:

DO NOT touch any part of the wound or any part of the dressing that will be in contact with the wound.

Bandages

A bandage can be used to:

- hold a dressing in place over an open wound

- apply direct pressure over a dressing to control bleeding
- prevent or reduce swelling
- provide support and stability for an extremity or joint

A bandage should be clean but need not be sterile.

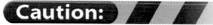

Caution:

DO NOT apply a bandage directly over a wound. Put a sterile dressing on first.

DO NOT bandage so tightly as to restrict blood circulation. Always check the extremity's pulse. If you cannot feel the pulse, loosen the bandage.

DO NOT bandage so loosely that the dressing will slip. This is the most common bandaging error. Bandages tend to stretch after a short time.

DO NOT leave loose ends. They might get caught.

DO NOT cover fingers or toes unless they are injured. They need to be observed for color changes that would indicate impaired circulation.

DO NOT use elastic bandages over a wound. There is a tendency to apply them too tightly.

DO NOT apply a circular bandage around a victim's neck—strangulation may occur.

DO NOT start a roller bandage above the wound. Instead, start below the wound and work upward.

Signs that a bandage is too tight:

- blue tinge of the fingernails or toenails
- blue or pale skin color
- tingling or loss of sensation
- coldness of the extremity
- inability to move the fingers or toes

Bandages should be applied firmly enough to keep dressings and splints in place but not so tightly that they will injure the part or impede blood circulation.

A square knot is preferred because it is neat, attractive, holds well, and can be easily untied. However, the type of knot is not important. If the knot or the bandage is likely to cause the victim discomfort, a pad should be placed between the knot or bandage and the body.

Types of Bandages

There are four basic types of bandages:

- *Roller bandages* come in various widths, lengths, and types of material. For best results, use different widths for different body areas:
  - 1-inch width for fingers
  - 2-inch width for wrists, hands, feet
  - 3-inch width for ankles, elbows, arms
  - 4-inch width for knees, legs
- *Self-adhering, conforming bandages* (▼Figure 8-4) come as rolls of slightly elastic, gauzelike material in various widths. Their self-adherent quality makes them easy to use.
- *Gauze rollers* are cotton, rigid, and nonelastic. They come in various widths (1, 2, and 3 inches) and usually are 10 yards long.
- *Elastic roller bandages* (▶Figure 8-5) are used for compression on sprains, strains, and contusions and come in various widths. Elastic bandages are not usually applied over dressings covering a wound.

  When commercial roller bandages are unavailable, you can make *improvised bandages* from belts, neckties, or strips of cloth torn from a sheet or other similar material.
- *Triangular bandages* (▶Figure 8-6) are available commercially or can be made from a 36- to 40-inch

Figure 8-4 Self-adhering conforming bandages of various sizes (3 on right). Gauze bandages (2 on left).

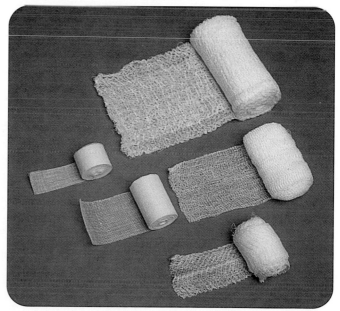

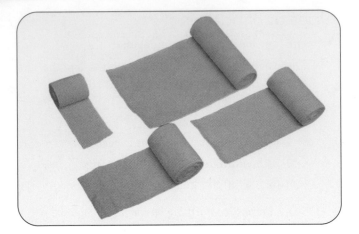

Figure 8-5 Elastic bandages of various sizes

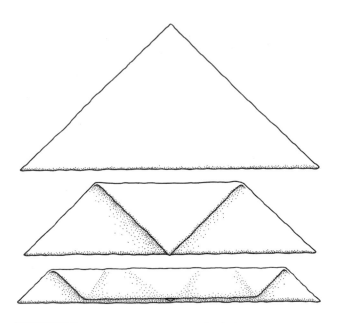

Figure 8-6 A triangular bandage folded into a cravat

square of preshrunk cotton muslin material. Cut the material diagonally from corner to corner to produce two triangular pieces of cloth. The longest side is called the *base*; the corner directly across from the base is the *point*; the other two corners are called *ends*. A triangular bandage may be applied two ways:

- Fully opened (not folded). Best used for an arm sling. When used to hold dressings in place, fully opened triangular bandages do not apply sufficient pressure on the wound.

- As a cravat (folded triangular). The point is folded to the center of the base and then the fabric is folded in half again from the top to the base to form a cravat. It is used to hold splints in

place, to hold dressings in place, to apply as a pressure bandage, or as a swathe (binder) around the victim's body to stabilize an injured arm in an arm sling.

- *Adhesive tape* comes in rolls and in a variety of widths. It is often used to secure roller bandages and small dressings in place. For those allergic to adhesive tape, use paper tape or special dermatologic tape.

Caution:

DO NOT apply adhesive tape over or to clothing or other material because it can slip. Adhesive tape should be applied directly to the skin.

- *Adhesive strips* are used for small cuts and abrasions and are a combination of a dressing and a bandage.

To apply an adhesive strip (▼Figure 8-7):

1. Remove the wrapping and hold the dressing, pad-side down, by the protective strips.

2. Peel back, but do not remove, the protective strips. Without touching the dressing pad, place it directly onto the wound.

3. Carefully pull away the protective strips. Press the ends and edges down.

Applying a Roller Bandage

With a little ingenuity, you can apply a roller bandage to almost any body part. Self-adhering, conforming roller bandages eliminate the need for many of the complicated

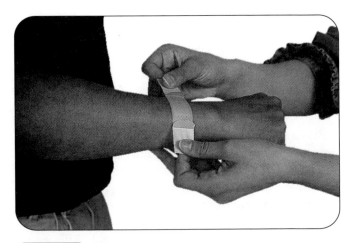

Figure 8-7 Applying an adhesive strip

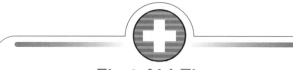
bandaging techniques that standard gauze roller, cravat, and triangular bandages require.

Circular Method: Forehead, Ear, Eyes (3- or 4-inch roller)

The roller bandage encircles the part with several layers of bandage on top of the previous ones. For an injured eye, cover both eyes to prevent the injured eye from moving.

What to Do

1. Place the end of the bandage over the dressing covering the wound (or eyes) and wrap the bandage around the head (▼Figure 8-8).

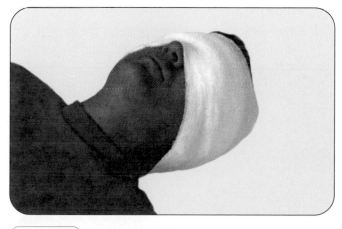

Figure 8-8 Bandaging both eyes stops eye movement.

2. When wrapping a roller bandage around the head, keep the bandage near the eyebrows and low on the back of the head to prevent the bandage from slipping.

Spiral Method: Arm or Leg (3-inch roller for arm; 4-inch roller for leg)

What to Do

1. Start at the narrow part of an arm or leg and wrap upward toward the wider part to make the bandage more secure. Start below and at the edge of the dressing (▼Figure 8-9, A–C).

2. Make two straight anchoring turns with the bandage.

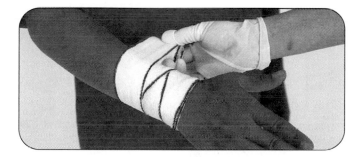

3. Make a series of turns, progressing up the arm or leg. Each turn should overlap the previous wrap. Wrap with a criss-cross (figure-eight) turns.

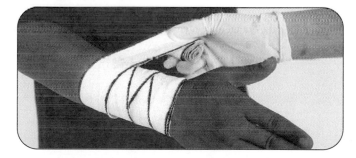

4. Finish with two straight turns and secure the bandage.

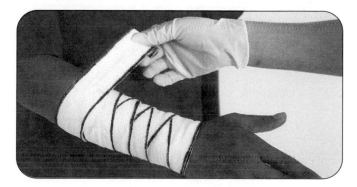

Figure-8 Method

Use this method of applying a roller bandage to hold dressings or to provide compression at or near a joint such as the ankle. The figure-8 method involves continuous spiral loops of bandage, one up and one down, crossing each other to form an "8" (▼**Figure 8-10, A–C**).

Elbow or Knee (3-inch roller for elbow; 4-inch roller for knee)

What to Do

1. Bend the elbow or knee slightly and make two straight anchoring turns with the bandage over the elbow point or kneecap.

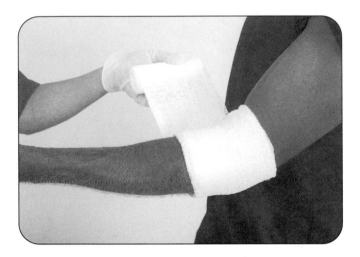

2. Bring the bandage above the joint to the upper arm or leg, and make one turn, covering half to three-fourths of the bandage from the first turn.

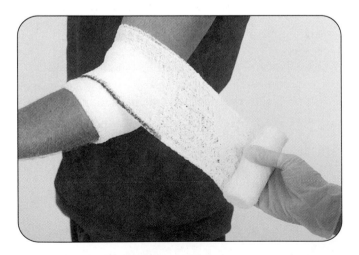

3. Bring the bandage just under the joint and make one turn around the lower arm or leg, covering half to three-fourths of the first straight turn.

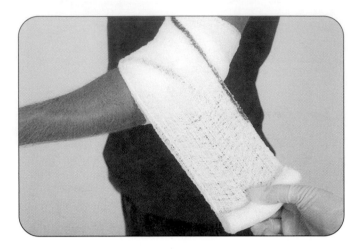

4. Continue alternating the turns in a figure-8 maneuver by covering only half to three-fourths of the previous layer each time.

5. Finish by making two straight turns and secure the end.

Hand (2- or 3-inch roller)

What to Do

Method 1

1. Make two straight anchoring turns with the bandage around the palm of the hand (▼**Figure 8-11, A–C**).

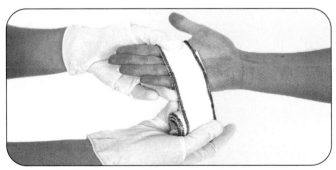

2. Carry the bandage diagonally across the back of the hand and then around the wrist and back across the palm.

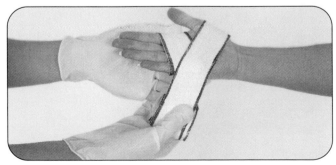

3. Complete several figure-8 turns, overlapping each by about three-fourths of the previous bandage width.

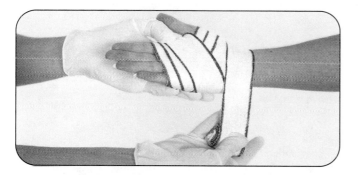

4. Make two straight turns around the wrist, and secure the bandage

Ankle or Foot (2- or 3-inch roller)

This wrapping will hold a dressing or apply pressure to treat a sprained ankle. It should not be used to support the ankle and foot during sports activity; that type of bandaging involves additional maneuvers.

What to Do

1. Make two straight anchoring turns with the bandage around the foot's instep.

2. Make a figure-8 turn by taking the bandage diagonally across the front of the foot, around the ankle, and again diagonally across the foot and under the arch.

3. Make several of these figure-8 turns, each turn overlapping the previous one by about three-fourths the width of the bandage. The bandage advances up the leg.

4. Finish with two straight turns around the leg and secure the bandage.

To securely fasten a roller bandage:

- Apply adhesive tape.
- Use safety pin(s).
- Use special clips provided with elastic bandages.
- Tie by either of these two methods:
  - *Loop method.* Reverse the direction of the bandage by looping it around a thumb or finger and continue back to the opposite side of the body part. Encircle the part with the looped end and the free end; tie them together.
  - *Split-tail method.* Split the end of the bandage lengthwise for about 12 inches, then tie a knot to prevent further splitting. Pass the ends in

opposite directions around the body part and tie.

Applying a Triangular Bandage

A triangular bandage can be used as a sling. Slings support and protect an arm. A sling is not a bandage but is used as a support for an injury to the shoulder, clavicle, scapula, upper arm, forearm, and hand when there are injuries to the upper extremity.

Arm Sling
What to Do

1. Support the injured arm slightly away from the chest, with the wrist and hand slightly higher than the elbow.

2. Place an open triangular bandage between the forearm and chest with its point toward the elbow and stretching well beyond it.

3. Pull the upper end over the shoulder on the uninjured side and around the neck to rest on the collarbone on the injured side.

4. Bring the lower end of the bandage over the hand and forearm and tie to the other end at the hollow above the collarbone.

5. Bring the point around to the front of the elbow, and secure it to the sling with a safety pin or twist it into a "pigtail," which can be tied into a knot or tucked away. Placing a swathe (binder) around the arm and body further stabilizes the arm.

6. Check for signs of circulation loss (eg, pulse, fingernail color). The hand should be in a thumbs-up position within the sling and slightly above the level of the elbow (about 4 inches).

Collarbone/Shoulder Sling
What to Do

1. Support the injured arm slightly away from chest with the wrist and hand slightly higher than the elbow.

2. Place an open triangular bandage between the forearm and chest with its point toward the elbow and stretching well beyond it.

3. Pull the upper end over the shoulder on the uninjured side.

4. Bring the lower end of the bandage over the forearm and under the armpit on the injured side.

5. Continue bringing the lower end of the bandage around the victim's back where it is tied to the

upper end of the triangular bandage. Placing a swathe (binder) around the arm and body further stabilizes the arm.

6. Check for signs of circulation loss (eg, pulse, finger-nail color). The hand should be in a thumbs-up position within the sling and slightly above the level of the elbow (about 4 inches).

Improvised Slings

- Place the hand inside a buttoned jacket.

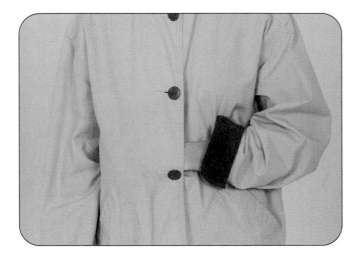

- Use a belt, necktie, or other clothing item looped around the neck and the injured arm.

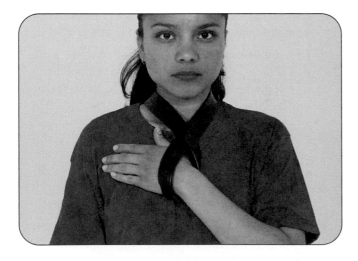

- Pin the sleeve of the shirt or jacket to the clothing in the desired position.

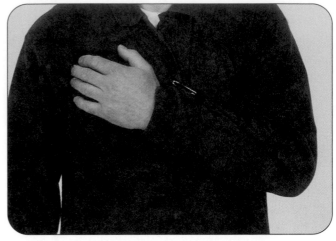

- Turn up the lower edge of the victim's jacket or shirt over the injured arm and pin it to the upper part of the jacket or shirt.

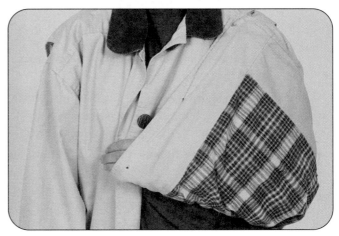

Skill Scan) Bandaging—Cravat

Cravat Bandage for Head, Ears, or Eyes

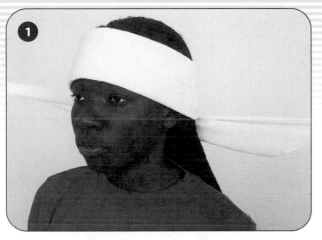

1. Place middle of bandage over the dressing covering the wound.

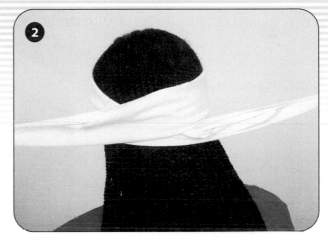

2. Cross the two ends snugly over each other.

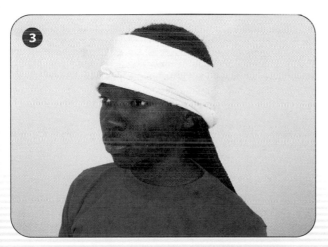

3. Bring the ends back around to where the dressing is and tie the ends in a knot.

Skill Scan Bandaging—Cravat

Cravat Bandage for Arm or Leg

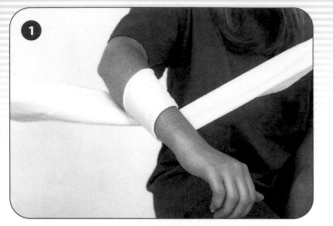

1. Wrap bandage over dressing.

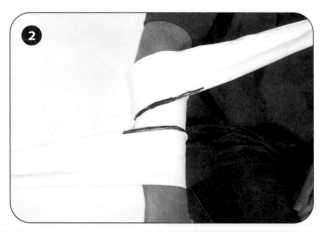

2. With one end make one turn going up the extremity and another turn going down.

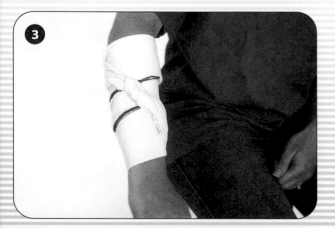

3. Tie the bandage off over the dressing.

Cravat for Palm of Hand

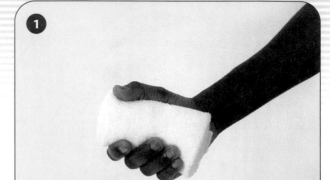

1. Fill palm with bulky dressings or pad.

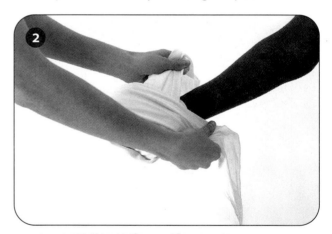

2. Wrap the bandage over the fingers and around the wrist.

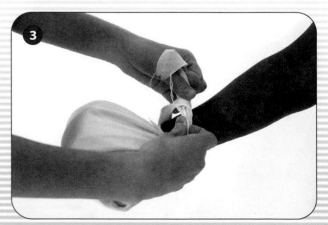

3. Tie the bandage off at the wrist.

Skill Scan

Bandaging—Roller (Self-adhering), Figure-8

Roller Bandage for Hand—Method 1

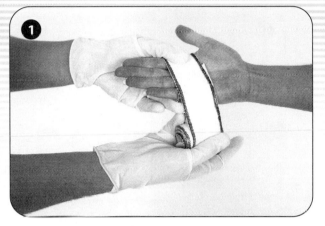

1. Anchor the bandage with one or two turns around the palm of the hand.

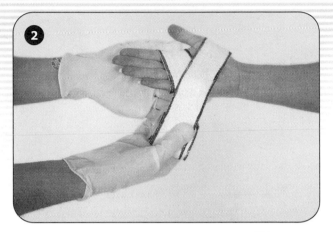

2. Carry it diagonally across the back of the hand and then around the wrist.

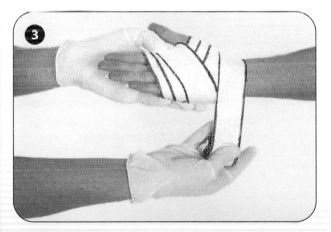

3. Repeat this figure-8 maneuver as many times as is necessary to cover the dressing, overlapping wraps to "stair-step" up the hand.

Skill Scan

Bandaging—Roller (Self-adhering), Figure-8

Roller Bandage for Elbow or Knee

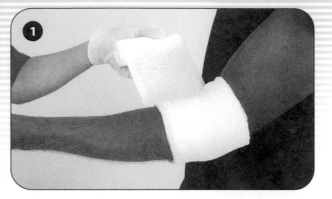

1. Bend arm. Wrap the bandage around the elbow several times.

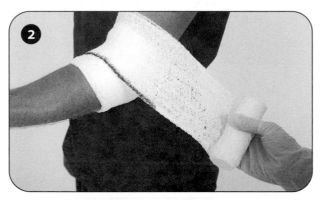

2. Make a diagonal turn to the upper arm covering the upper half of the bandage in step #1.

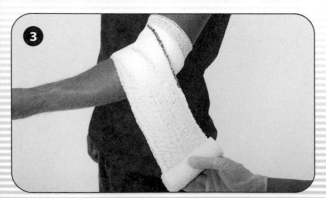

3. Take the bandage from the upper arm and make a diagonal turn around the forearm to cover the lower half of the bandage placed in step #1.

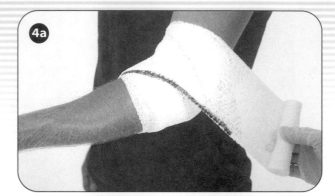

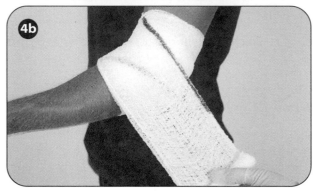

4. (a & b) Continue this figure-8 maneuver in steps #2 and #3 several times.

Skill Scan

Bandaging—Roller (Self-adhering), Figure-8

Roller Bandage for Ankle

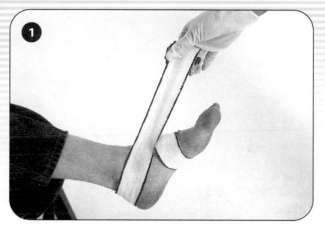

1. Anchor the bandage with one or two turns around the foot. Bring bandage diagonally across the top of the foot and around back of the ankle.

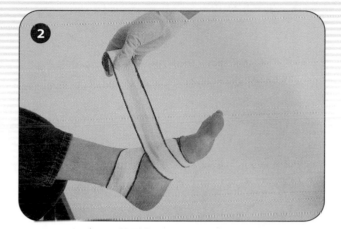

2. Continue bandage across the top of the foot and under the arch.

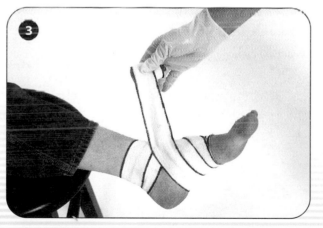

3. Continue figure-8 turns, with each turn overlapping the last turn and progressing up the ankle.

Skill Scan   Securing Roller Bandages

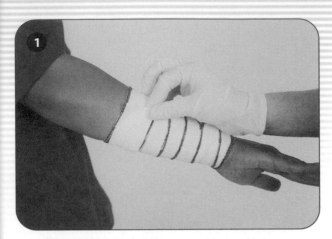

1. Apply adhesive tape to secure bandage

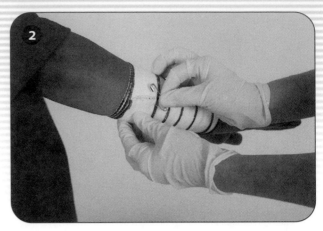

2. Use safety pin(s) to secure bandage

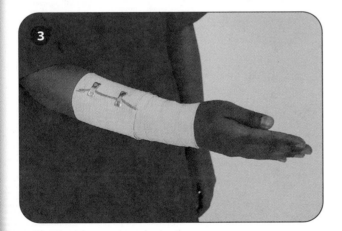

3. Use special clips provided with elastic bandages

Continued on next page

Skill Scan) Securing Roller Bandages

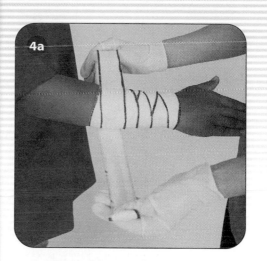

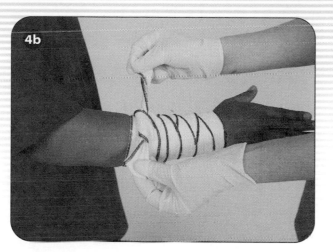

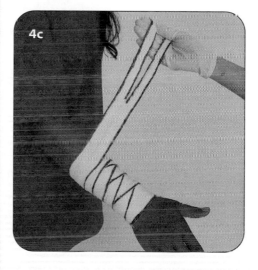

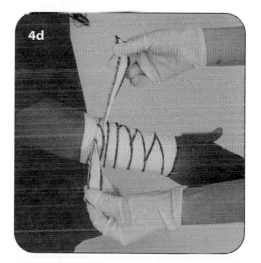

4. Tie by either of these two methods:
   Loop method. Reverse the direction of the bandage by looping it around a thumb or finger and continue back to the opposite side of the body part. Encircle the part with the looped end and the free end; tie them together (a-b).
   Split-tail method. Split the end of the bandage lengthwise for about 12 inches, then tie a knot to prevent further splitting. Pass the ends in opposite directions around the body part and tie (c-d).

Chapter Activities

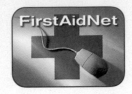

WEB Activities

Dressings and Bandages

Visit nsc.jbpub.com/FirstAidNet, then click on Web Activities, and select the appropriate chapter.

History of Bandages

A quick history lesson in the field of emergency care!
Learn how people cared for their wounds in ancient cultures.

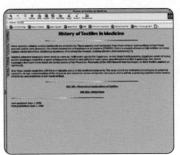

Chapter 9

Burns

Severe burns can be an overwhelming experience. An estimated 2 million burn injuries occur each year in the United States, resulting in 75,000 hospitalizations and more than 3,000 deaths. Burns occur in every age group, across all socioeconomic levels, at home and in the workplace, and in urban, suburban, and rural settings.

It has been estimated that about 70% of all burn injuries occur in the home, with house fires responsible for the majority of fire deaths. Most burn victims are injured as a result of their own actions.

The highest-risk age groups for burn injuries are children younger than 5 years and adults over 55 years of age. Both groups may have a limited ability to recognize and escape from a fire or burn incident. Their relatively thinner skin predisposes them to more serious injuries. Death and complications increase dramatically for burn victims older than 55 due to the likelihood of pre-existing health problems and their immune systems' decreased ability to fight infection.

Skin death and injury occur as the applied heat exceeds the body's ability to handle it. That point starts at about 113°F. The amount and depth of skin damage depend on the heat's intensity, the duration of contact, and the skin's thickness.

Burn injuries can be classified as thermal (heat), chemical, or electrical.

- *Thermal (heat) burns.* Not all thermal burns are caused by flames. Contact with hot objects, flammable vapor that ignites and causes a flash or an explosion, and steam or hot liquid are other common causes of burns. Just three seconds of exposure to water at 140°F can cause a full-thickness (third-degree) burn in an adult. At 156°F, the same burn occurs in one second.

- *Chemical burns.* A wide range of chemical agents can cause tissue damage and death on contact with the skin. As with thermal burns, the amount of tissue damage depends on the duration of contact, the skin thickness in the area of exposure, and the strength of the chemical agent. Chemicals will continue to cause tissue destruction until the chemical agent is removed. Three types of chemicals—acids, alkalis, and organic compounds—are responsible for most chemical burns. Alkalis produce deeper, more extensive burns than acids.

- *Electrical burns.* The injury severity from contact with electrical current depends on the type of current (direct or alternating), the voltage, the area of the body exposed, and the duration of contact.

  Electricity can induce ventricular fibrillation (a type of cardiac arrest), cause respiratory arrest, or "freeze" the victim to the electrical contact point with powerful muscle spasms that increase the length of exposure. Victims of low-voltage electrical injuries may have no skin burns at all yet suffer cardiac or respiratory arrest.

Historically, burns have been described as *first-degree*, *second-degree*, and *third-degree* injuries (▶Table 9-1). The terms *superficial*, *partial thickness*, and *full thickness* are often used by burn-care professionals because they are more descriptive of the tissue damage.

- **First-degree (superficial) burns** affect the skin's outer layer (epidermis) (▼Figure 9-1). Characteristics include redness, mild swelling, tenderness, and pain. Healing occurs without scarring, usually within a week. The outer edges of deeper burns often are first-degree burns.

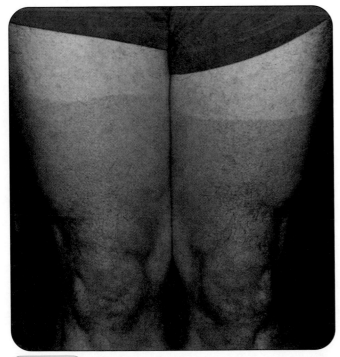

Figure 9-1 First-degree burn.

Table 9-1: Burn Severity

Minor Burns

First-degree burn covering less than 50% BSA* in adults (face, hands, feet, or genitals not burned)

Second-degree burn covering less than 15% BSA in adults

Second-degree burn covering less than 10% BSA in children/elderly persons

Third-degree burn covering less than 2% BSA in adults (face, hands, feet, or genitals not burned)

Moderate Burns

First-degree burn covering more than 50% BSA in adults

Second-degree burn covering 15% to 30% BSA in adults

Second-degree burn covering 10% to 20% BSA in children/elderly persons

Third-degree burn covering 2% to 10% BSA in adults (face, hands, or feet not burned)

Critical Burns

Second-degree burn covering more than 30% BSA in adults

Second-degree burn covering more than 20% BSA in children/elderly persons

Third-degree burn covering more than 10% BSA in adults

Third-degree burn covering more than 2% BSA in children/elderly persons

Third-degree burns of hands, face, eyes, feet, or genitalia; also most inhalation injuries, electrical injuries, and burns accompanied by major trauma or significant preexisting conditions

*BSA = body surface area
Source: Adapted from the American Burn Association categorization.

- **Second-degree (partial-thickness) burns** extend through the entire outer layer and into the inner skin layer (▶Figure 9-2). Blisters, swelling, weeping of fluids, and severe pain characterize these burns, which occur because the capillary blood vessels in the dermis are damaged and give up fluid into surrounding tissues. Intact blisters provide a sterile waterproof covering. Once a blister breaks, a weeping wound results and infection risk increases.
- **Third-degree (full-thickness) burns** are severe burns that penetrate all the skin layers, into the underlying fat and muscle (▶Figure 9-3). The skin looks leathery, waxy, or pearly gray and sometimes charred. It has a dry appearance, because capillary

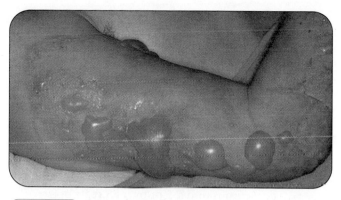

Figure 9-2) Second-degree burn blisters.

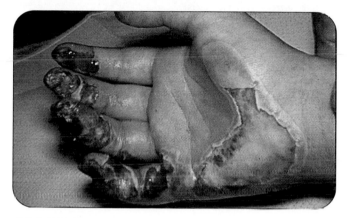

Figure 9-3) Third-degree burn.

blood vessels have been destroyed and no more fluid is brought to the area. The skin does not blanch after being pressed because the area is dead. The victim feels no pain from a third-degree burn because the nerve endings have been damaged or destroyed. Any pain felt is from surrounding burns of lesser degrees. A third-degree burn requires medical care, and the removal of the dead tissue and a skin graft to heal properly.

Respiratory-tract damage caused by heat associated with a burn remains the leading cause of death after a victim is hospitalized. Respiratory damage may result from breathing heat or the products of combustion; from being burned by a flame while in a closed space; or from being in an explosion. In those instances, even if there is no burn injury, there may be respiratory damage. It is rare that the upper respiratory tract or the lungs are actually burned. That is because they are constructed to cool or warm air to prepare it for inhalation. The superheated air from a flame or from a hot steam explosion will be absorbed by the upper respiratory tract (the area from the nose through to the trachea), resulting in inflammation. Swelling occurs in 2 to 24 hours, restricting or even

completely shutting off the airway so that air cannot reach the lungs. *All respiratory injuries must receive medical care.*

Burns can aggravate existing medical conditions such as diabetes, heart disease, and lung disease, as well as other medical problems. Concurrent injuries such as fractures, internal injuries, and open wounds increase the severity of a burn.

Thermal Burns

What to Do

1. Stop the burning! Burns can continue to injure tissue for a surprisingly long time. If clothing has ignited, have the victim roll on the ground using the "stop, drop, and roll" method. Smother the flames with a blanket or douse the victim with water. Stop a person whose clothes are on fire from running, which only fans the flames. The victim should not remain standing, because they are more apt to inhale flames. Once the fire is extinguished, remove all hot or smoldering clothing because the burning may continue if the clothing is left on. If possible, remove jewelry, since heat may be held near the skin and cause more damage.

2. Check ABCs.

3. Determine the depth (degree) of the burn. It can be difficult to tell a burn's depth because the destruction varies within the same burn. Even experienced physicians may not know the depth for several days after the burn. However, making an assessment of burn depth will help you decide whether to seek medical care for the victim.

4. Determine the extent of the burn. Skin will not ignite unless heated to thousands of degrees. However, if clothing ignites or skin is kept in contact with a heat source, such as scalding water, large areas of the skin will be injured. Determining the

Caution:

DO NOT remove clothing stuck to the skin. Cut around the areas where clothing sticks to the skin.

DO NOT pull on stuck clothing—pulling will further damage the skin.

DO NOT forget to remove jewelry as soon as possible—swelling could make jewelry difficult to remove later.

extent of a burn means estimating how much body surface area the burn covers. A rough guide known as the "rule of nines" (▼Figure 9-4) assigns a percentage value of total body surface area (BSA) to each part of an adult's body. The entire head is 9%, one complete arm is 9%, the front torso is 18%, the complete back is 18%, and each leg is 18%. The rule of nines must be modified to take into account the different proportions of a small child. In small children and infants, the head accounts for 18% and each leg is 14%.

For small or scattered burns, use the "rule of the palm." The victim's hand, excluding the fingers and the thumb, represents about 1% of his or her total body surface. For a very large burn, estimate the unburned area in number of hands and subtract from 100%.

5. Determine what parts of the body are burned. Burns on the face, hands, feet, and genitals are more severe than on other body parts. A circumferential burn (one that goes around a finger, toe, arm, leg, neck, or chest) is considered more severe than a noncircumferential one because of the possible constriction and tourniquet effect on circulation and, in some cases, breathing. All these burns require medical care.

6. Determine if other injuries or pre-existing medical problems exist or if the victim is elderly (over 55) or very young (under 5). A medical problem or belonging to one of those age groups increases a burn's severity.

(Figure 9-4) Rule of nines

4 1/2%

9% 9%

4 1/2% 4 1/2%

9% 9%

1%

9% 9% 9% 9%

9%

4 1/2% 4 1/2%

9%

9% 9%

Rule of Nines is used to calculate the extent of a burn

7. Determine the burn's severity. This forms the basis for how to treat the burned victim. After you have evaluated the burn according to Steps 3 through 6, use the American Burn Association (ABA) guidelines shown in Table 9-1 to determine the burn's severity. Most burns are minor, occur at home, and can be managed outside a medical setting. Seek medical attention for all moderate and severe burns, as classified by the ABA, or if any of the following conditions applies:

- The victim is under 5 or over 55 years of age.
- The victim has difficulty breathing.
- Other injuries exist.
- An electrical injury exists.
- The face, hands, feet, or genitals are burned.
- Child abuse is suspected.
- The surface area of a second-degree burn is greater than 15% of the body surface area.
- The burn is third degree.

Burn Care

Burn care aims to reduce pain, protect against infection, and prevent evaporation. All burn wounds are sterile for the first 24 to 48 hours after injury (►Table 9-2).

Care of First-Degree Burns

1. Immerse the burned area in cold water or apply a wet, cold cloth to reduce pain. Apply cold until the part is pain free both in and out of the water (usually in 10 minutes, but it may take up to 45 minutes). Cold also stops the burn's progression into deeper tissue. If cold water is unavailable, use any cold drinkable liquid to reduce the burned skin's temperature.

2. Give ibuprofen to relieve pain and inflammation. For children give acetaminophen (relieves pain but not inflammation).

3. Have victim drink as much water as possible without becoming nauseous.

4. After the burn has been cooled, apply an aloe vera gel or an inexpensive skin moisturizer lotion to keep the skin moistened and to reduce itching and peeling. Aloe vera has antimicrobial properties and is an effective analgesic.

5. Keep burned arm or leg raised to reduce swelling and pain.

Table 9-2: First Aid for Burns

Type of Burn	Do ...	Don't ...
First-degree Burn (redness, mild swelling, and pain)	... apply cold water and after cooled, apply aloe vera gel or a body lotion.	... apply butter, oleomargarine, etc.
Second-degree Burn (deeper injury; blisters develop)	... apply cold water. ... after cooled, apply bacitracin. ... treat for shock. ... obtain medical attention if severe.	... break blisters. ... remove shreds of tissue. ... use home remedy.
Third-degree Burn (deeper destruction; skin layers destroyed)	... cover burn with sterile cloth to protect it. ... treat victim for shock. ... watch for breathing difficulty. ... obtain medical attention quickly.	... remove charred clothing that is stuck to burn. ... apply ice. ... use home medication.
Chemical Burn	... remove chemical by flushing with large quantities of water for at least 20 minutes or longer. ... remove surrounding clothing. ... obtain medical attention.	

Caution:

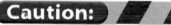

DO NOT apply cold to more than 20% of an adult's body surface (10% for children). Widespread cooling can cause hypothermia. Burn victims lose large amounts of heat and water.

DO NOT leave wet packs on wounds for long periods.

DO NOT use an ice pack unless it is the only source of cold. If you must use one, apply it for only 10 to 15 minutes, because frostbite and hypothermia can develop.

DO NOT apply salve, ointment, grease, butter, cream, spray, home remedy, or any other coating on a burn. Such coatings are unsterile and can lead to infection. They also can seal in heat, causing further damage.

DO NOT cover a first-degree burn.

DO NOT use anesthetic sprays because they may sensitize the skin to "-caine" anesthetics.

Care of Small Second-Degree Burns (< 20% BSA)

1. Immerse the burned area in cold water (►Figure 9-5) or apply a wet, cold cloth to reduce pain. Apply cold until the part is pain free both in and out of the water (usually in 10 minutes, but it may take up to 45 minutes). Cold also stops the burn's progression into deeper tissue. If cold water is unavailable, use any cold drinkable liquid to reduce the burned skin's temperature.

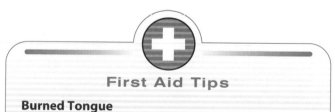

First Aid Tips

Burned Tongue
A few grains of sugar sprinkled on the tongue can relieve the misery of a tongue burned by hot food or drink. Repeat as often as needed. Sucking on ice chips or a Popsicle can cool the burn.

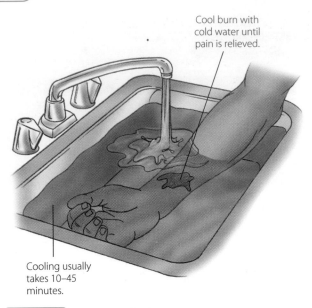

Cool burn with cold water until pain is relieved.

Cooling usually takes 10–45 minutes.

Figure 9-5 Immerse the burn

2. Give ibuprofen to relieve pain and inflammation. For children give acetaminophen (relieves pain but not inflammation).

3. Have the victim drink as much water as possible without becoming nauseous.

4. After a burn has been cooled, apply a thin layer of bacitracin ointment. Topical antibiotic therapy like bacitracin does not sterilize a wound, but it does decrease the number of bacteria to a level that can be controlled by the body's defense mechanisms and prevents the entrance of bacteria. Physicians may prescribe Silvadene™, which is the agent of choice for burn wounds. However, bacitracin works as well, does not require a physician's prescription, and is much less expensive.

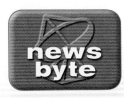

Topical Agents in Burn and Wound Care

Infection may occur with any open wound. Size and depth of the wound are critical factors in determining the infection risk of any wound. An infected wound not only heals more slowly, but there is also the risk of systemic infection and even death. Infected wounds also scar more severely and are associated with more prolonged rehabilitation. Topical therapeutic agents have been shown to be effective in the management of open skin wounds.

Source: Physical Therapy, Vol. 75, 1995.

5. Cover the burn with a dry, nonsticking, sterile dressing or a clean cloth. Covering the burn reduces the amount of pain by keeping air from the exposed nerve endings. The main purpose of a dressing over a burn is to keep the burn clean, prevent evaporative loss, and reduce the pain. If fingers or toes have been burned, place dry dressings between them.

6. Seek medical attention for second-degree burns covering more than 20% of the body surface area in adults or 10% to 20% in children or elderly victims.

Caution:

DO NOT cool more than 20% of an adult's body surface area (10% for a child) except to extinguish flames.

Care of Large Second-Degree Burns (> 20% BSA)

Do not apply cold on more than 20% BSA because it may cause hypothermia. Follow steps 2-6 of small second-degree burn care (<20% BSA). Seek medical attention for all victims with a large second-degree burn.

Care of Third-Degree Burns

It usually is not necessary to apply cold to third-degree burns since pain is absent. Any pain felt with a third-

Caution:

DO NOT break any blisters. Intact blisters serve as excellent burn dressings. Cover a ruptured blister with bacitracin ointment and a dry, sterile dressing.

DO NOT place a moist dressing over a burn since it will dry out quickly. A wet dressing over a large area can induce hypothermia. A cold wet pack can be used to cool a burn initially, but it should not serve as a dressing.

DO NOT use plastic as a dressing, because it will trap moisture and provide a good place for bacteria to grow (its only advantage is that it will not stick to the burn).

often full thickness. This type of injury is generally caused by abuse and is seen most often in children.

A **spill burn** occurs when a liquid spills, drops, or is thrown on a person. The pattern of this type of burn generally is irregular and may be scattered across large body areas. A spill burn usually is not as deep as an immersion burn.

Neglect and nonsupervison of children in the kitchen and the bathtub are frequent causes of spill burns in children. Scalds in adults are more often in the elderly population, who generally have decreased sensation. As a result, many elderly victims are scalded in their bath.

Sunburn

Sunburn is the skin's response to the trauma of ultraviolet radiation (UVR) that results mainly from exposure to ultraviolet B (UVB) radiation or, rarely, to UVA (ultraviolet A) radiation. Sunburn may be the most common burn suffered by humans, and probably all persons have had one at some time or another (▼Figure 9-6). True

degree burn comes from accompanying first- and second-degree burns, for which cold applications can be helpful.

1. Cover the burn with a dry, nonsticking, sterile dressing or a clean cloth.
2. Treat the victim for shock by elevating the legs and keeping the victim warm with a clean sheet or blanket.
3. Seek medical attention.

Scald Burns

Scald burns are the result of contact with hot liquids. Scald burns can be divided into two types: immersion burns and spill burns. An **immersion burn** results when an area of the body is fully immersed in a hot liquid. It generally has definite demarcations between healthy and injured tissue. This type of burn tends to be deep and is

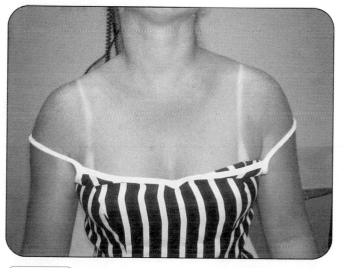

Figure 9-6 Sunburn

THERMAL BURNS

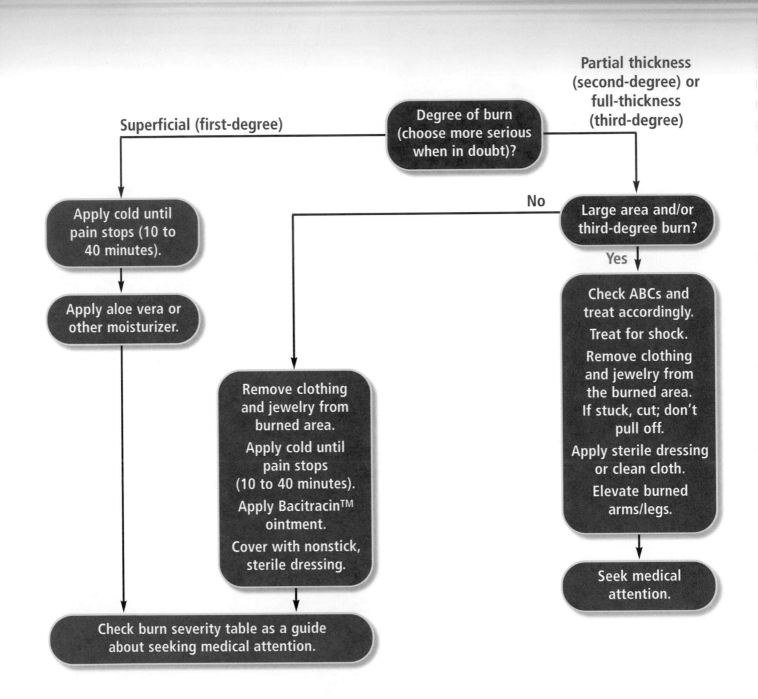

Degree of burn (choose more serious when in doubt)?

Superficial (first-degree)

Partial thickness (second-degree) or full-thickness (third-degree)

Apply cold until pain stops (10 to 40 minutes).

Apply aloe vera or other moisturizer.

Large area and/or third-degree burn?

No

Yes

Remove clothing and jewelry from burned area.
Apply cold until pain stops (10 to 40 minutes).
Apply Bacitracin™ ointment.
Cover with nonstick, sterile dressing.

Check ABCs and treat accordingly.
Treat for shock.
Remove clothing and jewelry from the burned area. If stuck, cut; don't pull off.
Apply sterile dressing or clean cloth.
Elevate burned arms/legs.

Seek medical attention.

Check burn severity table as a guide about seeking medical attention.

Sunburn Prevention

The best protection against the damaging effects of ultraviolet radiation (UVR) is to limit exposure to sunlight. That is done most easily with protective clothing, such as hats, long-sleeved shirts, and long pants. Wet, white cotton will transmit UVR light, so persons can be sunburned while wearing those clothes. People should avoid prolonged exposure during times of the day when radiation is most intense (usually between 10 a.m. and 2 p.m.) and apply effective sunscreens.

Sunscreens are readily available and offer the best protection against sunburn, developing skin cancers, and other long-term skin injury. The proper use of sunscreens will protect an individual from the harmful effects of the sun. Sunscreens must be applied correctly. That generally means applying the sunscreen at least 20 minutes before you go out, so it will "bond" to your skin, and reapplying it every few hours. Use waterproof sunscreen if you sweat a lot or if you are going to be in and out of the water. It is important to note that sunscreens do not promote tanning; they do, however, allow the user to tan gradually without serious burning.

To help consumers select an effective sunscreen, the system of rating products by the "skin protection factor" (SPF) has been developed. The higher the SPF number, the greater the protection against sunburn. However, a sunscreen that has an SPF of 30 is not twice as good as one with an SPF of 15. An SPF of 15 blocks out 95% of the most harmful rays; a sunscreen with an SPF of 30 gives you only another 3% of protection. But since most people usually use only half the amount of sunscreen that is effective, using a 15 SPF sunscreen probably affords protection equivalent to a 7.5 SPF sunscreen. If they use a sunscreen with a 30 SPF, they are probably getting the protection of a 15 SPF sunscreen.

Many "suntan lotions" have no sunscreen effect and serve only to keep the skin moist. Products such as baby oil and cocoa butter offer little protection against serious sunburn and may actually enhance burning.

---

sunburn reaction begins two to eight hours after UVR exposure. The amount of ultraviolet light the skin has received is difficult to gauge accurately. Not until after exposure (4 to 12 hours later) does the redness, tenderness, and discomfort of sunburned skin confirm the overexposure. Painful blistering and swelling peak about 24 hours later.

Sunburn results in first- or second-degree burns. A third-degree burn can occur from a sunburn, but it is rare. The redness of a sunburn is caused by the dilation of the small blood vessels. Blister formation comes from plasma leakage.

Human skin displays marked differences in its response to UVR exposure. Some individuals always burn and never tan, while others rarely experience a painful sunburn. The variability is largely attributed to the degree of pigmentation (melanin) that the skin contains. Darker-hued individuals generally are more resistant to the sun's rays than are those with light complexions, but all human beings eventually will burn if exposed to enough UVB. Other variables that contribute to individual sensitivity include the area of the body exposed, the underlying condition of the skin, the degree of tanning, and the role of various photosensitizing medicines.

Various skin types respond differently to ultraviolet light:

- Type I skin always burns easily and never tans. An example is Irish people, who often have blue eyes, red hair, and freckles.

- Type II skin burns easily, tans slightly.

- Type III skin sometimes burns, but always tans gradually and moderately.

CHEMICAL BURNS

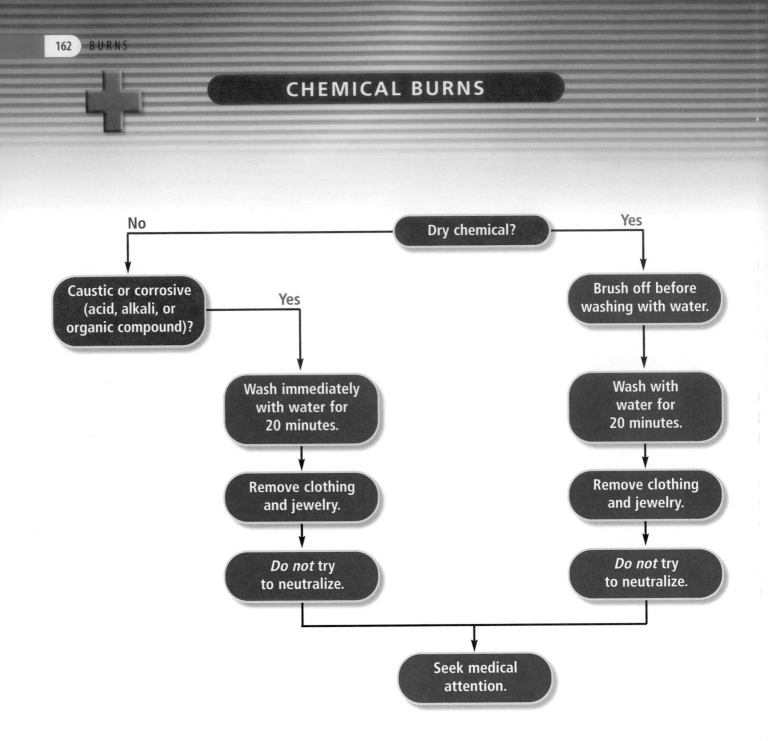

Dry chemical?

No → **Caustic or corrosive (acid, alkali, or organic compound)?**

Yes → **Wash immediately with water for 20 minutes.**

↓ **Remove clothing and jewelry.**

↓ ***Do not* try to neutralize.**

Yes → **Brush off before washing with water.**

↓ **Wash with water for 20 minutes.**

↓ **Remove clothing and jewelry.**

↓ ***Do not* try to neutralize.**

Seek medical attention.

- Type IV skin minimally burns and always tans well. Examples include people of Hispanic or Asian descent.

- Type V skin rarely burns and tans deeply. Examples include Middle Easterners and Indians (heavily pigmented).

- Type VI skin does not burn (although it can burn or peel with significant exposure). An example is people of African descent (deeply pigmented).

Cool compresses for up to 45 minutes are quite soothing to sunburned skin. Frequent cool showers or soaking in a tub may provide remarkable relief. Some experts advise against the use of topical analgesics, sprays, or lotions, especially those containing benzocaine. Benzocaine may sensitize the skin, resulting in contact dermatitis that compounds the original problem. Topical anesthetic sprays or lotions may provide temporary relief, but they are expensive and generally ineffective. Over-the-counter analgesics, such as aspirin and especially ibuprofen, should suffice in most cases because they reduce pain and inflammation. Drinking lots of water is also suggested.

First- and second-degree sunburns can be quite painful. When a large area of skin is involved, the individual may feel ill with chills and fever. After the pain of a first-degree sunburn has subsided, the use of aloe vera or another body lotion such as Noxzema™ can keep the skin moist. Do *not* use butter or petroleum jelly.

For aftercare of a second-degree sunburn, apply bacitracin (available as an over-the-counter medication) ointment in a thin layer. It is inexpensive, antimicrobial, widely available, easily applied, and adheres even to exposed areas such as the face.

If blisters break, thoroughly wash the area twice daily with soap and water and then cover with bacitracin and sterile gauze to prevent infection. If the burn becomes infected, contact a doctor. If the eyes are affected, contact a doctor.

Windburn resembles a first-degree sunburn. A greasy sunscreen can be used to prevent and treat it.

Caution:

DO NOT use topical over-the-counter burn ointments or sprays or anesthetic sprays because

- **some products may cause allergic reactions.**

- **most do not contain enough benzocaine or lidocaine to suppress pain.**

- **the duration of any possible relief is relatively short (30 to 40 minutes). More than three or four applications per day of products containing local anesthetics is discouraged because toxicity can occur if the agents are used too frequently.**

- **they seal in the heat.**

- **they are expensive.**

Figure 9-7 Chemical burn from sulfuric acid

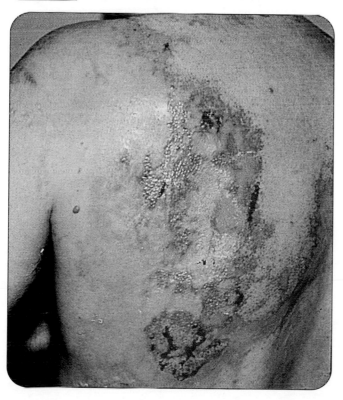

Chemical Burns

A chemical burn is the result of a caustic or corrosive substance touching the skin ◄Figure 9-7 . Because chemicals continue to "burn" as long as they are in contact with the skin, they should be removed from the victim as rapidly as possible.

First aid is the same for all chemical burns, except a few specific ones for which a chemical neutralizer has to be used. Alkalies such as drain cleaners cause more serious burns than acids such as battery acid because they penetrate deeper and remain active longer. Organic compounds like petroleum products are another type of chemical capable of burning.

What to Do

1. Immediately remove the chemical by flushing with water (▼Figure 9-8). If available, use a hose or a shower. Brush dry powder chemicals from the skin before flushing, unless large amounts of water are immediately available. Water may activate a dry chemical and cause more damage to the skin. Take precautions to protect yourself from exposure to the chemical.

2. Remove the victim's contaminated clothing while flushing with water. Clothing can hold chemicals, allowing them to continue to burn as long as they are in contact with the skin.

3. Flush for 20 minutes or longer. Let the victim wash with a mild soap before a final rinse. Dilution with large amounts of water decreases the chemical concentration and washes it away.

Caution:

DO NOT waste time! A chemical burn is an emergency!

DO NOT apply water under high pressure—it will drive the chemical deeper into the tissue.

DO NOT try to neutralize a chemical even if you know which chemical is involved—heat may be produced, resulting in more damage. Some product labels for neutralizing may be wrong. Save the container or the label for the chemical's name.

4. Cover the burned area with a dry, sterile dressing or, for large areas, a clean pillowcase.

5. If the chemical is in an eye, flood it for at least 20 minutes, using low pressure.

6. Seek medical attention immediately for all chemical burns.

Electrical Burns

Even a mild electrical shock can cause serious internal injuries (▶Figure 9-9, A–B). A current of 1,000 volts or more is considered high voltage, but even the 110 volts found in ordinary household current can be deadly.

There are three types of electrical injuries: thermal burn (flame), arc burn (flash), and true electrical injury (contact). A *thermal burn* (flame) results when clothing or objects in direct contact with the skin are ignited by an electrical current. These injuries are caused by the flames produced by the electrical current and not by the passage of the electrical current or arc.

An *arc burn* (flash) occurs from electricity jumping, or arcing, from one spot to another and not from the passage of an electrical current through the body. Although the duration of the flash may be brief, it usually causes extensive superficial injuries.

A *true electrical injury* (contact) happens when an electric current passes directly through the body. This type of injury is characterized by an entrance wound and an exit wound. The important factor with this type of injury is that the surface injury may be just the tip of the iceberg. High-voltage electrical currents passing through the body may disrupt the normal heart rhythm and cause cardiac arrest, burns, and other injuries.

During an electric shock, electricity enters the body at the point of contact and travels along the path of least re-

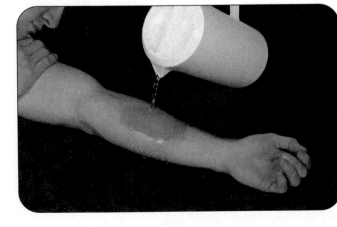

Figure 9-8 Flushing a chemical burn

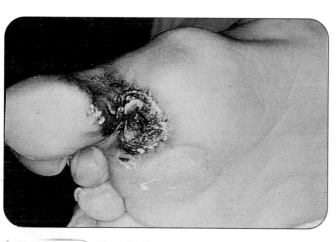

Figure 9-9A Electrical burn on toe

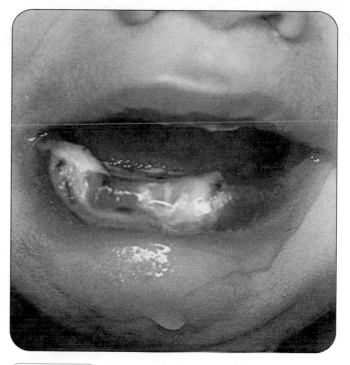

Figure 9-9B Elecrical burn caused by chewing through electrical cord

sistance (nerves and blood vessels). The major damage occurs inside the body—the outside burn may appear small. Usually, the electricity exits where the body is touching a surface or is in contact with a ground (eg, a metal object). Sometimes, a victim has more than one exit site.

What to Do

1. Make sure the area is safe. Unplug, disconnect, or turn off the power. If that is impossible, call the power company or EMS for help.
2. Check ABCs.
3. If the victim fell, check for a spinal injury.
4. Treat the victim for shock by elevating the legs 8 to 12 inches if no spinal injury is suspected, and prevent heat loss by covering the victim with a coat or blanket.
5. Seek medical attention immediately. Electrical injuries usually require treatment in a burn center.

Contact with a Power Line (Outdoors)

If the electric shock is from contact with a downed power line, the power *must* be turned off before a rescuer approaches anyone who may be in contact with the wire.

If a power line falls across a car containing a person, tell him or her to stay in the car until the power can be shut off. The only exception is if fire threatens the car. In that case, tell the victim to jump out of the car without making contact with the car or the wire.

If you feel a tingling sensation in your legs and lower body as you approach a victim, stop. The sensation signals that you are on energized ground and that an electrical current is entering through one foot, passing through your lower body, and leaving through the other foot. Raise one foot off the ground, turn around, and hop to a safe place.

If you can safely reach the victim, do not attempt to move any wires, even with wooden poles, tools with wood handles, or tree branches. Do not use objects with a high moisture content and certainly not metal objects. The reason for not using wood-handled rakes, brooms, or shovels is that if the voltage is high enough (you seldom will know how much voltage is involved) those objects can conduct electricity and the rescuer will be electrocuted. Do not attempt to move downed wires at all unless you are trained and are equipped with tools able to handle the high voltage.

Wait until trained personnel with the proper equipment can cut the wires or disconnect them. Prevent bystanders from entering the danger area.

ELECTRICAL BURNS

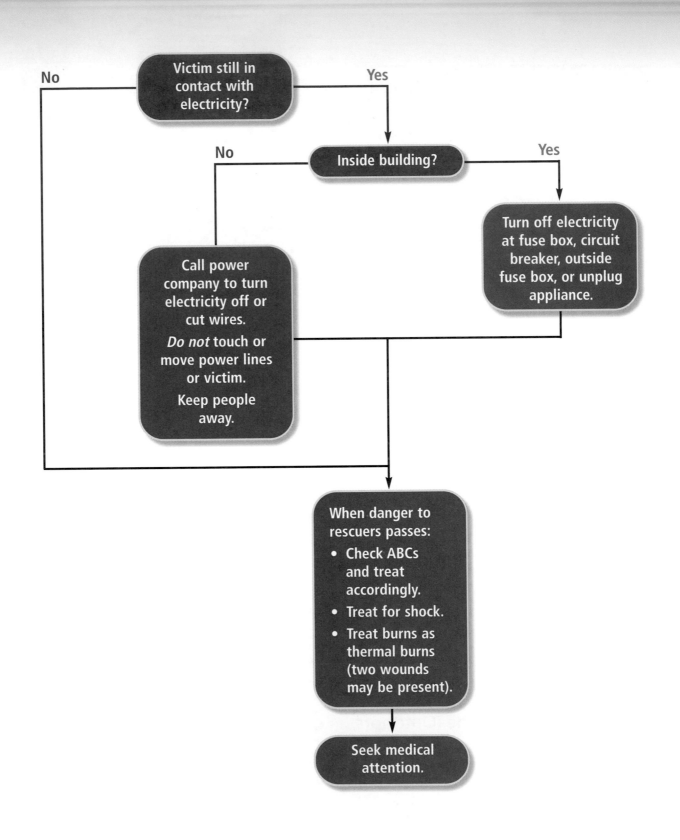

Victim still in contact with electricity?

No

Yes

Inside building?

No

Yes

Call power company to turn electricity off or cut wires.

Do not **touch or move power lines or victim.**

Keep people away.

Turn off electricity at fuse box, circuit breaker, outside fuse box, or unplug appliance.

When danger to rescuers passes:
- **Check ABCs and treat accordingly.**
- **Treat for shock.**
- **Treat burns as thermal burns (two wounds may be present).**

Seek medical attention.

Contact inside Buildings

Most electrical burns that occur indoors are caused by faulty electrical equipment or careless use of electrical appliances. Turn off the electricity at the circuit breaker, fuse box, or outside switch box or unplug the appliance if the plug is undamaged. Do not touch the appliance or the victim until the current is off.

Once there is no danger to rescuers, first aid can begin.

What to Do

1. Check ABCs and treat accordingly.
2. Check the victim for burns—most electrical burns are third-degree—and treat for shock by elevating the legs 8 to 12 inches and keeping the victim warm. Cover the burns with a sterile dressing.
3. Seek medical attention.

Electrical current flows quickly into the body's tissues, then exits. The surface injuries of the skin involve small surface areas (entrance and exit points); the major damage occurs deep under the skin. First aiders must keep that in mind when they treat anyone for electrical shock.

See Chapter 22 for lightning burns and their care.

STUDY
Questions ⑨

Name_____ Course_____ Date_____

Activities
Activity 1
Choose the best answer.

____ 1. What should you do first to ease the pain from a burn?
  a. Hold the injured part in a sink filled with warm water.
  b. Cover the burned area with a clean dressing.
  c. Cover the burn with petroleum jelly.
  d. Place the injured part in a sink filled with running cold water.

____ 2. How could you lessen a burn victim's pain while you seek medical assistance?
  a. Soak the burned area in warm water.
  b. Cover small burned areas with cool wet cloths.
  c. Pinch the areas.
  d. Immerse the burned area in cold saltwater.

____ 3. The type of burn characterized by reddening, blisters, and deep, intense pain is called a
  a. first-degree burn
  b. second-degree burn
  c. third-degree burn

____ 4. Which type of burn is characterized by little or no pain and skin that is usually charred black or has areas that are dry and white?
  a. first-degree burn
  b. second-degree burn
  c. third-degree burn

____ 5. Using the "rule of nines," what percentage of an adult's body is involved if one entire arm and the front of one leg are burned?
  a. 9%   b. 18%
  c. 27%   d. 36%

____ 6. Which body areas are especially sensitive to being burned?
  a. face   b. hands
  c. feet   d. all the above

____ 7. A victim's palm size represents what percentage of the body?
  a. 1%
  b. 5%
  c. 10%

Mark each action yes (Y) or no (N).
When giving first aid for a burn, you should

____ 8. Apply petroleum jelly on the burn.

____ 9. Pull off a piece of clothing that is stuck to a burn.

____ 10. Apply a clean dressing and secure it in place.

____ 11. Blow on a burned area to cool it.

____ 12. Use your fingers to remove pieces of burned skin.

____ 13. Open blisters before applying a dressing.

____ 14. Apply cool water to the burn.

Activity 2
Choose the best answer.

____ 1. All acids, alkalies, and organic compounds are best treated by
  a. neutralizing the chemicals
  b. applying a solvent to the burn
  c. washing the area with large quantities of water
  d. wrapping the area to keep out oxygen

____ 2. When washing chemicals from the body, it is best if the water is
  a. applied to the area under high pressure
  b. applied to the area under low pressure
  c. considerably warmer than normal body temperature
  d. kept in a large basin into which the part affected is submerged

____ 3. What type of chemical substances may be activated if flushed with water?
  a. dry chemicals
  b. petroleum products
  c. topical medications
  d. fluid or wet chemicals

STUDY
Questions 9

___ 4. Do not attempt to neutralize a chemical because the neutralization process may result in further damage due to
   a. mechanical irritation
   b. the electricity produced
   c. heat production
   d. radiation effects

___ 5. What is the first step in caring for dry chemicals spilled on the skin?
   a. Read the chemical container's label as to proper procedures.
   b. Flush with water.
   c. Brush off the substance before flushing with water.
   d. Cover the area with sterile gauze.

Activity 3
Choose the best answer.

___ 1. Household electricity, though damaging, is not deadly.
   a. Yes
   b. No

___ 2. When someone gets electrocuted, how many burn wounds usually occur?
   a. one
   b. two
   c. three or more

___ 3. If a victim is stranded in a car with a power line fallen across it, in most cases the victim should
   a. stay in the car
   b. climb out of the car's window
   c. jump from the car's window
   d. exit through the door

___ 4. If you ever feel a tingling sensation in your legs when near a downed electrical wire, you should
   a. raise a foot off the ground and hop to a safe place
   b. continue walking through the area
   c. run through the area
   d. be concerned since the tingling indicates low voltage

___ 5. If you are near a victim who is paralyzed by electrical current, you should
   a. try to move any wires with a wooden pole or handle
   b. try to pull the victim from any wires
   c. use wooden poles or handles to try to pull the victim from any wires
   d. wait until the power company can cut the wires or disconnect them

___ 6. Where does electricity produce the most damaging burns?
   a. on the skin   b. deep under the skin

___ 7. First aid for a victim of electrocution may include
   a. CPR   b. burn treatment
   c. shock treatment   d. all the above

Case Situations
Case 1
A 29-year-old male sustains burns on the front of both arms as a result of a leaf fire getting out of control. On arrival at the scene of the fire, you assess the depth of the burn and the extent of body surface involvement.

1. His burns have a reddened appearance and blisters are present. Classify the type of burn.

   _____

   _____

2. What is the rule of nines?

   _____

   _____

   _____

   _____

   _____

3. How would you describe the burns sustained by this man in terms of the rule of nines?

   _____

   _____

   _____

   _____

   _____

STUDY Questions 9

4. Describe each of the following burn classifications:

a. first-degree: _____

_____

b. second-degree: _____

_____

c. third-degree: _____

_____

5. Describe the appropriate first aid for a third-degree burn.

a. _____

_____

b. _____

_____

c. _____

_____

Case 2

A passerby pulls a victim from the burning wreckage of a car. She has burns on the front of both lower portions of the legs and the palms of both hands.

Choose the correct answer to each of the following questions.

___ **1.** First aid for burns that do not cover a large area of the body is as follows:

a. Soak the area in hot water until the pain subsides.

b. Apply a commercial ointment.

c. Submerge the area in cold water.

d. Apply butter or petroleum jelly.

___ **2.** Heat is applied to burns

a. until the pain is relieved

b. that do not cover a large area

c. to reduce swelling

d. to kill germs and reduce infection

e. never

___ **3.** To cover a painful burn, use

a. a burn ointment

b. first-aid cream

c. a dry dressing

d. a warm, moist dressing

___ **4.** A useful method for determining the extent of a burn is to use the victim's palm size, which is equivalent to what percentage of the victim's body area?

a. 1%   b. 5%

c. 9%   d. 11%

Case 3

A 24-year-old female working as a research chemist in a large industrial plant spills acid on her left hand. She starts to flood her hand with a large amount of water.

1. What is the normal first aid for the majority of chemical burns?

_____

_____

_____

_____

_____

_____

___ **2.** In dealing with powdered forms of chemicals, particularly lime, the initial emergency care procedure would be to:

a. wash the affected area with large amounts of water

b. do nothing, but transport immediately

c. brush the powdered chemical off, then wash the affected area with large amounts of water

___ **3.** What class of chemical inflicts the deepest and longest-lasting burns?

a. acids

b. alkalies

Case 4

At a chemical manufacturing company, an alkali product is accidentally splashed on the left upper body of a 47-year-old male. His left eye is also splashed with the solution.

1. What first aid would you give this worker?

a. _____

_____

b. _____

_____

c. _____

_____

STUDY
Questions 9

2. How long is it necessary to flush an acid- or alkali-burned area with water?

_____

_____

3. Would the above treatment be indicated for an alkali burn of the eye?

_____

_____

_____

Case 5

An 18-month-old child has bitten through a household electrical cord. He has a third-degree burn around his mouth.

1. What is the severity of this burn?

_____

_____

_____

2. Because electrical burns may result in paralysis of the breathing center in the brain and ventricular fibrillation of the heart, it may be necessary to start

_____

_____

_____

Case 6

A crane being used to unload lumber from a railroad flat car comes in contact with overhead power lines that run parallel to the railroad tracks. When you arrive, the crane appears to be energized, and the crane operator, although conscious and in the cab, shows signs of being injured.

1. What instructions should you give the crane operator in this situation?

_____

_____

_____

2. What is a general guideline that all first aiders should follow when confronted with rescue attempts involving high-voltage electrical power lines?

_____

_____

_____

____ **3.** What two types of injuries is the crane operator most likely to suffer?

    a. stroke

    b. electrical burns

    c. dislocations

    d. cardiac arrest

    e. fractures

Case 7

At a fast-food restaurant, a 16-year-old worker has been burned by hot grease that was accidentally splashed into his lap. A physical exam reveals burns to the front surfaces of both upper legs. The burned areas appear reddened with blisters.

____ **1.** This victim is suffering from ____ burns.

    a. first-degree

    b. third-degree

    c. second-degree

____ **2.** This victim has burns that involve what percentage of the body?

    a. 2% to 5%

    b. 8% to 10%

    c. 15% to 20%

    d. 18% to 24%

    e. more than 50%

____ **3.** Immediate care for this victim would include

    a. wrapping his legs in wet towels

    b. applying burn ointment to his legs

    c. applying butter to his legs

    d. removing clothing sticking to his burned legs

Chapter Activities

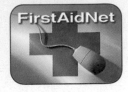

WEB Activities

Burns

Visit nsc.jbpub.com/FirstAidNet, then click on Web Activities, and select the appropriate chapter.

Caring for a Burn

After initial care, burns often require bandage changing for several days after the injury. Learn more about burn aftercare.

Risk of Skin Cancer

It is estimated that 1 out of 7 people in the United States will develop some form of skin cancer during their lifetime. One serious sunburn can increase your risk developing skin cancer by as much as 50%. Details about determining your skin type and preventing skin cancer can be found at this site.

UV Index

Developed by the National Weather Service and the Environmental Protection Agency, the UV Index is issued daily to help plan outdoor activities and prevent sunburn.

Chemical Burns

It is important to know which common household products are potential hazards for chemical burns, as there are many commercial products containing acids and bases. Check your household for these hazardous products.

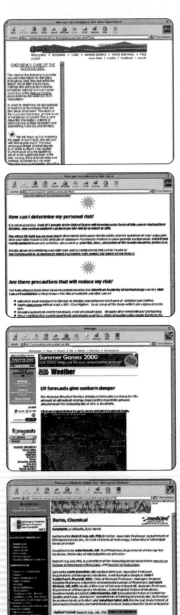

Chapter 10

Head and Spinal Injuries

Head Injuries

"Head injury" is an often misused term. To provide the right care it is important to distinguish the various types of head injuries—scalp wounds, skull fractures, and brain injuries.

Scalp Wounds

Scalp wounds bleed profusely because the scalp has a rich blood supply and the blood vessels there do not constrict. A profusely bleeding scalp wound does not affect the blood supply to the brain. The brain obtains its blood supply from arteries in the neck, not the scalp. A severe scalp wound may have an accompanying skull fracture, impaled object, or spinal injury.

What to Do

1. Control bleeding by gently applying direct pressure with a dry sterile dressing. If the dressing becomes blood-filled, do not remove it. Add another dressing on top of the first one.

2. If you suspect a skull fracture, apply pressure around the edges of the wound and over a broad area rather than on the center of the wound. Use a doughnut (ring) pad around the area.

3. Keep the head and shoulders slightly elevated to help control bleeding if no spinal injury is suspected.

Caution:

DO NOT remove an embedded object; instead, stabilize it in place with bulky dressings. If a skull fracture is suspected, do not clean a scalp wound or irrigate it since the fluid can carry debris and bacteria into the brain.

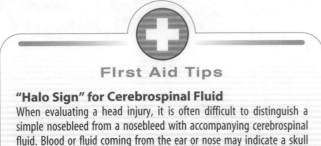

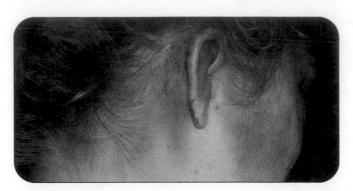

Figure 10-2 Battle's sign

Skull Fracture

A skull fracture is a break or a crack in the cranium (bony case surrounding the brain). Skull fractures may be open (with an accompanying scalp wound) or closed (without an accompanying scalp wound).

What to Look for

It is difficult to determine a skull fracture except by x-ray unless the skull deformity is severe. Signs and symptoms of a skull fracture include the following:

- Pain at the point of injury
- Deformity of the skull
- Bleeding coming from the ears or nose
- Clear, pink, watery fluid known as cerebrospinal fluid (CSF) leaking from an ear or the nose: A drop of CSF on a handkerchief, pillowcase, or other white or light-colored cloth will form a pink ring resembling a target around a slightly blood-tinged center; this is called the "halo sign" or "ring sign."
- Discoloration around the eyes ("raccoon eyes") appearing several hours after the injury
  ▼Figure 10-1

Figure 10-1 Raccoon eyes

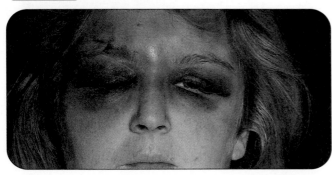

- Discoloration behind an ear (known as "Battle's sign"), appearing several hours after the injury
  ▲Figure 10-2
- Unequal-sized pupils
- Profuse scalp bleeding if skin is broken: A scalp wound may expose the skull or brain tissue.
- Penetrating wound such as from a bullet or impaled object

What to Do

1. Monitor ABCs.
2. Cover wounds with a sterile dressing.
3. Stabilize the victim's neck against movement.
4. Slightly elevate the victim's head and shoulders to help control bleeding.
5. To control bleeding apply pressure around the edges of the wound, not directly on it.

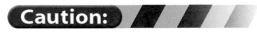

Caution:

DO NOT stop the flow of blood or cerebrospinal fluid (CSF) from an ear or nose. Blocking the flow could increase pressure within the skull.

DO NOT remove an impaled object from the head. Stabilize it in place with bulky dressings.

DO NOT clean an open skull fracture—infection of the brain could result.

DO NOT press on the fractured area.

Brain Injuries

Statistics from the insurance industry indicate that at least eight million head injuries are reported in the United States each year (▼Figure 10-3). It is not injury specifically to the head that causes most short- and long-term problems but injuries to the brain itself. Most head injuries come from motor vehicle accidents and falls. Many of these injuries are minor—shallow lacerations or localized bruising and swelling. However, 50,000 people die each year in the United States from head trauma, and twice that many suffer brain injuries that leave them with permanent damage.

The brain is a delicate organ. When the head is struck with sufficient force, the brain bounces against the inside of the skull. Brain injuries can be serious and difficult first aid emergencies to handle. The victim is often confused or unresponsive, making assessment difficult. Many brain injuries are life threatening. Mishandling a victim with a brain injury could result in permanent damage or death.

The brain, like other body tissues, will swell from bleeding and when injured. Unlike other tissues, however, the brain is confined in the skull where there is little room for swelling. Any swelling of brain tissue or accumulation of blood inside the skull will compress the brain, increase the pressure inside the skull, and interfere with brain functioning. Furthermore, because the skull is hard, both the brain and its surface blood vessels may be damaged if they strike the inside of the skull, which can occur when the head is struck directly or is rapidly accelerated or decelerated. The phenomenon of a person "seeing stars" when struck on the back of the head results because the occipital lobe of the brain (the part that controls vision) bangs against the back of the skull.

The nerve cells of the brain and the spinal cord, unlike most other cells in the body, are unable to regenerate. When those cells die, they are lost forever, and cannot even be replaced by transplantation.

Injuries to the brain can be caused by a penetrating foreign object, by bony fragments from a skull fracture, or by the brain's crashing into the inside of the skull after a person's head has hit a stationary object (such as the ground)—a *deceleration injury*—or been hit by something like a baseball bat or a teammate's knee—an *acceleration injury*.

Sometimes there will be two points of injury, one at the point of impact and one where the brain rebounds off the skull on the opposite side.

There are three types of commonly occurring brain injuries:

- A **concussion** is temporary loss of brain function, usually without permanent damage. No bleeding in the brain occurs, and there may not be any external cut or swelling. A person with a concussion can be "knocked out" (unconscious) or have memory loss (amnesia). A concussion can be dangerous even if the person is not knocked out because it affects the brain. The longer the victim is unconscious or the longer the memory loss lasts, the more serious the

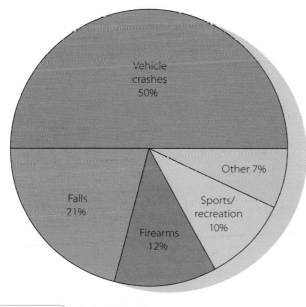

About 373,000 Americans are hospitalized annually for traumatic brain injuries. Their causes:

Vehicle crashes 50%
Other 7%
Falls 21%
Sports/recreation 10%
Firearms 12%

Figure 10-3 Brain Injury Dangers.
Source: Brain Injury Association

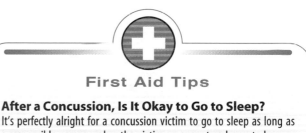

First Aid Tips

After a Concussion, Is It Okay to Go to Sleep?
It's perfectly alright for a concussion victim to go to sleep as long as a responsible person wakes the victim up every two hours to be sure the victim is as easy to wake up as he or she normally is. The victim should be able to recognize the person and recite such things as his or her own birth date, age, and telephone number. If the victim can't be easily awakened or does not answer the questions correctly, seek medical attention.

Table 10-1: Management of Concussion in Sports

Grades of Concussion

Grade 1

1. Transient confusion (inattention, inability to maintain a coherent stream of thought and carry out goal-directed movements).
2. No loss of consciousness
3. Concussion symptoms or mental status abnormalities on examination resolve in **less than 15 minutes**

Grade 2

1. Transient confusion
2. No loss of consciousness
3. Concussion symptoms or mental status abnormalities (including amnesia) on examination last **more than 15 minutes**

Grade 3

1. Any loss of consciousness
   a. Brief (seconds)
   b. Prolonged (minutes)

Management Recommendations

Grade 1

1. Remove from contest
2. Examine immediately and at 5-minute intervals for the development of mental status abnormalities or post-concussive symptoms at rest and with exertion
3. May return to contest if mental status abnormalities or post-concussive symptoms clear within 15 minutes

Grade 2

1. Remove from contest and disallow return that day
2. Examine on-site frequently for signs of evolving intracranial pathology
3. A trained person should reexamine the athlete the following day
4. A physician should perform a neurologic examination to clear the athlete for return to play after 1 full asymptomatic week at rest and with exertion.

Grade 3

1. Transport the athlete from the field to the nearest emergency department by ambulance if still unconscious of if worrisome signs are detected (with cervical spine immobilization, if indicated)
2. A thorough neurologic evaluation should be performed emergently, including appropriate neuroimaging procedures when indicated
3. Hospital admission is indicated if any signs of pathology are detected, or if the mental status of the athlete remains abnormal

When to Return to Play

Grade of Concussion:	Return to Play Only After Being Asymptomatic with Normal Neurologic Assessment at Rest and with Exercise:
Grade 1 Concussion	15 minutes or less
Multiple Grade 1 Concussions	1 week
Grade 2 Concussion	1 week
Multiple Grade 2 Concussions	2 weeks
Grade 3 - Brief Loss of Consciousness (seconds)	1 week
Grade 3 - Prolonged Loss of Consciousness (minutes)	2 weeks
Multiple Grade 3 Concussions	1 month or longer, based on decision of evaluating physician

Features of Concussion Frequently Observed

1. Vacant stare (befuddled facial expression)
2. Delayed verbal and motor responses (slow to answer questions or follow instructions)
3. Confusion and inability to focus attention (easily distracted and unable to follow through with normal activities
4. Disorientation (walking in the wrong direction; unaware of time, date and place)
5. Slurred or incoherent speech (making disjointed or incomprehensible statements)
6. Gross observable incoordination (stumbling, inability to walk tandem/straight line)
7. Emotions out of proportion to circumstances (distraught, crying for no apparent reason)
8. Memory deficits (exhibited by the athlete repeatedly asking the same question that has already been answered, or inability to memorize and recall 3 of 3 words or 3 of 3 objects in 5 minutes)
9. Any period of loss of consciousness (paralytic coma, unresponsiveness to arousal)

Sideline Evaluation

Mental Status Testing

Orientation:	Time, place, person, and situation (circumstances of injury)
Concentration:	Digits backward (i.e., 3-1-7, 4-6-8-2, 5-3-0-7-4) Months of the year in reverse order
Memory:	Names of teams in prior contest Recall of 3 words and 3 objects at 0 to 5 minutes Recent newsworthy events Details of the contest (plays, moves, strategies, etc.)

Exertional Provocative Tests

40 yard sprint
5 push-ups
5 sit-ups
5 knee-bends

Neurological Tests

Strength
Coordination and Agility
Sensation

Any appearance of associated symptoms is abnormal, e.g., headaches, dizziness, nausea, unsteadiness, photophobia, blurred or double vision, emotional lability, or mental status changes.

To purchase copies of this card, or the practice prameter, please call the American Academy of Neurology at 800-879-1960, or the Brain Injury Association at 703-236-6000.

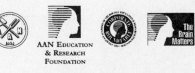
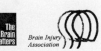

Quality Standards Subcommittee of the American Academy of Neurology. The Management of Concussion in Sports [practice parameter]. *Neurology* 1997; 48: 581-585.

concussion. Concussions usually are not serious, but occasionally they can result in permanent damage to the brain and even cause death.

- A **contusion** is a bruising of brain tissue.
- A **hematoma** is a localized collection of blood as a result of a broken blood vessel. A hematoma is the most serious type of brain injury.

Brain injuries produce varying degrees of local or generalized edema (swelling). As swelling increases or a hematoma expands, intracranial pressure increases. As pressure rises, it can compress swollen vessels, and shut off the blood supply, thus depriving brain tissue of oxygen. The brain stem can be squashed by the pressure, affecting heart and lung function.

Children are especially vulnerable to brain injuries. A young child has a relatively large head, supported by a weak neck, and positioned on a small trunk. A child's brain tissues are thinner, softer, and more flexible than an adult's. The tissues' flexibility diffuses the impact of an injury, but because they are fragile, they damage easily. Small children, overbalanced by their large heads, tend to run leaning forward and often run into things or fall over. Their immature motor development makes toddlers clumsy and liable to stumble over their own feet. Unattended infants can tumble from beds, highchairs, and changing tables.

What to Look for

After the first 6 to 18 hours, the following signs and symptoms indicate brain swelling.

- Altered mental status—levels V, P, or U on the AVPU scale (see page 47). Loss of responsiveness may be short or may persist for hours or days. The victim may alternate between periods of responsiveness and unresponsiveness or be responsive but disoriented, confused, and incoherent.
- Memory loss
- Vomiting and nausea
- Headache
- Vision disturbance: Victim sees "double," or eyes fail to move together.
- Unequal pupils
- Weakness, loss of balance, or paralysis
- Seizures
- Blood or CSF leaking from ears or nose

Recognizing Concussions

Signs and symptoms of a concussion frequently observed initially, according to the American Academy of Neurology and the Brain Injury Association:

- Confused facial expression
- Slow to answer questions or follow instruction
- Easily distracted and unable to follow through with normal activities
- Walking in the wrong direction; unaware of time, date, and place
- Making disjointed or incomprehensible statements
- Stumbling, inability to walk straight line
- Distraught, crying for no apparent reason
- Asking the same question that was already been answered, or inability to memorize and recall a series of three words or objects in 5 minutes
- Coma, unresponsiveness

- Combativeness: The victim strikes out randomly and with surprising strength at the nearest person.

Ask a responsive victim for his or her name and current location. If the victim cannot answer those questions, there may be a significant problem. Another useful test is having the victim recite the months of the year backward, starting with December. Inability to do so could indicate a concussion.

What to Do

1. Seek immediate medical attention for all brain-injury victims.
2. Suspect a spinal injury in an unresponsive victim until proved otherwise. Stabilize the victim's head and neck using one of the following methods:
   - Grasp the victim's head over the ears and hold the head and neck still until the EMS arrives.
   - If you anticipate a long wait for the EMS to arrive or if you are tired from holding the victim's head in place, kneel with the victim's head between your knees or place objects on each side of the victim's head to prevent it from rolling from side to side.

HEAD INJURIES

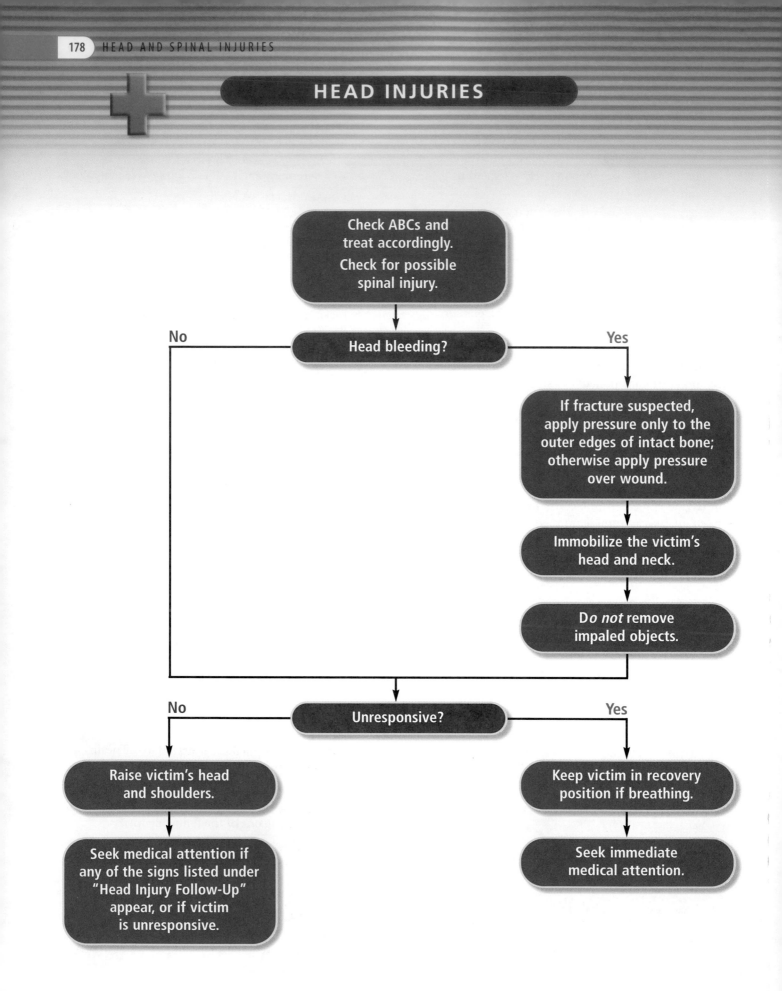

Check ABCs and treat accordingly. Check for possible spinal injury.

Head bleeding?

No

Yes

If fracture suspected, apply pressure only to the outer edges of intact bone; otherwise apply pressure over wound.

Immobilize the victim's head and neck.

D*o not* remove impaled objects.

Unresponsive?

No

Yes

Raise victim's head and shoulders.

Seek medical attention if any of the signs listed under "Head Injury Follow-Up" appear, or if victim is unresponsive.

Keep victim in recovery position if breathing.

Seek immediate medical attention.

3. Monitor ABCs.

4. Control scalp bleeding by covering wounds with sterile dressings as a barrier against infection. If you suspect a skull fracture, apply pressure around the wound edges, not directly on the wound. Do not try to clean a scalp wound if you suspect a skull fracture. Stabilize impaled objects in place. Do not try to stop blood or CSF draining from the ears or nose. Blocking either flow could increase pressure within the skull.

5. Brain-injury victims tend to vomit. Roll the victim onto his or her side and keep the neck stabilized to help drain vomit while maintaining an open airway.

6. If a spinal injury is not suspected, keep the victim in a slightly head-elevated position to prevent increased blood pressure on the brain. If the victim is unresponsive, roll him or her onto the left side to keep the airway open.

7. The victim's level of responsiveness or mental status is one of the best indicators of neurologic function. Observations over the first 24 hours may offer clues to problems. Using the mnemonic AVPU to assess and describe a victim's mental status is especially helpful with small children who don't talk.

   A: The victim is *alert* and can recognize and respond to people.

   V: The victim responds to *verbal* stimuli. The victim may appear sleepy or drowsy but responds to verbal questions by opening the eyes, moving, or waking up.

   P: The victim responds to *painful* stimuli. The victim is not awake and does not respond to verbal stimuli but does respond to painful stimuli by moving, opening the eyes, or groaning. To stimulate pain, pinch the victim's skin over the clavicle.

   U: The victim is *unresponsive* to voices or to painful stimulus.

Unfortunately, there is little a first aider can do for a brain injury. The victim must be transported to the care of a neurosurgeon who can relieve the pressure and stop intracranial bleeding. If the victim is wearing a helmet such as a motorcycle or football helmet, it should not be removed by a first aider unless:

- You suspect an obstructed airway.
- You see signs of a severe head injury.
- The helmet is so loose that you cannot stabilize the spine.

Head Injury Follow-Up

If any of the following signs appear within 48 hours of a head injury, seek medical attention:

+ **Headache:** Expect a headache. If it lasts more than one or two days or increases in severity, seek medical advice.

+ **Nausea, vomiting:** If nausea lasts more than two hours, seek medical advice. Vomiting once or twice, especially in children, may be expected after a head injury. Vomiting does not tell anything about the severity of the injury. However, if vomiting begins again hours after the initial episodes have ceased, consult a physician.

+ **Drowsiness:** Allow a victim to sleep, but wake the victim at least every two hours to check the state of consciousness and sense of orientation by asking his or her name and an information-processing question (e.g., "Recite the months of the year backwards starting with December"). If the victim cannot respond or appears confused or disoriented, call a physician.

+ **Vision problems:** If the victim "sees double," if the eyes fail to move together, or if one pupil appears to be larger than the other, seek medical advice.

+ **Mobility:** If the victim cannot use his or her arms or legs as well as previously or is unsteady in walking, seek medical care.

+ **Speech:** If the victim has slurred speech or is unable to talk, consult a doctor.

+ **Seizures or convulsions:** If the victim has a violent involuntary contraction (spasm) or series of contractions of the skeletal muscles, seek medical assistance.

Caution:

DO NOT stop the flow of blood or CSF from the ears or nose. Blocking either flow could increase pressure inside the skull.

DO NOT elevate the legs—that might increase pressure on the brain.

DO NOT clean an open skull injury—infection of the brain may result.

Eye Injuries

Of all the parts of the human body, an injured eye probably causes the most anxiety and concern in a victim. Eye injuries account for up to 10% of all bodily injuries.

The eyes—arguably the most important human sense organs—are easily damaged by trauma. A very slight penetration by a metal fragment, for example, means hospitalization. Medical treatment may include surgery; despite technical advances, blindness or the loss of an eye remains a possibility whenever there is an eye injury.

> ## Caution:
>
> **DO NOT** assume that any eye injury is innocent. When in doubt, seek medical attention immediately.

> ## Caution:
>
> **DO NOT** remove an object stuck in the eye or try to wash out an object with water.
>
> **DO NOT** exert pressure on an injured eyeball or a penetrating object.

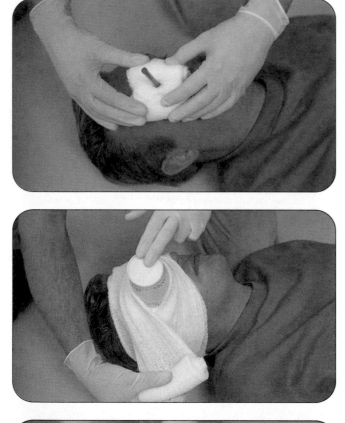

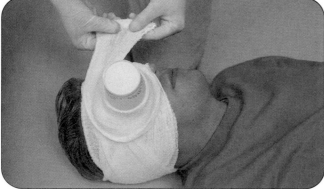

Figure 10-4 Protecting a long penetrating object against movement (using paper cup).

If you don't have a paper cup, a ring pad (see page 101) can be used to hold dressings in place.

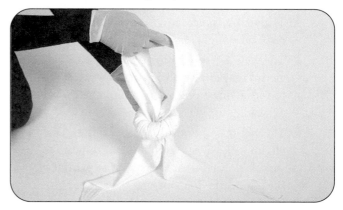

a. Pull a narrow cravat bandage through a ring pad. The large loop goes around the victim's head.

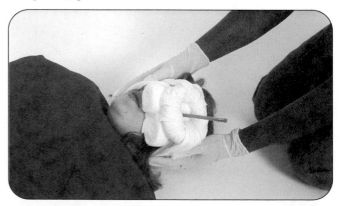

b. Stabilize the embedded object with bulky dressings. Bring the ends of the bandage around the head and tie.

Penetrating Eye Injuries

Penetrating eye injuries are severe injuries that result when a sharp object, such as a knife or a needle, penetrates the eye and then is withdrawn or when pieces from a tool enter the eye and lodge there as foreign bodies.

Any foreign body in the eye is hazardous, especially if it contains iron or copper. Those metals often dissociate, and their atoms or ions can gradually destroy the eye over a period of days or years.

Most penetrating injuries are obvious. Suspect penetration any time you see a lid laceration or cut.

What to Do

1. Seek immediate medical attention. Any penetrating eye injury should be managed in the hospital.

2. Stabilize the object. Stabilize a long protruding object with bulky dressings or clean cloths. You can place a protective paper cup or cardboard folded into a cone over the affected eye to prevent bumping of the object. For short objects, surround the eye without touching the object by using a doughnut-shaped (ring) pad held in place with a roller bandage (◀Figure 10-4, A-B).

3. Cover the undamaged eye. Most experts suggest that the undamaged eye should be covered to prevent sympathetic eye movement (▼Figure 10-5) (ie, the injured eye may move when the undamaged eye does, aggravating the injury). Remember that the victim is unable to see when both eyes are covered and may be anxious. Make sure you explain everything you are doing to the victim.

4. Seek immediate medical attention.

Blows to the Eye

Blows to the eye can range in severity from minor to sight threatening. One such injury is the common "shiner" or

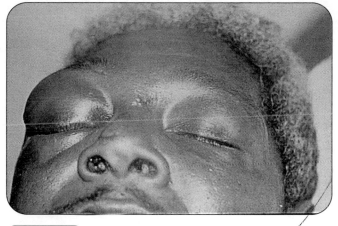

Figure 10-6 Blow to the eye.

"black eye," which occurs when some of the many delicate blood vessels around the eye rupture. The bleeding itself is insignificant and will disappear, but it may hide damage to the eyeball (▲Figure 10-6).

A fist, a ball, or other blunt object can break the bone around the eyeball. Symptoms that indicate such a break are double vision and the inability to look upward.

What to Do

1. Apply an ice pack immediately for about 15 minutes to reduce pain and swelling. Do not exert any pressure on the eye.

2. Seek medical attention immediately in cases of pain, reduced vision, or discoloration (a black eye). An eyeball could be ruptured.

Cuts of the Eye or Lid (▼Figure 10-7)
What to Do

1. Bandage both eyes lightly.

2. Seek medical attention immediately.

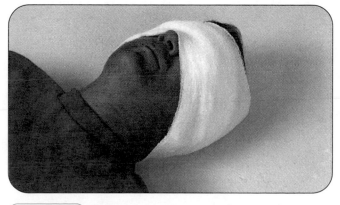

Figure 10-5 Bandaging both eyes stops sympathetic eye movement.

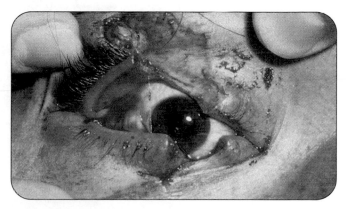

Figure 10-7 Lacerated eylid.

EYE INJURIES

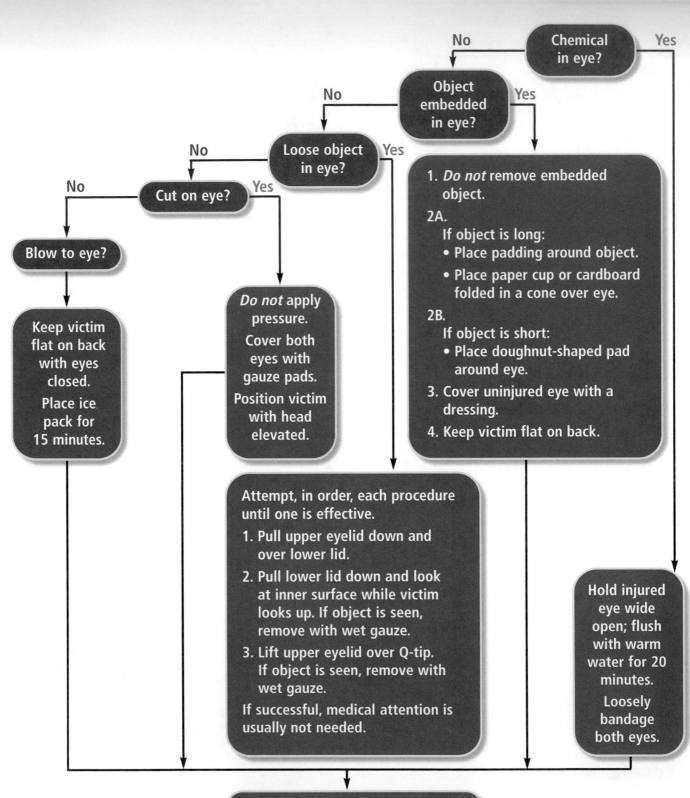

Chemical in eye? — No / Yes

Object embedded in eye? — No / Yes

Loose object in eye? — No / Yes

Cut on eye? — No / Yes

Blow to eye?

Keep victim flat on back with eyes closed. Place ice pack for 15 minutes.

Do not apply pressure. Cover both eyes with gauze pads. Position victim with head elevated.

1. *Do not* remove embedded object.
2A. If object is long:
   • Place padding around object.
   • Place paper cup or cardboard folded in a cone over eye.
2B. If object is short:
   • Place doughnut-shaped pad around eye.
3. Cover uninjured eye with a dressing.
4. Keep victim flat on back.

Attempt, in order, each procedure until one is effective.
1. Pull upper eyelid down and over lower lid.
2. Pull lower lid down and look at inner surface while victim looks up. If object is seen, remove with wet gauze.
3. Lift upper eyelid over Q-tip. If object is seen, remove with wet gauze.
If successful, medical attention is usually not needed.

Hold injured eye wide open; flush with warm water for 20 minutes. Loosely bandage both eyes.

Seek medical attention.

Chemical Burns of the Eye

Chemical burns of the eyes are extremely sight-threatening. First aid may determine the fate of the eye and vision.

Alkalies cause greater damage than acids because they penetrate deeper and continue to burn longer. Common alkalies include drain cleaners, cleaning agents, ammonia, cement, plaster, and caustic soda. Common acids include hydrochloric acid, nitric acid, sulfuric (battery) acid, and acetic acid.

Because damage can happen in one to five minutes, the chemical must be removed immediately (▼Figure 10-8).

Caution:

DO NOT try to neutralize the chemical. Water usually is readily available for eye irrigation.

DO NOT use an eye cup for a chemical burn.

DO NOT bandage eye tightly.

What to Do

1. Use your fingers to keep the eye open as wide as possible.
2. Flush the eye with water immediately. If possible, use warm water. If water is not available, use any nonirritating liquid.
   - Hold the victim's head under a faucet or pour water into the eye from any clean container for at least 20 minutes, continuously and gently. It is impossible to use too much water on these injuries.
   - Irrigate from the nose side of the eye toward the outside, to avoid flushing material into the other eye.
   - Tell the victim to roll the eyeball as much as possible to help wash out the eye.

Figure 10-8 Flushing eye for chemical burn

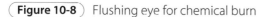
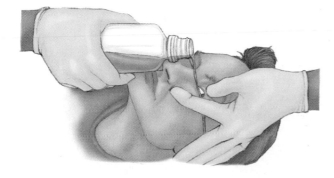

3. Loosely bandage both eyes with cold, wet dressings.
4. Seek immediate medical attention.

Eye Avulsion

A blow to the eye can avulse it (knock it out) from its socket.

What to Do

1. Cover the eye loosely with a sterile dressing that has been moistened with clean water. Do not try to push the eyeball back into the socket.
2. Protect the injured eye with a paper cup, a piece cardboard folded into a cone, or a doughnut-shaped pad made from a roller gauze bandage or a cravat bandage.
3. Cover the undamaged eye with a patch to stop movement of the damaged eye (known as sympathetic eye movement).
4. Seek medical attention immediately.

Foreign Objects in Eye

Foreign objects in the eye are the most frequent eye injury and can be very painful. Tearing is common because it is the body's way of trying to remove the object. Starting with the first suggestion below, try one or more techniques to remove the object.

Caution:

DO NOT wash eye out with water.

DO NOT try to remove an object stuck in the eye.

What to Do

1. Lift the upper lid over the lower lid, so that the lower lashes can brush the object off the inside of the upper lid. Have the victim blink a few times and let the eye move the object out. If the object remains, keep the eye closed.
2. Try flushing the object out by rinsing the eye gently with warm water. Hold the eyelid open and tell the victim to move the eye as it is rinsed.
3. Examine the lower lid by pulling it down gently. If you can see the object, remove it with a moistened sterile gauze or clean cloth.
4. Many foreign bodies lodge under the upper eyelid; however, it requires some expertise to evert the lid and remove the object (▶Figure 10-9). Examine the

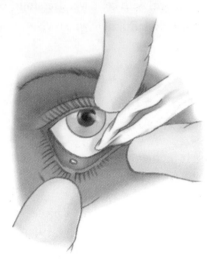 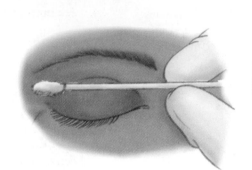 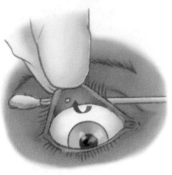

a. If tears or gentle flushing do not remove object, gently pull lower lid down. Remove an object by gently flushing with lukewarm water or a wet sterile gauze.

b. Tell the person to look down. Pull gently downward on upper eyelashes. Lay a swab or match stick across the top of the lid.

c. Fold the lid over the swab or matchstick. Remove an object by gently flushing with lukewarm water or a wet sterile gauze.

Figure 10-9 Removing foreign object from the eye

underside of the upper lid by grasping the lashes of the upper lid, placing a match stick or cotton-tipped swab across the upper lid and rolling the lid upward over the stick or swab. If you can see the object, remove it with a moistened sterile gauze or clean cloth.

5. If tears or gentle flushing do not remove object, gently pull lower lid down. Remove an object by gently flushing with lukewarm water or a wet sterile gauze.

6. Tell the person to look down. Pull gently downward on upper eyelashes. Lay a swab or match stick across the top of the lid.

7. Fold the lid over the swab or matchstick. Remove an object by gently flushing with lukewarm water or a wet sterile gauze.

Caution:

DO NOT allow the victim to rub the eye.

DO NOT try to remove an embedded foreign object.

DO NOT use dry cotton (cotton balls or cotton-tipped swabs) or instruments such as tweezers on an eye.

Eye Burns from Light

Burns can result if a person looks at a source of ultraviolet light such as sunlight, arc welding, bright snow, or tanning lamps. Severe pain happens one to six hours after exposure.

What to Do

1. Cover both eyes with cold, wet packs. Tell the victim not to rub the eyes.

2. Have the victim rest in a darkened room. Do not allow light to reach the victim's eyes.

3. Give pain medication, if needed.

4. Seek medical attention for advice.

An Unconscious Victim's Eyes

An unconscious victim may lose the reflexes such as blinking that protect the eye. Therefore, keep the victim's eyes closed either by taping them closed (use non-allergenic tape) or by covering them with moist dressings.

Contact Lenses

Determine if a victim is wearing contact lenses by asking, by checking a driver's license, or by looking for them on the eyeball, using a light shining on the eye from the side. In cases of chemical burns, lenses should be removed immediately. Usually the victim can remove the lenses.

Ear Injuries

Most ear problems are not life threatening. Fast action may be needed, however, to relieve pain and to prevent or reverse any hearing loss. Head trauma may involve the ear. In those cases, assess ABCDs and treat accordingly.

Foreign bodies in the ear canal usually produce overzealous removal attempts. Except for disk batteries (which damage moist tissue by creating a current) and live insects, few foreign bodies must be extracted immediately. First aiders should elect to seek medical attention for the victim because attempts to remove a foreign body from the ear can rupture the eardrum (membrane) or lacerate the ear canal.

A live insect crawling around in the ear canal can be very uncomfortable for the victim. Shine a small light into the ear. Sometimes the insect will crawl out toward the light. If it will not leave the ear, drown the insect by placing several drops of light mineral oil or vegetable oil (not motor oil) into the ear. Often the insect will crawl out before it dies. When it stops moving, and if the eardrum is intact and the insect is near the opening, carefully irrigate the ear with warm water. The insect should wash out. If that is unsuccessful, use a bulb syringe to suck the insect out.

Children insert all sorts of things into their ears that may be impossible for you to remove safely. If the object is near the ear canal opening and you feel it is safe, cautiously try to remove the object with tweezers. Small objects can sometimes be removed by irrigating the ear with warm water. Do not try irrigation if the object is near the eardrum, if it blocks the entire ear canal, if the eardrum has a hole in it, or if the object is vegetable matter such as a kernel of corn or a bean, which will swell when wet.

Nose Injuries

Nosebleeds

A severe nosebleed frightens the victim and often challenges the first aider's skill. Most nosebleeds are self-limiting and seldom require medical attention. In cases of accompanying head or neck injuries, stabilize the head and neck for protection. In some cases, loss of blood could cause shock.

There are two types of nosebleeds:

- Anterior (front of nose) is the most common type (90%). Blood comes out of the nose through one nostril.
- Posterior (back of nose) type involves massive bleeding backward into the mouth or down the back of the throat. A posterior nosebleed is serious and requires medical attention.

What to Do

To care for an anterior nosebleed, follow these guidelines from the American Academy of Otolaryngology:

1. Pinch the soft parts of the nose together between your thumb and two fingers (▶Figure 10-10).
2. Press firmly toward the face, compressing the pinched parts of the nose against the bones of the face.
3. Hold it for five minutes.

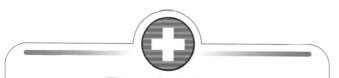

First Aid Tips

Insect in an Ear

Do not try to kill a lodged insect by poking something into the victim's ear. Insects are attracted to light, so it may be coaxed out with light. Outdoors, pull the ear lobe gently to straighten the canal and turn the ear toward the sun. Indoors, turn off all lights, then shine a flashlight into the ear while pulling gently on the ear lobe. This may induce the insect to crawl out toward the light.

If the light method fails, a little mineral oil may cause the insect to float out. Use this method only if you are absolutely sure that the foreign body in the ear is an insect. If the object is vegetable matter (eg, a bean, popcorn), the object may swell and be difficult to remove. Do not use mineral oil if there is any sign of eardrum rupture.

Do not go into the ear canal to remove foreign objects.

Care after a Nosebleed

After a nosebleed has stopped, suggest that the victim:

- ✚ Sneeze through an open mouth, if he or she needs to sneeze.
- ✚ Avoid bending over or too much physical exertion.
- ✚ Elevate the head with two pillows when lying down.
- ✚ Keep the nostrils moist by applying a little petroleum jelly just inside the nostril for a week; increase the humidity in the bedroom during the winter months with a cold-mist humidifier.
- ✚ Avoid picking or rubbing the nose.

NOSEBLEEDS

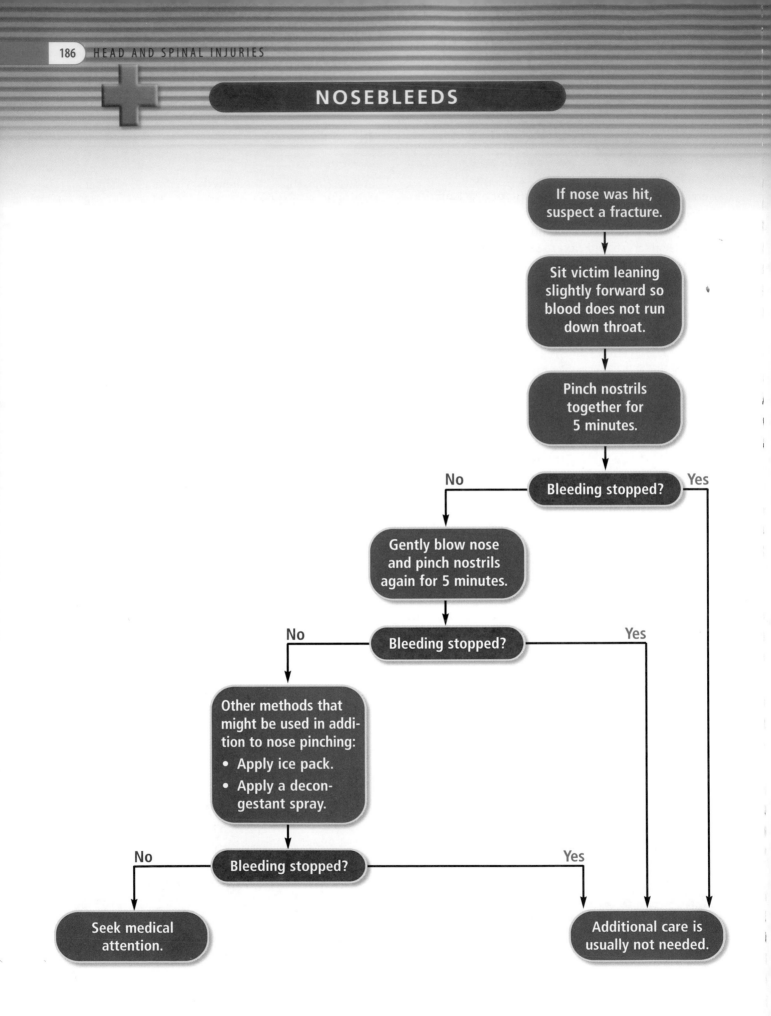

If nose was hit, suspect a fracture.

Sit victim leaning slightly forward so blood does not run down throat.

Pinch nostrils together for 5 minutes.

Bleeding stopped?

No — Gently blow nose and pinch nostrils again for 5 minutes.

Yes — Additional care is usually not needed.

Bleeding stopped?

No — Other methods that might be used in addition to nose pinching:
- Apply ice pack.
- Apply a decongestant spray.

Yes — Additional care is usually not needed.

Bleeding stopped?

No — Seek medical attention.

Yes — Additional care is usually not needed.

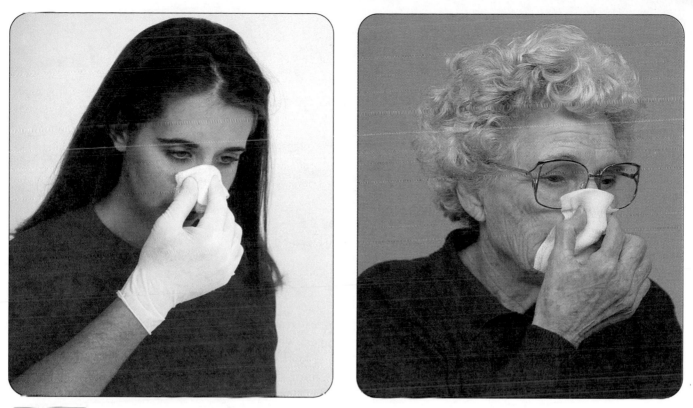

Figure 10-10 To control a nosebleed, have the victim lean forward and pinch both nostrils together or have the victim pinch his or her own nostrils.

4. Keep the head higher than the level of the heart. Have the victim sit and lean slightly forward or lie with the head elevated.

5. Apply ice (crushed in a plastic bag or washcloth) to the nose and cheeks.

If bleeding continues:

1. Clear the nose of all blood clots by gently blowing the nose.

2. If available, spray the nose on both sides with decongestant spray (such as Afrin™ or Neo-Synephrin™).

3. Pinch and press the nose toward the face again, as in Steps 1 to 3.

4. If the nosebleed continues, seek medical attention.

Seek professional medical help if:

- Bleeding cannot be stopped or keeps reappearing.
- Bleeding is rapid or if blood loss is large.
- Weakness or fainting are present.
- Blood begins to go down the back of the throat rather than out the front of the nose.

Caution:

DO NOT allow the victim to tilt the head backward.

DO NOT probe the nose with a cotton-tipped swab.

DO NOT move the victim's head and neck if a spinal injury is suspected.

Broken Nose

For a broken nose,

1. Seek medical attention.
2. If bleeding is present, give care as for a nosebleed.
3. Apply an ice pack to the nose for 15 minutes.
4. Do not try to straighten a crooked nose.

Foreign Objects

A foreign object in the nose is a problem mainly among small children, who seem to gain some satisfaction from putting peanuts, beans, raisins, and similar objects into their nostrils. Try one or more of these methods:

What to Do

1. Induce sneezing by having the victim sniff pepper or by tickling the opposite nostril.

2. Have the victim blow gently while you put compression on the opposite nostril.

3. Use tweezers to pull out an object that is visible. Do not probe or push an object deeper.

4. Seek medical attention if the object cannot be removed.

Dental Injuries

Because dental emergencies generally cause considerable pain and anxiety, managing them promptly can provide great relief to the victim.

What to Do

Objects Caught between Teeth

1. Try to remove the object with dental floss. Guide the floss carefully to avoid cutting the gums. Do not try to remove the object with a sharp or pointed instrument.

2. If unsuccessful, seek a dentist's attention.

Bitten Lip or Tongue

1. Apply direct pressure to the bleeding area with sterile gauze or a clean cloth.

2. If swelling is present, apply an ice pack or have victim suck on a Popsicle or ice chips.

3. If the bleeding does not stop, seek medical attention.

Loosened Tooth

Trauma can cause teeth to become loosened in their sockets. Applying pressure on either side of each tooth with the fingers can determine looseness. Any tooth movement, even if it is barely felt, indicates a possibly loose tooth.

1. Have the victim bite down on a piece of gauze to keep the tooth in place.

2. Consult a dentist or an oral surgeon.

Knocked-Out Tooth

A knocked-out tooth is a true dental emergency. It is also a common one. More than 90% of the two million teeth knocked out each year in the United States could be saved with proper treatment ▶Figure 10-11.

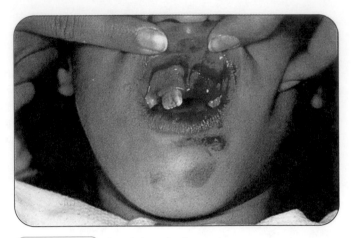

Figure 10-11 Tooth knocked out

Emergency care for knocked-out teeth has changed dramatically in recent years. The first question you want to ask when a tooth has been knocked out is, "Where is the tooth?" Time is crucial for successful reimplantation. A tooth that has been knocked out still has ligament fiber fragments attached to the tooth and the bone in the socket. These ligament fibers begin to die soon after the injury. Therefore, it is important to prevent the tooth from drying and to protect the ligament fibers from damage. Moisture alone is not sufficient because it does little to preserve the tooth's ligament fibers. Follow these steps to prevent dehydration and protect the fibers.

What to Do

1. Have the victim rinse his or her mouth, and put a rolled gauze pad in the socket to control bleeding.

2. Find the tooth and handle it by the crown, not the root, to minimize damage to the ligament fibers.

3. The best place for a knocked-out tooth is its socket. A tooth often can be successfully reimplanted if it is

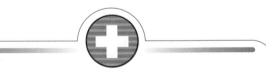

First Aid Tips

If you are in a remote area with no dentist nearby, you can make a temporary cap from melted candle wax or paraffin and a few strands of cotton. When the wax begins to harden but can still be molded, press a wad of it onto the tooth. Other improvisations include using ski wax or chewing gum (preferably sugarless).

replaced in its socket within 30 minutes after the injury; the odds of successful reimplantation decrease about 1% for every minute the tooth is absent from the socket.

Try to replace the tooth into the socket, using adjacent teeth as a guide. Push down on the tooth so the top is even with the adjacent teeth. Biting down gently on gauze is helpful.

Immediate reinsertion is not always possible, however. The victim may be reluctant to put the knocked-out tooth back into its socket, especially if it has fallen on the ground and is covered with debris. Or the tooth may repeatedly fall out, putting the victim at risk of inhaling or swallowing it. In victims with multiple trauma, the presence of more serious injuries may prevent reinsertion.

When immediate reinsertion is not feasible, one of the worst things you can do to a knocked-out tooth is to transport it dry. Consider using saliva for the short term (less than one hour). Milk is much better because of its calcium and magnesium concentrations. Ideally, the milk should be whole milk and kept cold to minimize bacterial growth. Do not use reconstituted powdered milk or milk by-products such as yogurt; they are damaging to the ligaments.

The best transport medium is Hank's solution, a balanced-pH cell-culture medium that helps restore the ligament fibers. The use of Hank's solution extends the viability of the ligament fibers for 6 to 12 hours. The solution, which is available commercially as the Save-a-Tooth™ kit, has been approved by the FDA for use up to 24 hours after an injury, and there is some evidence that using it enables successful reimplantation, even after 96 hours. The Save-a-Tooth™ kit is available in drugstores and deserves consideration as a standard item at schools and summer camps.

Some experts recommend that the tooth be placed in the victim's mouth to keep it moist until dental treatment is available. Do not use this method for children or others who may swallow the tooth.

4. Take the victim and the tooth to a dentist immediately.

Just getting the avulsed (knocked-out) tooth back into the socket, even if it is improperly placed, puts the tooth in a good physiologic environment that will only increase its viability.

Caution:

DO NOT handle a knocked-out tooth roughly.

DO NOT put a knocked-out tooth in water, mouthwash, alcohol, or Betadine.

DO NOT put a knocked-out tooth in skim milk, reconstituted powdered milk, or milk by-products such as yogurt.

DO NOT rinse a knocked-out tooth unless you are reinserting it in the socket.

DO NOT place a knocked-out tooth in anything that can dry or crush the outside of the tooth.

DO NOT scrub a knocked-out tooth or remove any attached tissue fragments.

DO NOT remove a partially extracted tooth. Push it back into place and seek a dentist so the loose tooth can be stabilized.

Broken Tooth

The front teeth are frequently broken by falls or direct blows. Such damage is not unusual in the victims of violent acts or automobile accidents. It is also common in children, especially those with an overbite (▼Figure 10-12).

What to Do

1. Gently clean dirt and blood from the injured area with a sterile gauze pad or a clean cloth and warm water.
2. Apply an ice pack on the face in the area of the injured tooth to decrease swelling.
3. If you suspect a jaw fracture, stabilize the jaw by wrapping a bandage under the chin and over the top of the head.
4. Seek a dentist immediately.

Figure 10-12 Broken teeth

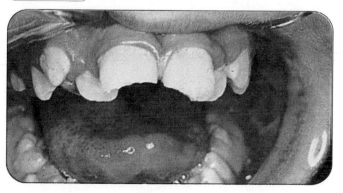

DENTAL INJURIES

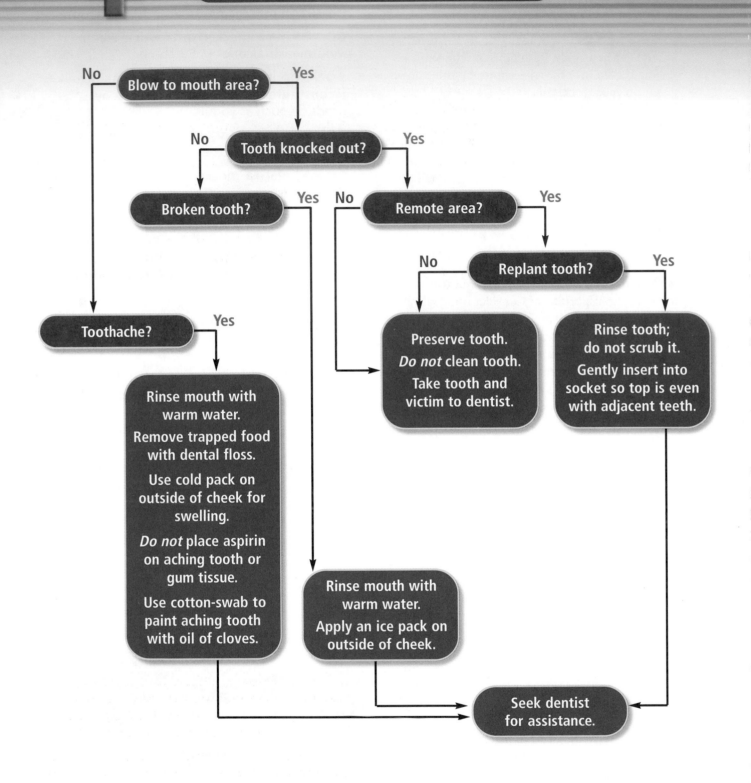

No — **Blow to mouth area?** — Yes

No — **Tooth knocked out?** — Yes

Broken tooth? — Yes

No — **Remote area?** — Yes

No — **Replant tooth?** — Yes

Toothache? — Yes

Rinse mouth with warm water.

Remove trapped food with dental floss.

Use cold pack on outside of cheek for swelling.

***Do not* place aspirin on aching tooth or gum tissue.**

Use cotton-swab to paint aching tooth with oil of cloves.

Preserve tooth.

***Do not* clean tooth.**

Take tooth and victim to dentist.

Rinse tooth; do not scrub it.

Gently insert into socket so top is even with adjacent teeth.

Rinse mouth with warm water.

Apply an ice pack on outside of cheek.

Seek dentist for assistance.

Dental Emergency Procedures

Toothache	Rinse the mouth vigorously with warm water to clean out debris. Use dental floss to remove any food that might be trapped between the teeth. **(Do not place aspirin on the aching tooth or gum tissues.)** See your dentist as soon as possible.
Orthodontic Problems (braces and retainers)	If a wire is causing irritation, cover the end of the wire with a small cotton ball, beeswax, or a piece of gauze until you can get to the dentist.
	If a wire is embedded in the cheek, tongue, or gum tissue, do not attempt to remove it. Go to your dentist immediately.
	If an appliance becomes loose or a piece of it breaks off, take the appliance and the piece and go to the dentist.
Knocked-Out Tooth	If the tooth is dirty, rinse it gently in running water. **Do not scrub it** or remove any attached tissue fragments.
	Gently insert and hold the tooth in its socket. If this is not possible, place the tooth in a container of milk or a special tooth-preserving solution.
	Go immediately to your dentist (within 30 minutes, if possible). Don't forget to bring the tooth.
Broken Tooth	Gently clean dirt or debris from the injured area by rinsing the mouth with warm water. Place cold compresses on the face, in the area of the injured tooth, to minimize swelling.
	Go to the dentist immediately.
Bitten Tongue or Lip	Apply direct pressure to the bleeding area with a clean cloth. If swelling is present, apply cold compresses. If bleeding does not stop, go to a hospital emergency room.
Object Wedged between Teeth	Try to gently remove the object with dental floss. Guide the floss and avoid cutting the gums. If not successful in removing the object, go to the dentist.
	Do not try to remove the object with a sharp or pointed instrument.
Possible Fractured Jaw	Immobilize the jaw by any means (necktie, dish towel). If swelling is present, apply cold compresses. Call your dentist or go immediately to a hospital emergency room.

Source: Copyright by the American Dental Association; reprinted with permission.

Toothache

The most common reason for toothaches is dental decay. Victims frequently complain of pain limited to one area of the mouth, although it can be more widespread—pain can also affect the ear, eye, neck, or even opposite side of the jaw. The tooth will be sensitive to heat and cold. Identify the diseased tooth by tapping the area with a spoon handle or similar object. A diseased tooth will hurt.

For pain relief, follow these steps:

1. Rinse the mouth with warm water to clean it out.

2. Use dental floss to remove any food that might be trapped between the teeth.

3. If you suspect a cavity, paint the tooth by using a small cotton swab soaked in oil of cloves (eugenol) to help suppress the pain. Take care to keep the oil off the gums, lips, and inside surfaces of the cheeks. If applicable, follow the same procedures as for a broken tooth.

4. Give the victim pain medication (aspirin, acetaminophen, or ibuprofen).

5. Seek a dentist immediately.

Caution:

DO NOT place pain medication (eg., aspirin, acetaminophen, or ibuprofen) on the aching tooth or gum tissues or allow them to dissolve in the mouth. A serious acid burn can result.

DO NOT cover a cavity with cotton if there is any pus discharge or facial swelling. See a dentist immediately.

DO NOT stick anything into an exposed cavity or into a softened exposed root.

Spinal Injuries

The spine is a column of vertebrae stacked one on the next from the skull's base to the tailbone. Each vertebra has a hollow center through which the spinal cord passes. The spinal cord consists of long tracts of nerves that join the brain with all the other body organs and parts.

If a broken vertebra pinches spinal nerves, paralysis can result. All unconscious victims should be treated as though they have a spinal injury. All conscious victims sustaining injuries from falls, diving accidents, or motor vehicle crashes should be carefully checked for a spinal injury before being moved. Suspect a spinal injury in all head-injury victims.

A mistake in the handling of a spinal injury victim could mean a lifetime in a wheelchair or a bed for the victim. Suspect a spinal injury whenever a significant mechanism of injury occurs.

What to Look for

Anytime there is a head injury, there may also be a spinal cord injury because the head may have been snapped suddenly in one or more directions. About 15% to 20% of head-injury victims also have a spinal injury. Other signs and symptoms include the following:

- Painful movement of the arms or legs
- Numbness, tingling, weakness, burning, or lessened sensation in the arms or legs
- Loss of bowel or bladder control
- Paralysis of the arms or legs
- Deformity (odd-looking angle of the victim's head and neck)

Ask a responsive victim these questions:

- *Is there pain?* Neck (cervical spine) injuries radiate pain to the arms; upper-back (thoracic spine) injuries radiate pain around the ribs; lower-back injuries usually radiate pain down the legs. Often, the victim will describe the pain as "electric."

- *Can you wiggle your fingers and squeeze my hand?* Moving the fingers is a sign that nerve pathways are intact. Ask the victim to grip your hand. A strong grip indicates that a spinal injury is unlikely.

- *Can you wiggle your toes and push your foot against my hand?* Moving the toes is a sign that nerve pathways are intact. Ask the victim to press a foot against your hand. If the victim cannot perform this movement or if the movement is extremely weak against your hand, the victim may have a spinal injury.

If the victim is unresponsive, do the following:

- Look for cuts, bruises, and deformities.

- Test responses by pinching the victim's hand (either palm or back of the hand) and bare foot (sole or top of the foot). No reaction could mean spinal cord damage.

Figure 10-13 Babinski test checks the nervous system (spinal cord and brain) for injury

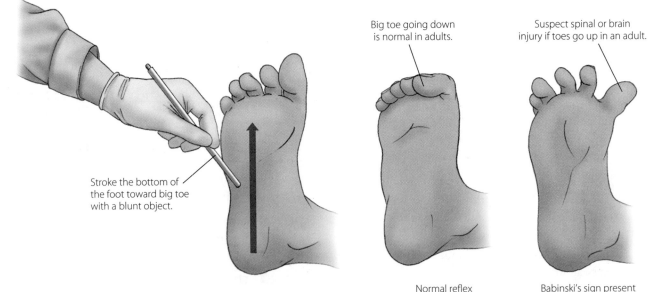

Stroke the bottom of the foot toward big toe with a blunt object.

Big toe going down is normal in adults.

Suspect spinal or brain injury if toes go up in an adult.

Normal reflex

Babinski's sign present

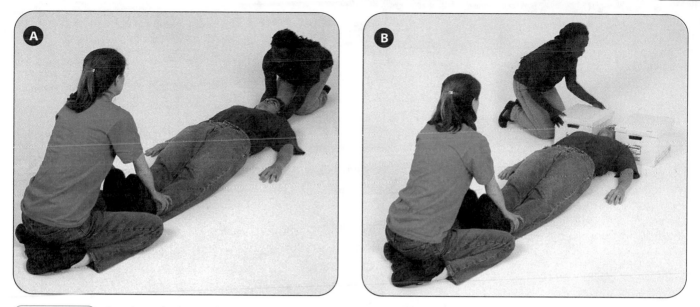

Figure 10-14 Steady and support the victim's head and neck as soon as possible. Have a bystander steady and support the feet. The head and feet should be continuously supported until medical help takes over.
A. Stabilize by holding head. Keep your arms steady by placing them on your thighs.
B. To free yourself to help others, place heavy objects on each side of the head

- Test the spinal cord by using the Babinski test: Stroke the bottom of the foot firmly toward the big toe with a key or similar sharp object. The body's normal response is to move the big toe down (except in infants). If the spinal cord or brain is injured, an adult's and child's big toe will flex upward (◀Figure 10-13).

- Ask bystanders what happened. If you still are not sure about a possible spinal injury, assume the victim has one until it is proved otherwise (▶Skill Scan).

What to Do

1. Check and monitor ABCs. For an unresponsive victim, use the procedures described on page 64 for opening the airway.

2. Stabilize the victim against any movement, using one of the following methods. Whichever method you use, tell the victim not to move.

- Grasp the victim's head over the ears and hold the head and neck still until the EMS arrives (▲Figure 10-14).

- If you anticipate a long wait for the EMS to arrive or if you are tired from holding the victim's head in place, kneel with the victim's head between your knees or place objects on each side of the victim's head to prevent it from rolling from side to side.

Caution:

DO NOT move the victim, even if the victim is in water. Wait for the EMS to arrive—they have the proper training and equipment. Victims with suspected spinal injury require cervical collars and stabilization on a spine board. It is better to do nothing than to mishandle a victim with a spinal injury.

SPINAL INJURIES

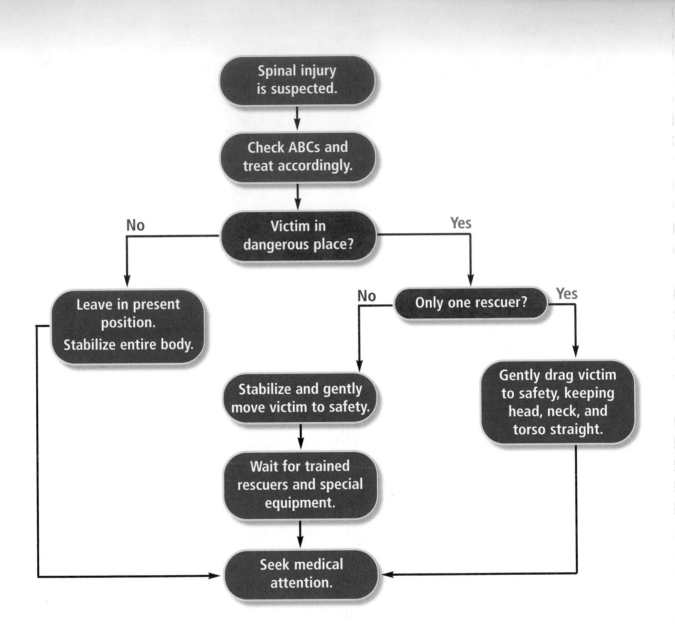

Skill Scan Checking for Spinal Injuries

Responsive Victim—Upper-Extremity Checks

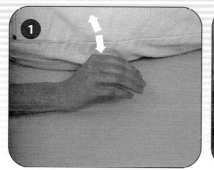 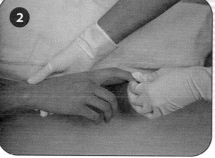 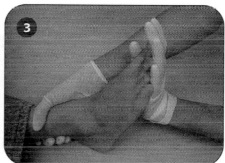

1. Victim wiggles fingers.

2. Rescuer squeezes fingers.

3. Victim squeezes rescuer's hand.

Responsive Victim—Lower-Extremity Checks Victim's failure to perform may mean spinal injury!

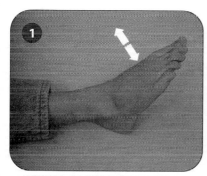 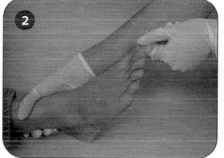 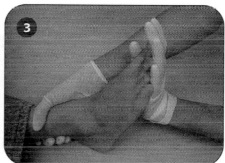

1. Victim wiggles toes.

2. Rescuer squeezes toes.

3. Victim pushes foot against rescuer's hand.

Unresponsive Victim

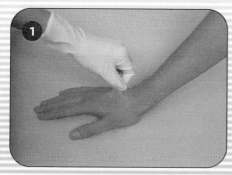 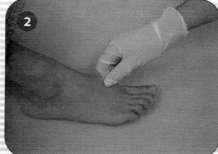

1. Pinch hand for response.

2. Pinch foot for response.

STUDY
Questions (10)

Name_____ Course_____ Date_____

Activities

Activity 1

Check (✓) the signs and symptoms of a skull fracture.

____ 1. pain at the injury site

____ 2. deformed skull

____ 3. fluid leaking from the ears or nose

____ 4. discoloration around the eye(s) (raccoon eyes)

____ 5. pupil of one eye larger than pupil of the other eye

Mark each sign yes (Y) or no (N).

After a head injury, which signs indicate a need for medical attention?

____ 6. Headache that lasts more than a day or increases in severity

____ 7. Vomiting that begins hours after the initial injury

____ 8. One pupil that appears larger than the other

____ 9. Convulsions or seizures

____ 10. "Seeing double"

Mark each statement as true (T) or false (F).

T F 11. A nosebleed victim should sit up with the head tilted back.

T F 12. A "halo sign" or "ring sign" results from a cerebrospinal fluid leak.

T F 13. Preserve a knocked-out tooth in mouthwash or rubbing alcohol.

T F 14. If it is necessary to bandage one eye, it is advisable to cover both eyes.

T F 15. If pupils are unequal in size, brain damage may exist.

T F 16. The first aider should not remove foreign objects embedded in an eyeball.

T F 17. To remove a foreign body from the surface of an eyeball, it is best to use cotton wrapped around a matchstick.

T F 18. Scalp wounds tend to bleed freely.

T F 19. Clear or blood-tinged fluid draining from the ears is a good indicator of a skull fracture.

T F 20. For a skull fracture, good first aid involves placing the victim's head lower than the rest of the body.

Check (✓) the signs and symptoms that indicate a possible spinal injury.

____ 21. description by the victim of pain down the arms or legs

____ 22. ability to strongly grip your hand and move a foot against your hand pressure

____ 23. a severe head injury

____ 24. inability of the victim to move fingers and toes when asked to do so

Mark each statement as true (T) or false (F).

T F 25. Do not move a victim unless extreme hazards exist (eg, burning building or car).

T F 26. Careless moving of a victim may permanently confine him or her to a wheelchair.

T F 27. Move a spinal injury victim as quickly as possible to a medical facility.

Activity 2

Mark each action yes (Y) or no (N).

Which is proper first aid for an object embedded in the eye?

____ 1. Use a damp sterile gauze or clean cloth to remove the object from the eyeball's surface.

____ 2. Use a toothpick or a matchstick to remove the foreign object.

____ 3. Use a paper cup or similar item over the eye but not touching the object.

____ 4. Allow the victim to see by leaving the uninjured eye uncovered.

Mark each statement as true (T) or false (F).

T F 5. Hitting the eye may cause a black eye.

T F 6. A victim with blurred vision should consult an ophthalmologist.

STUDY
Questions (10)

T F 7. For an eyeball knocked out of its socket, gently and carefully replace the eyeball in the socket and cover with a dressing.

T F 8. After a blow to the eye, apply a cold compress immediately for about 15 minutes to reduce pain and swelling.

Mark each action yes (Y) or no (N).

If a tree limb scrapes against an eye and cuts the eyeball, first aid, besides seeking medical help for the victim, would include:

___ 9. applying a dressing tightly over the injured eye

___ 10. holding the eyelids of the injured eye open

___ 11. applying direct pressure to the cut eyeball to control the bleeding

___ 12. loosely applying a dressing over both eyes

___ 13. tightly applying a dressing over both eyes

Choose the best answer.

___ 14. Corrosive acid has spilled into your co-worker's eyes, resulting in severe pain. What should you do first?
  a. Cover both eyes with dressings and immediately obtain medical aid.
  b. Allow tears to flush out the chemicals.
  c. Pour water into the eyes for about 20 minutes.

___ 15. Following your initial actions, what should you do?
  a. Place wet dressings over both eyes.
  b. Leave both eyes uncovered and seek medical attention.
  c. Allow the victim to rest for at least 30 minutes.
  d. Apply dressings over both eyes and seek medical attention.

Activity 3

In each pair, choose the better techniques for controlling most nosebleeds.

___ 1. a. Position victim in a sitting position.
     b. Position victim lying down.

___ 2. a. Keep the head tilted slightly backward.
     b. Keep the head tilted slightly forward.

___ 3. a. Pinch both nostrils for 5 minutes.
     b. Pinch only one nostril for 60 seconds.

___ 4. a. Always seek medical attention.
     b. Seek medical attention for victims taking blood thinners or large doses of aspirin and those with high blood pressure.

Case Situations
Case 1

During a football game, a player is knocked out for 10 minutes.

1. Define the term concussion.
_____
_____

2. List four signs of a concussion.
  a. _____
  b. _____
  c. _____
  d. _____

3. Give an example of a mental test you could use on a conscious victim.
_____
_____

4. When should the victim be allowed to return to activity?
_____
_____

Case 2

Several children are playing on a swing set. One child is hit on the forehead by another child coming back on a swing. The child is knocked several feet behind the swing set by the impact and appears dizzy, confused, and very weak. There is no bleeding. The child's pupils react slowly to light.

___ 1. You would most likely suspect
  a. a skull fracture
  b. a brain concussion
  c. both, since the signs and symptoms are almost identical

STUDY
Questions 10

2. First aid care for the child would include

a. _____
_____

b. _____
_____

c. _____
_____

d. _____
_____

_____ 3. With any head injury, always suspect:
a. The worst. Inform the parents the child may die.
b. Neck and spinal injury.
c. The best. No real emergency care is needed if there is no bleeding or other major sign of injury.

Case 3

During an automobile accident, a young female passenger is thrown from the back seat into the windshield. Her left eyelid is bleeding profusely, and the left eyeball appears to be bulging. Other injuries include a laceration of the forehead and bruises on her arms and legs.

1. What first aid should you provide to this victim?

a. _____
_____

b. _____
_____

c. _____
_____

d. _____
_____

2. Should both eyes be bandaged? (Explain why or why not.) yes _____ no _____

_____
_____
_____
_____

3. What special precautions should you take in caring for the avulsed eyeball?

a. _____
_____

b. _____
_____

Case 4

The victim of a motorcycle accident complains of loss of sensation in both lower extremities. You found him lying on his back with no other obvious injury. He is still wearing a helmet.

1. What should you suspect in this case?

_____
_____

2. What leads you to suspect this?

_____
_____

3. What is the correct first aid for this victim?

_____
_____

4. Should you move this victim?

_____
_____

5. When would you be justified in moving this victim?

_____
_____

Case 5

A child falls off a bike and knocks out a permanent tooth. The victim's dentist is minutes away. What are the proper procedures in this situation?

_____ 1. Rinse the child's mouth out with water and put a gauze pad on the socket to control bleeding.

_____ 2. Stick the tooth back in the child's tooth socket.

_____ 3. Scrub the dirt off the tooth in water and call your dentist.

_____ 4. Put the tooth in a glass of whole milk and take the child immediately to a dentist.

_____ 5. Depending on the child, have the child hold the tooth in his or her mouth with instructions not to swallow.

_____ 6. Place the tooth in a glass of mouthwash and take the child to a dentist.

_____ 7. Do not worry about the tooth, but take the child to a dentist.

STUDY
Questions (10)

Case 6

You and a friend have been cross-country skiing. Due to the sunlight reflection off the snow and not wearing dark goggles or glasses, your friend suffers light injuries to her eyes.

_____ 1. What other sources of light can produce this type of eye injury?

    a. looking at a welder's arc

    b. watching an eclipse of the sun

    c. reflection off large bodies of water

    d. all the above

_____ 2. Treatment for this injury would consist of

    a. applying moist dressings or eye patches to the closed eyes

    b. irrigating the eyes with a steady stream of water

    c. keeping both the victim's eyes closed

    d. irrigating the eyes with a saline solution

Chapter Activities

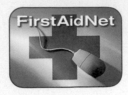

WEB Activities

Head and Spinal Injuries

Visit nsc.jbpub.com/FirstAidNet, then click on Web Activities, and select the appropriate chapter.

Brain Injury

Traumatic brain injury is one of the leading causes of injury and death among young people in the U.S. Severity can range from an athlete who has a minor concussion to a comatose state. Learn more about brain injury, including the signs and symptoms and the treatment.

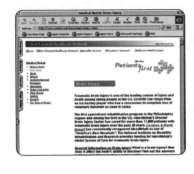

Spinal Injury

Spinal injuries can be devastating to both the victim and the victim's family. Learn about the physiological, psychological, and financial impact of spinal injury in America.

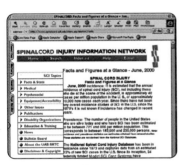

Chapter 11

Chest, Abdominal, and Pelvic Injuries

Chest Injuries

Chest injuries fall into two categories: those to the chest wall and those to the lungs. Injuries to the chest wall (the ribs) include:

- rib fracture
- flail chest

In a lung injury, one of the following conditions occurs:

- Blood fills up the chest, preventing complete lung expansion (**hemothorax**).
- Air fills a portion of the chest cavity (**pneumothorax**).
- Air in the chest cavity moves in and out; the lung does not expand (**open pneumothorax,** or "sucking chest wound").
- Air is pulled into the chest cavity but cannot exit, causing tension or pressures that reduce heart and lung function (**tension pneumothorax).**

All chest-injury victims should have their ABCs checked and rechecked. A responsive chest-injury victim should usually sit up or, if injury is on a side, be placed with the injured side down (▶Figure 11-1, A–B). That position prevents blood inside the chest cavity from seeping into the uninjured side and allows the uninjured side to expand.

Rib Fractures

The upper four ribs are rarely fractured because they are protected by the collarbone and the shoulder blades. Those ribs are so enmeshed by muscles that they rarely need to be splinted or realigned like other broken bones. The lower two ribs are hard to fracture because they are attached on only one end and have the freedom to move, which is why they are called "floating ribs". Broken ribs usually occur along the side of the chest. The main symptom of a rib fracture is pain at the injured rib site or when the victim breathes, coughs, moves, or when the area is touched.

CHEST INJURIES

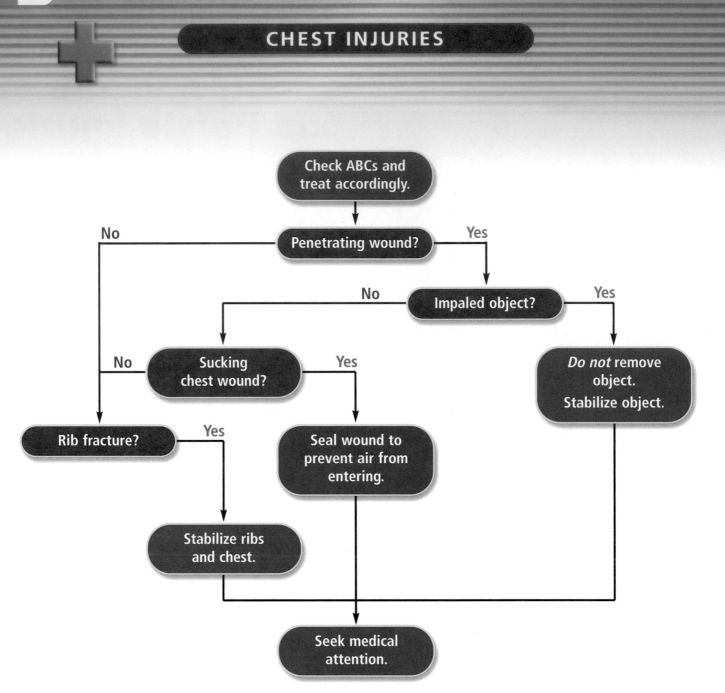

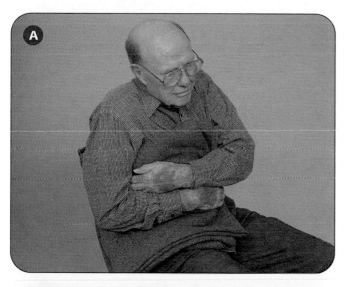

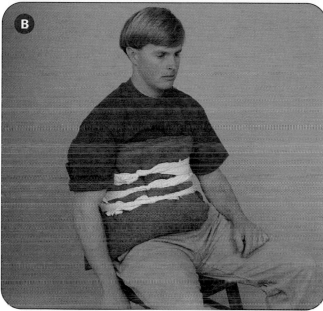

Figure 11-1, A–B Stabilize chest with soft object such as pillow, coat, or blanket (hold or tie). Tell victim to occasionally take a deep breath and to cough.

What to Do

1. Help the victim find a comfortable position. Stabilize the ribs by having the victim hold a pillow or other similar soft object against the injured area. Or use bandages to hold the pillow in place or tie an arm over the injured area. Do not apply tight bandages around the chest because this will restrict breathing.

2. Give pain medication.

3. Seek medical attention.

Flail Chest

A **flail chest** is a serious injury that involves several ribs in the same area broken in more than one place. The area over the injury may move in a direction opposite to that of the rest of the chest wall during breathing (known as "paradoxical movement"). This injury is very painful and makes breathing difficult.

What to Do

1. Support the chest by one of several methods:
   - Apply hand pressure. This is useful for a short time.
   - Place the victim on the injured side with a blanket or clothing underneath.

2. Monitor ABCs.

3. Seek medical attention.

Impaled Object in Chest
What to Do

1. Stabilize the object in place with several layers of bulky dressings or clothing. *Do not try to remove an impaled object*—bleeding and air in the chest cavity can result (▶Figure 11-2, A–B).

2. Seek medical attention.

Sucking Chest Wound

A sucking chest wound results when a chest wound allows air to pass into and out of the chest with each breath (▶Figure 11-3). Bubbles may be seen at the wound during exhalations and a sucking sound heard during inhalations.

What to Do

1. Seal the wound with anything available to stop air from entering the chest cavity. Plastic wrap or a plastic bag works well. Tape it in place, but leave one corner untaped. That creates a flutter valve to prevent air from being trapped in the chest cavity. If plastic wrap is not available, you can use your gloved hand.

2. If the victim has trouble breathing or seems to be getting worse, remove the plastic cover (or your hand) to let air escape, then reapply.

3. Seek medical attention.

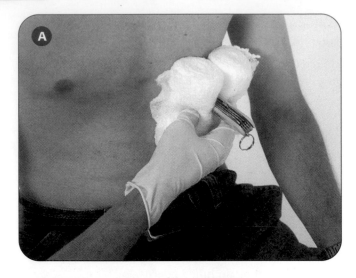

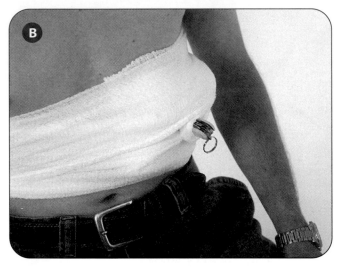

Figure 11-2, A–B Stabilize penetrating object with bulky padding. Secure padding and object.

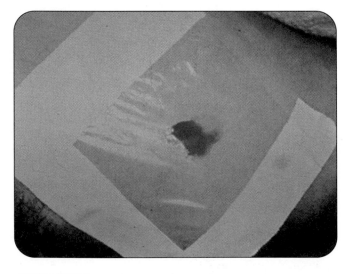

Figure 11-3 Sucking chest wound

Abdominal Injuries

Abdominal injuries have two components: what you can see (external or open) and what you cannot see (internal or closed). An internal abdominal injury is one of the most frequently unrecognized injuries; when missed, it becomes one of the main causes of death.

A hollow-organ rupture (eg, of the stomach or intestines) spills the contents of the organ into the abdominal cavity, causing inflammation. Solid-organ rupture (eg, of the liver or pancreas) results in severe bleeding.

Blow to the Abdomen

Bruising and damage to internal organs can result from a severe blow to the abdomen. Examine by gently pressing all four quadrants of the abdomen with your fingertips. Observe for pain, tenderness, muscle tightness, or rigidity. Normal abdomens are soft and not tender when pressed.

What to Do

1. Place the victim on one side in a comfortable position and expect vomiting. Do not give the victim any food or drink. If you are hours from a medical facility, allow the victim to suck on a clean cloth soaked in water to relieve a dry mouth.
2. Seek medical attention.

Penetrating Wound

Expect internal organs to be damaged.

What to Do

1. If the penetrating object is still in place, stabilize the object and control bleeding by using bulky dressings around it. ***Do not try to remove the object.***
2. Seek medical attention.

Protruding Organs
What to Do

1. Cover protruding organs with a moist sterile dressing or clean cloth.
2. Cover the area with a towel or blanket to maintain warmth.
3. Seek medical attention (►Figure 11-4).

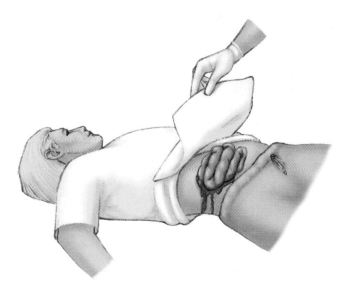

Figure 11-4 Do not reinsert protruding organs. Cover them with a moist, sterile dressing.

Pelvic Injuries

Pelvic fractures are usually caused by falls, crushing accidents, or sharp blows. Severe pain, shock, internal bleeding, and loss of the ability to use the lower extremities may be present. The bladder, as well as other organs that are protected by the pelvis, may be injured or ruptured. Victims may have massive internal bleeding.

If you must move the victim and are concerned about whether the victim's pelvis is fractured, gently press the sides of the pelvis downward and squeeze them inward at the iliac crests (upper points of the hips). A fractured pelvis will be painful. If the victim is already complaining of pain, do not apply pressure. If you suspect that the pelvis is fractured, there may also be a spinal injury.

What to Do

1. Treat the victim for shock.
2. Place padding between the victim's thighs, then tie the victim's knees and ankles together. If the knees are bent, place padding under them for support.
3. Keep the victim on a firm surface.
4. Seek medical attention.

Pelvic Fractures

A pelvic fracture should be suspected in anyone with pelvic pain on movement or with pushing and/or squeezing of the pelvis. Motor vehicle collisions, being struck by a motor vehicle, falls, and bicycle/motorcycle crashes are common causes of pelvic injury. It is important to suspect pelvic injuries because they can result in massive blood loss. Unstable pelvic bones can cause continued arterial and venous bleeding that can go unnoticed. Splinting is necessary. Laypersons should stabilize the victim and wait for the EMS ambulance with its trained personnel and equipment to transport the victim to a hospital emergency department.

Rib Fractures

Fractured ribs are a common injury and most frequently occur between ribs three and 10. The location for most fractures is on the sides of the body. The first two pairs of ribs are protected by the clavicles, while the last two pairs move freely and will give with an impact. Little can be done to assist the healing of broken ribs other than binding them to restrict movement. Tightly binding the chest limits breathing and because exhalation is inadequate, fluid accumulates in the air sacs (alveoli) and can result in pneumonia. This often explains pneumonia deaths in elderly persons.

ABDOMINAL INJURIES

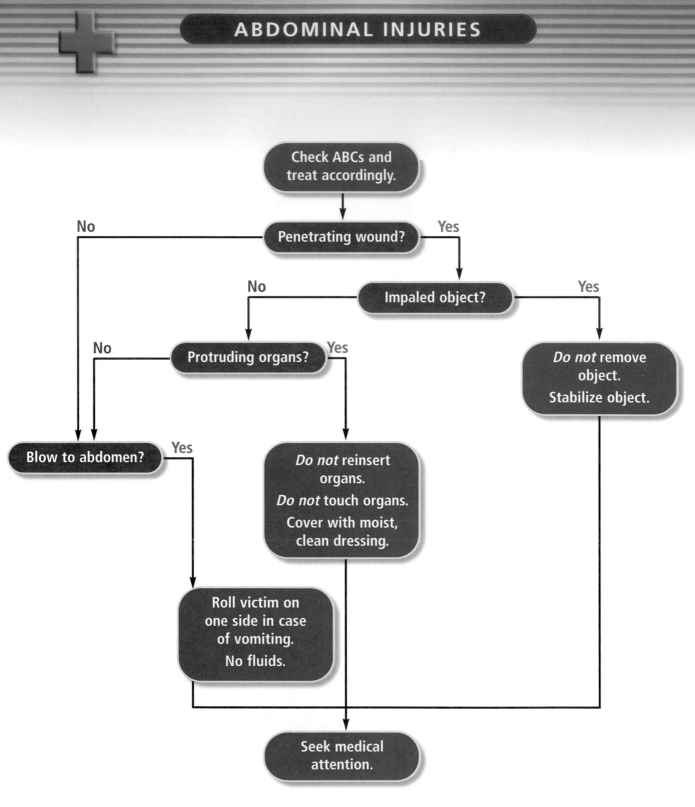

STUDY
Questions (11)

Name_____ Course_____ Date_____

Activities
Activity 1
Check (✓) the appropriate action(s).

1. Which of the following actions serve(s) as effective immediate first aid for a sucking chest wound?
   ____ **a.** Remove a penetrating object from the chest.
   ____ **b.** Apply a sterile or clean dressing loosely over the wound.
   ____ **c.** Leave the wound uncovered.
   ____ **d.** Tape a piece of plastic over the wound.

2. If the victim has trouble breathing after you have taped a piece of plastic over a sucking chest wound, you should:
   a. apply a second piece of plastic over the first.
   ____ **b.** make certain one side of the dressing is left untaped to allow air to escape from the chest cavity and then reapply.

____ 3. The first step in first aid for a sucking chest wound is to
   a. not cover the wound
   b. cover the hole immediately to prevent air from entering the chest

____ 4. First aid for a flail chest is to
   a. stabilize the injured chest wall
   b. not bind the injured chest since binding interferes with breathing

____ 5. Which of the following materials, when taped at the edges, would make an effective covering for a sucking chest wound?
   a. clear plastic wrap
   b. a large gauze dressing
   c. a wash cloth
   d. a pillow case

____ 6. Signs and symptoms of flail chest include:
   a. blood oozing from the injury site
   b. pain when breathing
   c. neck injury
   d. abnormal movement of part of the chest wall during breathing

Activity 2
Which is proper first aid for a blow to the abdomen if you suspect internal injuries?

____ 1. **a.** Place the victim on his or her back with a support on the abdomen.
   b. Place the victim on his or her side.

____ 2. **a.** Give the victim ice chips or sips of water to drink.
   b. Give the victim nothing to eat or drink.

Select the best first aid choice for treating an open abdominal wound resulting from a penetrating object.

____ 3. **a.** Remove the penetrating object.
   b. Leave the object in place and stabilize it.

When protruding organs appear through an abdominal wound, you should

____ 4. **a.** gently push the organs back into the abdomen
   b. not attempt to push them back into the abdomen

____ 5. **a.** cover the wound with a clean, moist dressing
   b. cover the wound with a cotton dressing

Mark each statement as true (T) or false (F).

T F 6. Reinsert any protruding intestines or organs into open wounds of the abdomen

T F 7. A dressing for exposed intestines should be kept dry if possible.

T F 8. In a penetrating wound of the chest, the object should be left in place.

Activity 3

1. List two procedures you would use to check for a pelvic fracture.
   a. _____
   b. _____

2. Name two things you can do for a person with a fractured pelvis.
   a. _____
   b. _____

Chapter Activities

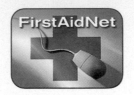

WEB Activities

Chest, Abdominal, and Pelvic Injuries

Visit nsc.jbpub.com/First AidNet, then click on Web Activities, and select the appropriate chapter.

Chest Trauma

Explore a case study of a 25 year old man who sustained a gunshot wound to the right chest. Learn more about the signs, symptoms, and treatment for life-threatening chest trauma.

Impaled Object

Examine a detailed case study of a 60 year old man involved in a motor vehicle crash in which a tree branch became impaled in his abdomen. Learn more about the treatment for impaled objects.

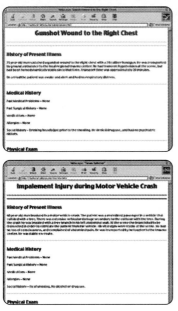

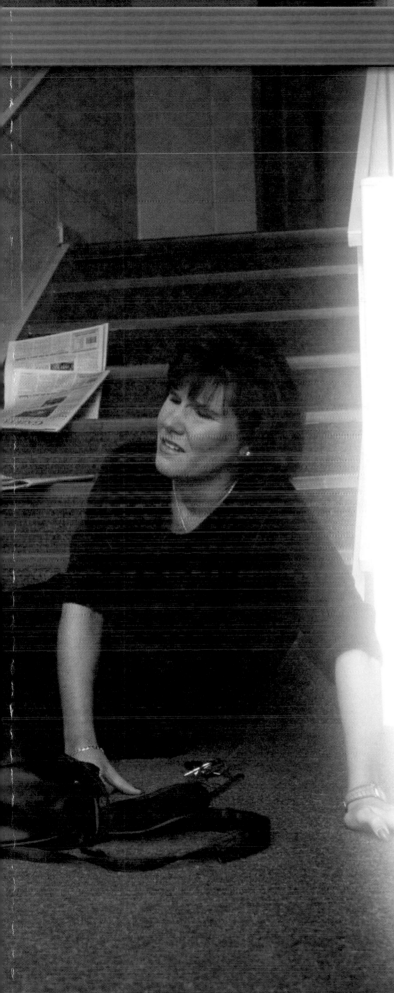

Chapter 12

Bone, Joint, and Muscle Injuries

Fractures

The real problems are not the broken bones themselves but the potential injury to the vital organs next to them. People do not die of broken bones. They die from airway obstructions, blood loss, and brain injuries. However, broken bones can be painful and debilitating, and can cause life-long aggravation, disability, and deformity.

The terms **fracture** and **broken bone** have the same meaning: a break or crack in a bone. There are two categories of fractures:

- **Closed (simple) fracture.** The skin is intact and no wound exists anywhere near the fracture site (▶Figure 12-1 A).
- **Open (compound) fracture.** The skin over the fracture has been damaged or broken. The wound may result from the bone's protruding through the skin or from a direct blow that cut the skin at the time of the fracture. The bone may not always be visible in the wound (▶Figure 12-1 B).

"The broken bone, once set together, is stronger than ever."

John Lyly Euphues

It is not possible to determine the exact nature of a broken bone outside a medical facility. It may be helpful, however, for first aiders to be familiar with the terminology that physicians use to describe fractures (▶Figure 12-2). A **transverse fracture** cuts across the bone at right angles to its long axis and is often caused by direct injury. **Greenstick fractures** are incomplete fractures that commonly occur in children, whose bones (like green sticks) are pliable. A spiral fracture usually results from a twisting injury, and the fracture line has the appearance of a spring. The fracture line of an **oblique fracture** crosses the bone at an oblique angle, or in a slanting direction. In an **impacted fracture**, the broken ends of the bone are jammed together and the bone may function as if no

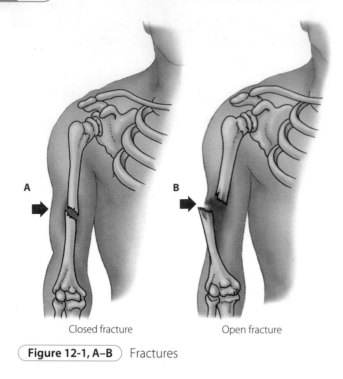

Closed fracture   Open fracture

Figure 12-1, A–B Fractures

fracture were present. A **comminuted fracture** is one in which the bone is fragmented into more than two pieces (ie, splintered or crushed).

What to Look for

It may be difficult to tell if a bone is fractured ▶**Figure 12-3** . When in doubt, treat the injury as

a fracture. Use the mnemonic DOTS in assessing for an injury—**D**eformity, **O**pen wound, **T**enderness, **S**welling.

- *Deformity* might not be obvious. Compare the injured part with the uninjured part on the other side.
- *Open wound* may indicate an underlying fracture.
- *Tenderness* and pain are commonly found only at the injury site. The victim usually will be able to point to the site of the pain. A useful procedure for detecting a fracture is to gently feel along the bone; a victim's complaint about pain or tenderness serves as a reliable sign of a fracture.
- *Swelling* caused by bleeding happens rapidly after a fracture.

Additional signs and symptoms include the following:

- *Loss of use* may or may not occur. "Guarding" occurs when motion produces pain; the victim refuses to use the injured part. Sometimes, however, the victim is able to move a fractured limb with little or no pain.
- A *grating sensation*, called **crepitus,** can be felt and sometimes even heard when the ends of the broken bone rub together. Do *not* move the injured limb in an attempt to detect it ▶**Figure 12-4** .
- *The history of the injury* can lead you to suspect a fracture whenever a serious accident has happened. The victim may have heard or felt the bone snap.

Figure 12-2 Types of fractures

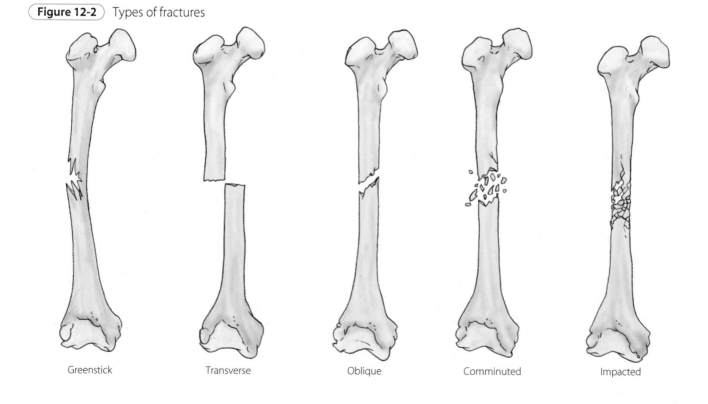

Greenstick   Transverse   Oblique   Comminuted   Impacted

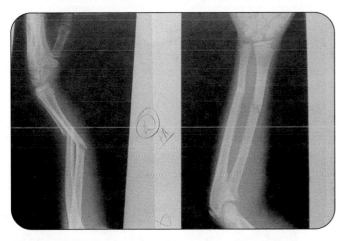

Figure 12-3 X-rays of victim with forearm fracture before and after setting

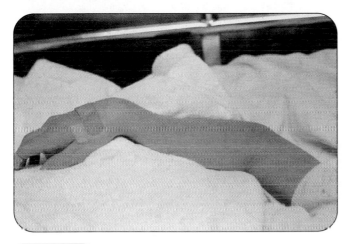

Figure 12-4 Forearm fracture

What to Do

1. Check and treat ABCs. A fracture, even an open fracture, seldom presents an immediate threat to life. Therefore, treatment should be deferred until after you have handled any life-threatening conditions such as opening an airway or controlling massive bleeding. A tourniquet is practically never necessary to treat an open fracture, even when an extremity has been mangled beyond all possibility of salvage or a limb has been amputated. Only when all life-threatening conditions have been dealt with is it appropriate to identify and stabilize fractures.

2. Determine what happened and the location of the injury.

3. Gently remove clothing covering the injured area. Cut clothing at the seams if necessary.

4. Examine the area by looking and feeling for DOTS previously described.

- Look at the injury site. Swelling and black-and-blue marks, which indicate escape of blood into the tissues, may come from either the bone end or associated muscular and blood vessel damage. Shortening or severe deformity (angulation) between the joints or deformity around the joints, shortening of the extremity, and rotation of the extremity when compared with the opposite extremity indicate a bone injury. Lacerations or even small puncture wounds near the site of a bone fracture are considered open fractures.

- Feel the injured area. If a fracture is not obvious, gently press, touch, or feel along the length of the bone for deformities, tenderness, and swelling ▼**Figure 12-5**.

5. Check blood flow and nerves. Use the mnemonic CSM (circulation, sensation, movement) as a way of remembering what to do Skill Scan.

- *Circulation.* For an arm injury, feel for the radial pulse (located on the thumb side of the wrist); use the posterior tibial pulse (located between the inside ankle bone and the Achilles tendon) for a leg injury. A pulseless arm or leg is a significant emergency that requires immediate surgical care. If there is no pulse, gently manipulate the extremity to try to restore the blood flow.

  If the victim is under 6 years of age, some experts recommend the capillary refill test. (Press on a fingernail or toenail, then release it. If circulation is normal, the nail bed should return to its normal color within two seconds.) Others, however, note that performing the capillary refill test in the dark or the cold may limit its accuracy.

- *Sensation.* This is the most useful early sign. Lightly touch or squeeze one of the victim's toes

Figure 12-5 Open tibia, fibula fracture

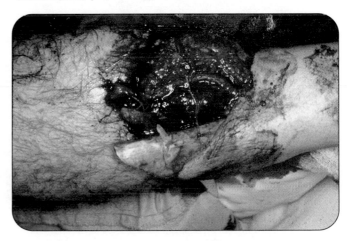

Skill Scan

Checking an Extremity's CSM

Check an Upper Extremity for:

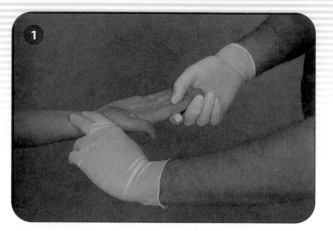

1. Circulation—radial pulse.

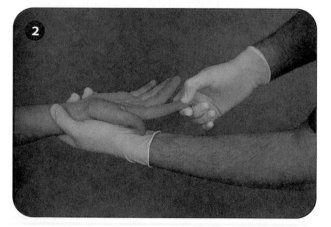

2. Sensation—squeeze fingers.

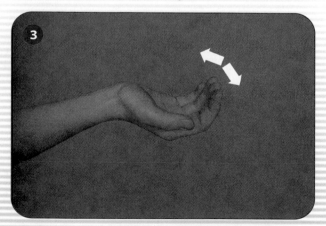

3. Movement—wiggle fingers.

Check a Lower Extremity for:

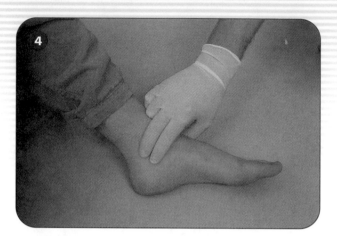

1. Circulation—posterial tibial pulse.

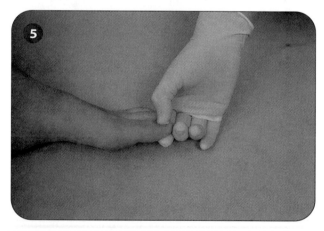

2. Sensation—squeeze toes.

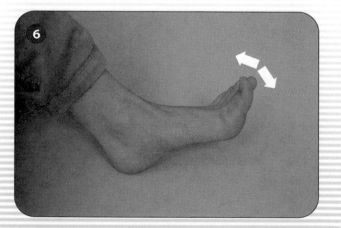

3. Movement—wiggle toes.

or fingers and ask the victim what he or she feels. Loss of sensation is an early sign of nerve damage.

- *Movement.* Inability to move develops later. Check for nerve damage by asking the victim to wiggle his or her toes or fingers. If the toes or fingers are injured, do not have the victim attempt to move them.

A quick nerve and circulatory check is very important. The most serious complication of a fracture is inadequate blood flow in an extremity. The major blood vessels of an extremity tend to run close to the bones, which means that any time a bone is broken, the adjacent blood vessels are at risk of being torn by bone fragments or pinched off between the ends of the broken bone. The tissues of the arms and legs cannot survive for more than two or three hours without a continuing blood supply. If you note any disruption in the nerve and circulatory supply, seek immediate medical attention. Major nerve pathways also travel close to bone and may be torn or pinched off between the ends of the broken bone.

6. Use the RICE procedures (see Chapter 13).
7. Use a splint to stabilize the fracture (see Chapter 14).
8. Give pain medication.
9. Seek medical attention.

Joint Injuries

A joint is where two or more bones come together.

Dislocations

A **dislocation** occurs when a joint comes apart and stays apart with the bone ends no longer in contact. The shoulders, elbows, fingers, hips, kneecaps (patellas), and ankles are the joints most frequently affected. Dislocations cause signs and symptoms similar to those of fractures: deformity, severe pain, swelling, and the inability of the victim to move the injured joint. The main sign of a dislocation is deformity. Its appearance will be different from an uninjured joint (▶Figure 12-6).

What to Do

1. Check the CSM (circulation, sensation, movement). If the end of the dislocated bone is pressing on nerves or blood vessels, numbness or paralysis may exist below the dislocation. Always check the pulses. If there is no pulse in the injured extremity, transport the victim to a medical facility immediately.

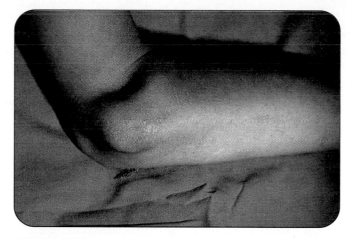

Figure 12-6 Dislocation

2. Use the RICE procedures (see Chapter 13).
3. Use a splint to stabilize the joint in the position in which it was found (see Chapter 14).
4. Do not try to **reduce** the joint (put the displaced parts back into their normal positions), because nerve and blood vessel damage could result. Experts in wilderness medicine have identified easy and safe ways to treat the following dislocations when medical help is more than one hour away: kneecap, fingers and toes, and anterior shoulder. See Chapter 22 for details.
5. Seek medical attention to reduce the dislocation.

Sprains

A **sprain** is an injury to a joint in which the ligaments and other tissues are damaged by violent stretching or twisting. The ankles and the knees are the joints most often sprained. In sports, 85% of all ankle injuries are sprains. Attempts to move or use the joint increase the pain. The skin around the joint may be discolored because of bleeding from torn tissues. It is often difficult to distinguish between a severe sprain and a fracture, because their signs and symptoms are similar (see page 210).

Ankle sprains most often occur when the foot turns inward and stress is placed on the outside (lateral side) of the ankle. A severe lateral ankle sprain, if not correctly treated, can result in a chronically unstable ankle that is prone to sprains. Any ligament or bone injury on the inner side of the ankle usually represents a serious problem and requires medical attention.

The goal of sprain care is to prevent further injury to the torn ligaments. Initial treatment consists of Rest, Ice, Compression, and Elevation (RICE; see Chapter 13). Swelling is like glue and can lock up a joint in a matter of hours. It is vitally important to keep a joint from swelling by using cold promptly; it is even more important to make the swelling recede as quickly as possible with a compression (elastic) bandage.

Muscle Injuries

Although muscle injuries pose no real emergency, first aiders have ample opportunities to care for them.

Strains

A normal, warmed-up muscle is much like a rubber band. When stretched, it will not snap. When a cold or tight muscle is stretched, however, there is a likelihood that it will tear. A muscle **strain,** also known as a muscle pull, occurs when a muscle is stretched beyond its normal range of motion, which tears the muscle. When muscle fibers tear, fluid from nearby tissues leaks out and starts to build up near the injury. The area becomes inflamed, swollen, and tender. Inflammation begins immediately after an injury, but it can take 24 to 72 hours for enough tissue fluid to build up to cause pain and stiffness.

What to Look for

Any of the following signs and symptoms may indicate a muscle strain:

- sharp pain
- extreme tenderness when the area is touched
- cavity, indentation, or bump that can be felt or seen
- severe weakness and loss of function of the injured part
- stiffness and pain when the victim moves the muscle

What to Do

Use the RICE procedures—Rest, Ice, Compression, and Elevation (see Chapter 13 for detailed discussion).

Contusions

A muscle **contusion,** or **bruise,** results from a blow to the muscle.

What to Look for

Any of the following signs and symptoms may occur in a muscle contusion:

- swelling
- pain and tenderness
- black-and-blue mark appearing hours later

What to Do

Use the RICE procedures—Rest, Ice, Compression, and Elevation (see Chapter 13 for detailed discussion).

Cramps

A cramp occurs when a muscle goes into an uncontrolled spasm and contraction, resulting in severe pain and restriction or loss of movement. Although scientific literature has yet to confirm the causes of muscle cramps, several factors are associated with them. For example, muscle cramping is associated with certain diseases such as diabetes and atherosclerosis. Muscle cramps are often, but not always, associated with physical activity and can be roughly divided into two categories: night cramps, which include any cramp occurring while an individual is at rest, and heat cramps, which are related to dehydration and electrolyte imbalance. (The electrolytes potassium and sodium carry an electric charge that helps trigger muscles to contract and relax.)

What to Do

There are many treatments for cramps. Try one or more of the following:

1. Have the victim gently stretch the affected muscle. Because a muscle cramp is an uncontrolled muscle contraction or spasm, a gradual extension of the muscle may help lengthen the muscle fibers and relieve the cramp.
2. Relax the muscle by applying pressure to it.
3. Apply ice to the cramped muscle to make it relax (unless you are in a cold environment).
4. Pinch the upper lip hard (an acupressure technique) to reduce calf-muscle cramping.
5. Drink lightly salted cool water (dissolve $1/4$ teaspoon salt in a quart of water) or a commercial sports drink.

> **Caution:**
>
> **DO NOT** give salt tablets to a person with muscle cramps. They can cause stomach irritation, nausea, and vomiting.
>
> **DO NOT** massage or rub the affected muscle. This only causes more pain and does not relieve the cramping.

STUDY
Questions (12)

Name_____ Course_____ Date_____

Activities

Activity 1

Mark each statement as true (T) or false (F).

T F   **1.** A strain is an overstretching of ligaments.

T F   **2.** Sprains involve joints.

T F   **3.** Dislocations involve joints.

Choose the best answer.

____   **4.** An open fracture is one in which
    a. there is bruising on the skin.
    b. an open wound exists.
    c. a traction splint is required.

____   **5.** First aid for strains is
    a. ice packs
    b. warm, wet packs
    c. warm, dry packs

____   **6.** First aid for a dislocated shoulder is
    a. repositioning
    b. stabilization
    c. bandaging
    d. traction

____   **7.** Fractures, dislocations, and sprains should be treated initially with
    a. a hot water bag
    b. an ice pack
    c. a saltwater solution
    d. a dressing

____   **8.** What is the main sign of a dislocation?
    a. deformity
    b. swelling
    c. an open wound
    d. tenderness

____   **9.** A complete rupture or tear of a ligament is a
    a. muscle strain
    b. dislocation
    c. sprain

____   **10.** Most ankle sprains occur when the foot turns _____ and stress is placed on the _____ of the ankle
    a. inward, outside
    b. inward, inside
    c. outward, outside
    d. outward, inside

11. List and briefly describe the two main types of fractures:
    a. _____
    b. _____

12. List five signs of a fracture:
    a. _____
    b. _____
    c. _____
    d. _____
    e. _____

13. What does the mnemonic CSM stand for? What should you do for each step?
    C – _____
    S = _____
    M = _____

14. What is the capillary refill test?
_____
_____

15. Why is it no longer recommended as a first aid procedure?
_____
_____

Activity 2

Mark each statement as true (T) or false (F).

T F   **1.** A muscle injury is a real emergency.

T F   **2.** A muscle strain and a muscle pull are the same injury.

T F   **3.** A muscle strain can involve the tearing of a muscle.

T F   **4.** The result of a blow to a muscle is also known as a bruise.

Check (✓) the appropriate actions to relieve leg muscle cramps.

____   **5.** Drink a commercial sports drink.

____   **6.** Take salt tablets.

____   **7.** Gently stretch the affected muscle.

____   **8.** Apply ice to the cramped muscle.

Chapter Activities

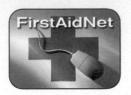

WEB Activities

Bone, Joint, and Muscle Injuries

Visit nsc.jbpub.com/FirstAidNet, then click on Web Activities, and select the appropriate chapter.

Broken Bones Quiz

Quiz yourself on broken bones, then read your results immediately! How did you do?

Growth Plate Injury

In a growing child, a serious injury to a joint is more likely to damage a growth plate, the area of developing tissue near the end of the long bones in children and adolescents. Injury to the growth plate can have serious consequences to the growing child. Learn more about growth plate injuries.

Shoulder Injuries and Surgery

The extreme range of motion of the shoulder makes it highly susceptible to injury. Learn more about the anatomy, signs and symptoms of injury, and emergency and hospital treatment of shoulder injuries.

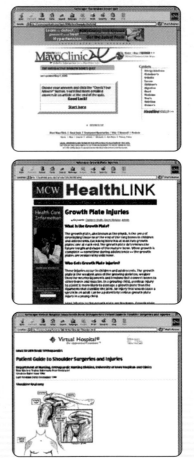

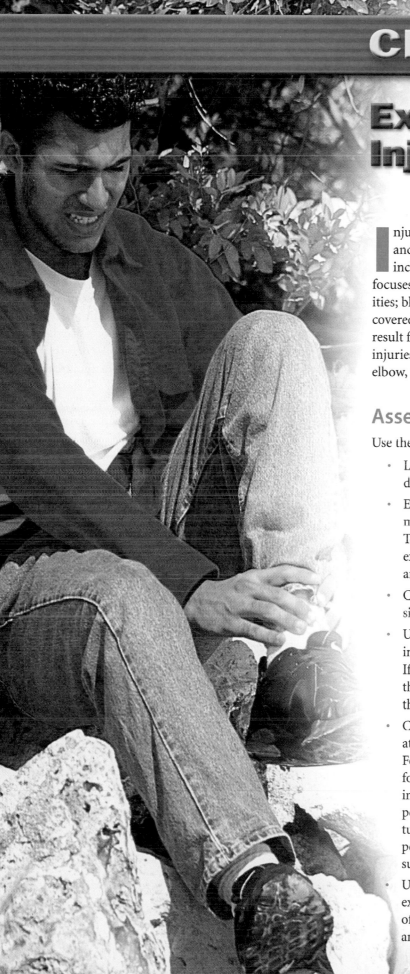

Chapter 13

Extremity Injuries

njuries to the extremities are common because more and more people are involved in active lifestyles that include sports and wilderness activities. This chapter focuses on bone, joint, and muscle injuries of the extremities; bleeding, wounds, and other soft-tissue injuries are covered elsewhere. Most of the conditions discussed here result from sudden trauma, although some chronic injuries incurred over a period of time, such as tennis elbow, are included.

Assessment

Use these guidelines to assess injuries to the extremities:

- Look for signs and symptoms of fractures and dislocations (see Chapter 12).

- Examine the extremities, keeping in mind the mnemonic D-O-T-S (Deformity, Open wound, Tenderness, Swelling). Look at and gently feel the extremity, starting at the distal end (fingers or toes) and working upward.

- Compare one extremity with the other to determine size and shape differences.

- Use the "rule of thirds" for extremity injuries. Imagine each long bone as being divided into thirds. If deformity, tenderness, or swelling is located in the upper or lower third of a long bone, assume that the nearest joint is injured.

- Consider the mechanism of injury (MOI) in evaluating the possibility of a fracture and its location. Forces that cause musculoskeletal injuries are direct forces (eg, a car bumper strikes a pedestrian's tibia), indirect forces along the long axis of bones (eg, a person falls onto his or her outstretched hand, fracturing the clavicle), and twisting forces (eg, a person's foot is fixed in one spot while the leg is suddenly twisted).

- Use the mnemonic CSM as a reminder to check the extremity for circulation, sensation, and movement of fingers or toes. Without adequate blood flow into an extremity, amputation may result.

Types of Injuries

There are many types of injuries to the extremities, ranging from simple contusions to complex open fractures:

- **contusions,** or bruising of the tissue
- **strains,** in which muscles are stretched or torn
- **sprains,** which involve tearing or stretching of the joints, causing mild to severe damage to the ligaments and joint capsules
- **dislocations,** in which bones are displaced from their normal joint alignment, out of their sockets, or out of their normal positions
- **fractures,** which are breaks in bones that may or may not be accompanied by open wounds
- **tendinitis,** which is inflammation of a tendon from overuse

First Aid

- Use the RICE procedures (see page 227) for injuries described in this chapter.
- Apply a splint to stabilize fractures and dislocations (see Chapter 14 for specific techniques).

Shoulder Injuries

Shoulder Dislocation (Separation)

Three bones come together at the shoulder: the scapula (shoulder bone), the clavicle (collarbone), and the humerus (upper arm bone). The shoulder is the most freely movable joint in the body. The extreme range of all its possible movements makes the shoulder joint highly susceptible to dislocation. A dislocation of the shoulder occurs when the different bones of the shoulder come apart as a result of a blow or a particular movement. Shoulder dislocation is second in frequency only to finger dislocations.

What to Look for

- In about 95% of shoulder dislocations, the victim holds the upper arm away from the body, supported by the uninjured arm. This position differentiates a dislocation from a fracture of the humerus, in which the victim holds the arm against the chest.
- The dislocated arm cannot be brought across the chest wall to touch the opposite shoulder (ie, in the sling position).

- The victim has extreme pain in the shoulder area.
- In a dislocation, the shoulder is squared off, rather than rounded.
- An injury to the shoulder resulting in complete loss of function is more apt to be a dislocation than a fracture.
- The victim may describe a history of previous dislocations.

Clavicle Fracture

Fractures of the clavicle (collarbone) are common and usually are the result of falling with the arm and hand outstretched. The victim falls onto his or her hand, and the force from the fall is transmitted to the shoulder. Most (80%) clavicle fractures occur in the middle third of the bone. Usually the fracture is easy to detect because the clavicle lies immediately under the skin and a deformity can be seen. You generally can feel a clavicle fracture by running a finger along the bone and noting a deformed, tender, or swollen area.

With a clavicle fracture, the victim usually holds the injured arm against the chest to stabilize the injury. The shoulder on the injured side may droop forward.

Contusions

Blows that cause contusions, or bruises, about the shoulder result in pain, swelling, sometimes black-and-blue marks, and restricted arm movement. Often called "shoulder pointers," contusions of this type may cause the victim severe discomfort.

Tendinitis (Painful Shoulder)

The general cause of tendinitis in the shoulder is continuous overuse. Repeated arm movement, as in many of the throwing sports such as baseball and in other sports where the shoulder is used extensively such as swimming, often results in painful shoulders.

Humerus (Upper-Arm) Fracture

The shaft of the humerus can be felt throughout its entire length along the inner side of the upper arm. Pain and tenderness at the fracture site and an obvious deformity may be present. The deformity may be hidden by swelling or by the large muscles surrounding the upper part of the arm. The victim may be unable to move the arm. The victim will be holding the upper arm against the chest for comfort.

Elbow Injuries

A deformity is obvious when a seriously injured elbow is compared with the uninjured elbow. Restricted, painful motion also is present.

All elbow injuries should be considered serious and treated with extreme care. Inappropriate care can result in injury to the nearby nerves and blood vessels.

Tennis Elbow

Tennis elbow results from sharp, quick twists of the wrist (not just from playing tennis). The muscles that bend the wrist back and straighten the fingers all begin in one spot, no bigger than a dime, on the outside bony protrusion, or bump, of the elbow. Tennis elbow, which is an inflammation of the tendons on this outer side of the elbow, can be very painful whenever the wrist and the elbow are used.

Little Leaguer's Elbow

This injury is the equivalent of the more common tennis elbow but with pain on the inside of the elbow. It is a tendinitis (inflammation) of the tendons attached to the bony protrusion, or bump, on the inside of the elbow.

Radius and Ulna (Forearm) Fractures

There are two large bones (radius and ulna) in the forearm, and either one or both bones may be broken. When only one bone is broken, the other acts as a splint and there may be little or no deformity. However, a marked deformity may be present in a fracture near the wrist. When both bones are broken, the arm usually appears deformed. In any fracture of the forearm, pain, tenderness, swelling, and inability to use the forearm may be present. Suspect a fracture if pain occurs when the victim rotates the palm up and down.

Wrist Fracture

The wrist usually is broken when the victim falls with the arm and hand outstretched. Generally, a lumplike deformity occurs on the back of the wrist, along with pain, tenderness, and swelling.

Hand Injuries

Crushed Hand

The hand may be fractured by a direct blow or by a crushing injury. There may be pain, swelling, loss of motion, open wounds, and broken bones.

Finger Injuries

The three bones that make up each finger are the most commonly broken bones in the body. Many of the tendons attached to the finger bones can tear with or without a fracture, and the three joints—the distal interphalangeal (DIP), the proximal interphalangeal (PIP), and the metacarpal phalangeal (MCP)—can also suffer injury. A so-called "finger sprain" may turn out to be a complicated fracture or dislocation.

Finger Fracture

Contrary to popular belief, broken bones—especially the fingers—can move when they are broken. When a finger is fractured, there is immediate pain, and the finger hurts with or without movement. Swelling occurs, and the finger has a twisted look.

Gently feel each bone of the injured finger. Pinpointed tenderness usually indicates a fracture. Ask the victim to make a half-fist with each hand and compare nail alignments for malrotation of the fingers, which could indicate a fracture.

Finger Dislocation

Finger dislocations are common. Motion of the joint usually is impossible, and there may be some loss of circulation and sensation. In a dislocation, the abnormal position of the two adjoining bones looks like a lump at the joint. There is pain, swelling, and shortening of the finger, and the victim may be unable to bend the finger in the injured area.

Sprained Finger

The upper joints of the fingers have a ligament on each side of the joint. A sprain can cause severe pain and swelling over a joint.

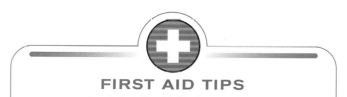

FIRST AID TIPS

Paper Cuts and Hangnails
Keeping a minor wound such as a paper cut or torn hangnail clean and dry can be difficult. Use one of these methods:
- Apply two thin coats of a flexible, waterproof, and durable clear nail polish to the surface of the wound, or
- Place a drop of "super glue" on the hangnail or paper cut and pinch the skin together. Avoid putting the glue inside the cut.

BONE INJURIES

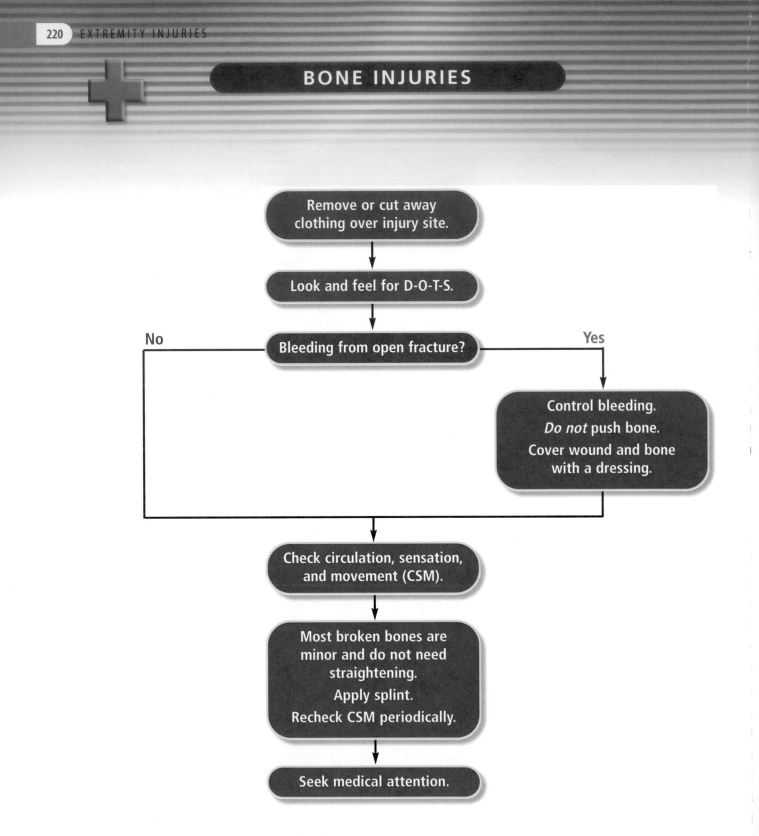

Feel both sides of the joints for tenderness. Pain will be directly over the side of the injured joint rather than above or below it.

Nail Avulsion

An injury in which a nail is partly or completely torn loose is known as a nail **avulsion.**

1. Secure the damaged nail in place with an adhesive bandage.

2. If part or all of the nail has been completely torn away, apply antibiotic ointment. Secure a partly torn loose nail with an adhesive bandage. Do not trim away the loose nail. Consult a physician for further advice.

Splinters

Remove a splinter in the skin by teasing it out with a sterile needle until the end can be grasped with tweezers or fingers.

If a splinter enters the skin under a nail and breaks off flush, cut a V-shaped notch in the nail to gain access to the splinter. Remove the embedded splinter by grasping its end with tweezers.

Blood under a Nail

When a fingernail has been crushed, blood collects under the nail. This condition usually is very painful because of the pressure of the blood pushing against the nail.

1. Immerse the finger in ice water or apply an ice pack with the hand elevated to reduce pain and swelling.

2. Relieve the pressure under the injured nail by one of the following methods (▼**Figure 13-1**):

   - Straighten the end of a metal (noncoated) paper clip or use the eye end of a sewing needle. Hold

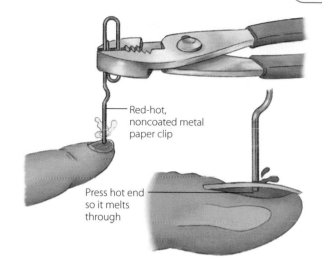

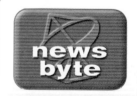
Red-hot, noncoated metal paper clip

Press hot end so it melts through

Figure 13-2) Making a hole in a fingernail.

the paper clip or needle with pliers and use a match or cigarette lighter to heat it until the metal is red hot. Press the glowing end of the paper clip or needle against the nail so it melts through. Little pressure is needed. The nail has no nerves, so it is painless (▲**Figure 13-2**).

   - Using a rotary action, carefully drill through the nail with the sharp point of a knife. This method may be painful, but less threatening than the previous method of using heat.

3. Apply a dressing to absorb the draining blood and to protect the injured nail.

Ring Strangulation

Sometimes an injured finger is so swollen that a ring cannot be removed. Ring strangulation can be a serious problem if it cuts off circulation long enough. Gangrene

Figure 13-1) Relieve pain by releasing blood under a nail.

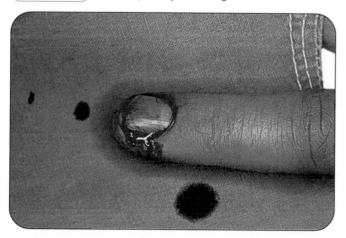

Blood Clot under a Fingernail

news byte

Blood clots are common problems. Relieving the pressure of blood under nails in 45 victims was successfully done using a heated object (first aiders could use a heated paperclip). All victims reported relief of pain after this procedure. No complications of infection or major nail deformities occurred. This method is preferred over removing the nail.

Source: D. C. Seaberg, et al: "Treatment of Subungual Hematomas with Nail Trephination." *American Journal of Emergency Medicine* 9(3):209–210.

may result within four or five hours. Try one or more of the following methods to remove a ring:

- Lubricate the finger with grease, oil, butter, petroleum jelly, or some other slippery substance, then try to remove the ring.

- Immerse the finger in cold water or apply an ice pack for several minutes to reduce the swelling.

- Massage the finger from the tip to the hand to move the swelling; lubricate the finger again and try removing the ring.

- Smoothly wind thread around the finger, starting about an inch from the ring edge and going toward the ring, keeping each round of thread touching the next. Wind smoothly and tightly right up to the edge of the ring. This action will push the swelling toward the hand. Slip the end of the thread under the ring with a matchstick or toothpick, then slowly unwind the thread on the hand side of the ring. You should be able to gently twist the ring over the thread and off the finger.

- Lubricate the finger well, then pass a rubber band under the ring. Hold both ends of the rubber band and, while maintaining tension on the rubber band toward the end of the finger, pull the rubber band around and around the finger.

- Cut the narrowest part of the ring with a ring saw, jeweler's saw, ring cutter, or fine hacksaw blade. Be sure to protect the exposed portions of the finger.

- Inflate an ordinary balloon (preferably a slender, tube-shaped one) about three-fourths full. Tie the end. Insert the victim's swollen finger into the end of the balloon until the balloon evenly surrounds the entire finger. In about 15 minutes, the air pressure in the balloon should return the finger to its normal size, and the ring can be removed.

- Liberally spray window or glass cleaner onto the finger, then try to slide the ring off.

Amputations

Fingers and toes are the most often amputated body parts. See Chapter 7 for amputation care.

Hip-Joint Injuries

Hip Dislocation

A hip can be dislocated by a fall, a blow to the thigh, or direct force to the foot or knee. The hip joint is a stable ball-and-socket joint that requires great force to dislocate. Often a hip is dislocated when the knee strikes the dashboard during a motor vehicle collision. There

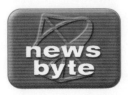

Ring Removal from an Extremely Swollen Finger

Rings on swollen fingers are not uncommon, but they must be removed or serious problems can result. Generally, the removal method is simply to cut the ring off the finger or to use one of several nondestructive removal methods using string or a rubber band. A new yet simple method that eliminates the swelling and permits the removal of a ring involves wrapping the entire finger starting at the nail and wrapping toward the ring distal with a tight, elastic band, which reduces the swelling and frees the ring.

Source: C. R. Cresap: "Removal of a Hardened Steel Ring from an Extremely Swollen Finger." *American Journal of Emergency Medicine* 13(3):318–320.

will be severe pain and loss of motion, and marked deformity may be present. The most common deformity has the victim's hip flexed and the knee bent and rotated inward toward the opposite hip. The foot may hang loose, and the victim is unable to flex the foot or lift the toes. It is difficult to differentiate a hip dislocation from a fracture.

Hip Fracture

A hip fracture is a fracture of the upper end of the femur (thighbone), not the pelvis. A fractured hip usually is caused by a fall. Elderly people, especially women, are susceptible to this type of injury because of brittle bones (osteoporosis). There is severe pain in the groin area, and the victim may not be able to lift the injured leg. The leg may appear shortened and be rotated with the toes pointing abnormally outward.

Thigh Injuries

Femur (Thighbone) Fracture

Because the femur is the largest bone in the body, considerable force is required to break it. Femur injuries can occur in any part of the femur, from the hip to just above the knee joint. A fracture of the femur usually is caused by a fall or a direct blow. There is severe pain, a shortening of the leg, deformity, and a grating sensation. The limb has a wobbly motion, and below the fracture there is a complete loss of control. Severe damage to the nerves and blood vessels may occur, resulting in swelling.

Femur fractures often include open wounds, and external bleeding may be severe. If the blood vessels are damaged, the victim may lose one or two quarts of blood into the thigh. There may be loss of blood circulation to the lower part of the extremity or nerve damage, especially with lower-third femur fractures.

Charley Horse

A charley horse is an injury of the thigh muscle, with bleeding inside the thigh. Look for tenderness, swelling, and possibly black-and-blue marks. It results from a direct blow to the the thigh.

Muscle Strain

The hamstring muscles (back of thigh) tear most commonly from the upper center of the muscle, but occasionally from the pelvic bone under the buttocks. Hamstring tears are mildly to severely disabling. The injury occurs most often in sports, especially track and field.

Knee Injuries

Knee injuries, of which there are many types, can be serious. You probably have seen a physician or an athletic trainer performing stress tests on a player's knee on the sidelines at a football game. Controversy exists as to the exact meaning and interpretation of many of the ligament stress tests. First aiders should not perform such tests unless they have the training and experience to do so.

Knee Fracture

A fracture of the knee generally occurs as a result of a fall or a direct blow. Besides the usual signs of a fracture, a groove in the kneecap may be felt. The victim will be

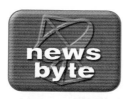

Thigh Muscle Injuries: Strain or Contusion?

Athletes often injure the large quadriceps muscles of their thighs. According to one report, strains (pulling of the muscle, which causes tears) should be treated first with ice, compression, elevation of the limb, nonsteroidal anti-inflammatory drugs, and use of crutches. After several days, start gentle stretching and knee extension but avoid straight leg raises. For thigh contusions (direct blow, causing bruising), immediately flex the knee and immobilize it in that position for 24 hours. Apply ice for the first half hour and intermittently thereafter, to slow bleeding and prevent swelling.

Source: C. C. Kaeding, et al: "Quadriceps Strains and Contusions." *Physician and Sportsmedicine* 23:59 (Jan. 1995).

FYI Did You Know?

Charley Horse

The term *charley horse* was derived from baseball players who experienced blows to muscles in the early twentieth century. At that time, the outfield grass of some major league ballparks was mowed by horses pulling lawn mowers. At Ebbet's Field in New York, the horse that did this chore—"Charley"—had a continual limp. When a baseball player was hit in the leg with a ball or, while sliding into base, received a blow to his leg muscle that subsequently caused him to limp, it was said that he was walking like Charley the horse. Consequently, the muscle blow and the contusion that caused an athlete's pain and limping were referred to as a charley horse injury. The term is still popular in America today.

---

unable to kick the leg forward, and the leg will drag if the victim tries to walk.

Knee Dislocation

A knee dislocation is a serious injury. Deformity will be grotesque. A first aider should be more concerned about possible injury to the popliteal artery (just behind the knee joint) than about any ligament damage. This major artery, which supplies the leg below the knee, can be lacerated or compressed by a displaced tibia.

Always check the ankle pulse in a knee dislocation. If an ankle pulse is absent, make one attempt to realign the leg to restore blood circulation. Try to gently straighten the knee *only once.* Then stabilize the knee in the position of deformity. Do not attempt to straighten any knee injury when an ankle pulse is present or when any attempt to realign the knee produces severe pain. In those cases, stabilize the knee in the position found. *Seek medical attention immediately.* Waiting longer than eight hours to reduce a knee dislocation can result in loss of the leg.

Do not confuse a knee dislocation with a patella dislocation. A knee dislocation is a much more serious injury.

Patella Dislocation

A dislocated patella (kneecap) can be a very painful injury and must be treated immediately. Some people have repeated kneecap dislocations, just as others have a tendency for shoulder dislocations.

When the patella is dislocated, a significant deformity appears, with the knee semiflexed and the patella on the outside (lateral side) of the joint. Compare it with the other kneecap.

MUSCLE INJURIES

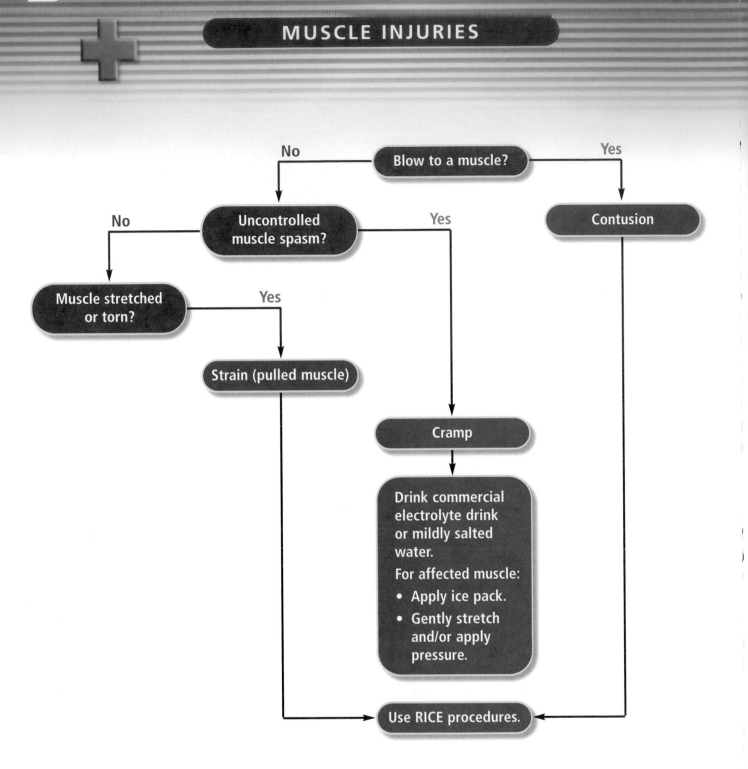

No ← **Blow to a muscle?** → Yes

No ← **Uncontrolled muscle spasm?** → Yes

Contusion

No ← **Muscle stretched or torn?** → Yes

Strain (pulled muscle)

Cramp

Drink commercial electrolyte drink or mildly salted water.

For affected muscle:
- Apply ice pack.
- Gently stretch and/or apply pressure.

Use RICE procedures.

Knee Sprain

Ligament injuries occur most often in sports. The knee is very prone to ligament injury, ranging from mild sprains to complete tearing. The knee will be swollen and painful and usually cannot be used normally.

Contusion

A knee bruise, or contusion, will be tender and swollen and may have black-and-blue marks.

Lower-Leg Injuries

Tibia and Fibula Fractures

Tibia and fibula injuries can occur at any place between the knee joint and the ankle joint. When both bones are broken, there is a marked deformity of the leg. When only one bone is broken, the other acts as a splint, and little deformity may be present. Some victims with a fibula fracture can walk on the injured leg. When the tibia (shin bone) is broken, an open fracture and severe deformity are likely to exist. Injuries to the blood vessels, caused by the extreme deformity, are common with injuries of the tibia and the fibula, and the pain usually is severe.

Contusion

Many contusions simply cause a black-and-blue mark and some soreness, then clear up with little attention.

Muscle Cramp

Muscle spasm or cramping usually occurs in the calf, sometimes in the thigh or hamstring. It is a temporary condition of little consequence. Refer to the section on heat cramps in Chapter 12 for more information.

What to Do

There are many treatments for cramps. Try one or more of the following:

1. Have the victim gently stretch the affected muscle. Because a muscle cramp is an uncontrolled muscle contraction or spasm, a gradual extension of the muscle may help lengthen the muscle fibers and relieve the cramp.

2. Relax the muscle by applying pressure to it.

3. Apply ice to the cramped muscle to make it relax. The exception might be in a cold environment.

4. Pinch the upper lip hard (an accupressure technique) to reduce calf-muscle cramping.

5. Drink lightly salted, cool water (dissolve $1/4$ teaspoon salt in a quart of water) or a commercial sports drink.

Caution:

DO NOT give salt tablets to a person with muscle cramps. They can cause stomach irritation, nausea, and vomiting.

DO NOT massage or rub the affected muscle. That only causes more pain and does not relieve the cramping.

Shin Splints

Experts disagree just what shin splints are, other than that they are pain in the shins and are caused by running and extensive walking. Pain and tenderness occur along the front edge of the shin where the muscles are attached.

Ankle and Foot Injuries

The ankle and the foot frequently get injured, mainly by twisting, which stretches or tears the supporting ligaments. Careless treatment can have consequences that include lifelong disability. In some cases, the damage requires surgical correction.

Most ankle injuries are sprains; about 85% of sprains involve the ankle's outside (lateral) ligaments and are caused by the ankle having turned or twisted inward ▼Figure 13-3 .

Figure 13-3 Sprained ankle

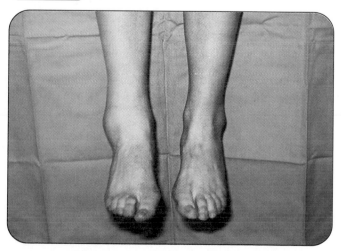

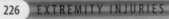

SPRAINS, STRAINS, CONTUSIONS, DISLOCATIONS

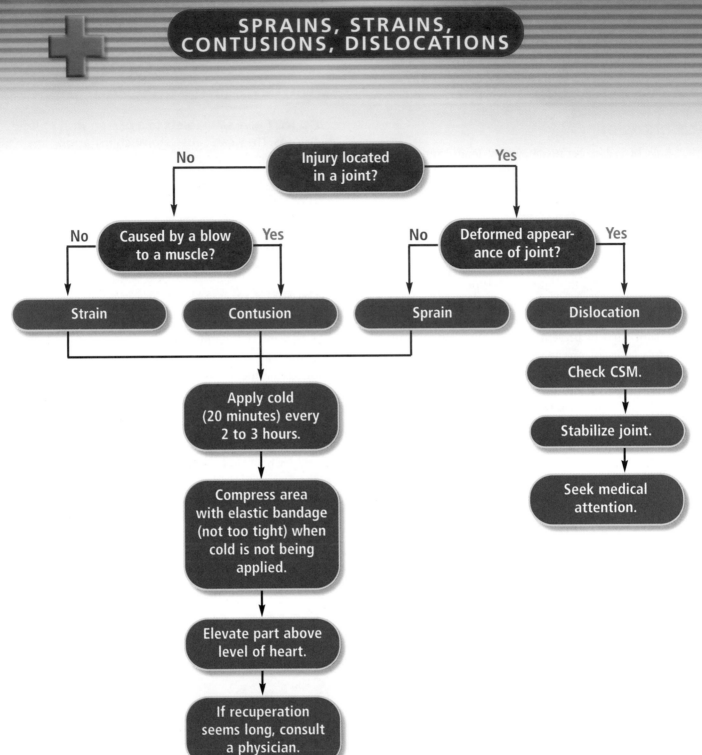

What to Look for

It is difficult to tell the difference between a severely sprained ankle and a fractured ankle. A useful two-part test can help determine whether the ankle or the midfoot needs to be x-rayed:

1. Press along the bones. Pain and tenderness over (a) the back edge or the tip of either of the ankle knob bones (malleolus bones) or (b) the midfoot's outside bone (fifth metatarsal) or inside bone (navicular) may indicate a broken bone.

2. Ask the victim, "Have you tried standing on it?" Putting some weight on the foot may hurt a little, but if the victim is able to do that and take four or more steps, most likely the ankle or foot is sprained. If it is broken, the victim will not want to put any weight on it and will not be able to take more than four steps.

A few additional signs and symptoms may help you determine whether an injured ankle or foot is sprained or fractured. These indicators are not hard-and-fast rules but rather useful guidelines to help you treat foot and ankle injuries.

- If the victim hops on the good foot and the injured ankle cannot tolerate the jarring, suspect a fracture.

- Some experts say that nausea right after an ankle injury indicates a fracture rather than a sprain.

- Foot injuries often are quite swollen. It has been observed that ankle sprains tend to swell on only one side of the foot (usually the lateral, or outer, side), whereas swelling on both sides of the foot usually accompanies fractures.

What to Do

Controversy exists about whether to remove a shoe from an injured foot. Those who favor leaving the shoe on believe it acts as a splint and helps retard swelling. However, taking off the shoe allows for a better examination, better checking of the foot's CSM (circulation, sensation, movement), and better care. A shoe that is left on often does not cover, and thus cannot compress, the injured area that is swelling. If a shoe does act as a compression device, it could also reduce blood circulation in the foot as swelling expands. In addition, footwear left in place will thwart efforts to apply an ice pack and elastic bandage.

Use the RICE procedures to limit swelling (see page below). Every minute RICE is delayed can add an hour to healing.

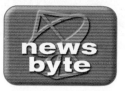

Ankle and Foot Injuries: Is Something Broken?

In a study of 1,500 people with ankle injuries, two symptoms were 100% accurate in predicting a broken ankle bone: (1) inability to bear weight and take four steps immediately after the injury; and (2) tenderness at the back edge or tip of either malleolus bone (the projections on each side of the ankle). Similar symptoms predicted whether a foot bone was broken: (1) pain in the midfoot or tenderness at the base of the fifth metatarsal bone at the outer edge of the foot or at the navicular bone at the inner edge, plus (2) inability to take four steps.

Source: I. G. Stiell, et al: "Decision Rules for the Use of Radiography in Acute Ankle Injuries." *Journal of the American Medical Association.* 269:1127.

Toe Injuries

A fractured toe usually is caused by a crushing injury or by kicking the foot against a hard object. There is pain and swelling, and a deformity may be present.

For nail avulsions, splinters, and blood under a nail, refer to the appropriate sections under "Finger Injuries."

RICE Procedure for Bone, Joint, and Muscle Injuries

RICE is the acronym for Rest, Ice, Compression, Elevation—the recommended immediate treatment for bone, joint, and muscle injuries (▶Skill Scan). What is done in the first 48 to 72 hours after an injury can do a lot to relieve, even prevent, aches and pains. **Treat all extremity bone, joint, and muscle injuries with the RICE procedure. In addition to RICE, fractures and dislocations should be splinted to stabilize the injured area. (See Chapter 14 for splinting techniques.)**

R = Rest

Injuries heal faster if rested. Rest means the victim stays off the injured part. Using any part of the body increases the blood circulation to that area, which can cause more swelling of an injured part. Crutches may be used to rest leg injuries.

I = Ice

An ice pack should be applied to the injured area as soon as possible after the injury for 20 to 30 minutes every 2 or

ANKLE INJURIES

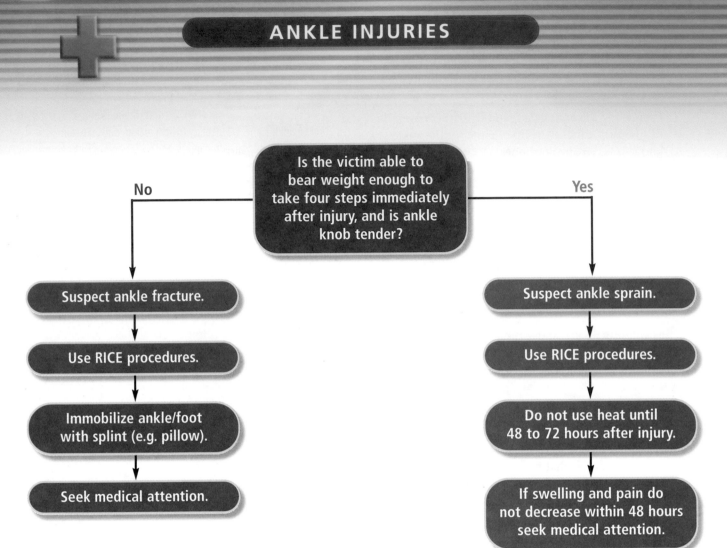

Is the victim able to bear weight enough to take four steps immediately after injury, and is ankle knob tender?

No

Suspect ankle fracture.

Use RICE procedures.

Immobilize ankle/foot with splint (e.g. pillow).

Seek medical attention.

Yes

Suspect ankle sprain.

Use RICE procedures.

Do not use heat until 48 to 72 hours after injury.

If swelling and pain do not decrease within 48 hours seek medical attention.

Skill Scan

RICE Procedures for an Ankle

1

R = Rest
Stop using the injured part. Continued use could cause further injury, delay healing, increase pain, and stimulate bleeding. Get the victim into a comfortable position, either sitting or lying down. This slows blood flow to the injured area.

1. R = Rest

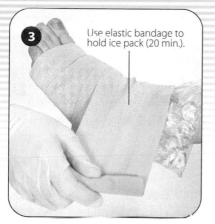
Place ice pack on area.

2. I = Ice

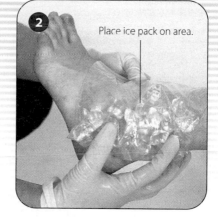
Use elastic bandage to hold ice pack (20 min.).

3. I = Ice

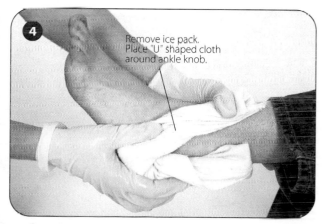
Remove ice pack. Place "U" shaped cloth around ankle knob.

4. C = Compression

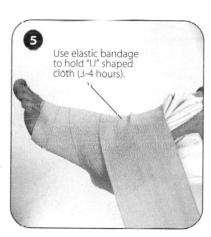
Use elastic bandage to hold "U" shaped cloth (3-4 hours).

5. C = Compression

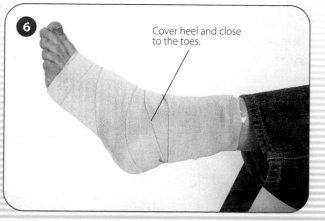
Cover heel and close to the toes.

6. C = Compression

7

E = Elevation
Elevating the injured part is another way to decrease swelling and pain. As you apply ice or compression, elevate the part in whatever way is most convenient. The aim of this step is to get the injured part higher than the heart, if possible.

7. E = Elevation

Aftercare of Ankle Injury

✛ **First 24 to 48 hours.** Use RICE treatment (see page 227).

✛ **Within three to seven days:** The victim should use a *contrast bath* if swelling persists. Submerge the ankle for one minute in cold water (45°F to 60°F) then for four minutes in warm water (100°F to 105°F). Continue to alternate cold and warm submersions for 15 minutes. Gently move the foot up and down for mobility. This should be done once or twice a day for one to two weeks.

The victim should avoid inward ankle movement. Once the initial swelling has decreased, discontinue immobilization and start range-of-motion exercises, even if the injured ankle cannot bear weight. Joint motion decreases swelling and stiffness and prevents fluid accumulation.

Begin with gentle exercises such as bending the ankle up and down 15 times, two or three times a day. Also, try sitting with the legs straight out in front. Place a towel around the ball of the foot and, sitting upright, hold the ends of the towel. Stretch the foot back toward you and hold for 10 seconds. Then point the toes away and hold for 10 seconds. Stop if pain is felt.

✛ **Within 7 to 14 days:** If there is no pain when the ankle is rotated and no swelling, the victim can begin to stretch and strengthen the calf and the ankle. Stretch calf muscles by leaning against a wall with one foot forward. Keep the back leg straight, heel down. Bend the front knee and lean into the wall. Hold for 10 seconds, then stretch with the other leg forward. This stretch can be done 5 to 10 times on each side, two or three times a day.

✛ **Avoiding reinjury:** Once the ankle has healed—typically within four to six weeks—consider taping it (after the first injury) or bracing it (more appropriate for chronic sprains). Bracing alternatives include lace-up, gel-filled, and air-stirrup devices. Also, firm high-top shoes may give added support. Continue to stretch and strengthen the ankle and calf muscles with exercises.

✛ **NSAIDs:** Nonsteroidal anti-inflammatory drugs (NSAIDs) greatly help to reduce pain and swelling. Examples of NSAIDs are ibuprofen, naproxen, and aspirin. Analgesics such as acetaminophen relieve only pain, not swelling.

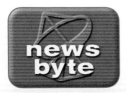

Coffee, Tea, or Frostbite? A Report of Inflight Freezing Hazard from Dry Ice

A passenger on a commercial airline flight suffered a third-degree frostbite due to the attempted therapeutic use of a cold pack. This cold pack was offered by the flight attendant and consisted of a section of dry ice used for cooling in the galley. The resulting injury consisted of a full-thickness cold injury of the left lumbar amounting to about 1.5% total body surface area.

Source: Aviation, Space and Environmental Medicine, September 1999

3 hours during the first 24 to 48 hours (▶**Table 13-1**). Skin treated with cold passes through 4 stages: cold, burning, aching, and numbness. When the skin becomes numb, usually in 20 to 30 minutes, remove the ice pack. After removing the ice pack, compress the injured part with an elastic bandage and keep it elevated (the "C" and "E" of RICE).

Cold constricts the blood vessels to and in the injured area, which helps reduce the swelling and inflammation while it also dulls the pain and relieves muscle spasms. Cold should be applied as soon as possible after the injury—healing time often is directly related to the amount of swelling that occurs. One minute's delay means an additional hour needed for healing. Heat has the opposite effect when applied to fresh injuries: it increases circula-

Table 13-1: Cold Applications

Effects — *Reduces:*

- Pain
- Swelling and inflammation
- Muscle spasm
- Injured tissues by reducing metabolic and oxygen needs

Contraindications:

- Circulatory disturbances (hypertension, Raynaud's)
- Cold allergy (urticaria)
- Prolonged application over superficial nerves (nerve palsy to peroneal nerve at head of fibula may cause foot drop)

Type	Description	Special Concerns	Duration	Expense
Crushed-ice bags	Crushed ice molds easily to body parts.	Apply wet cloth between bag and skin to avoid nerve damage or frostbite.	15–20 minutes	Inexpensive
Ice-water immersion	Uniform application of cold to extremity.	Carries the most risk of hypersensitivity reactions; does not allow elevation of extremity.	15–20 minutes	Inexpensive
Ice massage	Freeze water in foam cup, then peel back cup to expose ice; massage area as often as needed	Apply for short intervals to avoid frostbite; avoid excess pressure. Is not the best for acute injury because it does not cool as effectively as other methods.	5–10 minutes	Inexpensive
Chemical cold packs	Packets are squeezed or crushed to activate; convenient for emergency use.	Single use only. If pack ruptures, chemical burns can result from alkaline contents	15–20 minutes	Expensive
Reusable cold packs	Durable plastic packs containing silica gel that are available in many sizes and shapes.	Apply wet cloth between pack and skin to avoid nerve damage or frostbite.	20 minutes	Inexpensive
Vapo-coolant sprays	Portable.	Spray area for <6 seconds to avoid frostbite; dangerous in hands of untrained person. Use debatable; spray can harm Earth's ozone layer.	Multiple, brief sprays	Expensive

tion to the area and greatly increases both the swelling and the pain.

Use either of the following methods to apply cold to an injury:

- Put crushed ice (or cubes) into a double plastic bag, hot water bottle, or wet towel. Place the ice pack directly on the skin, and secure it in place with an elastic bandage for 20 to 30 minutes. Ice bags can conform to the body's contours.

- Use a chemical "snap pack," a sealed pouch that contains two chemical envelopes. Squeezing the pack mixes the chemicals, producing a chemical reaction that has a cooling effect. Although they do not cool as well as other methods, they are convenient to use when ice is not readily available. They lose their cooling power quickly, however, and can be used only once. Also, they may be impractical because they are expensive and easily breakable.

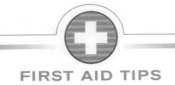

FIRST AID TIPS

Homemade Ice Packs

- Ice bags kept in a freezer freeze solid and cannot be shaped to fit the injured area. One part isopropyl (rubbing) alcohol to three parts water prevents freezing, and the ice bag can be easily molded. Bags can be reused for months.

- An unopened bag of frozen vegetables is inexpensive; keeps its basic shape (unlike ice chips, which melt); molds to the shape of the injured area; is reusable; and is packaged in a fairly puncture-resistant, water-tight bag.

- For cold therapy over a fairly large area, soak a face towel in cold water, wring it out, fold it, and place it in a large self-sealing plastic bag. Store the bag in the freezer. To use the cold pack, wrap it in a light cotton towel and apply for 20 minutes, after which it can be refrozen. A washcloth in a smaller bag can be used to treat a smaller area.

- Fill a plastic bag with snow.

- Fill a polystyrene plastic cup with water and freeze it. When you need an ice pack, peel the cup to below ice level; the remaining part of the cup forms a cold-resistant handle. Rub the ice over the injured area (movement is necessary to prevent skin damage). These ice "packs" are inexpensive, convenient, and take up little space.

- To fashion a funnel for filling an ice bag, push out the bottom of a paper cup and fit it into the neck of the ice bag. The ice will slide through the cup and into the bag.

Caution:

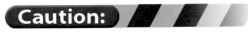

DO NOT apply an ice pack for more than 20 to 30 minutes at a time. Frostbite or nerve damage can result.

DO NOT apply an ice pack on the back outside part of the knee. Nerve damage can occur.

DO NOT apply cold if the victim has a history of circulatory disease, Raynaud's syndrome (spasms in the arteries of the extremities that reduce circulation), or abnormal sensitivity to cold, or if the injured part has been frostbitten previously.

DO NOT stop using an ice pack too soon. A common mistake is too early use of heat, which will result in swelling and pain. Use an ice pack three to four times a day for the first 24 hours, preferably up to 48 hours, before applying any heat. For severe injuries, using ice for up to 72 hours is recommended.

C = Compression

Compressing the injured area may squeeze some fluid and debris out of the injury site. Compression limits the ability of the skin and of other tissues to expand and reduces internal bleeding. Apply an elastic bandage to the injured area, especially the foot, ankle, knee, thigh, hand, or elbow. Fill the hollow areas with padding such as a sock or washcloth before applying the elastic bandage.

Elastic bandages come in various sizes, for different body areas:

- 2-inch width, used for the wrist and hand
- 3-inch width, used for the ankle, elbow, and arm
- 4-inch width, used for the knee and leg

Start the elastic bandage several inches below the injury and wrap in an upward, overlapping (about one-half to three-fourths of the bandage's width) spiral, starting with even and somewhat tight pressure, then gradually wrapping more loosely above the injury.

Applying compression may be the most important step in preventing swelling. The victim should wear the elastic bandage continuously for the first 18 to 24 hours (except when cold is applied). At night, have the victim loosen but not remove the elastic bandage.

For an ankle injury, place a horseshoe-shaped pad around the ankle knob and secure it with the elastic bandage. The pad will compress the soft tissues as well as the bones. Wrap the bandage tightest nearest the toes and loosest above the ankle. It should be tight enough to decrease swelling but not tight enough to inhibit blood flow.

For a contusion or a strain, place a pad between the injury and the elastic bandage.

Caution:

DO NOT apply an elastic bandage too tightly. If applied too tightly, elastic bandages will restrict circulation. Stretch a new elastic bandage to about one-third its maximum length for adequate compression. Leave fingers and toes exposed so possible color change can be easily observed. Compare the toes or fingers of the injured extremity with the uninjured one. Pale skin, pain, numbness, and tingling are signs of a too tight elastic bandage. If any of these symptoms appears, immediately remove the elastic bandage. Leave the elastic bandage off until all the symptoms disappear, then rewrap the area, but less tightly. Always wrap from below the injury and move toward the heart.

E = Elevation

Gravity slows the return of blood to the heart from the lower parts of the body. Once fluid gets to the hands or feet, the fluid has nowhere else to go and those parts of the body swell. Elevating the injured area, in combination with ice and compression, limits circulation to that area, which in turn helps limit internal bleeding and minimize swelling.

It is simple to prop up an injured leg or arm to limit bleeding. Whenever possible, elevate the injured part

FYI Medical Literature

Heat and Cold: When to Use Which?

Many people use heat devices or ice packs to speed recovery from sports injuries. But when is the right time to use each technique? Cold usually should be applied immediately after an acute injury, such as an ankle sprain. Putting ice chips in a plastic bag is a good way to apply cold. To avoid cold injury, ice should be applied for no more than 15 to 20 minutes at a time. At the same time, compression and elevation of the limb also should be used. Icing reduces pain, swelling, and muscle spasm immediately after injury, but its use should be discontinued after two or three days. Heat applications (heat packs, radiant heat, or whirlpool baths) can then be used to reduce muscle spasms and pain. In addition, heat increases blood flow and joint flexibility. Vigorous heat is used to treat chronic injuries, but mild heat can reduce muscle spasm. Heat is also effective for acute back pain, but ice massage is preferred if back pain persists for two weeks or more.

Source: M. P. Kaul and S. A. Herring: "Superficial Heat and Cold." *Physician and Sportsmedicine* 22:65 (Dec. 1994).

above the level of the heart for the first 24 hours after an injury. If a fracture is suspected, do not elevate an extremity until it has been stabilized with a splint.

Along with RICE, fractures and dislocations should be splinted. Chapter 14 describes splinting techniques for various parts of the body.

Thigh Injuries

Fractures lead the list of severe thigh injuries, and although a hip fracture technically occurs in the neck of the femur bone, it is a shaft fracture that is usually referred to in the thigh. Besides the disability experienced because a major bone has been broken, a bone that ordinarily supports much of the body's weight, these two fractures carry these complications:

+ A midshaft femur fracture may be associated with major blood loss—up to one or two pints of blood lost. If both thighbones are fractured at the same time, life-threatening shock can quickly occur.

+ A femur fracture above the knee (called a supracondylar fracture) may cause disruption of the artery to the leg, producing a cold foot. This is a circulatory emergency, and the fracture often requires surgery with pins, plates or screws). The leg is threatened with amputation if the lack of blood circulation to the leg goes beyond approximately three hours. Lesser thigh injuries include contusions (bruises), groin muscle pulls, and strains.

STUDY
Questions **13**

Name_____ Course_____ Date_____

Activities

Activity 1

Mark each answer as true (T) or false (F).

T F 1. A horseshoe-shaped pad under an elastic bandage is recommended for ankle sprains.

T F 2. Dislocations happen only in joints.

T F 3. After suffering a sprain or strain, you should immediately apply heat to the affected joint.

T F 4. Sprains are muscle injuries.

T F 5. Splint a fracture before moving a victim.

T F 6. The "rule of thirds" applies to the assessment of muscle injuries.

Activity 2

Check (✓) the appropriate answer(s).

Relieve the painful pressure caused by the accumulation of blood under a fingernail or toenail by

____ 1. placing the finger in hot water for several minutes

____ 2. drilling a hole through the nail with the point of a knife

____ 3. melting a hole through the nail to the site of the blood with a red-hot paper clip

Mark each technique yes (Y) or no (N).

Which techniques can be useful in removing a stuck ring?

____ 4. Lubricate the finger with oil, butter, or other slippery substance.

____ 5. Place the finger in hot water for several minutes.

____ 6. Use thread wrapped tightly around the finger.

____ 7. Cut the ring with a fine-toothed hacksaw.

____ 8. Cut the skin along the ring to relieve pressure.

Activity 3

Mark each statement as true (T) or false (F).

T F 1. The letters RICE represent the treatment for an ankle injury.

T F 2. When using ice, place it directly on the skin.

T F 3. A common mistake is the application of heat too soon.

T F 4. An elastic bandage, if used correctly, can help control swelling.

T F 5. Using an elastic bandage alone provides adequate compression.

T F 6. Controversy exists about whether to take a shoe off an injured ankle.

Activity 4

Those engaging in various types of sports may experience one of three different muscle injuries. Match the lettered types of muscle injury with the numbered definitions.

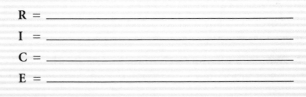

____ 1. strain   **a.** result of a blow

____ 2. contusion   **b.** uncontrolled spasm

____ 3. cramp   **c.** a tear

4. All muscle injuries can benefit from the RICE procedures. What do the letters represent?

R = _____

I = _____

C = _____

E = _____

STUDY
Questions (13)

5. How can compression be applied?

_____

_____

6. Give two sources of ice or cold.

a. _____

b. _____

7. How long and how often should cold be applied?

___ minutes every ___ hours for the first
___ hours.

8. Cold will decrease swelling and relieve

_____

9. It is best not to apply heat for ___ to ___ hours after an injury.

Case Situations

Case 1

A neighbor falls from a ladder. You find him lying down complaining about the pain. His lower leg looks deformed.

___ 1. How would you assess the leg?

   a. See whether the victim can stand on the leg.

   b. Ask the victim to wiggle his or her toes.

   c. Gently rotate the leg to check for a broken bone.

   d. With your fingers gently probe the leg for pain or tenderness and check for feeling and a pulse below the affected area.

___ 2. Which bones compose the lower leg?

   a. tibia, fibula
   b. radius, ulna
   c. radius, tibia
   d. fibula, ulna

___ 3. Proper splinting includes stabilizing the joint above and the joint below the fracture. In your neighbor's case, the joints to be stabilized would be the

   a. hip, knee

   b. shoulder, elbow

   c. knee, ankle

   d. hip, ankle

Case 2

At an ice skating rink, an 18-year-old male crashes through a gate and tumbles down a flight of stairs. You note that he is conscious but obviously intoxicated. You find deformity and swelling in the upper right leg. No other injuries are obvious.

___ 1. This victim is suffering from a fractured

   a. tibia

   b. humerus

   c. femur

   d. pelvis

___ 2. Which of the following pulse sites is used to assess blood flow into a lower extremity?

   a. posterior tibial

   b. femoral

   c. radial

   d. brachial

___ 3. Treatment for this victim would include

   a. placing him in a sitting position

   b. stabilizing the injured extremity by tying the legs together

   c. stabilizing the injured extremity by having a bystander hold the legs together

   d. raising the leg up to treat for shock

STUDY
Questions (13)

Case 3
During a pick-up basketball game, one of the players turns his ankle.

___ 1. What indicates a possible fractured ankle?

   a. Victim has pain over the ankle-knob bone when you press on it.

   b. Victim cannot take four steps.

   c. Victim refuses to stand on the injured ankle.

   d. All the above.

___ 2. For a suspected fracture, should you use the RICE procedures?

   a. yes

   b. no

___ 3. In which direction do most injured ankles turn?

   a. inward

   b. outward

Case 4
A 10-year-old boy suffers an injury to his forearm while riding double on a bicycle with his brother.

___ 1. What would indicate a fracture?

   a. deformity

   b. tenderness

   c. swelling

   d. all of these

___ 2. Which pulse would you check for blood flow in an arm?

   a. radial artery

   b. carotid artery

   c. femoral artery

Case 5
A 20-year-old softball player tips a ball off the end of her index finger.

___ 1. What test might indicate a broken finger?

   a. percussion test

   b. rule of nines

   c. rule of the palm

   d. rule of 50s

___ 2. Suspect a fracture if the test involves pain.

   a. true

   b. false

Case 6
A 20-year-old male is struck by a thrown baseball bat. A physical exam reveals deformity to the forearm with the bone ends protruding through the wound.

___ 1. This type of injury is known as a(n) ____ fracture.

   a. closed

   b. greenstick

   c. open

   d. impacted

___ 2. To determine the circulatory effectiveness in the injured arm, which of the following pulses should you check?

   a. carotid

   b. radial

   c. femoral

   d. brachial

___ 3. What should you apply to control the bleeding?

   a. direct pressure over the bleeding site

   b. pressure around the bleeding site

   c. pressure on the brachial artery

   d. a tourniquet

STUDY
Questions 13

Case 7

A motorcycle accident victim appears to have a closed fracture of the right femur. No other injuries are evident.

1. How can the circulation of a leg be checked?

_____

_____

_____

_____

___ 2. How much blood could be lost because of a femur fracture?

    a. 1 pint

    b. 1 to 2 quarts

    c. 1 gallon

Case 8

A mountain biker skids on loose rocks, catapults over the bike's handlebars, and lands on his shoulder.

1. What injuries would you suspect?

    a. _____

    b. _____

    c. _____

___ 2. Which injury involves the victim holding his or her arm away from the body?

    a. shoulder dislocation

    b. clavicle fracture

Chapter Activities

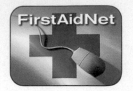

WEB Activities

Extremity Injuries

Visit nsc.jbpub.com/FirstAidNet, then click on Web Activities, and select the appropriate chapter.

Sprains and Strains

Participating in sports or other physical fitness activities can result in injury to the soft tissues of your body. Even simple everyday activities can sometimes lead to damaged ligaments, tendons, and muscles.

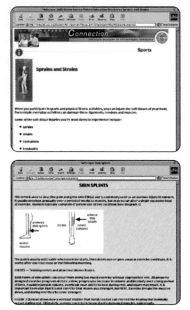

Shin Splints

Do your legs hurt when you run? Shin splints is a term used to describe pain along the shin (tibia). It is commonly seen as an overuse injury in runners. Learn more about the signs and treatment of this annoying ailment.

Chapter 14

Splinting Extremities

Most extremity fractures are minor. Until you can get medical care, stabilize the injury by splinting the extremity in the position it was found. Because medical help is usually nearby, the injury can be stabilized by splinting the extremity in the position it was found. To *stabilize* means to minimize further injury by holding a body part still to prevent movement. All fractures should be stabilized before a victim is moved. The reasons for splinting to stabilize an injured area are to:

- reduce pain
- prevent damage to muscle, nerves, and blood vessels
- prevent a closed fracture from becoming an open fracture
- reduce bleeding and swelling

All fractures are complicated to some degree by damage to the soft tissue and structures surrounding the bone. The major cause of tissue damage at a fracture site is movement by the end of the broken bone. The end of a broken bone is sharp, and it is important to prevent a fractured bone from moving into soft tissues.

Types of Splints

A **splint** is any device used to stabilize a fracture or a dislocation. Such a device can be improvised (eg, a folded newspaper), or it can be one of several commercially available splints (eg, SAM Splint™, air splint). Lack of a commercial splint should never prevent you from properly stabilizing an injured extremity. Splinting sometimes requires improvisation.

A rigid splint is an inflexible device attached to an extremity to maintain stability. It may be a padded board, a piece of heavy cardboard, or a SAM Splint™ molded to fit the extremity. Whatever its construction, a rigid splint must be long enough so that it can be secured well above and below the fracture site. A soft splint, such as an air

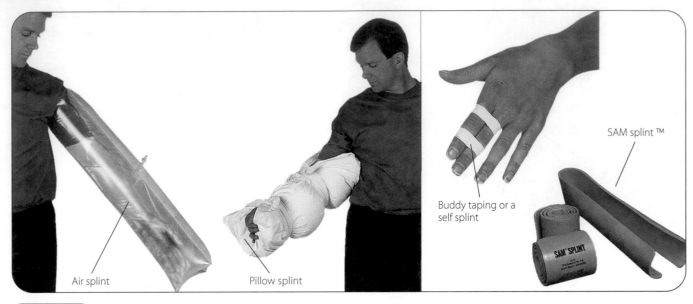

Figure 14-1 Examples of splints.

Air splint

Pillow splint

Buddy taping or a self splint

SAM splint ™

SAM SPLINT

splint or pillow, is useful mainly for stabilizing fractures of the lower leg or the forearm (▲Figure 14-1).

A self, or anatomic, splint is almost always available because it uses the body itself as the splint. A self splint is one in which the injured extremity is tied to an uninjured part (eg, injured finger to adjacent finger, legs together, injured arm to chest).

Splinting Guidelines

All fractures and dislocations should be stabilized before the victim is moved. When in doubt, apply a splint.

You should attempt to straighten a fracture only if you are in a remote location (more than one hour from medical care) *and* one of the following situations exists: (1) the extremity is severely deformed (angulated) from its normal anatomical position, or (2) the circulation-sensation-movement (CSM) check is negative. Use **traction**—a firm and steady pull to improve the position of a badly deformed, shortened, or angulated extremity—to achieve a more normal alignment. If you are not sure what the extremity should look like, check the correspond-ing undamaged part. Traction is not an attempt to pull the limb back in perfect alignment. That process, called **reduction** of a fracture, is done in a hospital with x-rays to assist medical personnel in visualizing the exact positions of the broken-bone ends. For first aid purposes, traction should be applied only for midshaft long-bone fractures to help prevent further soft-tissue injury, improve circulation, and relieve pain. If the victim shows increased pain or the extremity is resistant to traction, splint the extremity in the deformed position.

To apply traction, follow these steps:

1. Explain to the victim that straightening the fracture may cause a momentary increase in pain, but that the pain will be relieved once the fracture is straightened and splinted.

2. For an injured arm, grasp the arm firmly with one hand above and the other below the injury site. Exert steady, gentle traction in a line with the bone. Do not use excessive force. For an injured leg, pull on the leg below the injury with both hands while the victim's body acts as an anchor or another person holds the upper leg in place.

Caution:

DO NOT straighten dislocations or fractures of the spine, elbow, wrist, hip, or knee because of the proximity of major nerves and arteries. Instead, if the CSM is all right, splint joint injuries in the position found.

DO NOT apply traction on open fractures. Instead, cover the wound with a sterile dressing and apply a splint.

If the victim shows increased pain or you feel resistance, stop applying traction and splint the extremity as it is.

Medical experts disagree on whether an open fracture should be straightened. Traction usually is not recommended because dirt and bacteria can be pulled deeper into the wound. Instead, simply cover the open wound with a sterile dressing and splint the extremity. If, however, an open fracture has no CSM, you should attempt to straighten the extremity to restore blood flow.

1. Cover all open wounds, if any, with a dry, sterile dressing before applying a splint.

2. Check CSM in the extremity. If pulses are absent and medical help is hours away, straighten a midshaft long bone fracture to restore blood flow. Do *not* straighten dislocations or fractures involving the spine, elbow, hip, wrist, or knee. According to wilderness experts, if you are more than one hour from medical care, you can safely reduce three types of dislocations: anterior shoulder, patella (kneecap —not to be confused with the knee joint), and finger. See Chapter 22.

3. Determine what to splint by using the **"rule of thirds."** Imagine each long bone as being divided into thirds. If the injury is located in the upper or lower third of a bone, assume that the nearest joint is injured. Therefore, the splint should extend to stabilize the bones above and below the unstable joint. For example, for a fracture of the upper third of the tibia (shinbone), the splint must extend above the knee to include the upper leg, as well as the lower leg, because the knee is unstable.

   For a fracture of the middle third of a bone, stabilize the joints above and below the fracture (eg, wrist and elbow for fractured radius or ulna; shoulder and elbow for fractured humerus; knee and ankle for fractured tibia or fibula). In addition to splinting an upper extremity fracture, you should place the injured arm in an arm sling and a swathe (binder).

4. If two first aiders are present, one should support the injury site and minimize movement of the extremity until splinting is completed.

5. When possible, place splint materials on both sides of the injured part, especially when two bones are involved, such as in the lower arm with the radius and ulna or in the lower leg with the tibia and fibula. This "sandwich splint" prevents the injured extremity from rotating and keeps the two bones from touching. With rigid splints, use extra padding in natural body hollows and around any deformities.

6. Apply splints firmly but not so tightly that blood flow into an extremity is affected. Check CSM before and periodically after the splint is applied. If the pulse disappears, loosen the splint enough so you can feel the pulse. Leave the fingers or toes exposed so CSM can be checked easily.

7. Use RICE on the injured part. When practical, elevate the injured extremity after it is stabilized to promote drainage and reduce swelling. ***Do not, however, apply ice packs if a pulse is absent.***

If the victim has a possible spinal injury as well as an extremity injury, the spinal injury takes precedence. Splinting the spine is always a problem. Tell the victim not to move. Then stabilize the spine with rolled blankets or similar objects placed on each side of the neck and torso. In most cases, it is best to wait until the EMS arrives with trained personnel and proper equipment to handle spinal injuries.

Most fractures do not require rapid transportation. An exception is an arm or a leg without a pulse, which means there is insufficient blood flow to that extremity. In that case, ***immediate*** medical attention is necessary.

Seek medical attention for the following injuries or situations:

- Any open fracture
- Any dislocation (injury that causes joint deformity)
- Any joint injury with moderate to severe swelling
- Any injury in which there is deformity, tenderness, or swelling over the bone
- If the victim is unable to walk or bear weight after an ankle or knee injury
- If a "snap, crackle, or pop" was heard at the time of injury
- If the injured area, especially a joint, becomes hot, tender, swollen, or painful
- If you are unsure whether or not a bone was broken
- If the injury does not improve after two weeks of treatment

Slings

Slings support and protect the upper extremities. The sling is not a bandage, but is used as a support for any injury to the shoulder or arm.

Arm Slings

An arm sling supports the forearm and the hand when there are injuries to an upper extremity or the ribs. To apply an arm sling, follow these steps:

1. Support the injured arm slightly away from the chest, with the wrist and hand slightly higher than the elbow.

2. Place an open triangular bandage between the forearm and the chest, with the point of the bandage stretching well beyond the elbow.

Skill Scan Splinting—Upper Extremities

Arm Sling: Shoulder and Clavicle Injuries

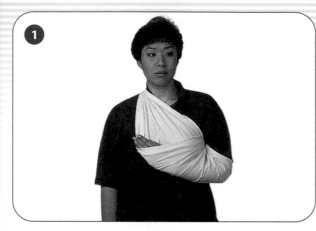

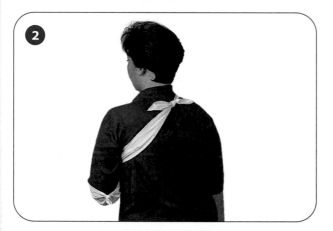

Arm Sling and Swathe for Upper Extremity Injuries (Swathe not shown)

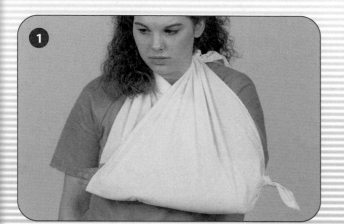

Upper Arm (Humerus)

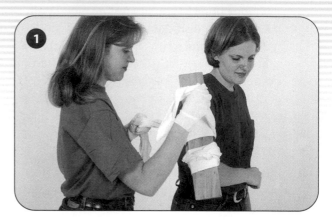

1. Gently place injured arm across the chest. If available, tie a rigid splint to the outside of the arm. If rigid splint is not available, go to step 2.

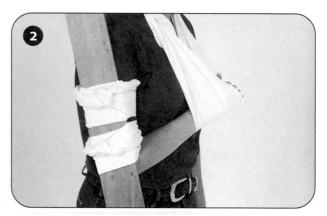

2. Place the arm in a sling.

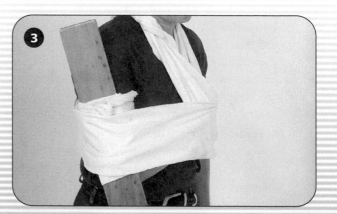

3. Secure the arm to the chest with a broad cravat bandage.

3. Pull the upper end of the bandage over the shoulder on the uninjured side and around the back of the neck to rest on the collarbone of the injured side.

4. Bring the lower end of the bandage over the hand and the forearm and tie it to the other end at the hollow above the collarbone.

5. Bring the point around to the front of the elbow and secure it to the sling with a safety pin or twist it into a "pigtail," which can be tied into a knot or tucked away.

6. Check the pulse and fingernail color for signs of circulation loss. The hand should be in a thumb-up position in the sling and above the level of the elbow.

Splinting Specific Areas ◀ Skill Scan
Shoulder

Shoulder injuries involve the clavicle (collarbone), the scapula (shoulder blade), or the head of the humerus (upper arm). To stabilize the shoulder and upper arm against movement with a shoulder sling, follow these steps:

1. Support the injured arm slightly away from the chest, with the wrist and hand higher than the elbow.

2. Place an open triangular bandage between the forearm and the chest, with the point stretching well beyond the elbow.

3. Pull the upper end of the bandage over the shoulder on the uninjured side.

4. Bring the lower end of the bandage over the forearm, under the armpit on the injured side, and around the victim's back.

5. Tie the upper and lower ends of the triangular bandage.

6. Check the pulse and fingernail color for signs of circulation loss.

The hand should be in a thumb-up position in the sling and slightly above the level of the elbow (▶Figure 14-2).

To further stabilize the arm, fold another triangular bandage to make a 3- to 4-inch-wide swathe. Tie one or two swathes (binders) around the upper arm and chest of the victim. This stabilizes the clavicle (collarbone) and most shoulder injuries, as well as upper humerus (upper arm) fractures.

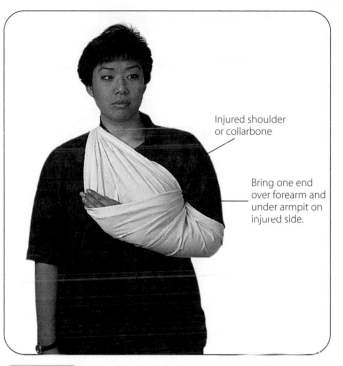

Injured shoulder or collarbone

Bring one end over forearm and under armpit on injured side.

Figure 14-2 Splinting a clavicle or shoulder injury.

If triangular bandages are not available, loop gauze or a belt around the victim's wrist and suspend the arm from the neck. Secure the arm gently, but firmly, to the chest wall with another length of gauze or belt. You can make a temporary splint by pinning a shirt or coat sleeve to the front of the coat or shirt or by pinning the shirt tail to the front of the shirt. See Chapter 8 for improvised slings.

Most shoulder dislocations (95%) are anterior, meaning that the top of the humerus pops out in front of the shoulder joint. The victim will hold the arm in a fixed position away from the chest wall. In these cases, the most comfortable splinting method is to place a pillow or rolled blanket between the involved arm and the chest. This fills the space created, and you can then use cravats or a roller bandage to secure the arm against the chest. If the injury occurs in a remote setting (more than one hour from medical attention), use one of the methods described in Chapter 22 to reduce an anterior shoulder dislocation.

Humerus (Upper Arm)

Fractures of the humerus (upper arm) should be stabilized with a rigid splint. Extend the splint along the outside of the humerus. Place padding between the arm and the chest. Then apply a sling and a swathe over the rigid splint, using the chest wall as an additional splint (▶Figure 14-3).

Skill Scan Splinting—Elbow

Elbow in Bent Position

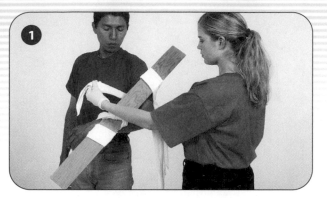

1. If injured elbow is bent, place rigid splint from upper arm to wrist.

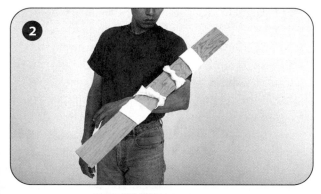

2. Tie rigid splint onto arm with cravat bandages.

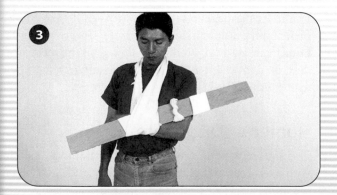

3. Place arm in a sling.

Elbow in Straight Position

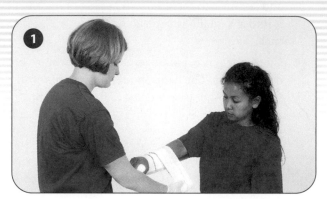

1. If injured elbow is straight, place a rigid splint along the inside of the arm from the hand to armpit.

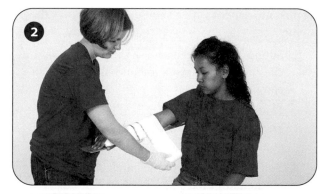

2. Secure with a roller bandage or several cravat bandages.

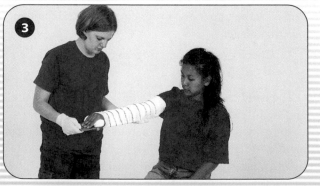

3. Placing in a sling is difficult. Splint elbow in position found. If straight, splint it straight. Rigid splint extends from hand to armpit.

Elbow ◄Skill Scan

An elbow must be stabilized in the position it is found: if bent, splint it bent; if straight, splint it straight. If the injured elbow is straight, place a rigid splint along the in-side of the arm from hand to armpit. Secure the splint with a roller bandage or several cravat bandages. For a bent elbow, apply a rigid splint diagonally, so that it extends from the humerus (near the armpit) to the wrist, to prevent motion of the elbow. Depending upon how bent the elbow is, you can also use a sling and a swathe (binder) for a bent elbow ▼Figure 14-4 A–C .

Figure 14-3 Splinting a humerus fracture.

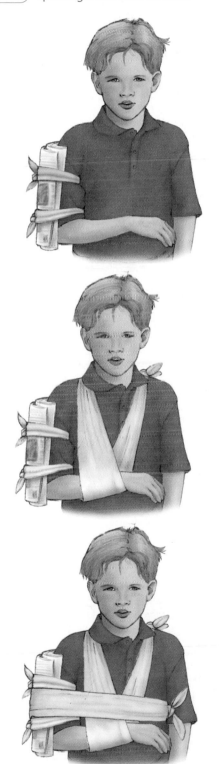

Figure 14-4 **A.** Splint elbow in position found. **B.** Completed splint for a bent elbow. **C.** Splint elbow in position found. If bent, splint it bent. If straight, splint it straight. Rigid splint extends from hand to armpit.

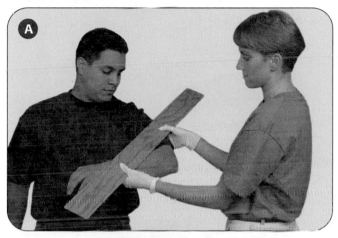

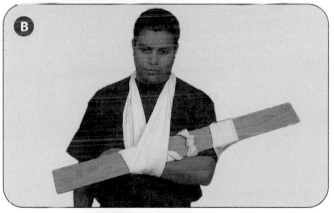

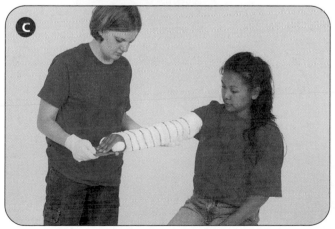

Skill Scan

Splinting—Upper Extremities

Forearm (Radius/Ulna)

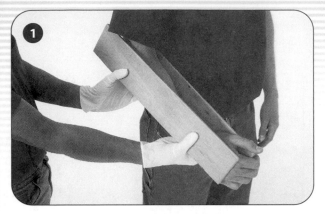

1. Place splints on both sides of a forearm to prevent rotation of the forearm.

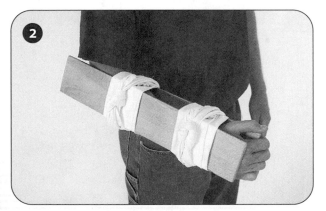

2. Secure with cravat or roller bandage.

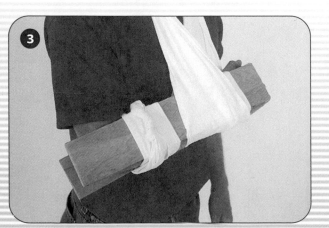

3. Place arm in sling. A binder or swathe around the body is recommended. Keep thumb in upright position

Fingers and Hand (Position of Function)

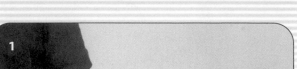

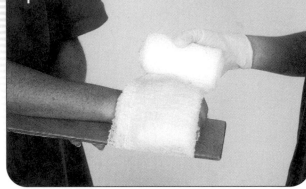

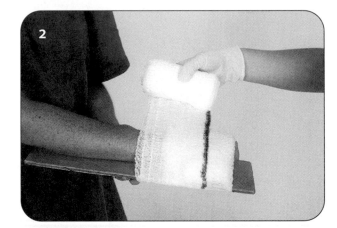

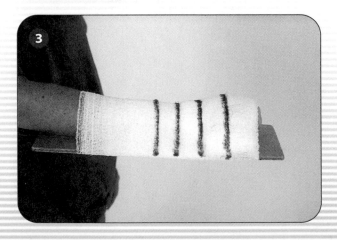

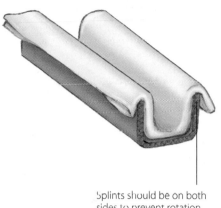

Splints should be on both sides to prevent rotation (shows use of cardboard).

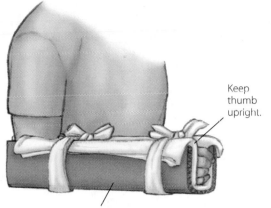

Keep thumb upright.

Rigid splint from palm to out past elbow.

Figure 14-5 Splinting a forearm fracture.

Forearm ◀ Skill Scan

To stabilize a forearm fracture, use one rigid splint extending from the palm of the hand out past the elbow, and a second one on the opposite side of the arm. Placing splints on both sides of the injured part ("sandwich splint") keeps the forearm from twisting or rotating (▲ Figure 14-5). Keep the victim's thumb in an upright position so that the two bones in the forearm (the radius and the ulna) won't touch each other. Secure the splint with either a roller bandage or several cravats. A pillow or a rolled, folded blanket also can be secured onto the arm. Put the arm in a sling and secure it with a swathe (binder) around the body (▼ Figure 14-6).

Figure 14-6 An arm sling can help stabilize upper-extremity injuries.

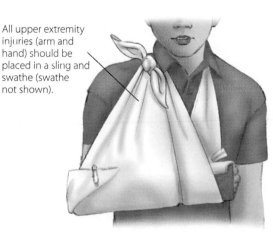

All upper extremity injuries (arm and hand) should be placed in a sling and swathe (swathe not shown).

Wrist, Hand, and Fingers

To stabilize the wrist, hand, and fingers, use either of two methods.

* Place the injured hand in the "position of function" (hand looks like it is holding a baseball) by placing a rolled pair of socks or a roller bandage in the palm. Then attach a rigid splint that extends past the tips of the fingers along the forearm (▶ Figure 14-7, A–C), or

* Place the hand in the position of function, mold a pillow around the hand and forearm, and tie the pillow in place with cravats or a roller bandage.

Then place the arm in a sling and a swathe (binder), with the thumb in an upright position.

Another way to splint fingers is to tape them together ("buddy taping"), with gauze separating the fingers.

Pelvis and Hip

If you suspect a pelvic or hip fracture, stabilize the victim as you found him or her. Treat the victim for shock, do not lift the legs, and wait for the EMS ambulance to arrive. Pelvic and hip fractures require a long backboard (spine board).

Femur (Thigh)

A fractured femur is best splinted with a traction splint, which requires special training to use. Traction splints are seldom available except on ambulances.

Skill Scan Splinting—Knee

Knee in Bent Position

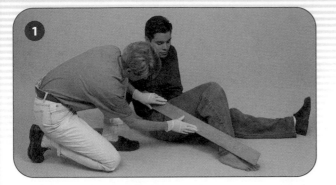

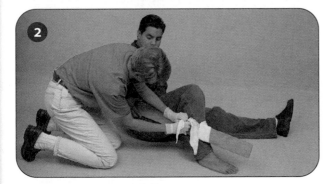

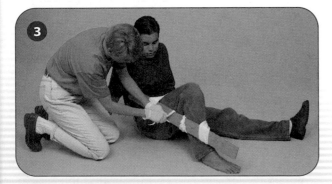

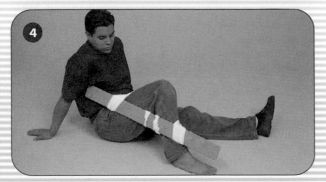

Knee in Straight Position

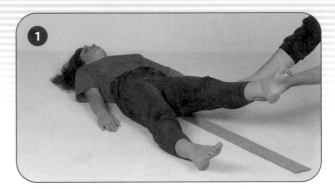

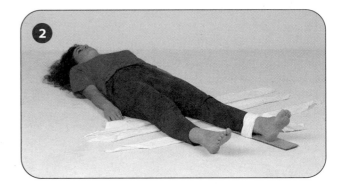

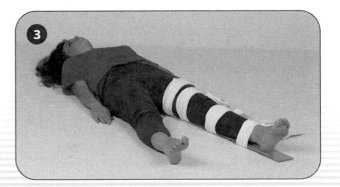

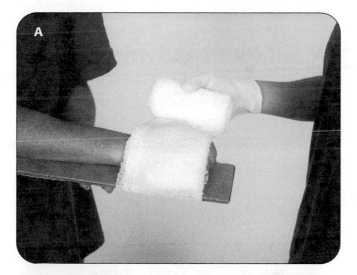

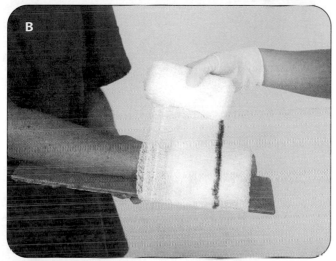

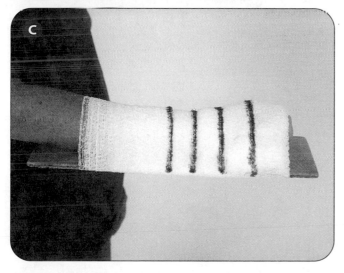

First aiders can use one of two methods to splint a fractured femur:

- Place a folded blanket or pillows between the victim's legs for padding, then tie the injured leg to the uninjured leg with several cravats or bandages, or
- Place one board long enough to extend from the groin to the foot between the victim's legs. Place another board, long enough to extend from the armpit to the foot, along the victim's side. The boards must be well padded along their entire lengths. Tie the boards securely. This will stabilize the hip and the knee against movement (▼Figure 14-8).

Knee (◄Skill Scan)

Always stabilize an injured knee in the position that you find it. If the knee is straight, splint it straight; if it is bent, splint it bent (►Figure 14-9, A–B). For a straight knee, you have three options. You can tie one long, padded board that extends from the hip to the ankle underneath the leg. Or you can tie two boards on either side of the leg, one placed between the victim's legs that extends from the groin to the foot and the other on the outer side that extends from the hip to the foot. Finally, you can tie the injured leg to the uninjured one

For a bent knee, tie a long board extending from just below the hip to just above the ankle, to prevent motion of the knee. Or, place a pillow or a rolled blanket beneath the knee and tie the injured leg to the uninjured leg.

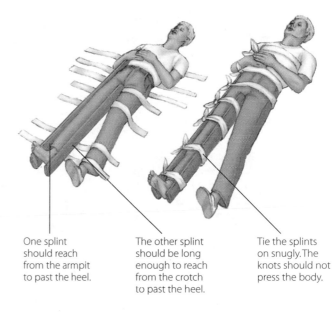

One splint should reach from the armpit to past the heel.

The other splint should be long enough to reach from the crotch to past the heel.

Tie the splints on snugly. The knots should not press the body.

Figure 14-7 A–C   **A.** Splinting a wrist, hand, or finger fracture **B.** Use gauze roller bandage. Apply roller working up the elbow. **C.** Overlap previous layer by one-half to three-quarters.

Figure 14-8   Splinting a femur fracture.

Skill Scan) Splinting—Lower Extremities

Lower Leg (Tibia/Fibula)

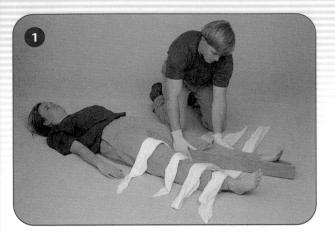

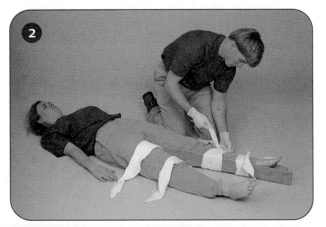

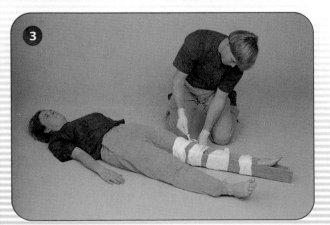

Thigh (Femur)

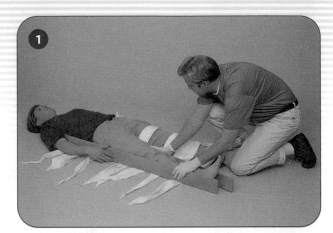

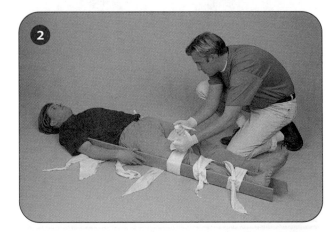

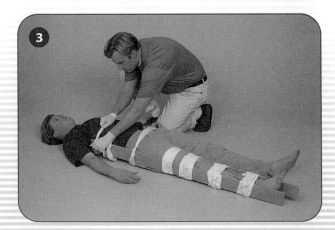

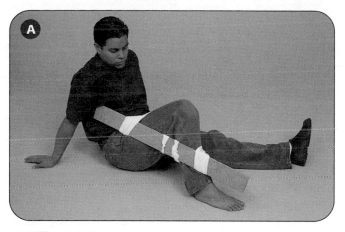

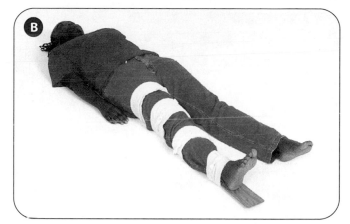

Figure 14-9 A–B **A.** Splint knee in position found. If bent, splint it bent.

B. Splint knee in position found. If straight, splint it straight.

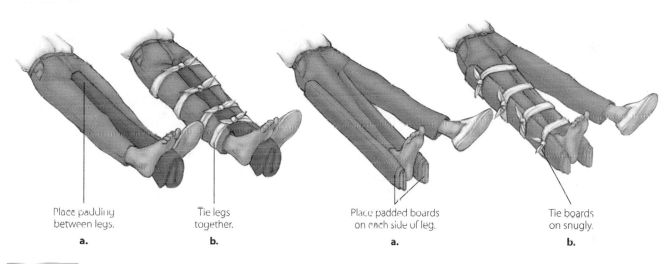

Place padding between legs.
a.

Tie legs together.
b.

Place padded boards on each side of leg.
a.

Tie boards on snugly.
b.

Figure 14-10 Two methods of splinting tibia and fibula fractures: self-splint (left) and two boards (right).

Lower Leg ◄Skill Scan

Stabilize the lower leg with two boards that extend from the upper thigh to the bottom of the foot. Or place a folded blanket or pillow between the victim's legs for padding and then tie the injured leg to the uninjured leg with several swathes, cravats, or bandages ▲Figure 14-10).

Ankle and Foot ►Skill Scan

Treat ankle and foot injuries with the RICE procedures (see Chapter 13). To further stabilize an ankle, wrap a pillow or folded blanket around the ankle and foot and tie with cravats ►Figure 14-11).

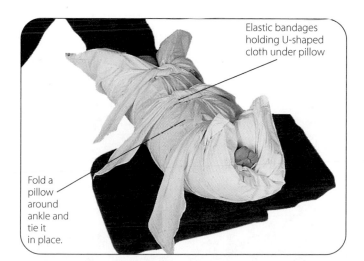

Elastic bandages holding U-shaped cloth under pillow

Fold a pillow around ankle and tie it in place.

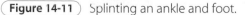
Figure 14-11 Splinting an ankle and foot.

Skill Scan — Splinting—Lower Extremities

Ankle/Foot

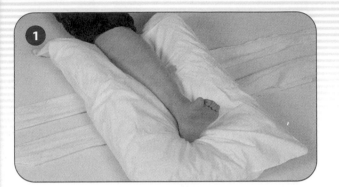

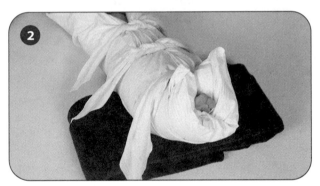

Self-Splint: Fingers/Toes

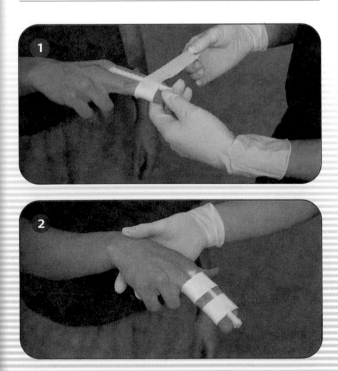

Self-Splint: Leg

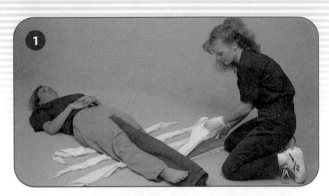

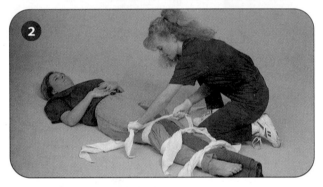

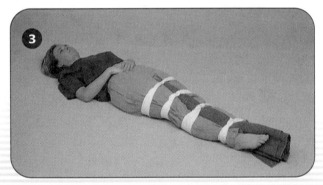

STUDY
Questions (14)

Name_____ Course_____ Date_____

Activities

Activity 1

Mark each statement as true (T) or false (F).

T F **1.** An uninjured body part can provide support for an injured extremity.

T F **2.** Applying splinting materials on both sides of an injured forearm or lower leg prevents the bones from rotating.

T F **3.** Do not apply an ice pack over a suspected broken bone.

T F **4.** A pillow can serve as a splint.

T F **5.** A splint for a fractured lower leg should extend from below the knee to above the heel.

T F **6.** Generally victims with a fracture need rapid transportation to medical care.

T F **7.** While in an arm sling, the hand should be in a thumb-up position.

T F **8.** A victim with a shoulder dislocation usually holds the affected arm close to the chest.

T F **9.** Splint an injured elbow or knee in the position it is found.

T F **10.** A broken femur is best splinted with one long board.

Choose the best answer.

____ **11.** Care for an open fracture by:
  a. applying pressure to push the bone back into place.
  b. flushing the wound with water
  c. applying an antiseptic into the wound
  d. covering with a dry, sterile dressing before splinting

____ **12.** A splint's purpose is to:
  a. decrease pain
  b. prevent motion
  c. reduce bleeding
  d. all of these

Activity 2
Matching:

Fracture	Recommended Type of Splint
____ **13.** Foot	**a.** "buddy taping"
____ **14.** Lower leg	**b.** pillow
____ **15.** Finger	**c.** sling and swathe (binder) only
____ **16.** Forearm	**d.** 2 rigid splints (eg, 2 boards)
____ **17.** Shoulder	**e.** 1 rigid splint (eg, 1 board)
____ **18.** Wrist, hand	

Case Situations

Case 1

A college student hit a roadside curb and fell from his bicycle. He landed on his outstretch arm. His forearm is deformed and painful.

____ **1.** What do you suspect?
  a. fracture
  b. dislocation
  c. contusion
  d. sprain

____ **2.** Which could you apply for this victim?
  a. pillow
  b. folded blanket
  c. boards
  d. any of these

____ **3.** What should the splints try to prevent?
  a. need to seek medical care
  b. rotation of the bones
  c. need to call 9-1-1

Chapter Activities

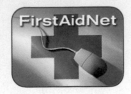

WEB Activities

Splinting the Extremities

Visit **nsc.jbpub.com/FirstAidNet**, then click on **Web Activities, and select the appropriate chapter.**

Cast Care

Many people, at one time or another, have worn a cast to aid in healing a broken bone. For successful therapy, learn how to properly care for a cast.

Medical Emergencies

Part 5

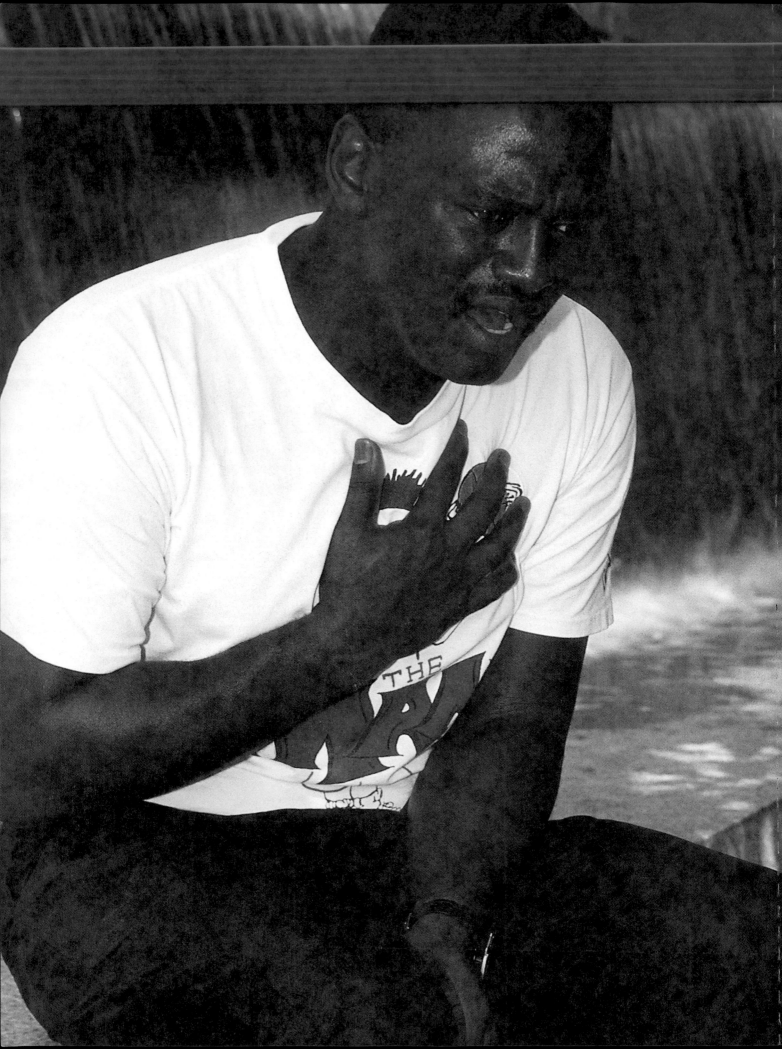

Chapter 15

Sudden Illnesses

Heart Attack

A heart attack, or **acute myocardial infarction (AMI),** happens when the blood supply to part of the heart muscle is severely reduced or stopped. That occurs when one of the coronary arteries (the arteries that supply blood to the heart muscle) is blocked by an obstruction or a spasm (▶Figure 15-1).

"A man is as old as his arteries."

—Pierre J. G. Cabanis

What to Look for

A heart attack is difficult to determine. Because medical care at the onset of a heart attack is vital to survival and the quality of recovery, if you suspect a heart attack for any reason, seek medical attention *at once* (▶Figure 15-2).

The possible signs and symptoms of a heart attack include:

- uncomfortable pressure, fullness, squeezing, or pain in the center of the chest that lasts more than a few minutes or that goes away and comes back
- pain spreading to the shoulders, neck, or arms
- chest discomfort with lightheadedness, fainting, sweating, nausea, or shortness of breath

Not all of these warning signs occur in every heart attack. It is difficult to determine if someone is having a heart attack. Many victims will deny that they might be experiencing something as serious as a heart attack. Don't take "no" for an answer. Delay can seriously increase the risk of major damage. Insist on taking prompt action.

Victims with heart attack symptoms who are brought to a hospital by ambulance receive clot-dissolving drugs (thrombolytics) sooner than those arriving by other means (▶Figures 15-3 and 15-4). Reducing the time from the onset of a heart attack to the administration of thrombolytic drugs is beneficial and decreases the amount of heart damage.

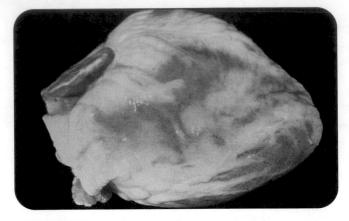

Figure 15-1 Healthy heart.

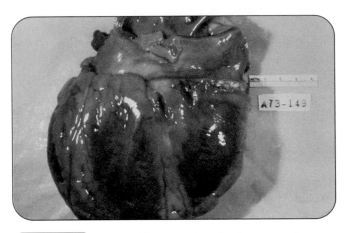

Figure 15-2 Heart with artery clot after heart attack.

What to Do

1. Call the EMS or get to the nearest hospital emergency department that offers 24-hour emergency cardiac care.

2. Monitor ABCs. Give CPR if necessary and if you are properly trained.

3. Help the victim to the least painful position, usually sitting. Loosen clothing around the neck and midriff. Be calm and reassuring ▶**Figure 15-5**.

4. Find out whether the victim has coronary heart disease and is using nitroglycerin. Nitroglycerin tablets or spray under the tongue or nitroglycerin ointment on the skin may relieve chest pain from angina but not heart attack. Nitroglycerin dilates the coronary arteries, which increases blood flow to the heart muscle. It also lowers blood pressure and dilates the veins, thus decreasing the work of the heart and the heart muscle's need for oxygen.

   Caution: Because nitroglycerin lowers blood pressure, the victim should be sitting or lying down.

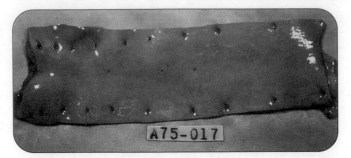

Figure 15-3 Normal artery (aorta).

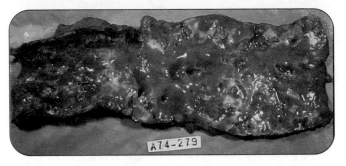

Figure 15-4 Inside of atherosclerotic artery (aorta).

Nitroglycerin normally may be repeated for a total of three doses in 10 minutes if the first dose does not relieve the pain. Keep in mind, though, that the victim may have already taken some nitroglycerin. Also, nitroglycerin is prescribed in different strengths—three tablets of one strength may be a

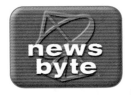

No Chest Pain in 1/3 of Heart Attacks

A study of hundreds of thousands of heart attack victims has found that as many as a third suffered no chest pain and that these people were less likely to seek help and twice as likely to die.

The study found that women, non-white, people older than 75, and those with previous heart failure, stroke, or diabetes were most likely to have "painless" heart attacks. Though doctors have long known about painless heart attacks, many said they didn't realize the number was so high.

Patients with chest pain were more than twice as likely to be diagnosed upon admission and to get either clot-busting drugs or angioplasty to open clogged arteries.

Source: J.G. Canto, et al. (2000) "Prevalence, Clinical Characteristics, and Mortality Among Patients with Myocardial Infarction Presenting Without Chest Pain," *Journal of the American Medical Association,* 283:3223-3229.

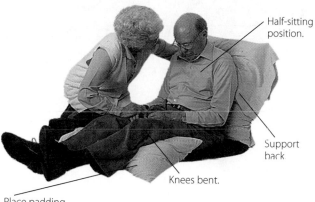

Half-sitting position.

Support back

Knees bent.

Place padding under knees.

Figure 15-5 Help the victim into a relaxed position to ease strain on heart.

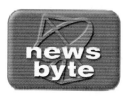

Dangerous Morning Hours

The chances of suffering cardiac arrest are higher in the morning hours than at any other time of day. A study of 1,019 consecutive cardiac arrest cases that occurred in Houston during a one-year period found that out-of-hospital cardiac arrest was more common among—and more likely to be survived by—men. Women victims, however, tended to be older than the men.

The study revealed that cardiac arrest events were least common during the night hours, and their occurrence began to increase at around 6 a.m. The incidence of cardiac arrest peaked in the late morning (around 10 or 11) and then declined for the rest of the day. Cardiac arrest may be tied to the circadian rhythm cycle, changes in blood pressure, ability of platelets to aggregate, or fluctuations in epinephrine levels.

Source: R. L. Levine et al: "Prospective Evidence of a Circadian Rhythm for Out-of-Hospital Cardiac Arrests." *Journal of the American Medical Association,* 267:2935–2937 (June 3, 1992).

Risk Factors for Heart Disease

Several factors contribute to an increased risk of heart attack and stroke. The more risk factors present, the greater the possibility that a person will develop heart disease.

Risk factors you cannot change:

+ Heredity. Tendencies appear in family lines.

+ Gender. Men have a greater risk, although heart attack is still the leading cause regarding death among women.

+ Age. Most heart attack victims are 65 or older.

Risk factors you can change:

+ Cigarette smoking. Smokers have more than twice the risk of heart attack as nonsmokers.

+ High blood pressure. This condition adds to the heart's workload.

+ High blood cholesterol level. Too much cholesterol in the blood can cause a buildup on the walls of the arteries.

Other risk factors you can change or control:

+ Diabetes. This condition affects the blood's cholesterol and triglyceride levels.

+ Obesity. Being overweight influences blood pressure and blood cholesterol, can result in diabetes, and can put an added strain on the heart.

+ Physical inactivity. Inactive people have twice the risk of heart attack as active people.

+ Stress. All people feel stress but react in different ways. Excessive, long-term stress may create problems in some people.

mild dose, while three tablets of another strength may be a very high dose.

5. If the victim is unresponsive, check ABCs and start CPR if needed.

Angina

Chest pain called **angina pectoris** can result from coronary heart disease just as a heart attack does (►**Table 15-1**).

Angina happens when the heart muscle does not get as much blood as it needs (which means a lack of oxygen).

Angina is brought on by physical exertion, exposure to cold, emotional stress, or the ingestion of food. It seldom lasts longer than 10 minutes and almost always is relieved by nitroglycerin. In contrast, chest pain from a heart attack is as likely to happen at rest as during activity; the pain lasts longer than 10 minutes and is not relieved by nitroglycerin. As previously discussed, nitroglycerin is the drug most often used to dilate coronary arteries to increase the blood supply to the heart. As a result, it is often prescribed by physicians for their patients with angina.

HEART ATTACK

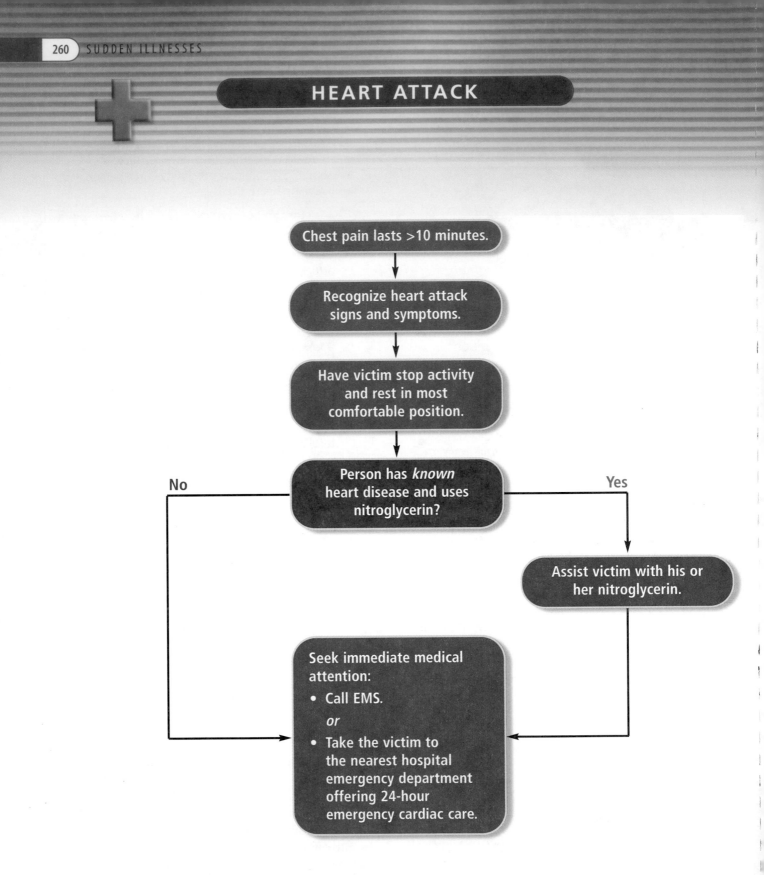

Chest pain lasts >10 minutes.

Recognize heart attack signs and symptoms.

Have victim stop activity and rest in most comfortable position.

Person has *known* heart disease and uses nitroglycerin?

No

Yes

Assist victim with his or her nitroglycerin.

Seek immediate medical attention:
- Call EMS.

  or
- Take the victim to the nearest hospital emergency department offering 24-hour emergency cardiac care.

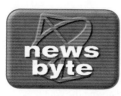

Inflammation May Cause Heart Attacks

Inflammation that builds up over years in blood vessels appears to play a significant role in heart attacks and strokes. If this finding is confirmed by further research, antibiotics, vaccines, or anti-inflammatory drugs could be used to treat or prevent heart disease.

The finding helps explain why aspirin is effective at cutting heart attack risk. Aspirin prevents blood clots and reduces inflammation.

Heart disease causes 42% of all deaths in the United States.

Source: P.M. Ridker, et al: "Inflammation, Aspirin, and the Risk of Cardiovascular Disease in Apparently Healthy Men." *New England Journal of Medicine,* April 1997 Vol 336 #14, p. 973.

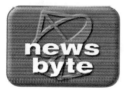

Why Don't They Call?

A study of heart attack victims who waited for more than 20 minutes before getting help were asked why they delayed. Their answers included the following:

- They thought the symptoms would go away.
- The symptoms were "not severe enough."
- They thought it was a different illness.
- They were worried about medical costs.
- They were afraid of hospitals.
- They feared being embarrassed.
- They wanted to wait for a better time.
- They did not want to find out what was wrong.

The average time that elapsed between symptom onset and hospital arrival was two hours; 28% waited at least one hour, 33% waited one to three hours, 15% waited three to six hours, and 23% waited more than six hours. The researchers noted that the main reason for victim delay appeared to be uncertainty in interpreting heart attack symptoms. Most victims reported they were not sure their symptoms were severe enough to merit such drastic action as calling 9-1-1.

The same study concluded that one way to shorten out-of-hospital delay is to encourage victims with heart-related symptoms to use the emergency medical service rather than slower transportation methods.

Source: H. Meischke et al: "Reasons Patients with Chest Pain Delay or Do Not Call 911." *Annals of Emergency Medicine* 25:193–197 (February 1995).

What to Do

1. ***If a victim has his or own nitroglycerin, assist the victim in using it appropriately. Refer to the Caution under the Heart Attack Section.***
2. If the pain does not quickly subside (5-10 minutes) suspect a heart attack and care for the victim accordingly.

Many causes of chest pain have nothing to do with the heart:

- Muscle or rib pain from exercise or injury: The victim can reproduce the pain by movement, and often the area of complaint is tender when pressed. Rest and aspirin or ibuprofen relieve the pain.
- Respiratory infections such as pneumonia, bronchitis, pleuritis, or lung injury: Chest pain from these conditions usually worsens when the victim coughs or breathes deeply. Fever and colored sputum may be present.

Table 15-1: Chest Pain

Cause of Pain	Characteristics	Care
Muscle or rib pain from exercise or injury	Reproduced by movement Tender spot when pressed	Rest Aspirin or ibuprofen
Respiratory infection (pneumonia, bronchitis, pleuritis)	Cough Fever Sore throat Production of sputum	Antibiotics
Indigestion	Belching Heartburn Nausea Sour taste	Antacids
Angina pectoris	Lasts <10 minutes	Rest Victim's nitroglycerin
Heart attack (myocardial infarction) of chest	Lasts >10 minutes Pressure, squeezing, or pain in center position Pain spreads to shoulders, neck, or arms Lightheadedness, fainting, sweating, nausea, shortness of breath	Call EMS Check ABCs Rothberg Victim's nitroglycerin

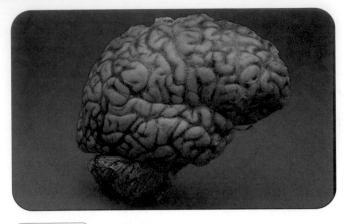

Figure 15-6 Healthy brain.

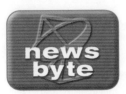

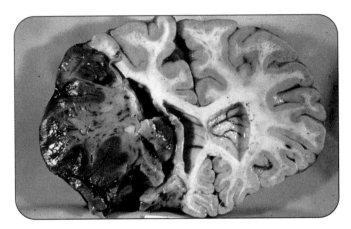

Figure 15-7 Stroke resulting from a severe hemorrhage.

- Indigestion, usually accompanied by belching, heartburn, nausea, and a sour taste in the mouth. This type of pain is relieved by antacids.

Stroke (Brain Attack)

A **stroke,** also referred to as a **cerebrovascular accident (CVA)** or **"brain attack,"** occurs when blood vessels that deliver oxygen-rich blood to the brain rupture or become plugged, so part of the brain does not get the blood flow it needs (▲**Figure 15-6**). Deprived of oxygen, nerve cells in the affected area of the brain cannot function and die within minutes. Because dead brain cells are not replaced, the devastating effects of strokes often are permanent (▲**Figure 15-7**). Each year, approximately 500,000 Americans suffer a stroke and approximately one-third of these victims die, making it the third leading cause of death.

The risk factors for a stroke include:

- age (greater than 50 years old)
- taking birth control pills *and* being over 30 years old
- overweight
- hypertension (high blood pressure)
- high blood cholesterol levels
- diabetes
- heart disease
- sickle cell disease
- substance abuse, particularly of crack cocaine
- family history of strokes or transient ischemic attacks

The most common type of stroke (about 80%) is *ischemic,* that is, a clot either forms in a brain artery (thrombotic stroke) or travels from the heart to the brain and plugs the artery (embolic stroke). In about 20% of cases, a blood vessel ruptures (hemorrhagic stroke). Other causes include tumors pressing on blood vessels, blood vessel spasms, and **aneurysms** (ballooning out of blood vessels).

Transient ischemic attacks (TIAs) are closely associated with CVAs. Because TIAs have many of the same signs and symptoms, they often are confused with strokes. The main difference between a TIA and a stroke is that the symptoms of TIA are transient, lasting from several minutes (75% last less than five minutes) to several hours, with a return to normal neurologic function. TIAs are "mini-strokes." A TIA should be considered a serious

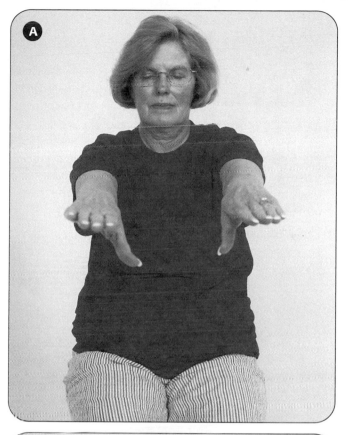

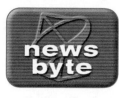

Los Angeles Stroke Screen

Los Angeles paramedics use a proven method for quickly identifying stroke victims, and so can first aiders. When you suspect a stroke, apply these three simple tests for one-side paralysis:

1. **Arm strength** (both arms): person closes eyes and holds both arms out with palms down. Slowly count to five. If one arm does not move and the other drifts down, suspect a stroke (►Figure 15-8, A-B).

2. **Facial smile:** person smiles or shows teeth. If one side of face does not move as well as the other side, suspect a stroke.

3. **Hand grip** (both hands): person grips two of your fingers at the same time. If grip strength is not equal, suspect a stroke.

warning sign of a potential stroke—about one-third of all TIA patients will suffer a CVA two to five years after their first TIA. Any signs and symptoms of a TIA should be reported to a physician.

What to Look for

The next time you think about stroke, think "brain attack." The symptoms of stroke should have the same alarming significance that acute chest pain has in identifying a heart attack:

- weakness, numbness, or paralysis of the face, an arm, or a leg on one side of the body (►Figure 15-8, A–B)

- blurred or decreased vision, especially in one eye

- problems speaking or understanding

- dizziness or loss of balance

- sudden, severe, and unexplained headache

- deviation of the eyes from PEARL (**P**upils **E**qual **A**nd **R**eactive to **L**ight), which may mean the brain is being affected by lack of oxygen

What to Do

First aid for a stroke victim is limited to supportive care:

1. Call EMS. Hospitals staffed with teams trained to treat acute stroke offer the best treatment for stroke. Minimize brain damage by getting the victim to a hospital.

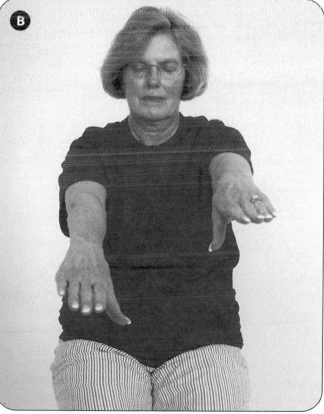

Figure 15-8 One-sided weakness (stroke test). **A.** Arms straight out. **B.** One arm dropped.

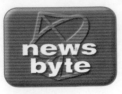

Get Immediate Medical Attention for Stroke Symptoms

Two studies urge people experiencing stroke symptoms to get immediate medical attention in order to increase their eligibility for potentially beneficial therapy. The studies found that most stroke patients arrive at the emergency department too late to receive tissue-type plasminogen activator (tPA), a clot-busting therapy shown to reduce the consequences including neurologic damage of this debilitating, but now treatable, disease.

Source: N. Azia, et. Al., "The effect of FDA Approval of Thrombolytic Therapy on the Management of Acute Stroke in the Emergency Department, *Annals of Emergency Medicine*, 32:42 December 1998.

2. If the victim is unresponsive, check ABCs: keep the airway open and check breathing and pulse. If there is no pulse, give CPR. If there is a pulse but no breathing, perform rescue breathing.

3. If the victim is conscious, lay the victim down with the head and shoulders slightly elevated. Place a victim who is unresponsive but breathing in the recovery position to keep the airway open and to permit secretions and vomit to drain from the mouth.

Caution:

DO NOT give a stroke victim anything to drink or eat. The throat may be paralyzed, which restricts swallowing.

Asthma

Asthma is a chronic, inflammatory lung disease characterized by repeated breathing problems. People with asthma have acute episodes (some sufferers call them "attacks" or "flares") when the air passages in their lungs get narrower, and breathing becomes more difficult. The problems are caused by an oversensitivity of the lungs' airways, which overreact to certain triggers and become inflamed and clogged. Asthma affects an estimated 10 million people in the United States and accounts for an annual death toll of 6,000.

The condition is most common in children and young adults and tends to improve or resolve with age. Asthma is the number one prehospital emergency in children. It can happen in infants who are as young as a few weeks; about one-half of all children with asthma experience the condition in their first two years of life. Viral infections are a common cause of acute asthma onset in children younger than six months. Adult-onset asthma tends to be chronic.

Asthma has three components: airway obstruction, airway inflammation, and overly sensitive airways. Some of the known triggers of asthma include:

- respiratory tract infection
- exposure to temperature extremes, especially cold air
- strong odors, perfumes, talcum powder, deodorizers, paint
- occupational exposures: dust, fumes, smoke
- certain drugs: aspirin, nonsteroidal anti-inflammatory drugs (NSAIDs), yellow dye #5, beta blockers
- exercise
- emotional stress
- allergens: pollen, mold, dust mites, animal dander, tobacco smoke
- air pollution: ozone, sulfur dioxide

What to Look for

Asthma varies a great deal from one person to another. Symptoms can range from mild to moderate to severe and can be life threatening. The episodes may come occasionally or often. The signs of an asthma attack include

- coughing
- cyanosis (bluish skin color)
- inability to speak in complete sentences without pausing for breath
- nostrils flaring with each breath
- difficulty breathing, including wheezing

Not all persons with these signs have asthma. Other causes include foreign body aspiration, lung cancer, cystic fibrosis, congestive heart failure, upper-airway obstruction or inflammation, and pneumonia. Some victims of asthma attack may have little or no wheezing.

What to Do

1. Keep the victim in a comfortable upright position and leaning slightly forward.

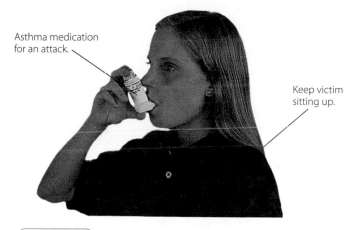

Asthma medication for an attack.

Keep victim sitting up.

Figure 15-9 Keep an asthma victim comfortable.

This is known as the "tripod" position. Generally the victim will dictate what position is most tolerable, usually sitting up since that makes it easier to breathe.

2. Check and monitor ABCs.

3. Ask the victim about any asthma medication he or she may be using. Most asthma sufferers will have some form of asthma medication, usually administered through physician-prescribed, hand-held inhalers(▲Figure 15-9).

4. If the victim does not respond well to his or her inhaled medication or is having an extreme asthma attack (known as **status asthmaticus**), seek medical attention immediately.

Asthma is common and is treated fairly easily. Although asthma is a complex condition that may warrant use of several different medications, the preferred method of initial care for both children and adults is use of their inhaled bronchodilators.

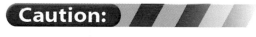

Caution:

DO NOT wait too long to get medical help for the victim of a severe asthma attack.

Hyperventilation

Fast, deep breathing, called hyperventilation, is common during emotional stress. The victim may be hysterical or quite calm. Other factors that can cause rapid breathing

include untreated diabetes, severe shock, certain poisons, and brain swelling from injury or high altitude.

What to Look for

- dizziness or lightheadedness
- numbness
- tingling of the hands and feet
- shortness of breath
- breathing rates faster than 40 per minute

What to Do

1. Calm and reassure the victim.

2. Encourage the person to breathe slowly, using the abdominal muscles: inhale through the nose, hold the full inhalation for several seconds, then exhale slowly.

Chronic Obstructive Pulmonary Disease (COPD)

Chronic obstructive pulmonary disease (COPD) is a broad term applied to emphysema, chronic bronchitis, and related lung diseases. The incidence of COPD is very high in North America, and the most common causative factor is cigarette smoking.

Chronic obstructive pulmonary disease (COPD) describes a disease that makes it hard for a person to breathe because the normal flow of air into and out of the person's lungs is partially obstructed.

Because COPD takes many years to develop before a person notices difficulty breathing, COPD is usually

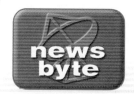

news byte

Breathing into a Paper Bag

If you are advised to breathe into a paper bag—a popular remedy for anxiety-related hyperventilation (fast breathing)—don't do it. Tests on normal, healthy people show that bag rebreathing rarely restores blood gas balance but often causes dangerous stress to the heart and respiratory system, especially in people with a chronic respiratory disease.

Source: M. Callaham: "Hypoxic Hazards of Traditional Paper Bag Rebreathing in Hyperventilating Patients." *Annals of Emergency Medicine,* 18:622.

considered a disease of older adults and is most commonly diagnosed in people over the age of 60.

Chronic bronchitis is caused by chronic infection which can be brought on by irritations such as tobacco smoke. The bronchi become thick, unable to stretch, and partially blocked. Early symptoms include a "cigarette cough" or cough due to a cold. Later, more severe symptoms include difficult breathing, increased sputum, and severe coughing.

Emphysema often occurs with chronic bronchitis. The alveoli of the lungs are partially destroyed and the lungs have lost their elasticity, making it difficult for the victim to exhale. Common symptoms include coughing, wheezing, and shortness of breath. Breathing is extremely difficult for emphysema victims.

COPD signs and symptoms are similar to those of asthma. Most victims will wheeze; coughing and shortness of breath may be more prominent in COPD than in asthma. Many COPD victims depend on a constant low level of artificially supplied oxygen to maintain breathing.

What to Do

1. Persons with COPD usually will have their own physician-prescribed medications. Assist the victim in taking any prescribed medications.

2. Place the victim in the sitting position that provides the greatest comfort.

3. Encourage the victim to cough up any secretions.

4. Encourage the victim to drink fluids.

5. For acute breathing distress, obtain immediate medical assistance. The victim may need oxygen, which is available from EMS ambulances and at hospital emergency departments.

Altered Mental Status

A quick neurologic assessment can determine a victim's level of responsiveness or mental status. The AVPU method describes whether the victim is

    A – **A**lert

    V – responsive to **V**erbal stimuli

    P – responsive to **P**ainful stimuli

    U – **U**nresponsive

With the AVPU method, you can assess a victim's mental status in seconds. For example, a victim in a coma would have a depressed mental state with no responses to verbal or physical stimuli. On the AVPU scale, that victim would be in the unresponsive category.

Altered mental status can be caused by a variety of conditions. If you encounter a victim with altered mental status (V, P, or U category), use the following mnemonics to narrow down what may be causing the condition:

- **AEIOU** (vowels)

  Alcohol, **A**irway blocked, **A**naphylaxis

  Epilepsy, **E**lectrocution

  Insulin reaction (diabetes)

  Oxygen (lack of), **O**verdose of drugs

  Underdose of insulin

- **TIPS**

  Trauma (brain), **T**emperature (heatstroke, hypothermia)

  Infection (meningitis)

  Psychogenic fainting, **P**oisoning

  Stroke, **S**eizure, **S**hock

What to Do

1. Check ABCs. Gather additional information through a rapid physical exam and collect the victim's history from any family members or other bystanders who may be knowledgeable about the victim's condition. Use the scene survey, your victim assessment, and relevant information from family, friends, or bystanders about the possible causes (AEIOU—TIPS) to determine necessary care.

2. If the victim is breathing, keep the airway open by placing the victim in the recovery position. This may be the most important care. If the victim is not breathing, perform rescue breathing. If the victim is without a pulse, perform CPR.

3. Seek medical attention.

For specific information on some of the more common problems that can cause altered mental status or unresponsiveness and their first aid, refer to the appropriate sections of this book:

Alcohol	Page 288
Airway blocked	Page 75
Anaphylaxis	Page 107
Epilepsy	Page 269
Electrocution	Page 164
Lightning	Page 402

Fainting

A sudden brief loss of consciousness not associated with a head injury is known as **syncope,** simple fainting, or **psychogenic shock.**

Simple fainting is a common and benign sign of hypoperfusion shock that can have either physical or emotional causes. Fainting happens when the brain's blood flow is decreased. The nervous system dilates blood vessels to three to four times their normal size and allows blood to pool in the legs and lower body.

Syncope or simple fainting can be precipitated by unpleasant emotional stimuli such as the sight of blood or strong fear. It usually occurs when the victim is in the upright position.

Most fainting episodes are associated with decreased blood flow causing deficient oxygen or glucose to the brain. The decreased blood flow may be caused by low blood sugar (**hypoglycemia**), slow heart rate (vagal reaction, in which the vagus nerve, which slows the heart rate, is overstimulated by fright, anxiety, drugs, fatigue), heart-rhythm disturbances, dehydration, heat exhaustion, anemia, or bleeding.

Sitting or standing for a long time without moving, especially in a hot environment, can cause blood to pool in dilated vessels. That results in a loss of effective circulating blood volume, which causes the blood pressure to drop. As the brain's blood flow decreases, the person loses consciousness and collapses.

What to Look for

A person who is about to faint usually will have one or more of the following signs and symptoms:

- dizziness
- weakness
- seeing spots
- visual blurring
- nausea
- pale skin
- sweating

What to Do

If a person appears about to faint,

1. Prevent the person from falling.
2. Help the person lie down and raise the legs 8 to 12 inches. This position increases venous blood flow back to the heart, which in turn pumps more blood to the brain.
3. Loosen tight clothing at the neck and waist.
4. Stay with victim until he or she recovers.

If fainting has happened or is anticipated,

1. Check ABCs.
2. Loosen tight clothing and belts.
3. If the victim has fallen, check for any sign of injury.
4. If injuries allow, turn victim into recovery position.
5. After recovery, have the victim sit for a while and, when he or she is able to swallow, give cool, sweetened liquids to drink, and slowly help the victim regain an upright posture.
6. Fresh air and a cold, wet cloth for the face usually aid recovery.

Most fainting episodes are not serious, and the victim recovers quickly. Seek medical attention, however, if the victim

- has had repeated attacks of unconsciousness
- does not quickly regain consciousness
- loses consciousness while sitting or lying down
- faints for no apparent reason

FAINTING

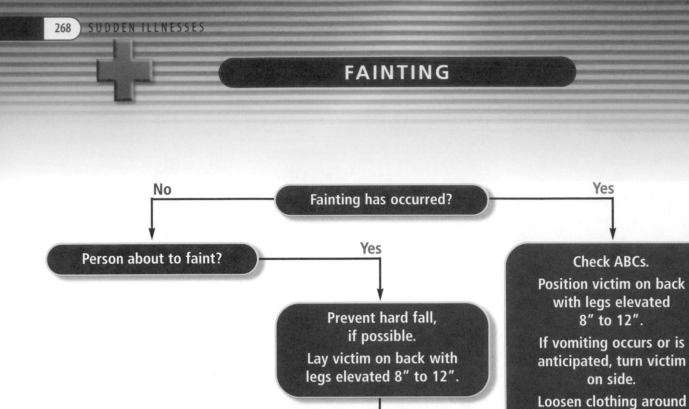

Fainting has occurred?

No → **Person about to faint?**

Yes

Person about to faint? → Yes

Prevent hard fall, if possible.
Lay victim on back with legs elevated 8" to 12".

↓

If vomiting occurs or is anticipated, turn victim on side.
Loosen clothing around victim's neck.
Wipe victim's forehead with cool, wet cloth.

Fainting has occurred? → Yes

Check ABCs.
Position victim on back with legs elevated 8" to 12".
If vomiting occurs or is anticipated, turn victim on side.
Loosen clothing around victim's neck.
Wipe victim's forehead with cool, wet cloth.

↓

Seek medical attention if victim
- **has repeated attacks of unresponsiveness**
- **loses consciousness while sitting or lying down**
- **faints for no apparent reason**
- **does not quickly regain consciousness**

Caution: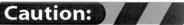

DO NOT splash or pour water on the victim's face.

DO NOT use smelling salts or ammonia inhalants.

DO NOT slap the victim's face in an attempt to revive him or her.

DO NOT give the victim anything to drink until he or she has fully recovered and can swallow.

Seizures

A seizure is the result of an abnormal stimulation of the brain's cells. A variety of medical conditions increase the instability or irritability of the brain and can lead to seizures, including the following:

- epilepsy
- heatstroke
- poisoning
- electric shock
- hypoglycemia
- high fever in children
- brain injury, tumor, or stroke
- alcohol withdrawal, drug abuse/overdose

Most people with seizures have idiopathic epilepsy, that is, the cause of the seizures is not known.

There are four types of seizures. Because seizure types are so different, they require different first aid actions, and some require no action at all (▶Table15-2).

- Generalized motor seizures (**grand mal seizures**) are characterized by loss of consciousness, muscle contraction, and sometimes tongue biting, loss of bladder control, and mental confusion. The grand mal seizure is often frightening to witness. The seizure usually is followed by a period of coma or drowsiness.
- **Focal motor seizures** usually cause one part of the body such as one side of the face or an arm to twitch.
- **Psychomotor (temporal-lobe) seizures** are characterized by an altered personality state and are often preceded by dizziness or a peculiar metallic taste in the mouth. In some people, temporal-lobe seizures may cause sudden, unexplained attacks of rage; in

others, these seizures are manifested by automatic (involuntary) types of behavior.

- **Petit mal seizures** usually occur in children and are rarely an emergency. They are characterized by a brief loss of consciousness. The child suddenly stares off into space for a few seconds and then returns immediately to consciousness.

Because of the nature of the electrical discharge in the brain, grand mal seizures usually follow a typical sequence. Many victims experience an aura, a strange sensation lasting a few seconds. The aura may consist of auditory or visual hallucinations, a peculiar taste in the mouth, or a painful sensation in the abdomen. The victim then loses consciousness and has contractions of the muscles of the extremities, trunk, and head. The attack usually lasts two to five minutes. It may be followed by deep sleep, headache, and muscle soreness.

The following information is important to obtain from the seizure victim, the family, or bystanders:

- Does the victim have a history of seizures? Does the victim take medication for seizures? Has the victim been taking the medication according to instructions?
- What did the seizure look like? How long did the seizure last? Was the seizure preceded by an aura?
- Does the victim have a recent or remote history of head injury? Trauma can irritate parts of the brain, causing seizures. More than half the victims of acute head injuries will experience a seizure within one year following the injury.
- Does the victim abuse alcohol or drugs? Seizures often occur during withdrawal from alcohol and barbiturates.
- Has the victim recently had a fever, headache, or stiff neck? These signs and symptoms could indicate meningitis.
- Does the victim have a history of diabetes, heart disease, or stroke?

Epilepsy is not a mental illness, and it is not a sign of low intelligence. It also is not contagious. Between seizures, a person with epilepsy can function as normally as a nonepileptic.

What to Do

The Epilepsy Foundation lists the following first aid procedures for convulsions and grand mal seizures:

1. Cushion the victim's head; remove items that could cause injury if the person bumped into them.

2. Loosen any tight clothing, especially around neck.

3. Roll the victim onto his or her side.

4. Look for a medical-alert tag (bracelet or necklace).

5. As the seizure ends, offer your help. Most seizures in people with epilepsy are not medical emergencies.

They end after a minute or two without harm and usually do not require medical attention.

6. Call EMS if:

- A seizure happens to someone who is not known to have epilepsy (eg, there is no "epilepsy" or

Table 15-2: Seizures: Recognition and First Aid

Seizure Type	What It Looks Like	What It Is Not	What to Do	What Not to Do
Generalized Seizure (also called grand mal)	Sudden cry, fall, rigidity, followed by muscle jerks, shallow breathing or temporarily suspended breathing, bluish skin, possible loss of bladder or bowel control; usually lasts a couple of minutes. Normal breathing then starts again. There may be some confusion and/or fatigue, followed by return to full consciousness.	• Heart attack • Stroke	Look for medical-alert tag. Protect from nearby hazards. Loosen tie or shirt collars. Protect head from injury. Turn on side to keep airway clear. Reassure when consciousness returns. If single seizure lasted less than 5 minutes, ask if hospital evaluation is wanted. If multiple seizures, or if one seizure lasts longer than 5 minutes, call an ambulance. If person is pregnant, injured, or diabetic, call for aid at once.	Don't put any hard implement in the mouth. Don't try to hold tongue. It can't be swallowed. Don't try to give liquids during or just after seizure. Don't use rescue breathing unless breathing is absent after muscle jerks subside or unless water has been inhaled. Don't restrain.
Absence Seizure (also called petit mal)	A blank stare, lasting only a few seconds; most common in children. May be accompanied by rapid blinking, some chewing movements of the mouth. Child is unaware of what's going on during the seizure but quickly returns to full awareness once it has stopped.	• Daydreaming • Lack of attention • Deliberate ignoring of adult instructions	No first aid necessary, but if this is the first observation of the seizure(s), seek medical evaluation.	
Simple Partial Seizure	Jerking may begin in one area of the body, arm, leg, or face. Can't be stopped, but patient stays awake and aware. Jerking may proceed from one area of the body to another and sometimes spreads to become a convulsive seizure. Partial sensory seizures may not be obvious to an onlooker. Patient experiences a distorted environment. May see or hear things that aren't there, may feel unexplained fear, sadness, anger, or joy. May have nausea, experience odd smells, and have a generally "funny" feeling in the stomach.	• Acting out, bizarre behavior • Hysteria • Mental illness • Psychosomatic illness • Parapsychological or mystical experience	No first aid necessary unless seizure becomes convulsive, then first aid as above. No action needed other than reassurance and emotional support. Medical evaluation should be recommended.	

"seizure disorder" identification). It could be a sign of serious illness.

- A seizure lasts more than five minutes.

- The victim is slow to recover, has a second seizure, or has difficulty breathing afterward.

- The victim is pregnant or has another medical condition.

- There are any signs of injury or illnesses.

Status epilepticus is defined as two or more seizures without an intervening period of consciousness.

Table 15-2: Seizures: Recognition and First Aid (continued)

Seizure Type	What It Looks Like	What It Is Not	What to Do	What Not to Do
Complex Partial Seizure (also called psychomotor or temporal lobe)	Usually starts with blank stare, followed by chewing, followed by random activity. Person appears unaware of surroundings, may seem dazed and mumble. Unresponsive. Actions clumsy, not directed. May pick at clothing, pick up objects, try to take clothes off. May run, appear to be afraid. Same set of actions usually occur with each seizure. Lasts a few minutes, but postseizure confusion can last substantially longer. No memory of what happened during seizure period.	• Drunkenness • Drug intoxication • Mental illness • Disorderly conduct	Speak calmly and reassuringly to patient and others. Guide gently away from obvious hazards. Stay until person is completely aware of environment. Offer to help get person home.	Don't grab or hold person unless sudden danger (such as a cliff edge or an approaching car) threatens. Don't shout. Don't expect verbal instructions to be obeyed.
Atonic Seizure (also called drop attack)	Person suddenly collapses. After 10 seconds to a minute, person recovers, regains consciousness, and can stand and walk again.	• Clumsiness • Normal childhood "stage" • In a child, lack of good walking skills • In an adult, drunkenness, acute illness	No first aid needed (unless fall results in injury), but child should be given a thorough medical evaluation.	
Myoclonic Seizure	Sudden brief, massive muscle jerks that may involve the whole body or parts of body. May cause person to drop things or fall off a chair.	• Clumsiness • Poor coordination	No first aid needed but should be given a thorough medical evaluation.	
Infantile Spasms	Clusters of quick, sudden movements that start between 3 months and 2 years. If child is sitting up, head will fall forward, and arms will flex forward. If lying down, knees will be drawn up, with arms and head flexed forward as if baby is reaching for support.	• Normal movements of the baby • Colic	No first aid, but doctor should be consulted.	

Source: © Epilepsy Foundation; reprinted with permission.

SEIZURES

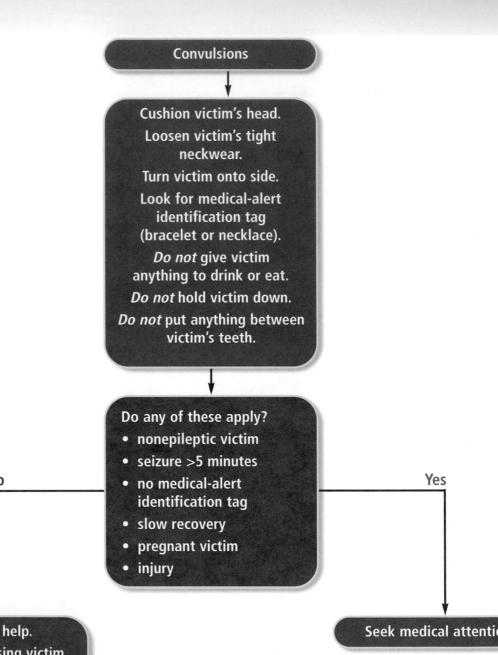

Convulsions

Cushion victim's head.

Loosen victim's tight neckwear.

Turn victim onto side.

Look for medical-alert identification tag (bracelet or necklace).

Do not give victim anything to drink or eat.

Do not hold victim down.

Do not put anything between victim's teeth.

Do any of these apply?
- nonepileptic victim
- seizure >5 minutes
- no medical-alert identification tag
- slow recovery
- pregnant victim
- injury

No

Yes

Offer your help.

Avoid embarrassing victim.

Most seizures are not medical emergencies, end in 1 to 2 minutes, and do not require medical attention.

Seek medical attention.

Status epilepticus is an emergency situation and requires immediate medical attention. Repeated uncontrolled seizures can lead to aspiration, brain damage, fractures, and severe dehydration. In adults, the most common cause of status epilepticus is failure to take prescribed medicines for epilepsy.

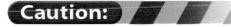

Caution:

DO NOT give the victim anything to eat or drink.

DO NOT restrain the victim.

DO NOT put anything between the victim's teeth during the seizure.

DO NOT splash or pour any liquid on the victim's face.

DO NOT move the victim to another place (unless it is the only way to protect the victim from injury).

Diabetic Emergencies

Diabetes is a condition in which **insulin,** a hormone produced by the pancreas that helps the body use the energy in food, is either lacking or ineffective. Insulin is needed to take sugar from the blood and carry it into the cells to be used. When excess sugar remains in the blood, the body cells must rely on fat as fuel. Blood sugar is a major body fuel, and when it cannot be used, it builds up in the blood and overflows into the urine and passes out of the body unused—the body loses an important source of fuel. Diabetes develops. Diabetes is not contagious.

There are two types of diabetes:

- *Type I: juvenile-onset or insulin-dependent diabetes.* Type I diabetics require external (not made by the body) insulin to allow sugar to pass from the blood into cells. When deprived of external insulin, the diabetic becomes quite ill.

- *Type II: adult-onset or non–insulin-dependent diabetes.* Type II diabetics tend to be overweight. They are not dependent on external insulin to allow sugar into cells. However, if their insulin level is low, the lack of sugar in the cells increases sugar production and sugar in the blood to very high levels. That causes glucose to spill into the urine, which draws fluid with it, resulting in dehydration.

Table 15-3: Diabetic Emergencies		
	Diabetic Coma	**Insulin Shock**
Cause	Not enough insulin; too much sugar	Too much insulin; not enough sugar
Insulin level	Insufficient	Excessive
Onset of symptoms	Gradual	Sudden
Skin	Flushed, dry, warm	Pale, clammy
Breath	Fruity odor	Normal
Thirst	Severe	Normal
Urination	Frequent	Normal
Behavior	–	Appearance of intoxication; combativeness, bad temper, anger; confusion, disorientation
Other symptoms	Drowsiness, vomiting, heavy breathing, eventual stupor or unconsciousness	Sudden hunger, eventual stupor or unconsciousness
First aid	• If in doubt, give sugar. • Give fluids to fight dehydration. • Take victim to hospital.	• Give sugar. • Seek medical attention.

Gestational diabetes occurs in some pregnancies. It usually ends after a baby is born, but women with gestational diabetes may develop Type II diabetes when they get older. Gestational diabetes results from the body's resistance to the action of insulin. This resistance is caused by hormones the placenta produces during pregnancy. Gestational diabetes is usually treated with diet. Some women may need insulin.

The body is continuously balancing sugar and insulin. Too much insulin and not enough sugar leads to low blood sugar, possibly insulin shock. Too much sugar and not enough insulin leads to high blood sugar, possibly diabetic coma (▲Table 15-3) (▶Figure 15-10).

Low Blood Sugar

Very low blood sugar, called hypoglycemia, is sometimes referred to as an "insulin reaction." This condition can

DIABETIC EMERGENCIES

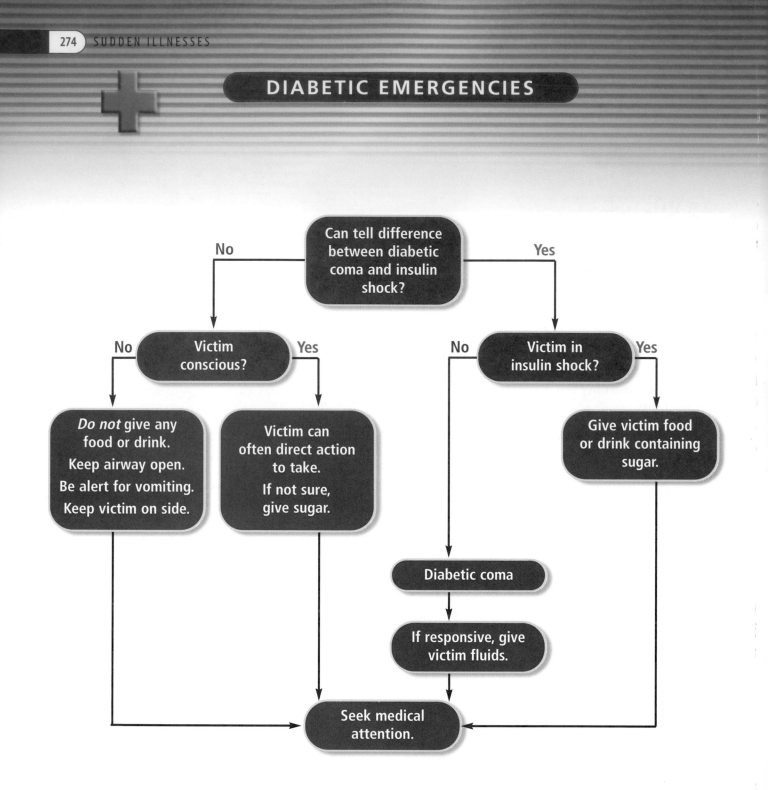

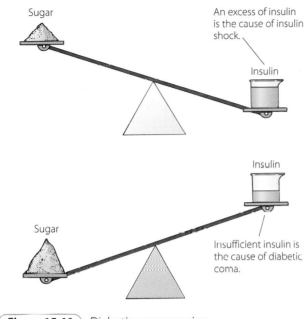

Figure 15-10 Diabetic emergencies

An excess of insulin is the cause of insulin shock.

Insufficient insulin is the cause of diabetic coma.

be caused by too much insulin, too little or delayed food, exercise, alcohol, or any combination of these factors.

The American Diabetes Association lists the following signs and symptoms of insulin reaction and hypoglycemia as diabetic emergencies requiring first aid:

- sudden onset
- staggering, poor coordination
- anger, bad temper
- pale color
- confusion, disorientation
- sudden hunger
- excessive sweating
- trembling
- eventual unconsciousness

What to Do

Give sugar using the "rule of 15s" for insulin reaction if all three conditions are present:

- The victim is a known diabetic, and
- The victim's mental status is altered, and
- The victim is awake enough to swallow.

Fast-acting sugars of 10-15 grams:

- one tube of glucose gel
- two to five glucose tablets ▶**Figure 15-11**

"Rule of 15s" for Insulin Reaction (Hypoglycemia)

1. Give 15 grams of carbohydrate (sugar).
2. Wait 15 minutes.
3. If no improvement, give 15 more grams of carbohydrate.
4. If no improvement, seek medical attention.

- two large lumps or teaspoons of sugar
- one half can of regular soda
- 4 oz. of orange juice
- two tablespoons of raisins
- five to seven Lifesavers™
- six jellybeans
- 10 gumdrops
- 6 to 8 oz. of skim or 1% milk
- two teaspoons of honey or corn syrup

An injectable medication called glucagon, available by a physician's prescription, raises blood sugar quickly. A family member or friend should learn when and how to inject glucagon in an emergency.

High Blood Sugar

Hyperglycemia—also known as diabetic coma—is the opposite of hypoglycemia. Hyperglycemia occurs when the body has too much sugar in the blood. This condition may be caused by insufficient insulin, overeating, inactivity, illness, stress, or a combination of these factors.

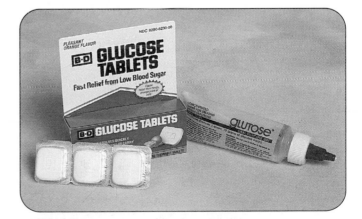

Figure 15-11 Glucose tablets and gel

The American Diabetes Association lists the following signs and symptoms of diabetic coma, hyperglycemia, and acidosis as diabetic emergencies requiring first aid:

- gradual onset
- drowsiness
- extreme thirst
- very frequent urination
- flushed skin
- vomiting
- fruity breath odor
- heavy breathing
- eventual unconsciousness

What to Do

1. If you are uncertain whether the victim has high or low blood-sugar level, give the person sugar-containing foods or drinks.

2. If improvement is not seen in 15 minutes, take the victim to the hospital.

Abdominal Distress

People with gastrointestinal problems usually complain of one or more of the following symptoms:

- *Abdominal pain that is aching, cramping, sharp, or dull.* It may be constant, or it may come and go. The pain may indicate a mild problem or an acute one requiring immediate surgery.
- *Nausea and vomiting.* Vomiting is the ejection of the stomach's contents through the mouth. Nausea is a feeling of the need to vomit.
- *Diarrhea or constipation.* Diarrhea is the frequent passage of loose, watery stools. Constipation is the opposite of diarrhea; stools are infrequent, hard, and difficult to pass.

Abdominal Pain

The abdomen is the area between the nipple line and the groin. Abdominal organs are either hollow or solid. Hollow organs are tubes, such as the stomach and the intestines, through which material passes, conducting food through the body. Solid organs are solid masses of tissue where much of the chemical work of the body takes place. The liver, spleen, and gallbladder are solid organs. The peritoneum is a thin membrane lining the entire abdominal cavity. Irritation of the peritoneum is called **peritonitis.**

There are many possible causes of abdominal pain, some not so serious and some life threatening. They often can be serious enough to require emergency surgery. Illnesses that affect the abdomen have one thing in common: they are very painful.

Abdominal problems are so difficult to diagnose that even skilled physicians may have trouble pinpointing an exact cause. It is neither feasible nor useful for a first aider to distinguish among the many causes of abdominal pain because first aid usually will be similar regardless of the cause.

What to Look for

- When did the pain start? Where is it located?
- Is the pain constant, or does it come and go? Constant pain may be more serious than a cramping pain. Constant abdominal pain suggests inflammation of an organ; cramping suggests obstruction of a hollow organ.
- Does belching or passing gas relieve the pain? That suggests the intestine is affected.
- Does the victim feel nauseated, or does he or she have a good appetite?
- Is there diarrhea or vomiting?
- Does the victim feel warm (feverish)?
- Does anyone in the group have similar symptoms?
- For a female, is there any chance of pregnancy? Any pain with pregnancy should be treated as an emergency.
- Is the abdomen rigid to touch? That may be a sign of an emergency condition.

What to Do

1. Give the victim only clear fluids (anything you can see through, except alcohol and caffeine). Have the victim slowly sip the fluids.

2. Give the victim an antacid.

3. If feasible, place a hot-water bottle against the victim's abdomen or have the victim soak in a warm bath.

4. Recognize the possibility of vomiting and be prepared for it. Keep the victim on the left side to help prevent vomiting.

5. Keep the victim in a comfortable position, usually lying down with knees bent (unless the victim is nauseated).

6. Seek medical care if any of the following applies:

- Pain is constant for more than six hours.
- The victim is unable to drink fluids.
- The victim is or may be pregnant.
- Abdomen is rigid and painful.
- Abdomen is swollen.
- After you press your fingers on the victim's abdomen and suddenly release it, more pain occurs.
- There is bloody, blood-stained, or black stool.
- The victim has a fever.
- Pain began around the belly button and later moved to the lower right abdomen.

Caution:

DO NOT give enemas and laxatives, which may worsen the condition or cause complications such as a ruptured appendix.

DO NOT give fluids other than clear ones as long as the pain continues.

DO NOT give solid foods.

DO NOT give milk products.

Nausea and Vomiting

Nausea (upset stomach) and vomiting (throwing up) often occur with conditions such as mild altitude sickness, motion sickness, brain injury, intestinal viruses, eating or drinking too much, and being emotionally upset. In minor illnesses, nausea and vomiting should clear up in a couple of days. Persistent nausea and vomiting may signal more serious illnesses such as appendicitis, food poisoning, or bowel obstruction. In general, if the condition lasts longer than one or two days, the victim may become dehydrated (lose too much fluid). Young children and the elderly may be more seriously affected.

What to Look for

- Is there abdominal pain?
- Is there blood or brown, grainy material in the vomit?
- Is there diarrhea? Vomiting and diarrhea together *usually* indicate a self-limited viral infection.

- Are there signs of dehydration (ie, victim is dizzy when standing; has dry, cracked lips; is very thirsty)?
- Does anyone else in the group have similar symptoms?
- Has the victim had a recent head injury?

What to Do

1. Give the victim small amounts of clear fluids (eg, sports drinks, clear soups, flat soda, apple or cranberry juice), except alcohol and caffeine.

2. If the victim is able to keep fluids down, offer carbohydrates (eg, bread, cereal, pasta) first—they are easier to digest. Avoid milk products and meats for 48 hours.

3. Have the victim rest and avoid exertion until he or she is able to eat solid foods easily.

4. Prevent inhalation of vomit by positioning the victim on his or her side to allow drainage. Inhaled vomit can result in severe pneumonia.

5. Seek medical care if:

- Blood or brown, grainy material appears in the vomit.
- There is constant abdominal pain.
- The victim faints when standing.
- The victim is unable to keep fluids down for more than 24 hours.
- The victim has severe, projectile vomiting (vomit shoots out in large quantities).
- The vomiting follows a recent head injury.

Caution:

DO NOT give solid foods until the victim can take fluids without vomiting and starts to feel hungry.

DO NOT give milk products.

What to Do for Motion Sickness

1. If the victim is prone to motion sickness, he or she should sit near the midsection of a plane, boat, bus, train, or car and close his or her eyes. Those susceptible to motion sickness should not read, should look far ahead to the horizon, not to the sides, and should avoid overeating.

2. Try Dramamine™ (works on the ears) or Bonine™ (works on the stomach) one hour before traveling (follow label directions).

Diarrhea

Diarrhea is the frequent (usually more than four times a day) passage of loose, watery, or unformed stools. Diarrhea may be a symptom of intestinal infection (bacterial, viral, or parasitic), food poisoning, or food sensitivity/allergy, among other ailments. Dehydration can occur if the body loses too much fluid through the stool and the victim cannot drink enough fluid to keep up with the fluid losses from the diarrhea. The elderly and the very young are especially prone to dehydration, which can result in dangerous chemical imbalances. Replacing fluids and electrolytes such as sodium and potassium is of primary importance for any diarrhea victim.

Diarrhea flushes bacteria and parasites out of the body. Letting diarrhea run its course is best because then bacteria or parasites are not trapped in the intestines.

What to Look for

- Was the victim recently exposed to untreated, possibly contaminated water or food?
- Is there blood or mucus in the stool? That may signal more serious problems.
- Are there signs of dehydration (ie, victim is dizzy when standing; has dry, cracked lips; is very thirsty)?
- Does victim have cramping abdominal pain?
- Does victim lose bowel control (sometimes)?
- Is the victim feverish (sometimes)?
- Do others in the group have similar symptoms?

What to Do

1. Have victim drink lots of clear fluids (8 to 10 eight-ounce glasses daily). This is the single most important treatment.
2. When the victim can tolerate clear fluids, give mild foods such as soup and gelatin. Later, the BRAT diet—**b**ananas, **r**ice, **a**pplesauce, **t**oast—is recommended.
3. Bismuth (eg, Pepto-Bismol™) can help in most cases (follow label directions). Be aware that Pepto-Bismol can turn the stool and the tongue black. Those sensitive to aspirin should not use it.

If the victim must, for some reason, be in control of his or her bodily functions, over-the-counter Imodium A-D™, Kaopectate II™, Maalox Anti-Diarrheal Caplets™, or Pepto Diarrhea Control™ will tighten up the bowel, thus reducing movement of food through the intestines.

4. Seek medical care if:
   - The victim has bloody stools, which may appear black (keep in mind that Pepto-Bismol can cause black stools).
   - There is no improvement after 24 hours.
   - The victim has a fever.
   - The victim has severe, constant abdominal pain.
   - The victim is severely dehydrated.

Caution:

DO NOT give milk products and meats for 48 hours after diarrhea stops.

DO NOT give caffeine, which stimulates the intestine and causes urination, furthering dehydration.

Constipation

Constipation is the passage of hard, dry stools. Most physicians define constipation as two or fewer bowel movements a week, of which 25% require straining. Constipation is rarely more than a passing discomfort in otherwise healthy people. Normal bowel movements may occur three times a day or once every three days. Minor changes in diet, fluid intake, activity, or emotional state can cause bowel movement changes. Rectifying any of those changes will also relieve constipation in most cases. Bowel stimulants or laxatives are rarely needed.

What to Look for

- Bloating sensation of abdomen. A very painful or visibly swollen abdomen is a more serious problem than simple constipation.
- Hard, dry stools. Small strings of blood are not unusual if the stool was painful to evacuate.

Appendicitis

The possibility of appendicitis can occur in any age group—fortunately, it is rare. While surgery is the best choice, probably as many as 70% of people not treated with surgery or antibiotics can survive this problem. Appendicitis causes a vague feeling of discomfort around the umbilicus (navel). Temperature may be low grade, 99.6° to 100°F (37°C) at first. Within a matter of 12 hours the discomfort turns to pain and localizes in the right lower quadrant, most frequently at a point two-thirds of the way between the navel and the very top of the right pelvic bone (iliac crest). Ask the victim two questions: Where did you first start hurting? (navel). Now where do you hurt? (right lower quadrant). Those answers mean appendicitis until it is ruled out. It is possible but unusual to have diarrhea with appendicitis. Diarrhea usually means that the victim does not have appendicitis. Those with appendicitis will walk with rather careful, short steps, bent slightly forward in pain. Anyone with springy steps most likely does not have appendicitis. Never give the victim a laxative when appendicitis is suspected. This could lead to massive abdominal infection (peritonitis).

What to Do

1. Have the victim eat more fiber (fresh or dried fruits, vegetables, bran). Fiber causes the colon to contract. Over-the-counter fiber products such as Metamucil™ or Citrucel™ can be used, but follow label directions.

2. Make sure the victim drinks plenty of fluids (8 to 10 eight-ounce glasses daily). Excessively hard stools often are the result of dehydration.

3. Encourage the victim to remain active. Activity such as walking stimulates colon contractions.

Gall Bladder

Nausea associated with pain in the right upper quadrant of the abdomen may be from a gall bladder problem. No burning is associated with gall bladder pain, and this discomfort is typically made worse by eating greasy foods. While drinking milk would help the pain of an ulcer or gastritis, it causes immediate pain if the gall bladder is involved. Treatment is avoidance of fatty foods. The onset of fever is an important indication of infection of the blocked gall bladder. This demands immediate medical attention.

4. If there is no improvement, try one of the following:
   - milk of magnesia (a mild laxative and stool softener)
   - caffeine, which stimulates colon contractions
   - mineral oil to coat the stool for easier passage, although this takes six to eight hours to work (This method is debatable).

5. Seek medical care if the victim experiences any of the following:
   - severe abdominal pain
   - visibly swollen or very painful abdomen
   - fever
   - vomiting

Caution:

DO NOT give laxatives such as Epsom salts to those with severe abdominal pain or vomiting.

DO NOT give alcohol.

DO NOT give "binding" foods, such as bananas, cheese, applesauce.

STUDY
Questions (15)

Name_____ Course_____ Date_____

Activities

Activity 1

Mark each question as true (T) or false (F).

T F 1. A person having a heart attack will find it easier to breathe while lying flat.

T F 2. A squeezing or crushing sensation can be a sign of a heart attack.

T F 3. Heart attack victims should be kept in a sitting position.

T F 4. Angina occurs when the heart's need for oxygen exceeds the supply.

T F 5. Angina can be treated with physician-prescribed nitroglycerin.

T F 6. Stroke victims may have difficulty with speech or vision.

T F 7. One side of the body becoming suddenly weak or numb may indicate a stroke.

T F 8. Only heart attacks and angina cause chest pain.

T F 9. When taking nitroglycerin, the person should be sitting or lying down.

T F 10. An "aura" may accompany a grand mal seizure.

T F 11. Call the EMS for seizures that last longer than 5 minutes.

T F 12. When an artery in the heart becomes blocked, the part of the heart muscle it serves dies.

T F 13. A feeling of crushing pressure in the chest is one sign of a heart attack.

T F 14. Diabetes is a condition in which the body is unable to use sugar normally.

T F 15. Insulin permits sugar to pass from the body cells into the bloodstream.

T F 16. Sugar may save the life of a person in diabetic coma.

T F 17. If you are in doubt about whether someone is in insulin shock or diabetic coma, always give sugar to a conscious victim.

T F 18. Place a blunt object between the teeth of a person having a seizure.

T F 19. For hyperventilation, have the victim breathe into and out of a paper bag.

Case Situations

Case 1

Your father complains of tightness in his chest and shortness of breath.

____ 1. What do you suspect?
   a. stroke
   b. heart attack
   c. seizure
   d. diabetic emergency

____ 2. What can you do for him?
   a. Have him lie down for 30 minutes to see if the symptoms go away.
   b. Begin performing CPR.
   c. Call 9-1-1.

____ 3. An acute myocardial infarction (AMI) is caused by
   a. injury or death of the brain tissue
   b. tearing of the aorta
   c. severe constriction of peripheral arteries
   d. a clot or spasm blocking a coronary artery

Case 2

Your elderly grandmother appears dazed and disoriented and complains of weakness and numbness on one side of her body.

____ 1. What is your grandmother likely to have suffered?
   a. stroke
   b. heart attack
   c. asthma
   d. seizure

STUDY
Questions 15

____ **2.** What should you do for her?
  a. Have her sit down and rest for a few minutes.
  b. Check to see if her pupils are dilated.
  c. Have her lie down and massage the numb area until feeling returns.
  d. Call 9-1-1 or take her immediately to the hospital.

Case 3

A 23-year-old female is short of breath after cleaning the dust-filled living room of her grandmother's house. She is sitting bolt upright on the steps outside the house. She is experiencing obvious respiratory distress and is unable to speak in full sentences. The grand mother says that her granddaughter is allergic to a number of things and suffers from "a breathing condition."

____ **1.** This victim is most likely experiencing
  a. an acute asthma attack
  b. anaphylaxis
  c. a respiratory infection
  d. angina

Check what you should do for this victim:

____ **2.** Have her take two aspirin tablets.

____ **3.** Reassure her.

____ **4.** Seek immediate medical care.

____ **5.** Have her use her physician-prescribed inhaler.

____ **6.** Have her breathe into a paper sack.

____ **7.** Give her an ammonia inhalant.

Case 4

A 19-year-old male has been found unconscious in the hallway of a college dormitory. According to his roommate, he has a history of diabetes.

____ **1.** This victim is most likely experiencing
  a. insulin shock
  b. crack cocaine overdose
  c. a head injury
  d. alcohol intoxication

____ **2.** Treatment for this victim includes
  a. giving CPR
  b. giving milk
  c. giving Pepto-Bismol
  d. giving sugar

____ **3.** Diabetes is caused by
  a. a lack of glucose in the body
  b. excessive calcium in the bones
  c. a lack of red blood cells
  d. a lack of insulin in the body

____ **4.** Hyperglycemia is
  a. too much plasma in the blood
  b. an eating disorder in which too much food is ingested
  c. an accumulation of carbon dioxide
  d. an excessive amount of glucose in the blood

Case 5

During a high school gym class, a 16-year-old male collapses while playing basketball. He is responsive but is having difficulty answering your questions. He remembers his name but not where he is, the date, or the time. You find a medical-alert bracelet indicating that he has diabetes and takes insulin daily.

____ **1.** This victim is most likely experiencing
  a. diabetic coma
  b. drug overdose
  c. insulin shock
  d. a seizure

____ **2.** Treatment for this victim includes
  a. using an ammonia inhalant to arouse him
  b. having him rebreathe into a paper sack
  c. giving him oral glucose or other form of sugar
  d. performing rescue breathing

Chapter Activities

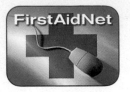

WEB Activities
Sudden Illnesses

Visit nsc.jbpub.com/FirstAidNet, then click on Web Activities, and select the appropriate chapter.

Stroke Quiz

Learn the facts and risk factors associated with strokes. Recognizing the early warning signs can greatly help a first aider treat a stroke victim.

Insulin Reaction

Insulin reactions can occur in a matter of seconds, so acting quickly to help someone suffering from an attack is very important.

Fainting

Fainting, although more common than other "sudden illnesses," is still a serious condition. When should a fainting victim seek the advice of a doctor?

Asthma

Over 14 million people in the United States have asthma. Learn more about asthma and what to do for an asthma attack.

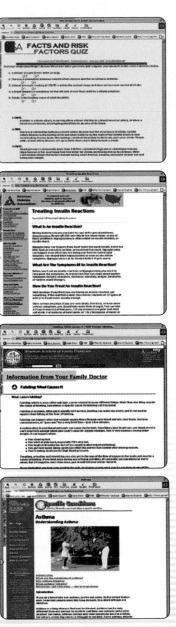

Chapter 16

Poisoning

Types of Poisons

Poisons are classified by how they enter the body:

- Ingested (swallowed)—through the mouth
- Inhaled (breathed)—through the lungs
- Absorbed (contact)—through the skin
- Injected—through needle-like device (eg, snake's fangs)

Ingested (Swallowed) Poisons

Swallowing nonfood substances is so common among children that it is unusual for a child to reach the age of five without ingesting a nonfood substance at least once. Although many nonfood substances such as dirt or paper are not harmful, others present definite health threats. Some have the potential to block an airway. Others are poisonous. Hundreds of thousands of poisonings occur in the United States each year, but only a small percentage progress to severe or life-threatening conditions.

Household cleaning agents account for the largest category of poisoning exposures. Drugs, both prescription and nonprescription, miscellaneous chemicals, and cosmetics also are frequently implicated. Basically, any substance that is accessible to a child is a potential poison. Analgesic products that contain acetaminophen, for example, are involved in poisoning incidents more often than other analgesics, not because acetaminophen is more toxic but because products that contain acetaminophen outsell products that contain other analgesics (▶Figure 16-1).

It is important not to confuse poisoning frequency with poisoning severity. Plants and mushrooms, for example, account for about 5.5% (over 100,000 cases) of the total poisoning exposures reported each year. However, plant and mushroom ingestion result in only 0.02% of serious poisonings and one death each year. Therefore, most exposures to plants are minor, with harmless effects. On the other hand, gun-blueing products (agents containing

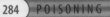

SWALLOWED POISON

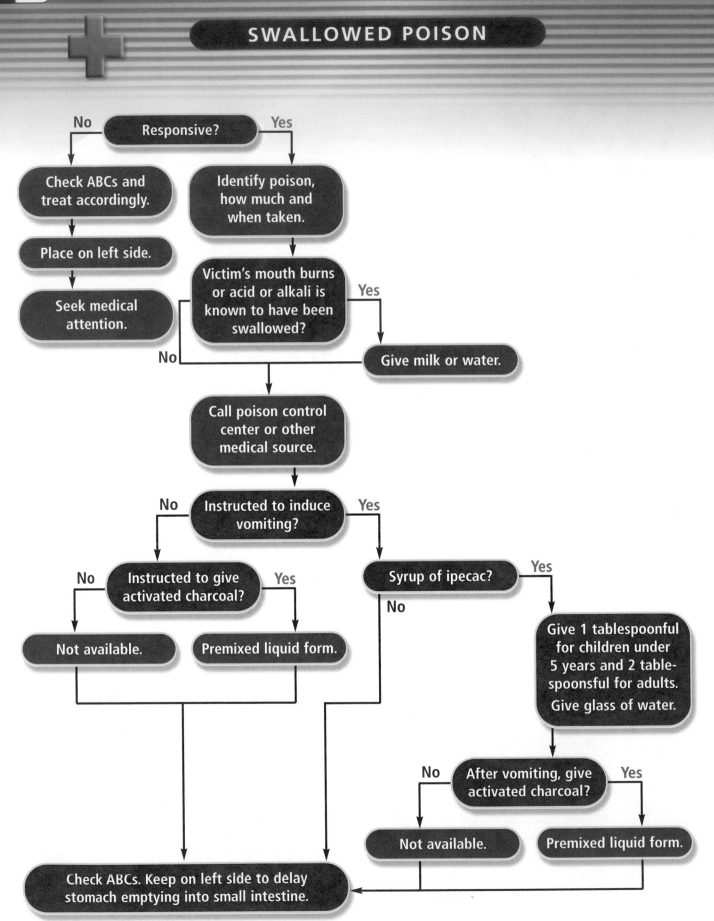

Responsive? — No → **Check ABCs and treat accordingly.** → **Place on left side.** → **Seek medical attention.**

Responsive? — Yes → **Identify poison, how much and when taken.** → **Victim's mouth burns or acid or alkali is known to have been swallowed?**

Victim's mouth burns or acid or alkali is known to have been swallowed? — Yes → **Give milk or water.**

Victim's mouth burns or acid or alkali is known to have been swallowed? — No → **Call poison control center or other medical source.** → **Instructed to induce vomiting?**

Instructed to induce vomiting? — No → **Instructed to give activated charcoal?**

Instructed to give activated charcoal? — No → **Not available.**

Instructed to give activated charcoal? — Yes → **Premixed liquid form.**

Instructed to induce vomiting? — Yes → **Syrup of ipecac?**

Syrup of ipecac? — No

Syrup of ipecac? — Yes → **Give 1 tablespoonful for children under 5 years and 2 tablespoonsful for adults. Give glass of water.** → **After vomiting, give activated charcoal?**

After vomiting, give activated charcoal? — No → **Not available.**

After vomiting, give activated charcoal? — Yes → **Premixed liquid form.**

Check ABCs. Keep on left side to delay stomach emptying into small intestine.

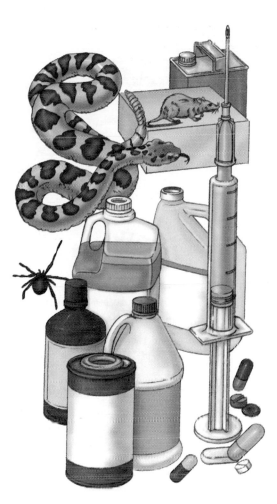

Figure 16-1 Sources of poisons

Table 16-1: Substances Most Frequently Involved in Human Exposures

Substance	Annual Number	Percentage of Total Exposures*
Cleaning substances	229,500	10.2
Analgesics	215,067	9.6
Cosmetics and personal care products	210,224	9.4
Plants	122,578	5.5
Foreign bodies	103,696	4.6
Cough and cold preparations	99,924	4.5
Bites/envenomations	92,182	4.1
Insecticides/pesticides (includes rodenticides)	86,289	3.9
Topicals	83,455	3.7
Food products, food poisoning	78,690	3.5
Sedatives/hypnotics/ antipsychotics	70,982	3.2
Antidepressants	67,872	3.0
Hydrocarbons	66,623	3.0
Antimicrobials	62,034	2.8
Chemicals	61,061	2.7
Alcohols	55,246	2.5

NOTE: Despite a high frequency of involvement, these substances are not necessarily the most toxic, but rather may only be the most readily accessible.

*Percentages are based on the total number of human exposures rather than the total number of substances.

Source: American Association of Poison Control Centers

selenious acid that are used to maintain the blue color of gun barrels) were involved in 100 poisoning episodes and resulted in four deaths (death rate of 4%). So although there are fewer exposure episodes, the potential for harm is much greater.

Fortunately, most poison ingestions involve products with low toxicity or amounts so small that severe poisoning rarely occurs. However, the potential for severe or fatal poisoning is always present.

Swallowed poisons usually remain in the stomach only a short time, and the stomach absorbs only small amounts. Most absorption takes place after the poison passes into the small intestine.

What to Look for

- abdominal pain and cramping
- nausea or vomiting
- diarrhea
- burns, odor, or stains around and in mouth
- drowsiness or unconsciousness
- poison containers nearby

What to Do

1. Determine critical information:
   - Age and size of the victim?
   - What was swallowed (container label; save vomit for analysis)?
   - How much was swallowed (eg, a "taste," half a bottle, a dozen tablets)?
   - When was it swallowed?

2. If a corrosive or caustic (ie, acid or alkali) substance was swallowed, immediately dilute it by having the victim drink at least one or two eight-ounce glasses of water or milk. (*Cold* milk or water tends to absorb heat better than room-temperature or warmer liquids.)

Caution:

DO NOT give water or milk to dilute poisons other than caustic or corrosive substances (acids and alkalis) unless told to do so by a poison control center. Fluids may dissolve a dry poison such as tablets or capsules more rapidly and fill up the stomach, forcing the stomach contents (the poison) into the small intestine, where it will be absorbed faster.

3. For a responsive victim, call a poison control center *immediately*. Some poisons do not cause harm until hours later, while others damage immediately. More than 75% of poisonings can be treated through instructions taken over the telephone from a poison control center. The center also will advise you if medical attention is needed. Poison control centers routinely follow up calls to check whether additional symptoms or unexpected effects are occurring. The inside front covers of telephone directories contain the number for the local poison control center.

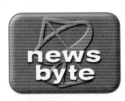

Poisoning: Where Can You Call for Help?

If someone swallows poison, do not call the hospital emergency room. Call the local poison control center. Researchers who made 156 "test calls" to 52 hospital emergency departments in Illinois found that the advice given was correct only 64% of the time. Calls to the same emergency department on different days for the same problem did not consistently produce the same advice. In contrast, poison control centers gave correct advice in 17 out of 18 test calls (94%).

Source: H. N. Wigder et al: "Emergency Department Poison Advice Telephone Calls." *Annals of Emergency Medicine,* 25:349 March 1995.

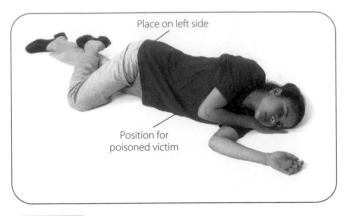

Place on left side

Position for poisoned victim

Figure 16-2 The left-side position delays the poison from advancing into the small intestine.

4. For an unresponsive victim, check the victim's ABCs and treat accordingly, and call 9-1-1 or the local emergency number.

5. Place the victim on his or her side (recovery position) **▲Figure 16-2**. For ingested poisoning, the *left*-side position is best since it positions the end of the stomach where it enters the small intestine (pylorus) straight up. Gravity will delay the poison's advance into the small intestine, where absorption into the victim's circulatory system is faster, by as much as two hours. The side position also helps prevent aspiration (inhalation) into the lungs if vomiting begins.

6. Induce vomiting *only* if a poison control center or a physician advises it. Induced vomiting with syrup of ipecac and within 30 minutes of swallowing the poison removes 30% to 50% of the poison from the stomach, which means that 50% to 70% of the poison remains in the stomach.

   If you are instructed by a poison control center or a physician to induce vomiting, use syrup of ipecac. It can be purchased without a prescription and is easily given. Follow the directions carefully. Ipecac will not work unless sufficient water also is given.

7. Give activated charcoal, if a poison control center advises **▶Figure 16-3**. It is the single most effective agent in prehospital settings for most swallowed poisons. Activated charcoal acts like a sponge to bind and keep the poison in the digestive system, thus preventing its absorption by the blood. Doses of activated charcoal every two to six hours have been shown to increase the elimination of certain drugs faster than does a single dose.

   Activated charcoal is a black, tasteless, odorless, insoluble, inert powder that is the product of or-

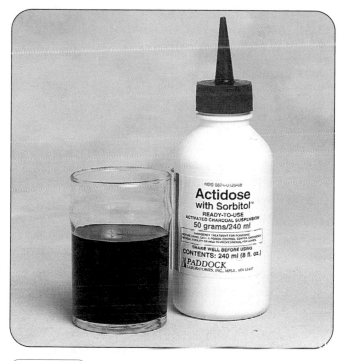

Figure 16-3 Activated charcoal

ganic vegetable matter, usually wood pulp, burned at high temperatures and then exposed to steam and strong acids. A network of tiny pores on each particle increases the surface area enormously, which enables activated charcoal to bind many commonly ingested toxic materials. Although acti vated charcoal may appear similar to burnt-toast scrapings and charcoal briquettes, they *cannot* be used interchangeably.

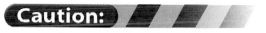

Caution:

DO NOT gag or tickle the back of the victim's throat with a finger or a spoon handle. That method is usually ineffective in causing vomiting, and any vomiting produced is not very forceful.

DO NOT give dish soap, raw eggs, or mustard powder. They are not effective.

DO NOT use syrup of ipecac and activated charcoal at the same time. Charcoal will bind the ipecac and may prevent vomiting. Many toxicologists now recommend the use of activated charcoal rather than ipecac.

Caution:

DO NOT induce vomiting unless advised to do so by a poison control center or a physician. Reasons for *not* using syrup of ipecac include:

- Waiting for vomiting to begin may take 20 to 30 minutes, during which time some poison may pass into the small intestine.
- Additional treatment will be delayed until vomiting stops.
- The victim could inhale the vomitus.
- Vomiting caused by syrup of ipecac removes up to 30% to 50% of the poison from the stomach but leaves 50% to 70%.

DO NOT induce vomiting if:

- The victim is having seizures.
- The victim is unconscious or drowsy.
- The victim is in the third trimester (last 3 months) of pregnancy.
- The victim has a history of advanced heart disease or is likely to suffer a heart attack.
- The victim swallowed a corrosive or caustic substance such as drain cleaner.
- The victim swallowed a petroleum product, (eg, lighter fluid, furniture polish, or gas).
- The victim swallowed strychnine (rat poison).
- The victim is less than six months old.

DO NOT use saltwater to induce vomiting. It is dangerous and can kill a small child.

However, activated charcoal does not absorb all drugs well. Acids and alkalies (eg, bleach, ammonia), potassium, iron, alcohol, methanol, kerosene, cyanide, DDT, malathion, and ferrous sulfate will require different treatment.

Major drawbacks of activated charcoal are its grittiness and its appearance. Trying to improve the taste or consistency by adding chocolate syrup, sherbet, ice cream, milk, or other flavoring agents only decreases the charcoal's binding capacity. Place the charcoal mixture in an opaque container and have the victim sip it through a straw to make it more palatable. First aiders should give only the pre-mixed form.

Although activated charcoal is an inexpensive, safe, and effective means for decreasing poison absorption, pharmacies do not routinely stock it.

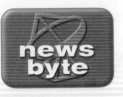

Activated Charcoal Useful

Of 361 drug overdose patients identified in emergency department records, 60% could have benefited from the administration of activated charcoal. The researchers stressed the need for more aggressive use of activated charcoal.

Source: P.M. Was and D.J. Cobaugh, "Prehospital Gastrointestinal Decontamination of Toxic Ingestions: A Missed Opportunity."*American Journal of Emergency Medicine*, 16:114-116, March 1998.

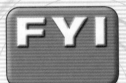

According to the American Association of Poison Control Centers the "Top 5" most commonly ingested plants are:

1. **Ornamental pepper**
   - *Capsicum annuum*
   - Frequency: 5,374
   - Symptoms: Painful but harmless burning sensation of lips, mouth, tongue

2. **Philodendron**
   - *Philodendron* spp.
   - Frequency: 4,061
   - Symptoms: Burning in mouth and throat, swelling of mouth and/or tongue, nausea, vomiting, diarrhea

3. **Holly**
   - *Ilex* spp.
   - Frequency: 3,441
   - Symptoms: Nausea, persistent vomiting, diarrhea

4. **Peace lily**
   - *Spathiphyllum* spp.
   - Frequency: 3,350
   - Symptoms: Same as philodendron

5. **Poinsettia**
   - *Euphorbia pulcherrima*
   - Frequency: 3,296
   - Symptoms: Skin irritation and blistering, abdominal pain, nausea and/or vomiting, diarrhea

Caution:

DO NOT follow the first aid procedures or recommendations on a container label without first getting confirmation from a medical source. Many labels are incorrect or out of date.

DO NOT try to neutralize a poison. Giving weak acids, such as lemon juice or vinegar, is not safe, contrary to the advice given on many drain cleaner and lye-product labels. Chemical neutralization releases large quantities of heat that can burn sensitive tissues.

DO NOT think that a specific antidote exists for most poisons. An *antidote* is a substance that counteracts a poison's effects. Few poisons have specific antidotes that will effectively block their toxic effects.

DO NOT think that there is a "universal antidote." No product is effective in treating most or all poisons.

8. Save poison containers, plants, and the victim's vomit to help medical personnel identify the poison.

Alcohol and Drug Emergencies

Alcohol Intoxication

Alcohol is a depressant, not a stimulant. It affects a person's judgment, vision, reaction time, and coordination. In very large amounts, it can cause death by paralyzing the respiratory center of the brain.

Alcohol is the most commonly used *and* abused drug in the United States, possibly even the world (▶**Figure 16-4**). It is also one of the most lethal, because it is implicated as a cofactor in 40% of drownings, about 50% of traffic deaths, 67% of homicides, and 25% of successful suicides. It directly affects more than 12 million people annually (10% of all males and 3% of all females) and causes more than 200,000 deaths. **Alcohol abuse is a major national health problem, ranking with heart disease and cancer.** Lack of data makes it difficult to assess the actual number of alcohol-related injuries. It is estimated, however, that 20% to 25% of patients treated in many urban hospital emergency departments are intoxicated.

Helping an intoxicated person is often difficult because the individual may be belligerent and combative. Also, personal hygiene is sometimes less than optimal.

However, it is important that alcohol abusers be helped and not just labeled as "drunks." Their condition may be quite serious, even life threatening.

Occasionally, a person will have consumed so much alcohol that there are signs that the central nervous system is depressed. In such cases, complete respiratory support may be necessary. Death can result from the excessive consumption of alcohol.

What to Look for

Although some of these symptoms can also mean illness or injury other than alcohol abuse, such as diabetes or heat injury, the following are generally signs of alcohol intoxication:

- the odor of alcohol on a person's breath or clothing
- unsteady, staggering walking
- slurred speech and the inability to carry on a conversation
- nausea and vomiting
- flushed face

Alcohol-induced seizures, from either alcohol ingestion or alcohol withdrawal, are usually brief and self-limiting. The consumption of alcohol is deeply imbedded in our society. Because of alcohol's widespread use, those whose lives are affected directly or indirectly by alcohol abuse should be educated so they can recognize problems and know what to do in an emergency.

What to Do

First aid for an intoxicated person includes these steps:

1. Look for any injuries. Alcohol can mask pain.
2. Check ABCs and treat accordingly.

Figure 16-4 Drunk driving

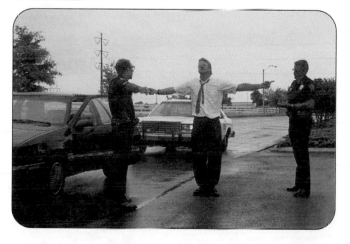

Preventing Poisoning

Follow these precautions to reduce the risk of poisoning:

1. Household products and medicines should be kept out of reach and out of sight of children, preferably in a locked cabinet or closet. When an adult leaves the room even briefly, he or she should move these containers to a safe place.

2. Medicines should be stored separately from other household products and kept in their original containers—never in cups or soft-drink bottles.

3. All products should be properly labeled, and the label should be read before use.

4. A light should be turned on when giving or taking medicine.

5. Because children tend to imitate adults, adults should avoid taking medications in their presence.

6. Medicines should be referred to by their correct names. They are not candies.

7. Medicine cabinets should be cleaned out periodically. Old medicines should be disposed of by flushing them down the drain, rinsing the container with water, and discarding it.

8. Use household substances in child-resistant packaging. Prescription medicines should be kept in safety packaging.

To avoid poisonings among elderly persons:

1. Always read the label and follow instructions when taking medicine.

2. Turn on a light at night when taking medicine.

3. Never mix medicines and alcohol, and never take more than the prescribed amount of medicine.

4. Do not "borrow" a friend's medicine or take old medicines.

5. Inform the physician what other medicines are being taken to avoid the risk of adverse drug interactions.

Source: U.S. Consumer Product Safety Commission

Caution:

DO NOT let an intoxicated person sleep on his or her back.

DO NOT leave an intoxicated person alone.

DO NOT try to handle a hostile drunk by yourself. Find a safe place, then call the police for help.

3. If the intoxicated person is lying down, place him or her in the recovery (left-side) position, to reduce the likelihood of vomiting and aspiration of vomit and to delay the alcohol's absorption into the bloodstream. Be sure to check that the victim is breathing and does not have a spinal injury before you move him or her. The recovery position can be used for both responsive and unresponsive persons.

4. Call the poison control center for advice or the local emergency number for help. It may be best to let EMS personnel decide if the police should be alerted.

5. If the victim becomes violent, leave the scene and find a safe place until police arrive.

6. Provide emotional support.

7. Assume that an injured or unconscious victim has a spinal injury and needs to be stabilized against movement. Because of decreased pain perception, an intoxicated victim cannot be assessed reliably. If you suspect a spinal injury, wait for EMS to arrive. They have the proper equipment and training to stabilize and move a victim.

8. Because many intoxicated individuals have been exposed to the cold, suspect hypothermia and move the person to a warm place. Remove wet clothing and cover the individual with warm blankets. Handle a hypothermic victim gently, because rough handling could induce a heart attack.

Drugs

Drugs are classified according to their effects on the user:

- **Uppers** are stimulants of the central nervous system. They include amphetamines, cocaine, and caffeine (▶**Figure 16-5**).

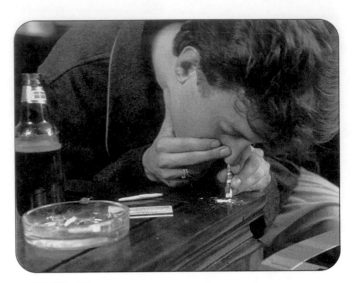

Figure 16-5) Cocaine

- **Downers** are depressants of the central nervous system. They include barbiturates, tranquilizers, marijuana, and narcotics.

- **Hallucinogens** alter and often enhance the sensory and emotional information in the brain centers. They include LSD, mescaline, peyote, and PCP (angel dust). Marijuana also has some hallucinogenic properties (▼**Figure 16-6**).

Figure 16-6) Marijuana

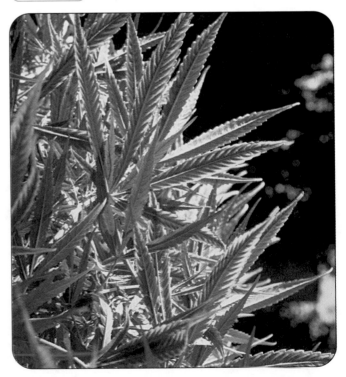

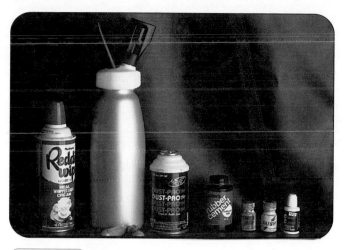

Figure 16-7 Inhalants

- **Volatile chemicals** usually are inhaled and can cause serious damage to many body organs. They include plastic model glue and cements, paint solvents, gasoline, spray paint, and nail polish remover ▲**Figure 16-7** .

Amphetamines and Cocaine

Amphetamines and cocaine provide relief from fatigue and a feeling of well-being. Blood pressure, breathing, and general body activity are increased. Some users take a "speed run" of repeated high doses. Results are hyperactivity, restlessness, and belligerence. Such persons need to be protected from hurting themselves and others. Acute cases need medical attention.

Hallucinogens

Hallucinogens produce changes in mood and sensory awareness—a person may "hear" colors and "see" sounds. They can cause hallucinations and bizarre behavior that may make users dangerous to themselves or to others. Acute cases need medical attention. Users should be protected from hurting themselves.

Marijuana

Marijuana provides a feeling of relaxation and euphoria. Users report distortions of time and space. In some people, marijuana can cause a reaction similar to a bad LSD trip.

Barbiturates

Barbiturates induce relaxation, drowsiness, and sleep. Overdose can produce respiratory depression, coma, and death. Withdrawal can cause anxiety, tremors, nausea, fever, delirium, convulsions, and ultimately death.

Tranquilizers

Tranquilizers are used to calm anxiety. High doses and withdrawal produce the same effects as barbiturate overdose and withdrawal.

Inhaled Substances

Inhaling glue or other solvents (gasoline, lighter fluid, nail polish) produces effects similar to those from ingesting alcohol. Persons who "sniff" these substances can die from suffocation. In addition, some inhalants can cause death by changing the rhythm of the heartbeat.

Opiates

Opiates, or narcotics, are used medicinally to relieve pain and anxiety. Overdoses can result in deep sleep (coma), respiratory depression, and death. The pupils of opiate users are described as "pinpoint" in size. Withdrawal symptoms include intense agitation, abdominal discomfort, dilated pupils, increased breathing and body temperature, and a strong craving for a "fix."

What to Do

1. Check ABCs.
2. Call the poison control center for advice or the EMS for help.
3. Check for injuries.
4. Keep the person on the *left* side to reduce the likelihood of vomiting and aspiration of vomit and to delay absorption.
5. Provide reassurance and emotional support.
6. If the person becomes violent, seek safety until the police arrive. Let law enforcement officers handle dangerous situations.
7. Seek medical attention.

Carbon Monoxide Poisoning

Carbon monoxide (CO) is not the most dangerous poison around, but its common presence in our environment, along with its insidious nature, makes it the leading cause of poisoning death in the United States each year. According to a report from the Centers for Disease Control and Prevention, CO poisoning kills at least 1,500 people and sends 10,000 more to the hospital annually.

People who ride long distances in older, poorly maintained cars are at increased risk. Rust is a major factor in

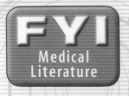

FYI
Medical Literature

Carbon Monoxide Poisoning

Riding in the back of an open pickup truck is extremely dangerous. Every year, people are maimed or killed when they are thrown out of the vehicle in which they are riding or when the truck rolls over. A recent report now maintains that riding in the enclosed back of a pickup exposes children to another danger: carbon monoxide poisoning.

Investigators at Seattle's Virginia Mason Medical School found that 20 out of 68 pediatric patients treated for carbon monoxide poisoning had been passengers in the back of pickup trucks. In 17 cases, the rear was enclosed by a rigid cap, and in three incidents, the children had been riding beneath tarpaulins. In all cases, exhaust fumes had built up in the enclosed space. One child died from cerebral edema, and one had permanent neurologic damage. The remaining patients apparently recovered well. Several states specifically outlaw riding in the back of pickup trucks.

Source: N. B. Hampson and D. M. Norkool: "Carbon Monoxide Poisoning in Children Riding in the Back of Pickup Trucks." *Journal of American Medical Association* 267:538–540 (January 22, 1992).

What to Look for

It is difficult to tell if a person is a CO victim. Sometimes, a complaint of having the "flu" is really a symptom of CO poisoning. Although many symptoms of CO poisoning resemble those of the flu, there are differences. For example, CO poisoning does not cause low-grade fever or generalized aching or involve the lymph nodes.

The traditionally cited sign of CO poisoning is a cherry-red color of the skin and the lips. This sign is uncommon, however, and occurs only at death; therefore, it is a poor initial indicator of CO poisoning. The following conditions are earmarks of possible CO poisoning:

- The symptoms come and go.
- The symptoms worsen or improve in certain places or at certain times of the day.
- People around the victim have similar symptoms.
- Pets seem ill.

The signs and symptoms of CO poisoning are as follows:

- headache
- ringing in the ears (tinnitus)
- chest pain (angina)
- muscle weakness
- nausea and vomiting

damaging an automobile's exhaust system and creating holes in the car's body through which CO can enter. Many deaths involve people sleeping inside a running car, often because of drinking. Many deaths also involve parking in remote areas for romantic purposes.

Persons in a closed room where there is cigarette smoking experience mild increases in the level of CO in their blood. Less familiar, and therefore more dangerous, sources of CO are faulty furnaces, water heaters, and kerosene heaters. Recreational fires, whether open-flame, charcoal, sterno, or hibachi grills, also give off CO.

CO victims are often unaware of its presence. The gas is invisible, tasteless, odorless, and nonirritating. It is produced by the incomplete burning of organic material such as gasoline, wood, paper, charcoal, coal, and natural gas.

CO poisons its victims by causing **hypoxia,** or lack of oxygen, in two ways. First, red blood cells (hemoglobin) are about 200 times more likely to bind to CO than to oxygen if both are present in the blood; thus, even a small amount of CO can greatly reduce the amount of oxygen carried in the bloodstream. Second, CO does not allow the cells to use what little oxygen is delivered. In short, CO deprives the body parts that need oxygen the most—the heart and the brain.

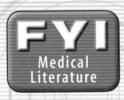

FYI
Medical Literature

Carbon Monoxide Detectors Can Save Lives

The U.S. Consumer Product Safety Commission recommends that consumers purchase and install carbon monoxide (CO) detectors with labels showing they meet the requirements of the Underwriters Laboratories, Inc. (UL) voluntary standard (UL 2034). The standard requires detectors to sound an alarm when exposure to CO reaches potentially hazardous levels over a period of time.

Properly working CO detectors can provide an early warning before the deadly gas builds up to a dangerous level. Exposure to a low concentration over several hours can be as dangerous as exposure to high carbon monoxide levels for a few minutes. The new detectors will detect both conditions. Each home should have at least one CO detector in the area outside individual bedrooms. CO detectors are as important to home safety as smoke detectors are.

Source: U.S. Consumer Product Safety Commission

- dizziness and visual changes (blurred or double vision)
- unconsciousness
- respiratory and cardiac arrest

What to Do

1. Remove the victim from the toxic environment and into fresh air *immediately*.

2. Call the EMS, which will be able to give the victim 100% oxygen, improving oxygenation and disassociating the linkage between the CO and the hemoglobin. For a responsive victim, it takes four to five hours with ordinary air (21% oxygen) or 30–40 minutes with 100% oxygen to reverse the effects of CO poisoning.

3. Monitor ABCs.

4. Place an unresponsive victim on one side.

5. Seek medical attention. All suspected CO victims should obtain a blood test to determine the level of CO.

Plant-Induced Dermatitis: Poison Ivy, Poison Oak, and Poison Sumac

Fifty percent of the United States population is sensitive to poison ivy, and with more people venturing into the outdoors, episodes of dermatitis caused by exposure to poison ivy (▼**Figure 16-8**), poison oak (▶**Figure 16-9**), and poison sumac (▶**Figure 16-10**) are increasing. (Actually, more than 60 plants can cause allergic reactions, but these three are by far the most common offenders.) Of

those who do react, 15% to 25% will have incapacitating swelling and blistering eruptions (▼**Figure 16-11**) that require medical treatment with systemic corticosteroids.

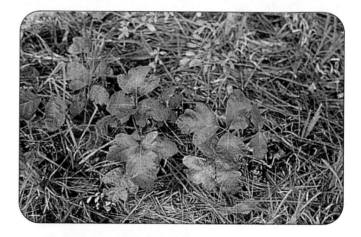

Figure 16-9   Poison oak

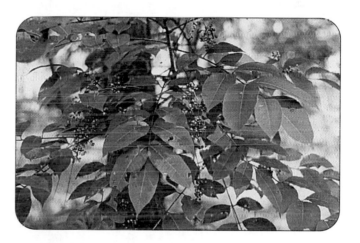

Figure 16-10   Poison sumac

Figure 16-8   Poison ivy, found in all 48 contiguous U.S. states

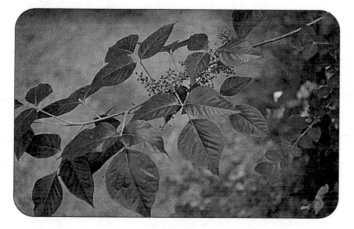

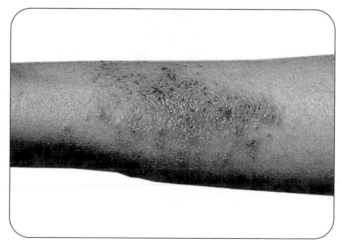

Figure 16-11   Poison ivy dermatitis

POISON IVY, OAK, AND SUMAC

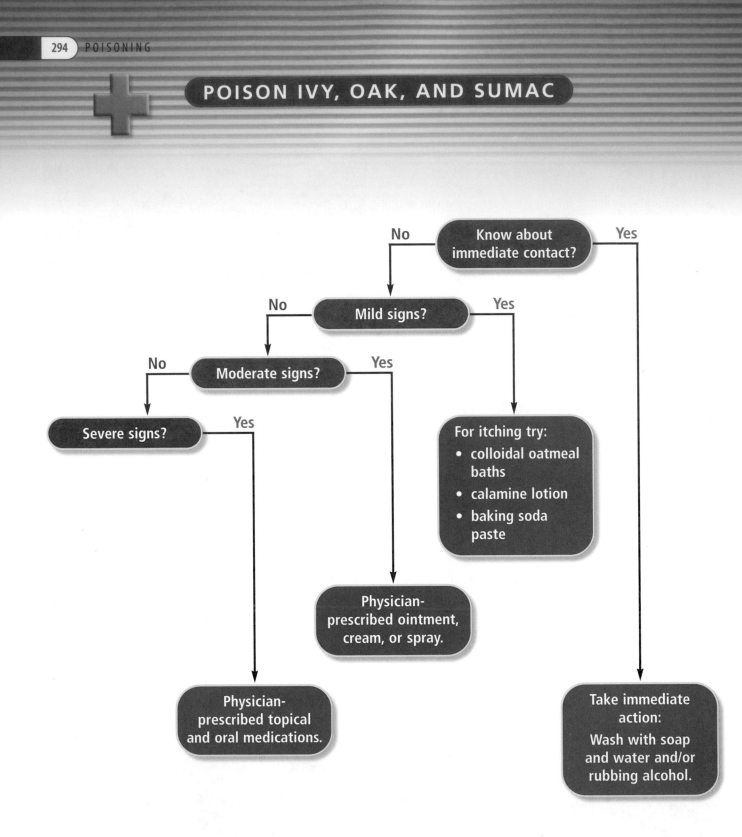

Know about immediate contact?

No → **Mild signs?**

Yes →

No → **Moderate signs?**

Yes →

No → **Severe signs?**

Yes →

For itching try:
- colloidal oatmeal baths
- calamine lotion
- baking soda paste

Physician-prescribed ointment, cream, or spray.

Physician-prescribed topical and oral medications.

Take immediate action:

Wash with soap and water and/or rubbing alcohol.

Did You Know?

Poison Ivy, Oak, and Sumac

+ Most common allergy in the country, affecting half the population.
+ Sensitivity to urushiol can develop at any time.
+ Solutions or cures are those that annihilate urushiol.
+ Everyone appears to react slightly differently to all the remedies.
+ Covered by workers compensation in some states (CA, for example).
+ First published records of poison ivy in North America date back to 1600s.
+ Poison ivy coined by Captain John Smith in 1609.
+ Western poison oak discovered by David Douglas (1799-1834) on Vancouver Island; The Douglas fir tree was also named after him.

There is no routine test to determine an individual's degree of sensitivity—a history of past dermatitis is the most reliable indicator.

The resin (urushiol) of these plants is a colorless or slightly yellow, light oil. It runs in resin canals just under the surface, from the roots through the stems, into the leaves and flowers, and just under the surface of the fruit. It is not present in the nectar. The leaves of the plants are fragile and easily ruptured by high winds or by humans or animals brushing against them. The oil immediately oozes onto the surface.

The light oil generally is not visible on human skin. On the sole of a shoe, on the palm of a hand or glove, or on the surface of an animal's fur, it can be spread by direct contact. On some objects, the oil can stay in an active form for months or years. Smoke from burning plants can produce severe dermatitis. Firefighters and picnickers downwind from a campfire often are affected by airborne oil.

Most people cannot identify these irritating plants. Poison ivy and poison oak are low bushes or climbing vines with waxy, broad, green leaves in the summer that change to a brown-to-red color in the fall. The leaflets of poison ivy and poison oak grow in groups of three (three leaves radiating from a single attachment point), giving rise to the warning "Leaves of three, let them be." Poison ivy flourishes throughout most of the United States, except in Alaska and Hawaii, while poison oak is found in the West and East Coasts and some South Central areas of the U.S. Poison sumac is found chiefly in damp, swampy areas in the eastern United States. These plants tend not to grow at elevations above 5,000 feet or in hot, dry deserts. A helpful method of identifying these plants is the "black-spot test." When the sap is exposed to the air, it turns brown in a matter of minutes and black the next day.

Allergic people can come in contact with the urushiol of these plants from their clothes or shoes, pet fur, or the smoke from burning plants. Contrary to popular belief, no one can develop a rash by touching the fluid from the blisters (their own or others'), since the fluid does not contain the oily resin. Any apparent spreading is actually a delayed reaction to contact with the resin.

Facts and Myths

Myth	Fact
Poison ivy is contagious.	Rubbing the rashes won't spread poison ivy to other parts of your body (or to another person). You spread the rash only if urushiol oil—the sticky, resinlike substance that causes the rash—has been left on your hands.
You can catch poison ivy simply by being near the plants.	Direct contact is needed to release urushiol oil. Stay away from forest fires, direct burning, or anything else that can cause the oil to become airborne such as a lawnmower, trimmer, etc.
Leaves of three, let them be.	Poison sumac has 7 to 13 leaves on a branch, although poison ivy and oak have three leaves per cluster.
Do not worry about dead plants.	Urushiol oil stays active on any surface, including dead plants, for up to five years.
Breaking the blisters releases urushiol oil that can spread.	Not true. But your wounds can become infected and you may make the scarring worse. In very extreme cases, excessive fluid may need to be withdrawn by a doctor.

What to Look for

Most people do not realize they have come in contact with a poisonous plant until the rash erupts. Reactions can range from mild to severe:

- mild: itching
- mild to moderate: itching and redness
- moderate: itching, redness, and swelling
- severe: itching, redness, swelling, and blisters

Severity is important, but so is the amount of skin affected. The greater the amount of skin affected, the greater the need for medical attention. A day or two is the usual time between contact and the onset of signs and symptoms.

What to Do

1. Those who know they have been in contact with a poisonous plant should decontaminate the skin as soon as possible (within five minutes for sensitive people, up to one hour for moderately sensitive individuals). Unfortunately, most victims do not know about their contact until several hours or days later, when the itching and rash begin. Use soap and water to clean the skin of the oily resin or apply rubbing (isopropyl) alcohol liberally (not in swab-type dabs). If too little isopropyl alcohol is used, the oil will actually be spread to another site and enlarge the injury. Other solvents such as paint

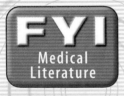

Black-Spot Test

Most poison ivy dermatitis victims fail to recognize the plant. Poison ivy and poison oak leaves have three leaflets; poison sumac has 7 to 13 leaflets per leaf. The mature fruit is an off-white berry. These botanical characteristics explain the axioms "Leaflets three, let it be" and "Berries white, poisonous sight!"

The "black-spot test" is another means of identifying these plants. To check a suspicious plant, grasp a leaf with a piece of white paper (do not touch the leaf) and crush it with a rock. The clear sap of poison ivy, poison oak, and poison sumac on the paper will turn dark brown in 10 minutes and turn black in a day.

Source: J. D. Guin: "The Black Spot Test for Recognizing Poison Ivy and Related Species." *Journal of the American Academy of Dermatology* 2:332–333, February 1980.

Preventing Poisonous-Plant Dermatitis

To reduce the likelihood of developing poisonous-plant dermatitis, follow these steps:

- Avoid the plants.
- Wear protective clothing and use appropriate commercial barrier preparations.
- Replenish the barrier protection every four to six hours, if practical.
- Decontaminate after known exposure with liberal amounts of soap and water and then reapply the barrier preparation.
- Decontaminate at the end of the day with isopropyl alcohol and a water rinse.
- Dispose of all contaminated clothing and equipment.

thinner can be used, but they are hard on the skin. Rinse with water to remove the solubilized material. Water removes urushiol from the skin, oxidizes and inactivates it, and does not penetrate the skin as do solvents.

2. For the mild stage, have the victim soak in a luke-warm bath sprinkled with one to two cups of col-loidal oatmeal such as Aveeno™. Colloidal oatmeal makes a tub slick, so take appropriate precautions. Or, apply any of the following:

- wet compresses soaked with Burow's solution (aluminum acetate) for 20 to 30 minutes three or four times a day
- calamine lotion (calamine ointment if the skin becomes dry and cracked) or zinc oxide
- baking soda paste: one teaspoon of water mixed with three teaspoons of baking soda

To control itching, immerse or run hot water over the area. The water should be hot enough to redden the skin but not burn it. Do not use soap. Heat re-leases histamine, the substance in the skin's cells that causes severe itching. A hot shower or bath causes intense itching as the histamine is released. That depletes the cells of histamine, and the victim will then get up to eight hours of relief from itching.

3. For the mild to moderate stage, care for the skin as you would for the mild stage and use a physician-prescribed corticosteroid ointment.

4. For the severe stage, care for the skin as you would for the mild and moderate stages and use a physician-prescribed oral corticosteroid such as prednisone. Apply a topical corticosteroid ointment or cream, cover it with a transparent plastic wrap, and lightly bind the area with an elastic or self-adhering bandage.

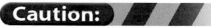

Caution:

DO NOT use nonprescription hydrocortisone creams, ointments, and sprays in strengths of less than 1%. They offer little benefit.

DO NOT use over-the-counter anti-itch lotions like Caladryl™ because they may cause further skin irritation. Oral antihistamines such as Benadryl™ often are used in conjunction with prescription creams to help decrease itching.

DO NOT let the victim rub or scratch the rash or itching skin.

Stinging Nettle

The stinging nettle plant has stinging hairs on its stem and leaves. The stinging hair is a fine, hollow tube with a bladder at its base that contains a chemical irritant. When the stinging hair is touched, a fine needlepoint is formed that penetrates the skin and injects an irritating chemical.

What to Look for

Stinging nettle affects almost all people. Its effects are not an allergic response, as with poison ivy, but rather are due to a direct irritant effect of the plant's sap. The effects are limited to the exposed area, and the response is usually immediate.

Stinging nettle produces some degree of redness, burning, and itching for an hour or more, depending on the area of the body exposed to the plant. For example, the thicker skin on the soles and the palms retards the stinging hairs better than areas of thinner skin, such as the backs of the hands and the arms. Humans vary in sensitivity when the plant actually contacts exposed skin.

The typical response to contact with stinging nettle is a rapid, intense burning sensation at the site of the injection. The area then may itch for an hour or more. Usually, no systemic (whole-body) effects are noted.

What to Do

1. Wash the exposed area with soap and water to remove irritant chemicals.

2. Apply a cold, wet pack to help soothe the painful itching. Other treatments might include a paste of colloidal oatmeal, an over-the-counter hydrocortisone cream (1%), or calamine lotion.

3. Take Benadryl™, an over-the-counter antihistamine, if desired. Be sure to follow package directions and be aware that it causes drowsiness.

The duration of the stinging nettle reaction is measured in hours rather than days, so little therapy is needed.

Carbon Monoxide Poisoning Deaths Associated with Camping

Carbon monoxide (CO) is an odorless, colorless, nonirritating gas produced by the incomplete combustion of carbon-based fuels. CO exposure is responsible for more fatal unintentional poisonings in the U.S. than any other agent, with the highest incidence occurring during the cold-weather months. Although most of these deaths occur in residences or motor vehicles, two incidents among campers in Georgia illustrate the danger of CO in outdoor settings.

✦ Case 1

A 51-year-old man, his 10-year-old son, a 9-year old body, and a 7-year-old girl were found dead inside a zipped-up, 10-foot by 14-foot, 2-room tent at their campsite in southeast Georgia (a pet dog also died). A propane gas stove, still burning, was found inside the tent; the stove apparently had been brought inside to provide warmth.

✦ Case 2

A 34-year-old man and his 7-year-old son were found dead inside their zipped-up tent at a group camping site in central Georgia. They were discovered by other campers. A charcoal grill was found inside the tent; the grill apparently had been brought inside to provide warmth after it had been used outside for cooking.

During 1990-1994, in the U.S., portable fuel-burning camp stoves and lanterns were involved in 10 to 17 CO poisoning deaths each year, and charcoal grills were involved in 15 to 27 deaths each year. During this same time, an annual average of 30 fatal CO poisonings occurred inside tents or campers.

Source: *CDC MMWR Weekly;* 48(32):705-706 (August 20, 1999)

STUDY Questions (16)

Name_____ Course_____ Date_____

Activities

Activity 1

Mark each question as true (T) or false (F).

T F **1.** The "black-spot test" can help identify poison ivy.

T F **2.** Carbon monoxide has an odor.

T F **3.** Automatically dilute any swallowed poison with water or milk.

T F **4.** If the poison victim is conscious, first call the emergency telephone number.

T F **5.** Use syrup of ipecac only when directed by a poison control center.

T F **6.** Charcoal scraped from burnt toast is effective for treating a swallowed poison.

T F **7.** Attempt to neutralize a corrosive-acid poison.

Case Situations

Case 1

A 25-year-old male complains of a rash on his arms and legs. He has no known allergies and has never had a similar rash. The rash began earlier in the day, and he cannot associate it with any new medications, soaps, foods, or colognes. He did, however, just return from a two-day camping trip. The rash is red, with mild swelling, itching, and blisters.

Check (✓) the appropriate action(s) that may be useful in alleviating itching caused by poison ivy, poison oak, or poison sumac.

____ **1.** Apply rubbing alcohol to the rash and all affected areas.

____ **2.** Apply calamine lotion to the affected areas.

____ **3.** Take an antihistamine.

____ **4.** Apply hot water (not hot enough to burn), even though it will initially intensify the itching.

Case 2

A 39-year-old female attempted suicide by leaving her car running in a closed garage. Bystanders have removed her from the garage just as you arrive. Your assessment reveals she is unconscious and pulseless.

____ **1.** This victim is suffering from
    a. carbon dioxide overload
    b. cyanide poisoning
    c. carbon monoxide poisoning
    d. freon exposure

____ **2.** Treatment for this victim would include
    a. giving CPR
    b. giving only chest compressions to avoid the gas involved
    c. giving syrup of ipecac
    d. giving the Heimlich maneuver

Check (✓) the statements that apply to carbon monoxide poisoning:

____ **3.** Victims need 100% oxygen as quickly as possible.

____ **4.** Symptoms of carbon monoxide poisoning can be confused with those of the flu.

____ **5.** Carbon monoxide is easily recognized by its odor.

____ **6.** A headache can be an early symptom of carbon monoxide poisoning.

Case 3

You arrive at a scene in which a car has crashed into a building. The driver, a 45-year-old male, is awake but appears to be confused and unable to think clearly. You are able to determine that he and his family were out for a ride in their newly purchased used car when he experienced an intense headache and lost control of the vehicle. Both passengers, the driver's 38-year-old wife and his 14-year-old son, are unconscious but breathing. The driver states that they fell asleep just before the accident. All three are cyanotic about the lips.

____ **1.** These victims are most likely suffering from
    a. carbon monoxide poisoning
    b. severe head injuries
    c. diabetic coma
    d. seizures

STUDY
Questions 16

____ 2. Care for them would involve
   a. calling the EMS
   b. placing them with their legs elevated
   c. flushing them with large amounts of water
   d. having them rebreathe their exhaled air
      from a paper sack

Case 4

A frantic young mother fears that her two-year-old son has eaten some rat poison. Unfortunately, the toddler is too young to reliably tell what he has done. No unusual signs of symptoms are immediately present.

1. What action would you take first for this type of poisoning?

   _____

   _____

   _____

2. What should you do next?

   _____

   _____

   _____

3. What critical information would it be useful for you to have before calling the emergency telephone number?

   _____

   _____

   _____

4. What is the telephone number of the poison control center nearest your home?

   _____

____ 5. For which type of swallowed poison should you automatically give the victim water or milk?
   a. caustics or corrosives
   b. pills
   c. tablets
   d. plants

____ 6. In what position should you place a person who has swallowed poison?
   a. left side
   b. right side
   c. prone
   d. supine (on the back)

7. What two substances can you give at home for a swallowed poison?
   a. _____
   b. _____

8. Before you give either of the substances in the preceding question, what should you obtain?

   _____

   _____

Chapter Activities

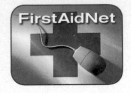

WEB Activities

Poisoning

Visit nsc.jbpub.com/FirstAidNet, then click on Web Activities, and select the appropriate chapter.

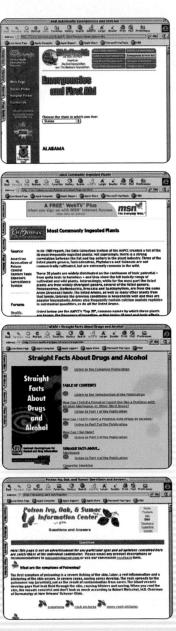

1. Poison Control Center

One of the first things to do when encountering a poisoning is call the poison control center. Locate your nearest poison control center telephone number.

2. Ingested Plants

As there are no sure-fire ways to determine if a plant is poisonous, it is best to assume that all plants contain toxins that are dangerous to the human body if ingested. Do you know any of the top 20 poisonous plants?

3. Drugs and Alcohol

The more you know about drugs and alcohol, the better prepared you will be to help a person who is suffering from a drug and alcohol–related problem.

4. Poison Ivy, Oak, and Sumac

Poison Ivy, oak, or sumac can be found in almost every part of the United States. Being able to recognize these plants before contact is made can greatly alleviate any discomfort associated with a case of poison ivy, oak, or sumac.

Chapter 17

Bites and Stings

Animal Bites

It is estimated that one of every two Americans will be bitten at some time by an animal* or by another person (▶ Figure 17-1). Dogs are responsible for about 80% of all animal-bite injuries. Of the nearly five million dog bites that occur yearly, 80% are trivial or minor, and medical attention is not required or sought, which demonstrates the importance of knowing first aid. The remainder account for about 1% of all emergency department and physician office visits. Each year, 10 to 20 dog bite–related fatalities occur in the United States (▶ Table 17-1). Animal bites represent a major, largely unrecognized public health problem.

Two concerns result from an animal bite: immediate tissue damage and later infection from microorganisms. A dog's mouth may carry more than 60 different species of bacteria, some of which are dangerous to humans. Two examples of infection—tetanus and rabies—have been almost eradicated by medical advances, but they still pose a potential problem.

Though less mutilating, cat bites are common, about 400,000 bites annually in the United States. Cat bites have a much higher rate of infection than dog bites. Cats have very sharp teeth, which can create deep puncture wounds and involve muscle, tendon, and bone.

Another pet especially likely to bite children is the ferret. These animals are often unpredictable and can cause severe facial injury to infants. Ferrets sometimes unleash frenzied, rapid-fire bite-and-slash attacks on infants, usually on their heads and throats, and can inflict hundreds of bites.

Besides children, elderly persons and invalids are especially prone to animal bites since they are sometimes unable to detect or prevent a dangerous situation. Many of the animal-related deaths occurred when the victim was left alone with the offending pet. Contrary to popular belief, wild or stray dogs seldom are involved in fatal attacks.

---

*As is commonly interpreted, the term animal bite in this section refers to a bite by a mammal, not an insect or reptile.

ANIMAL BITES

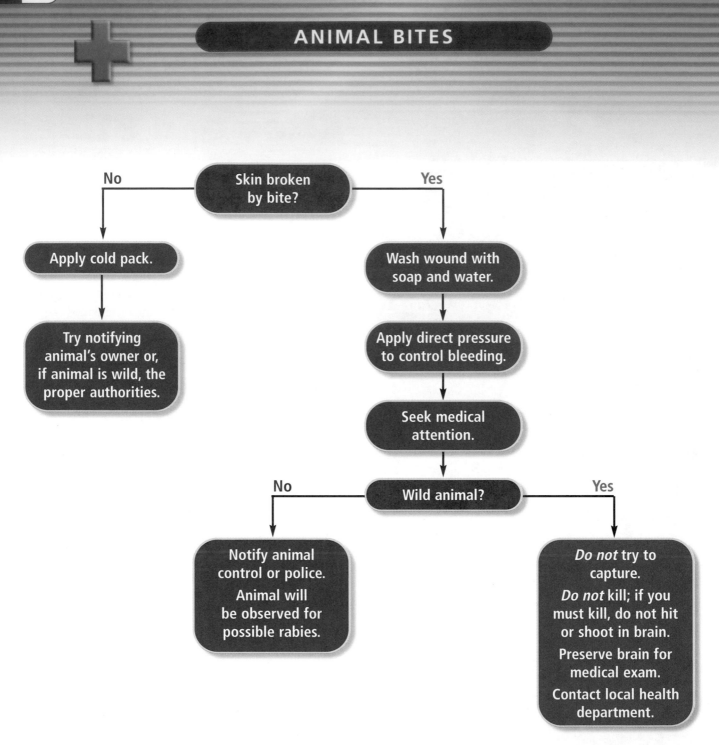

Skin broken by bite?

No → Apply cold pack. → Try notifying animal's owner or, if animal is wild, the proper authorities.

Yes → Wash wound with soap and water. → Apply direct pressure to control bleeding. → Seek medical attention. → Wild animal?

No → Notify animal control or police. Animal will be observed for possible rabies.

Yes → *Do not* try to capture. *Do not* kill; if you must kill, do not hit or shoot in brain. Preserve brain for medical exam. Contact local health department.

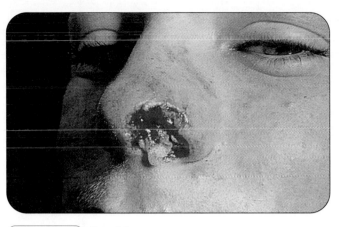

Figure 17-1 Dog bite

Damage mostly occurs on the hands (48% to 59% of all bites), the arms (16% to 26%), the legs (15%), and the face (8% to 30%). A damaged face presents several problems because the proximity of blood vessels to the skin surface make it susceptible to copious bleeding. Facial disfigurement and scarring can result in emotional trauma. Complete or partial loss of an eye can also happen. See Chapter 22 for wild animal attack information.

Rabies

Rabies is one of the most ancient and feared of diseases (▶**Figure 17-2**). Although human rabies rarely occurs in the United States or in other industrialized nations, it remains a scourge in developing countries. A virus found in warm-blooded animals causes rabies and spreads from one animal to another in the saliva, usually through a bite or by licking. Bites from cold-blooded animals such as reptiles do not carry the danger of rabies. (Such bites can

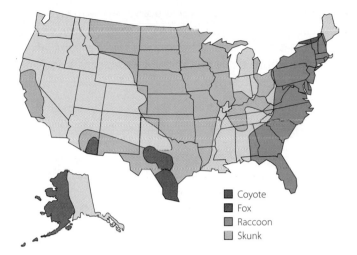

Figure 17-2 Distribution of major terrestrial reservoirs of rabies in the United States, 1996 (Centers for Disease Control and Prevention).

- ■ Coyote
- ■ Fox
- ■ Raccoon
- ■ Skunk

become infected, however, and should be washed well and watched for signs of infection.)

Although there have been 12 human rabies infections since 1966 in the United States caused by rabid dogs, the exposures themselves were outside the continental United States.

Of all rabies cases in the United States, 90% come from skunks, raccoons, bats, and foxes (▼**Figure 17-3**). About 100 rabid dogs are reported annually, but those dogs do not always bite someone. Because there is no cure for rabies, it is fatal once symptoms develop. Three humans who were infected but who were treated promptly survived the disease in the 1970s, but no survivors have been reported since.

A bite or a scratch is considered a significant rabies exposure if it penetrates the skin. Unprovoked attacks are more likely to have been inflicted by a rabid animal than

Figure 17-3 Cases of rabies in animals

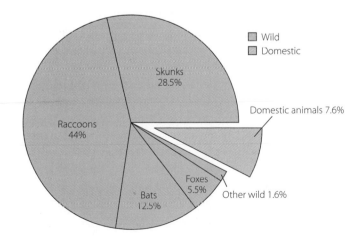

- ■ Wild
- ■ Domestic

Skunks 28.5%

Domestic animals 7.6%

Raccoons 44%

Foxes 5.5%

Other wild 1.6%

Bats 12.5%

Table 17-1: Human Deaths Caused by Animals in the United States, 1996	
Species Causing Deaths	**Number of Deaths**
Humans (homicides)	20,917
Farm animals	46
Hornets, wasps, bees	45
Dog bites	23
Venomous snakes, spiders	13
Unspecified venomous animal	10
Unspecified animal	84

Source: National Safety Council, *Injury Facts,* 1999

are provoked attacks. Bites that occur during the feeding or handling of apparently healthy animals generally are regarded as unprovoked. Nonbite exposure consists of contamination of wounds, including scratches, abrasions, and weeping skin rashes.

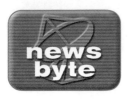

Rabies

Between 1990 and 1998, 27 human rabies cases occurred in the United States, approximately 3 per year. This can be compared to the more than 8,000 cases of animal rabies cases reported each year. Although 20 of the 27 human cases were attributed to bat-associated variants of the rabies virus, a definitive history of a bat bite was established for only one case. Although bat-associated rabies virus variants theoretically can be secondarily transmitted from terrestial mammals, an unrecognized bat bite is the most likely explanation for these cases.

Source: Centers for Disease Control and Prevention, United States Rabies Surveillance Data, 1998.

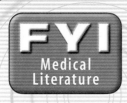

Dog Bites

During the past few years, there has been a rash of news stories about vicious attacks by pit bull terriers. The public hysteria has spurred some communities to such action as outlawing pit bulls.

The Centers for Disease Control undertook a study of fatalities related to dog bites. The researchers found 157 fatalities during a 10-year period. Pet dogs were responsible for almost 70% of fatalities, strays were involved in 27% of cases, and police or guard dogs in only 2.8% of the deaths. No significant "obvious" seasonal trends were noted, except that strays seemed to be involved more often in the fall, while pets were involved more often in the winter. The victims were primarily children under 10 years of age (70%), with a "particularly high" death rate noted for infants less than one month old.

Pit bulls were implicated in more than 40% of the fatalities, "almost three times more than German shepherds, the next most commonly reported breed." Deaths attributed to pit bulls increased from 20% to 62% during the period. The researchers concluded that dog bite fatalities had been underestimated and suggested "strong animal control laws, public education regarding dog bites, and more responsible dog ownership."

Source: J. J. Sacks et al: Dog Bite–Related Fatalities from 1979 through 1988." *Journal of the American Medical Association,* 262:1489–1492.

Consider an animal as possibly rabid if any of the following applies:

- The animal made an unprovoked attack.
- The animal acted strangely, that is, out of character (eg, a usually friendly dog is aggressive, or a wild fox seems docile and "friendly").
- The animal was a high-risk species (skunk, raccoon, or bat).

What to Do

1. If the victim was bitten in the United States (except for the area along the border with Mexico) by a healthy domestic dog or cat, the animal should be confined and observed for 10 days. Any illness during confinement should be evaluated by a veterinarian. If rabies is suspected, a veterinarian should humanely kill the animal and ship its head under refrigeration to a qualified laboratory. (Examination for rabies cannot be reliably performed on decomposed brain tissue.) If the offending animal is a stray or unwanted dog or cat, it should be killed immediately and its head submitted for rabies examination. If feasible, only a veterinarian should kill an animal (domesticated or wild) and decapitate it for sending the head to a laboratory. If the animal is dead, transport the entire body; do not attempt decapitation (precautions must be taken to prevent exposure to potentially infected tissues and saliva).

   No one in the United States has died of rabies when the attacking animal has remained healthy after 10 days of observation. If an attacking dog or cat is rabid or suspected to be rabid, treatment should be started at once. Report animal bites to

Dog Bites: Which Breeds Are Most Dangerous?

Researchers who checked Denver records during a recent year found 178 reports of dog bites to people outside the dog owners' households (this is more common than bites to family members). They also identified 178 nonbiting dogs from the same neighborhoods. Results showed that male dogs (especially unneutered males), German shepherds, and Chow Chows were the most likely to bite outsiders, especially children. Children under age 12 were the victims in 51% of cases. Too few pit bulls, Akitas, and collies were involved in this study to rate their risks.

Source: K. A. Gershman et al. "Which Dogs Bite? A Case-Control Study of Risk Factors." *Pediatrics,* June 1994, 93:913-917.

Animal Rabies Within the United States

Raccoons

Raccoons remain the most frequently reported rabid animal in the United States. The raccoon rabies reservoir extends throughout the southeastern, mid-Atlantic, and northeastern states. No other reservoirs of raccoon rabies have been identified. Rabid raccoons occasionally detected outside of the reservoir area have been found to have non-raccoon variants of the rabies virus, suggesting that they were infected by other species.

Skunks

Skunks are the second most frequently reported rabid animal in this country. Three virus variants are responsible for rabies in skunks. There are two large geographically distinct reservoirs of skunk rabies due to three different variants of the virus: one in California; the other in the central US from Montana to Texas. Rabid skunks reported in eastern states outside the reservoir areas apparently were infected by raccoons rather than by other skunks.

Foxes

Two variants of the rabies virus are associated with persistent reservoirs of rabies in foxes. One long-standing reservoir involves arctic and red foxes in Alaska (and Canada) and to a lesser extent, areas of New York, Vermont, New Hampshire, and Maine. A different variant of the virus has been associated with gray foxes, resulting in reservoirs in Texas and Arizona.

Coyotes

A rabies variant found in domestic dogs along the Texas-Mexico border is currently present in coyotes in southern Texas. Northward spread of this reservoir has been limited by an aggressive (and expensive) airdrop vaccination program.

Bats

Rabid bats of many different species have been found in all of the 48 contiguous states. To date, only one rabid bat has ever been identified in Alaska—in the southeastern part of the state. No rabid bats (or other rabid animals) have ever been identified in Hawaii.

Rodents/small mammals

Providers are often asked about the risks associated with small wild mammals—such as rats, mice, squirrels, chipmunks, rabbits, and hares. Rodent bites are common, so rodents are often tested for rabies in the US. Despite the large number of rodents examined, it is exceedingly uncommon for one to be infected with rabies virus. It has been postulated that these animals are so small that they are unlikely to survive an attack of a larger rabid animal (such as a raccoon, skunk, or fox). Furthermore, although there have been several case reports of humans infected by rabid rodents in other countries, no transmission of rabies from a rodent to a human (or any other mammal) has ever been documented in the United States.

Other wild animals

Other wild animals in the US are occasionally found to be rabid. Most are infected with virus strains associated with terrestrial animal species, rather than bats. In 1996, 87 rabid non-reservoir wild animals were reported from the 50 states, including 43 groundhogs and 23 bobcats.

Source: Washington State Health Department

the police or animal control officers; they should be the ones to capture the animal for observation. If the dog or cat escapes and is not suspected to be rabid, consult local public health officials.

If the victim was bitten in the United States by a skunk, raccoon, bat, fox, or other mammal, it should be considered a rabies exposure and treatment started *immediately.* The only exception is when the bite occurred in a part of the continental United States known to be free of rabies. If the wild animal is captured, it should be killed by a veterinarian and its head shipped to a qualified laboratory *immediately.* In developing countries, except for those few areas where rabies does not occur, all attacking animals that elude capture should be considered rabid.

Ferret Attacks on Infants

news byte

A study identified three infants attacked by pet ferrets resulting in severe facial injuries. Two of the children had their ears bitten off and required reconstructive surgery. The attacks were unprovoked. Two of the children were asleep in their cribs when they were bitten. Although ferrets are increasingly popular pets, medical experts believe that they are not suitable pets for families with small children. Ferrets may unpredictably injure infants and small children. There is no effective rabies vaccine for ferrets yet available.

Source: J.A. Applegate and M. F. Walhout, "Childhood Risk from the Ferret," *Journal of Emergency Medicine,* May 1998, 16:425-427.

Facts About Dog Bites

+ Carefully choose your pet dog. Evaluate your environment and lifestyles and speak with a professional to determine the appropriate type of pet.

+ Dogs should be neutered to reduce aggressive tendencies.

+ Never leave infants or young children alone with a dog. Be sensitive to cues that a child is fearful or apprehensive about a dog.

+ Teach children basic safety around dogs and review regularly.

+ Dogs with histories of aggression are inappropriate for families with children.

+ Do not play aggressive games with your dog; for example, wrestling.

+ Never approach an unfamiliar dog. Immediately report stray dogs or dogs displaying unusual behavior.

+ Remain motionless when approached by an unfamiliar dog—never run or scream.

+ Do not disturb a dog that is sleeping, eating, or caring for puppies.

+ If knocked down by a dog, lie still and remain in a ball.

+ If bitten by a dog, immediately report the bite.

Source: Centers for Disease Control and Prevention.

Caution:

DO NOT try to capture the animal yourself.

DO NOT get near the animal.

DO NOT kill the animal unless absolutely necessary. If it must be killed, protect the head and brain from damage so they can be examined for rabies. Transport a dead animal intact to limit exposure to potentially infected tissues or saliva. The animal's remains should be refrigerated to prevent decomposition.

DO NOT handle the animal without taking appropriate precautions. Infected saliva may be on the animal's fur, so wear heavy gloves or use a shovel if you have to move a dead animal.

2. Thoroughly cleanse the bite wound with soap and water under pressure *immediately.* For best results, clean the wound with a soap solution, rinse it completely, then irrigate the area with water under pressure. If available, use diluted Betadine to rinse the wound.

3. Stop the bleeding and give wound care.

4. Seek medical attention for further wound cleaning and a possible tetanus shot. The physician will determine if sutures are needed to close the wound. If needed, a vaccination against rabies will be started. The old series of 20 painful abdominal injections has been replaced by a five-shot vaccine, which is given in the deltoid muscle of the arm.

Human Bites

After dogs and cats, the animal most likely to bite humans is another human. Human bites can cause severe injury, often more so than other animal bites. The human mouth contains a wide range of bacteria, so the chance of infection is greater from a human bite than from bites of other warm-blooded animals.

Most human bites are inflicted by fighting youths, by children at play, by people in mental institutions, or during sexual assaults. Embarrassment sometimes causes a victim not to seek medical attention immediately, which greatly increases the risk of infection.

Although most human bites occur during acts of violence, about one-fourth are (1) accidental or sports related, (2) sustained by hospital workers trying to restrain children or seizure patients, or (3) self-inflicted during nail chewing or thumb sucking.

Men are more often victims than women, mostly during aggressive altercations, with the peak age being 25. The most common injury location is the hand, sustained on a closed fist as the result of a punch.

Types of Human Bites

There are two types of human bites. **True bites** occur when any part of the body's flesh is caught between teeth, usually deliberately. True bites happen during fights and in cases of abuse. Mandatory-reporting laws apply if spousal or child abuse is involved. A "schoolyard bite," with one child biting another, generally is not reportable.

Transmission of HIV by a bite has not been documented and is unlikely.

Much worse than a true bite is the **clenched-fist injury,** which results from cutting a fist on teeth. It is associated with a high likelihood of infection. The injury is usually a laceration over the knuckles. Although clenched-fist injuries usually result from a fight, unintentional injury can happen during sports and play.

What to Do

1. If the wound is not bleeding heavily, wash it with soap and water (under the pressure from a faucet) for 5 to 10 minutes. Avoid scrubbing, which can bruise tissues.

2. Rinse the wound thoroughly with running water under pressure. If available, use diluted Betadine™ to rinse the wound. This helps kill any bacteria.

3. Control bleeding with direct pressure. See Chapter 6 for details.

4. Cover the wound with a sterile dressing. Do *not* close the wound with tape or butterfly bandages. That traps bacteria in the wound, increasing the chance of infection.

5. Seek medical attention for possible further wound cleaning, a tetanus shot, and sutures applied to close the wound.

Snakebites

Throughout the world, about 50,000 people die each year from snakebites. Each year in the United States, 40,000 to 50,000 people are bitten by snakes, 7,000 to 8,000 of them by venomous snakes (▶**Figure 17-4, A–B**). Amazingly, fewer than a dozen Americans die each year from snakebites. Victims who die from snakebites in the United States usually do so in the first 48 hours.

Only four snake species in the United States are poisonous: rattlesnakes (▶**Figure 17-5**) (which account for about 65% of all venomous snakebites and nearly all the snakebite deaths in the United States), copperheads (▶**Figure 17-6**), water moccasins (also known as cottonmouths) (▶**Figure 17-7**), and coral snakes (▶**Figure 17-8**). The first three are pit vipers, which have three characteristics in common (▶**Figure 17-9**):

- triangular, flat heads wider than their necks
- elliptical pupils ("cat's eyes")
- a heat-sensitive "pit" between the eye and the nostril on each side of the head

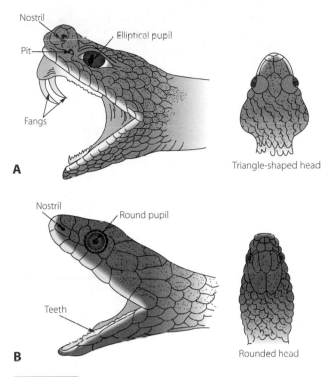

Figure 17-4 Characteristic features of poisonous snakes (pit vipers) and of harmless snakes

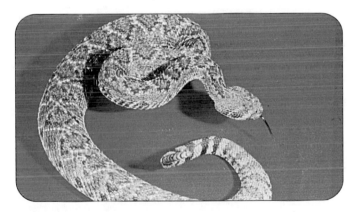

Figure 17-5 Rattlesnake

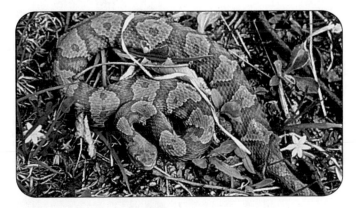

Figure 17-6 Copperhead snake

SNAKE BITES

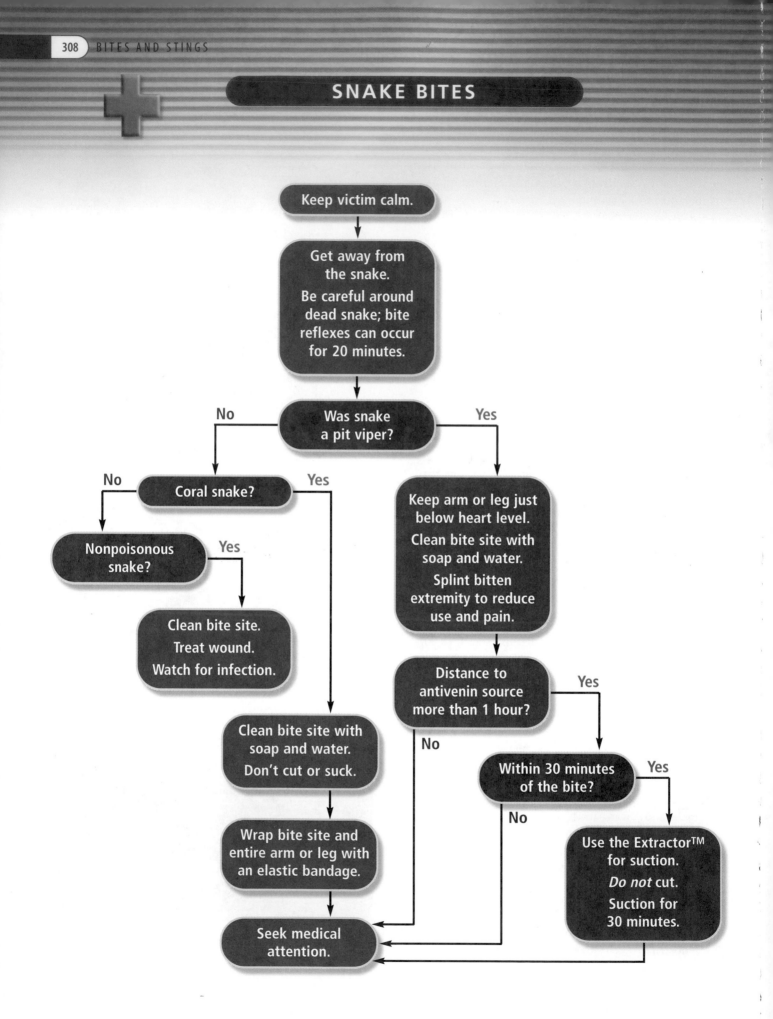

Keep victim calm.

↓

Get away from the snake.

Be careful around dead snake; bite reflexes can occur for 20 minutes.

↓

Was snake a pit viper?

No ← | → Yes

No ← **Coral snake?** → **Yes**

Nonpoisonous snake? — **Yes** →

Clean bite site. Treat wound. Watch for infection.

Keep arm or leg just below heart level.
Clean bite site with soap and water.
Splint bitten extremity to reduce use and pain.

↓

Distance to antivenin source more than 1 hour? — **Yes** →

No

Clean bite site with soap and water. Don't cut or suck.

Within 30 minutes of the bite? — **Yes** →

No

↓

Wrap bite site and entire arm or leg with an elastic bandage.

Use the Extractor™ for suction.
***Do not* cut.**
Suction for 30 minutes.

↓

Seek medical attention.

The coral snake is small and colorful, with a series of bright red, yellow, and black bands around its body (every other band is yellow). It also has a black snout.

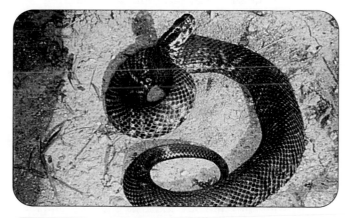

Figure 17-7 Water moccasin (cottonmouth)

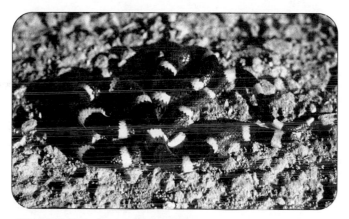

Figure 17-8 Coral snake, America's most venomous snake

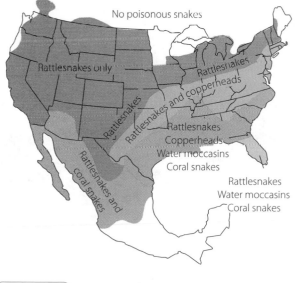

Figure 17-9 Location of venomous snakes

Exotic snakes, whether imported legally or smuggled into the United States and found in zoos, schools, snake farms, and amateur and professional collections, account for at least 15 bites a year.

Little information can be found describing the circumstances surrounding snakebites (such as what the victim was doing to get bitten by a rattlesnake **▼Figure 17-10, A–B**). A "legitimate" snakebite is one in which the victim was bitten before the encounter with a snake was recognized or while trying to move away from the snake. They most often involve the lower extremities and are "accidental."

An "illegitimate" snakebite means that, before being bitten, the victim recognized the encounter with a snake but did not attempt to move away from the snake. Most illegitimate bites occur on the upper extremities. Most bites of this type happen when the victim tries to kill, capture, play with, or move a snake.

Adult snakes deliver more serious bites because they inject more venom than do young snakes, even though a young snake's venom is two to three times more toxic than an adult's.

Pit Viper Bites
What to Look for

- severe burning pain at the bite site
- two small puncture wounds about one-half inch apart (some cases may have only one fang mark)

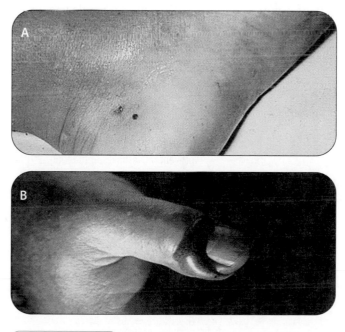

Figure 17-10 A–B **A** Rattlesnake bite (note two fang marks). **B** Copperhead bite two hours after bite.

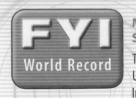

Most Venomous Snake in the U.S.

The most venomous snake in the United States is the coral snake. In a standard LD99-100 test, it took just 0.55 grain of venom per 2.2 lbs. of mouse weight injected intravenously to kill 99% to 100% of all mice injected. In this test, the smaller the dosage, the more toxic the venom. However, the teeth of the coral snake point back into its mouth; therefore, it cannot inject the venom until it has a firm hold on the victim.

Source: The Guinness Book of Records, New York: Bantam Books, 1995, p. 72

- swelling (happens within five minutes and can involve an entire extremity)
- discoloration and blood-filled blisters possibly developing in 6 to 10 hours
- in severe cases, nausea, vomiting, sweating, and weakness

In about 25% of poisonous snakebites, there is no venom injection, only fang and tooth wounds (known as a "dry" bite).

What to Do

Most snakebites occur within a few hours of a medical facility, where antivenin is available. Bites showing no sign of venom injection require only a possible tetanus shot and care of the bite wounds. Identifying the type

of pit viper is of minimal importance, since the same antivenin is used to counteract all North American pit viper venom.

The Wilderness Medical Society lists the following guidelines for dealing with bites by pit vipers.

1. Get the victim and bystanders away from the snake. Snakes have been known to bite more than once. Pit vipers can strike about one-half their body length. Be careful around a decapitated snake head—head reactions can persist for 20 minutes or more.

2. Keep the victim quiet. If possible, carry the victim or have the victim walk very slowly to help.

3. Gently wash the bitten area with soap and water.

4. If you are more than one hour from a medical facility with antivenin or if the snake was large and the victim's skin is swelling rapidly, immediately apply suction with the Extractor™ (from Sawyer Products (▼**Figure 17-11**)). It does not require an incision (cutting). If the Extractor™ is applied within three minutes of the bite and left on for 30 minutes, it will remove up to 30% of the venom. This procedure is seldom necessary because of the close proximity of medical facilities.

5. Seek medical attention *immediately*. This is the most important thing to do for the victim. Antivenin

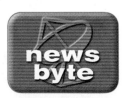

Dead Snakes Can Still Bite

Data collected at the Good Samaritan Regional Medical Center in Phoenix show that fatal injuries do not prevent rattlesnakes from biting humans. Of the 34 patients admitted to the Phoenix Center for Rattlesnake Bites in a recent 11-month period, five were bitten by snakes that had been fatally injured and were presumed dead. One patient was bitten on the index finger after picking up a snake he had bludgeoned in the head and assumed was dead. Another was bitten after picking up a snake he had shot, then decapitated.

Source: J.R. Suchard and F. LoVecchio, "Envenomations by Rattlesnakes Thought to Be Dead," New England Journal of Medicine, 34(24):1930, June 17, 1999.

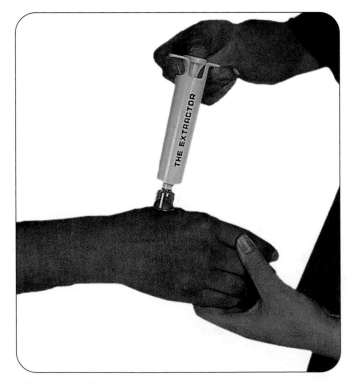

Figure 17-11 Extractor™ use does not require cutting the skin.

must be given *within four hours* of the bite (not every venomous snakebite requires antivenin). Antivenin is found only in hospitals for several reasons: (1) it has a short shelf life; (2) the victim needs to be tested for sensitivity to horse serum (an allergic person will develop anaphylaxis); (3) the minimum dose is 5 to 10 vials for each incident; and (4) it is very expensive, over $100 per vial.

Caution:

DO NOT apply cold or ice to a snakebite. It does not inactivate the venom and poses a danger of frostbite.

DO NOT use the "cut-and-suck" procedure—you could damage underlying structures (eg, blood vessels, nerves).

DO NOT apply mouth suction. Your mouth is filled with bacteria, increasing the likelihood of wound infection.

DO NOT apply electric shock. No medical studies support this method.

Coral Snake Bites

The coral snake is America's most venomous snake, but it rarely bites people. The coral snake has short fangs and tends to hang on and "chew" its venom into the victim rather than to strike and release, like a pit viper. Coral-snake venom is neurotoxic, and symptoms may begin one to five hours after the bite.

What to Do

1. Keep the victim calm.
2. Gently clean the bite site with soap and water.
3. Apply mild pressure by wrapping several elastic bandages (eg, Ace™ bandage) over the bite site and the entire arm or leg. Applying mild pressure is recommended only for bites from elapid snakes like the coral snake, not pit vipers. The technique originated in Australia, where it has been very successful. Do *not* cut the victim's skin (▶Figure 17-12) or use an Extractor™.
4. Seek medical attention for antivenin. No deaths have occurred since 1961 with the development of an antivenin.

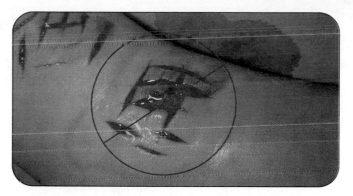

Figure 17-12 Do not excise the skin for a snakebite.

Preventing Snakebites

Follow these guidelines to prevent snakebites:

+ Do not handle venomous snakes.
+ Avoid hiking and camping in snake-infested areas; avoid exploring caves, rock crevices, dens, lairs, stone walls, and wood piles.
+ Know the outdoor terrain and be alert for snakes in thick foliage.
+ Watch where you sit, step, and stretch; do not reach into holes or hidden ledges.
+ Wear protective gear such as boots, trousers, long pants, long-sleeved shirts, and gloves when you are in possible snake habitats.
+ Take a friend with you; it may save your life.
+ Do not alarm a sleeping snake (even a newborn snake) or tease or molest an awake snake.
+ Do not keep poisonous snakes as pets; zoos are better qualified to care for them. A 16% reduction in bites from rattlesnakes would occur if they were not kept as pets.
+ When you are in snake country, carry a Sawyer Extractor™ device.
+ Don't sit on or step over logs until you closely scrutinize the area.
+ Don't handle a dead venomous snake. The reflex action of the jaws can still inflict a wound 20 minutes or more after the snake has died.
+ Don't surprise or corner a snake. Use a walking stick to prod uncleared ground and make noise so a snake can sense you coming.
+ Researchers suggest that more than one-half of all rattlesnake bites would be eliminated if people simply moved away from the snake.

INSECT STINGS

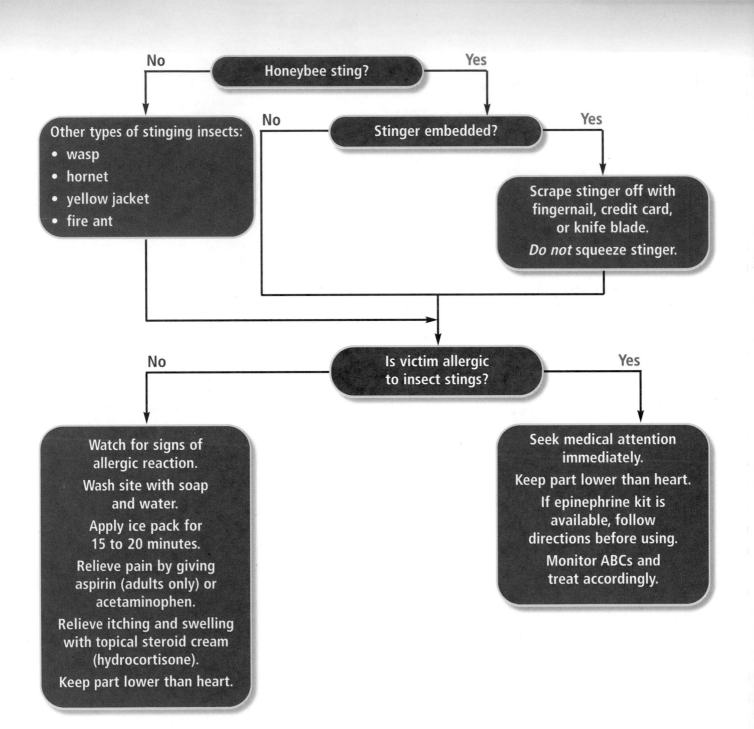

Honeybee sting?

No → **Other types of stinging insects:**
- wasp
- hornet
- yellow jacket
- fire ant

Yes → **Stinger embedded?**

No

Yes → **Scrape stinger off with fingernail, credit card, or knife blade.**

Do not squeeze stinger.

Is victim allergic to insect stings?

No → **Watch for signs of allergic reaction.**

Wash site with soap and water.

Apply ice pack for 15 to 20 minutes.

Relieve pain by giving aspirin (adults only) or acetaminophen.

Relieve itching and swelling with topical steroid cream (hydrocortisone).

Keep part lower than heart.

Yes → **Seek medical attention immediately.**

Keep part lower than heart.

If epinephrine kit is available, follow directions before using.

Monitor ABCs and treat accordingly.

Nonpoisonous Snakebites

A nonpoisonous snake leaves a horseshoe shape of tooth-marks on the victim's skin. If you are not positive about a snake, assume it was venomous. Some so-called non-poisonous North American snakes such as the hognose and garter snakes have venom that can cause painful local reactions but no systemic (whole-body) symptoms.

What to Do

1. Gently clean the bite site with soap and water.
2. Care for the bite as you would a minor wound.
3. Seek medical advice.

Insect Stings

The stinging insects belonging to the order of *Hymenoptera* include honeybees (▶ **Figure 17-13, A–D**), bumblebees, yellow jackets, hornets, wasps, and fire ants (▶ **Table 17-2**).

Hymenopterans kill between 50 and 100 people in the United States each year. The actual number is probably higher because an unknown number of deaths due to hymenopteran-caused anaphylaxis are mistakenly attributed to cardiac arrest. These insects account for more deaths and illnesses each year than all other venomous animals combined. About 1 in every 200 people is dangerously allergic to Hymenoptera venom. Fortunately, localized pain, itching, and swelling—the most common consequences of an insect bite—can be treated with first aid.

Generally, venomous flying insects are aggressive only when threatened or when their hives or nests are disrupted. Under such conditions, they sting, sometimes in swarms. Honeybees and bumblebees have barbed stingers that become embedded in the victim's skin during the sting. After injecting its venom, the bee flies away, tearing and leaving behind the embedded stinger and venom sac, causing it to die. Honeybees and bumblebees do not release all their venom during the initial injection; some remains in the stinger left embedded in the victim's skin. If the stinger and venom sac are not removed properly, additional venom may be released and worsen the victim's reaction.

In contrast, the stingers of wasps, yellow jackets, and hornets are not barbed and do not become embedded in the victim. Thus, these insects can sting multiple times, and most species (with a few exceptions, such as some yellow jacket species) do not die as a result of the stinging.

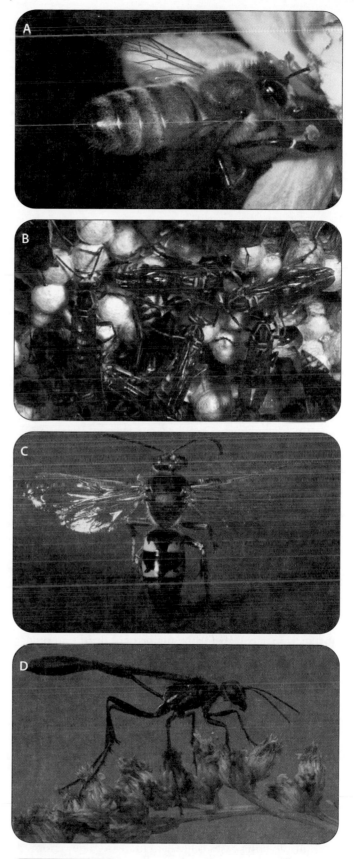

(**Figure 17-13 A–D**) **A.** Honeybee. **B.** Yellow jacket. **C.** Hornet. **D.** Wasp.

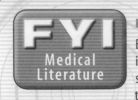

Honeybee Venom Delivery

Envenomation by a honeybee is initiated by the insertion of the stinging apparatus or stinger into the victim's skin. Researchers found that at least 90% of the venom contents were delivered within 20 seconds of the initiation of the sting and that venom delivery was completed within one minute. This suggests that a bee stinger must be removed within a few seconds to prevent anaphylaxis in an allergic person.

Source: M. J. Schumacher et al: "Rate and Quantity of Delivery of Venom from Honeybee Stings." *Journal of Allergy and Clinical Immunology*, 92:831–835.

Most stings cause only self-limited, local inflammatory reactions consisting of pain, itching, redness, and swelling. These reactions are usually more a nuisance than a medical emergency. However, local reactions can be extensive, involving the victim's entire arm. When that occurs, the swelling and redness may peak two to three days after the sting and last a week or longer. Signs and symptoms of life-threatening reactions include nausea, vomiting, bronchospasm, wheezing, fever, or drippy nose. A victim may go into anaphylaxis almost immediately or first progress through a variety of symptoms. Most people who have anaphylactic reactions have no history of them. In a study of 400 fatal bee stings, only 15% of the victims had a known sensitivity.

Reactions generally happen within a few minutes to one hour after the sting. Bee-sting victims who have anaphylactic reactions develop throat swelling and bronchospasm, which are manifested by difficulty in speaking, tightness in the throat or chest, wheezing, shortness of breath, and chest pain. Respiratory-tract obstruction accounts for the majority of deaths among victims of flying-insect stings.

For the severely allergic person, a single sting may be fatal within minutes. And although accounts exist of individuals who have survived some 2,000 stings at one time, 500 stings will usually kill even those people who are not allergic to stinging insects.

Massive multiple stings are rare. Such a case might happen if a person stumbled into a hive, or if a truck carrying a load of hives crashed. With the slow migration of Africanized bees (so-called "killer bees") from South and Central America into the United States, the number of multiple-sting cases is likely to increase. The venom of the Africanized bee is no more potent than that of the European type; it is just that the African type is extremely aggressive and thus more likely to be involved in multiple

stings. A number of child deaths have resulted from the multiple stings of fire ants, which are common in the southeastern United States.

What to Look for

A rule of thumb is that the sooner symptoms develop after a sting, the more serious the reaction will be.

- Usual reactions are momentary pain, redness around the sting site, itching, and heat.
- Worrisome reactions include skin flush, hives, localized swelling of lips or tongue, a "tickle" in the throat, wheezing, abdominal cramps, and diarrhea.
- Life-threatening reactions are bluish or grayish skin color, seizures, unconsciousness, and an inability to breathe due to swelling of the vocal cords.

About 60% to 80% of anaphylactic deaths are caused by the victim's not being able to breathe because swollen airway passages obstruct airflow to the lungs. The second

Preventing Insect Stings

People who know they are allergic to insect stings need to exercise extra care to avoid being stung. They should carry a bee-sting kit and follow these guidelines:

- Wear long pants and long-sleeved shirts.
- Insects are attracted to bright colors and floral patterns. Wear white, green, tan, and khaki—the least attractive colors to insects.
- Wear shoes outdoors.
- Avoid yardwork and other activities where insect contact is frequent.
- Keep garbage cans away from the house.
- Remove insect-attracting plants from inside and the immediate proximity of the house.
- Do not use scented soaps, lotions, or perfumes.
- Keep car windows closed.
- If you are confronted by an insect, avoid quick movements and do not provoke it. Turn away, lower your face, and walk away slowly. Do not run about wildly or move erratically when bees are nearby.
- Do not eat when bees are nearby.
- Have insect nests around the house removed by professional exterminators.

most common cause of death is shock, caused by insufficient blood circulating through the body.

One of the difficulties in dealing with stings is the lack of uniformity in victims' responses. One sting is not necessarily equivalent to another, even within the same species, because the amount of venom injected varies from sting to sting.

A person who goes into anaphylactic shock after being stung by a hornet may respond to a bee sting with only a small amount of swelling. One person may have a local reaction involving an entire limb, although the more typical response is a small circle of redness and swelling that disappears without incident in a few days. In bee-keepers, for whom stings are an accepted occupational hazard, the response is likely to be even less than in most other people, because they have become tolerant to the toxins in the venom from having been stung many times on different occasions. There seems to be no easy way to predict how a person may react. Most people who get stung, however, do have local reactions: redness, swelling, and pain.

Stings to the mouth or eye tend to be more dangerous than stings to other body areas. Also, victims tend to react more severely to multiple stings, especially 10 or more.

The most dangerous single stings in nonallergic individuals are those inside the throat, which can result from swallowing an insect that has dropped into a soft drink can or from inhaling one that flies into the victim's open mouth. A sting in the mouth or throat can cause swelling that obstructs the airway even in a person who is not allergic to insect stings. If the sting is not life threatening, have the victim suck on ice or flush his or her mouth with cold water. For a bee sting, dissolve a teaspoon of baking soda in a glass of water. Have the victim rinse his or her mouth and then hold the water in the mouth for several minutes.

What to Do

Most people who have been stung can be treated on site, and everyone should know what to do if a life-threatening allergic reaction (anaphylaxis) occurs. In particular, those who have had a severe reaction to an insect sting should be instructed on what they can do to protect themselves. They also should be advised to wear a medical-alert identification tag identifying them as insect allergic.

1. Look at the sting site for a stinger and venom sac embedded in the skin. Bees are the only stinging insects that leave their stingers and venom sac behind. If the stinger is still embedded, remove it or it will continue to inject poison for two or three minutes. Scrape the stinger and venom sac away

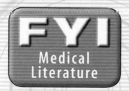

FYI
Medical
Literature

Doctors Not Giving Aftercare Instructions to Sting Anaphylaxis Victims

A survey of 124 emergency department or urgent care center physicians found that 58% of them never provided written avoidance instructions to those suffering anaphylaxis from an insect sting. Physicians did deliver other types of aftercare instructions: 24% provided or prescribed medical-alert identification bracelets, 44% referred all their patients to an allergist for further evaluation, and 73% reported prescribing an Epi-Pen™ or Anakit™ to all hymenoptera sting anaphylaxis victims. However, 24% of physicians did not know where to obtain anaphylaxis identification bracelets. This survey demonstrated that a substantial number of physicians practicing emergency medicine are not providing appropriate aftercare instructions to patients.

Source: L. McDougle et al: "Management of Hymenoptera Sting Anaphylaxis." *Journal of Emergency Medicine* 13(1):9–13 (January 1995)

with a hard object such as a long fingernail, credit card (▼Figure 17-14), scissor edge, or knife blade. If applied in the first three minutes, a Sawyer Extractor™ can remove a portion of the venom.

2. Wash the sting site with soap and water to prevent infection.

3. Apply an ice pack over the sting site to slow absorption of the venom and relieve pain. Use a commercial "sting stick" containing a topical anesthetic like Xylocaine (unless the victim is known to be allergic to the drug). Because bee venom is acidic, a paste made of baking soda and water can help. Sodium

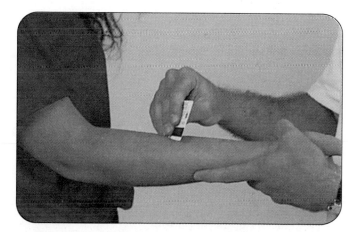

Figure 17-14 Scraping stinger away with credit card

bicarbonate is an alkalinizing agent that draws out fluid and reduces itching and swelling. Wasp venom, on the other hand, is alkaline, so apply vinegar or lemon juice.

A paste made of unseasoned meat tenderizer can help a bee sting victim if it comes in direct contact with the venom. That generally is not possible, however, because the bee will have injected the venom through too small a hole and too deeply into the victim's skin.

4. To further relieve pain and itching, use aspirin (adults only), some type of acetaminophen, or ibuprofen. A topical steroid cream, such as hydrocortisone, can help combat local swelling and itching. An antihistamine may prevent some local symptoms if given early, but it works too slowly to counteract a life-threatening allergic reaction.

5. Observe the victim for at least 30 minutes for signs of an allergic reaction. For a person having a severe allergic reaction, a dose of epinephrine is the only effective treatment. A person with a known allergy to insect stings should have a physician-prescribed emergency kit that includes prefilled syringes of epinephrine (Anakit™) or a spring-loaded device that automatically injects epinephrine. (The spring-loaded device, Epi-Pen™, is useful for those reluctant to use a syringe with a visible needle.) The allergic person should take along the kit whenever he or she is going someplace where stinging insects are known to exist. (Appendix B describes these kits in more detail.) Because epinephrine is short-acting, watch the victim closely for signs of returning anaphylaxis. Inject another dose of epinephrine as often as every 15 minutes if needed.

Do *not* use epinephrine to treat a sting unless the victim has a severe allergic reaction. Epinephrine has a shelf life of one to three years, or until it turns brown.

Watch for signs and symptoms of a delayed allergic reaction, especially in the first 6 to 24 hours. If the victim develops difficulty in breathing, facial swelling, fever, chills, or dizziness, call the local emergency telephone number.

Spider Bites

Most spiders are venomous, which is how they paralyze and kill their prey. However, most spiders lack an effective delivery system—long fangs and strong jaws to bite a human. About 60 species of spiders in North America are capable of biting humans although only a few species have produced significant poisonings (▶Figure 17-15).

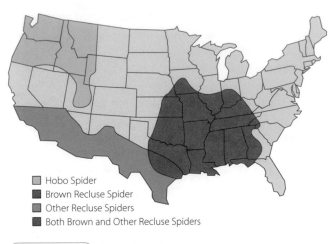

■ Hobo Spider
■ Brown Recluse Spider
■ Other Recluse Spiders
■ Both Brown and Other Recluse Spiders

Figure 17-15 Map of spider range.

Most bites are by female spiders. Male spiders are almost always smaller than females and have fangs that are too short and fragile to bite humans. Death occurs rarely and only from bites by brown recluse and black widow spiders.

The number of deaths from spider bites is not accurately known. A spider bite is difficult to diagnose, especially when the spider was not seen or recovered, because the bites typically cause little immediate pain. In a study of 600 suspected spider bites, 80% were caused by other arthropods (eg, kissing bugs, ticks, fleas, mites, bedbugs) and 10% by disease states (eg, poison ivy, diabetic ulcer, bedsore, Lyme disease, gonococcus). Spiders rarely bite more than once, and they do not always release venom.

Black Widow Spiders

Black widow spiders (▼Figure 17-16) are also commonly known as brown widow spiders and red-legged spiders, depending on the species. The term *black widow*

Figure 17-16 Black widow spider. Note red hourglass configuration on abdomen.

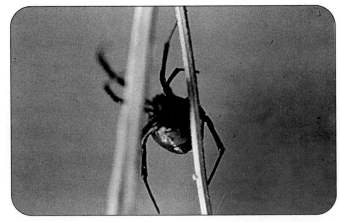

is actually inaccurate, because only three of the five species of widow spider are actually black, the others are brown and gray. Newly hatched spiders are almost entirely red. Males have white stripes along the outside of the abdomen.

The female black widow spider is one of the largest spiders, with a body that ranges up to one-half inch in length and a leg span of up to two inches. It is precisely her large size that allows the female black widow's fangs to be large and strong enough to penetrate human skin.

The female black widow may live as long as three years. Black widow spiders have round abdomens that vary in color from gray to brown to black, depending on the species. In the female black widow, the abdomen is shiny black with a red or yellow spot (often in the shape of an hourglass) or white spots or bands.

The male is only one-third the size of the female. Contrary to popular myth, the male usually mates safely with the female. Because of his small size, the male's fangs are incapable of penetrating human skin, so bites are from

Table 17-2: Facts About Troublesome Insects

Description	Habitat	Problem	Severity	Treatment	Protection
Chigger					
Oval with red velvety covering. Sometimes almost colorless. Larva has six legs. Harmless adult has eight legs and resembles a small spider. Very tiny—about $\frac{1}{20}$ inch long.	Found in low damp places covered with vegetation: shaded woods, high grass or weeds, fruit orchards. Also lawns and golf courses. From Canada to Argentina.	Attaches itself to the skin by inserting mouthparts into a hair follicle. Injects a digestive fluid that causes cells to disintegrate. Then feeds on cell parts. It does not suck blood.	Itching from secreted enzymes results several hours after contact. Small red welts appear. Secondary infection often follows. Degree of irritation varies with individuals.	Lather with soap and rinse several times to remove chiggers. If welts have formed, dab antiseptic on area. Severe lesions may require antihistamine ointment.	Apply proper repellent to clothing, particularly near uncovered areas such as wrists and ankles. Apply to skin. Spray or dust infested areas (lawns, plants) with suitable chemicals.
Bedbug					
Flat oval body with short broad head and six legs. Adult is reddish brown. Young are yellowish white. Unpleasant pungent odor. From $\frac{1}{8}$ to $\frac{1}{4}$ inch in length.	Hides in crevices, mattresses, under loose wallpaper during day. At night travels considerable distance to find victims. Widely distributed throughout the world.	Punctures the skin with piercing organs and sucks blood. Local inflammation and welts result from anticoagulant enzyme that bug secretes from salivary glands while feeding.	Affects people differently. Some have marked swelling and considerable irritation; others aren't bothered. Sometimes transmits serious diseases.	Apply antiseptic to prevent possible infection. Bug usually bites sleeping victim, gorges itself completely in three to five minutes, and departs. It's rarely necessary to remove one.	Spray beds, mattresses, bed springs, and baseboards with insecticide. Bugs live in large groups. They migrate to new homes on water pipes and clothing.
Brown Recluse Spider					
Oval body with eight legs. Light yellow to medium dark brown. Has distinctive mark shaped like a fiddle on its back. Body from $\frac{3}{8}$ to $\frac{1}{2}$ inch long, $\frac{1}{4}$ inch wide, $\frac{3}{4}$ inch from toe-to-toe.	Prefers dark places where it's seldom disturbed. Outdoors: old trash piles, debris, and rough ground. Indoors: attics, storerooms, closets. Found in southern and midwestern United States.	Bite produces an almost painless sting that may not be noticed, at first. Shy, it bites only when annoyed or surprised. Left alone, it won't bite. Victim rarely sees the spider.	In two to eight hours pain may be noticed, followed by blisters, swelling, hemorrhage, or ulceration. Some people experience rash, nausea, jaundice, chills, fever, cramps, or joint pain.	Summon doctor. Bite may require hospitalization for a few days. Full healing may take from six to eight weeks. Weak adults and children have been known to die.	Use caution when cleaning secluded areas in the home or using machinery usually left idle. Check firewood, inside shoes, packed clothing, and bedrolls—frequent hideaways.

(continued)

the female. Black widow spiders produce one of the most potent venoms known in terms of volume. The venom is chiefly a neurotoxin in humans, with symptoms most often manifested as severe muscle pain and cramping.

Black widow spiders are found throughout the world. In the western hemisphere, these spiders are found from southern Canada, throughout every state in the continental United States, to the tip of South America, and in Hawaii.

The web of the black widow spider is an extensive, irregular, shaggy trap for the insects she normally eats. The black widow rarely leaves the web and stays close to her egg mass. She aggressively defends the egg mass and bites if it is disturbed. When she is not guarding eggs, the spider often attempts to escape rather than bite.

Frequent cleaning to remove spiders and their webs from buildings, outbuildings, and outdoor living areas decreases the chance of accidental contact with black

Table 17-2: Facts About Troublesome Insects (Continued)

Description	Habitat	Problem	Severity	Treatment	Protection
Black Widow Spider Color varies from dark brown to glossy black. Densely covered with short microscopic hairs. Red or yellow hourglass marking on the underside of the female's abdomen. Male does not have this mark and is not poisonous. Overall length with legs extended is $1\frac{1}{2}$ inches. Body is $\frac{1}{4}$ inch wide.	Found with eggs and web. Outside: in vacant rodent holes, under stones, logs, in long grass, hollow stumps, and brush piles. Inside: in dark corners of barns, garages, piles of stone, wood. Most bites occur in outhouses. Found in southern Canada, throughout United States, except Alaska.	Bites cause local redness. Two tiny red spots may appear. Pain follows almost immediately. Larger muscles become rigid. Body temperature rises slightly. Profuse perspiration and tendency toward nausea follow. It's usually difficult to breathe or talk. May cause constipation, urine retention.	Venom is more dangerous than a rattlesnake's but is given in much smaller amounts. About 5% of bite cases result in death. Death is from asphyxiation due to respiratory paralysis. More dangerous for children; to adults its worst feature is pain. Convulsions result in some cases.	Use an antiseptic such as alcohol on the bitten area to prevent secondary infection. Keep victim quiet and call a doctor. Do not treat as you would a snakebite since this will only increase the pain and chance of infection; bleeding will not remove the venom.	Wear gloves when working in areas where there might be spiders. Destroy any egg sacs you find. Spray insecticide in any area where spiders are usually found, especially under privy seats. Check them out regularly. General cleanliness, paint, and light discourage spiders.
Tick Oval with small head; the body is not divided into definite segments. Gray or brown. Measures from $\frac{1}{4}$ to $\frac{3}{4}$ inch when mature.	Found in all United States areas and in parts of southern Canada, on low shrubs, grass, and trees. Carried around by both wild and domestic animals.	Attaches itself to the skin and sucks blood. After removal there is danger of infection, especially if the mouthparts are left in the wound.	Sometimes carries and spreads Rocky Mountain spotted fever, Lyme disease, Colorado tick fever. In a few rare cases, causes paralysis until removed.	Gently remove with tweezers so none of the mouthparts are left in skin. Wash with soap and water; apply antiseptic.	Cover exposed parts of body when in tick-infested areas. Use proper repellent. Remove ticks attached to clothes, body. Check neck and hair. Bathe.
Mosquito Small dark fragile body with transparent wings and elongated mouthparts. From $\frac{1}{8}$ to $\frac{1}{4}$ inch long.	Found in temperate climates throughout the world where the water necessary for breeding is available.	Bites and sucks blood. Itching and localized swelling result. Bite may turn red. Only the female is equipped to bite.	Sometimes transmits yellow fever, malaria, encephalitis, and other diseases. Scratching can cause secondary infections.	Don't scratch. Lather with soap and rinse to avoid infection. Apply antiseptic to relieve itching.	Destroy available breeding water to check multiplication. Place nets on windows and beds. Use proper repellent.

(continued)

widow spiders. Insecticides may decrease the population of the food for the black widows but do not usually affect the spiders themselves.

What to Look For

If the spider is trapped against the skin or crushed, it will bite. It is difficult to determine if a person has been bitten by a black widow spider or, for that matter, by any spider.

- The victim may feel a sharp pinprick when the spider bites, but some victims are not even aware of the bite. Within 15 minutes, a dull, numbing pain develops in the bite area.

- Two small fang marks might be seen as tiny red spots.

- Within 15 minutes to 4 hours, muscle stiffness and cramps occur, usually affecting the abdomen when

Table 17-2: Facts About Troublesome Insects (Continued)

Description	Habitat	Problem	Severity	Treatment	Protection
Scorpion					
Crablike appearance with clawlike pincers. Fleshy post-abdomen or "tail" has five segments, ending in a bulbous sac and stinger. Two poisonous types: solid straw yellow or yellow with irregular black stripes on back. From 2½ to 4 inches long.	Spends days under loose stones, bark, boards, floors of outhouses. Burrows in the sand. Roams freely at night. Crawls under doors into homes. Lethal types are found only in the warm desert-like climate of Arizona and adjacent areas.	Stings by thrusting its tail forward over its head. Swelling or discoloration of the area indicates a nondangerous, though painful, sting. A dangerously toxic sting doesn't change the appearance of the area, which does become hypersensitive.	Excessive salivation and facial contortions may follow. Temperature rises to over 104°F. Tongue becomes sluggish. Convulsions, in waves of increasing intensity, may lead to death from nervous exhaustion. First three hours most critical.	Apply ice pack. Keep victim quiet and call a doctor immediately. Do not cut the skin or give painkillers. They increase the killing power of the venom. Antitoxin, readily available to doctors, has proved to be very effective.	Apply a petroleum distillate to any dwelling places that cannot be destroyed. Cats are considered effective predators, as are ducks and chickens, though the latter are more likely to be stung and killed. Don't go barefoot at night.
Bee					
Winged body with yellow and black stripes. Covered with branched or feathery hairs. Makes a buzzing sound. Different species vary from ½ to 1 inch in length.	Lives in aerial or underground nests or hives. Widely distributed throughout the world wherever there are flowering plants—from the polar regions to the equator.	Stings with tail when annoyed. Burning and itching with localized swelling occur. Usually leaves venom sac in victim. It takes two to three minutes to inject all the venom.	If a person is allergic, more serious reactions occur—nausea, shock, unconsciousness. Swelling may occur in another part of the body. Death may result.	Gently scrape (don't pluck) the stinger so venom sac won't be squeezed. Wash with soap and antiseptic. If swelling occurs, contact doctor. Apply ice pack.	Have exterminator destroy nests and hives. Avoid wearing sweet fragrances and bright clothing. Keep food covered. Move slowly or stand still in the vicinity of bees.
Tarantula					
Large dark "spider" with a furry covering. From 6 to 7 inches in toe-to-toe diameter.	Found in southwestern United States. The tropical varieties are poisonous.	Bites produce pinprick sensation with negligible effect. It will not bite unless teased.	Usually no more dangerous than a pinprick. Has only local effects.	Wash and apply antiseptic to prevent the possibility of secondary infection.	Harmless to man, the tarantula is beneficial since it destroys harmful insects.

Source: National Safety Council, *Family Safety,* Spring 1980, pp. 20–21.

SPIDER BITES AND SCORPION STINGS

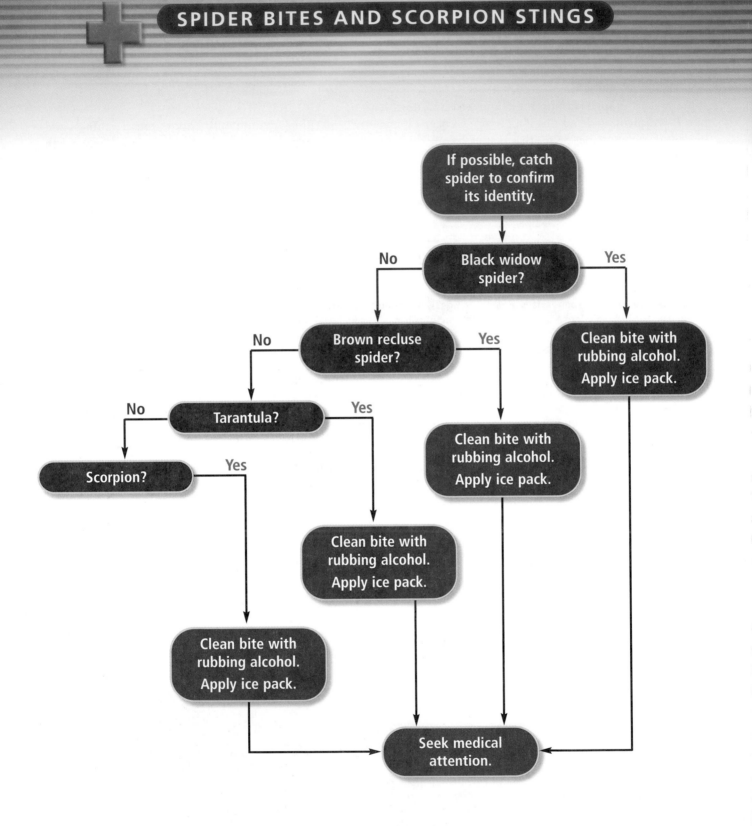

the bite is on a lower part of the body and the shoulders, back, or chest when the bite is on an upper part. Victims often describe the pain as the most severe they have ever experienced.

- Headache, chills, fever, heavy sweating, dizziness, nausea, and vomiting appear next. Severe pain around the bite site peaks in two to three hours and can last 12 to 48 hours.

Brown Recluse Spiders

Brown recluse spiders are also known in North America as fiddle-back and violin spiders. They have a violin-shaped figure on their backs (several other spider species have a similar configuration on their backs (▼**Figure 17-17A**)). Color varies from fawn to dark brown, with darker legs. Both male and female spiders are venomous.

Brown recluse spiders are found primarily in the southern and midwestern states, with other less toxic related spiders throughout the rest of the country. They are absent from the Pacific Northwest.

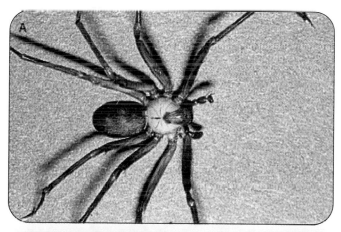

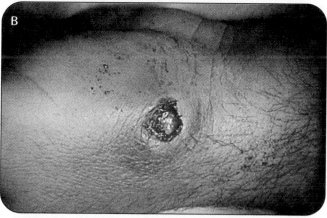

Figure 17-17 A–B **A** Brown recluse spider. Note violin or fiddle configuration on back. **B** Brown recluse spider bite. Note bull's-eye appearance.

What to Look For

The brown recluse spider bites only when it is trapped against the skin.

- A local reaction usually occurs within two to eight hours with mild to severe pain at the bite site and the development of redness, swelling, and local itching.

- In 48 to 72 hours, a blister develops at the bite site, becomes red, and bursts. During the early stages, the affected area often takes on a bull's-eye appearance, with a central white area surrounded by a reddened area, ringed by a whitish or blue border (◄**Figure 17-17B**). A small, red crater remains, over which a scab forms. When that scab falls away in a few days, a still larger crater remains. That too scabs over and falls off, leaving a yet larger crater. The craters are known as *volcano lesions*. This process of slow tissue destruction can continue for weeks or even months. The ulcer sometimes requires skin grafting.

- Fever, weakness, vomiting, joint pain, and a rash may occur.

- Stomach cramps, nausea, and vomiting may occur. Death is rare.

Tarantulas

Tarantulas (▼**Figure 17-18**) bite only when vigorously provoked or roughly handled. The bite varies from almost painless to a deep throbbing pain lasting up to one hour. The tarantula, when upset, will roughly scratch the lower surface of its abdomen with its legs and flick hairs onto the invader's skin. The hairs cause itching and hives that can last several weeks. Treatment is cortisone cream and antihistamines.

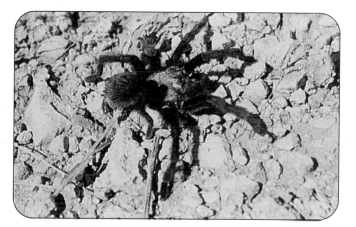

Figure 17-18 Tarantula

Common Aggressive House Spider

Another biter is the common aggressive house spider, or hobo spider. It arrived in the Pacific Northwest in 1936 and slowly made its way across Washington state and into surrounding states. In those areas, the hobo spider is the most common large spider. The signs and symptoms of its bite are similar to those of the brown recluse.

What to Do (for All Spider Bites)

1. If possible, catch the spider to confirm its identity. Even if the body has been crushed, save it for identification (although most spider-bite victims never see the spider). The species helps determine the treatment, so the dead spider (if it can be found) should be taken with the victim to the hospital.

2. Clean the bite area with soap and water or rubbing alcohol.

3. Place an ice pack over the bite to relieve pain and delay the effects of the venom.

4. Monitor the ABCs.

5. Seek medical attention immediately. For black widow spider bites, an antivenin exists. It is usually reserved for children (under 6 years), the elderly (over 60 and with high blood pressure), pregnant women, and victims with severe reactions. The antivenin will give relief within one to three hours. Antivenin for brown recluse and other spider bites is not currently available.

Scorpion Stings

Scorpions look like miniature lobsters, with lobster-like pincers and a long upcurved "tail" with a poisonous stinger (▶**Figure 17-19**). Several species of scorpions inhabit the southwestern United States, but only the bark scorpion poses a threat to humans. Severe cases, which usually appear only in children, may include paralysis, spasms, or breathing difficulties. Death from scorpion stings in the United States is rare.

The bark scorpion is found in the desert Southwest. There are rare colonies on the north side of the Colorado River in Nevada and Utah and occasional colonies in New Mexico. Rare stings have been reported in other parts of the United States, after the scorpions traveled from Arizona as "hitchhikers" in luggage or in car trunks. The bark scorpion is pale tan in color and is $3/4$ to $1^1/_4$ inches long, not including the so-called tail.

Stings to adult victims usually are not life threatening. Stings to small children, however, are often dangerous.

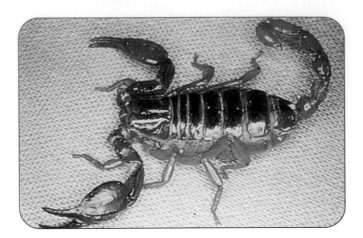

Figure 17-19 Scorpion

When a child is stung, every effort should be made to get the victim to a medical facility as quickly as possible. Pay close attention to making sure the victim's airway is open and that he or she is breathing.

What to Look for

The most frequent symptom of a scorpion sting, especially to an adult victim, is local, immediate pain and burning around the sting site. Later, numbness or tingling occurs. There is no swelling or blanching. Tapping a finger over the sting site may cause pain (the "tap test") and may serve to indicate a scorpion sting. More severely affected individuals will experience pain along the stung arm or leg, even paralysis. In even more serious stings, uncontrolled jerking movements of the legs or arms and facial twitching may occur.

Victims with a severe reaction will have a fast heart rate, will salivate, and will experience breathing distress. Symptoms begin from within minutes to half an hour and reach their height within the first few hours. Symptoms usually last from 6 to 24 hours.

What to Do

1. Monitor the ABCs.

2. Gently clean the sting site with soap and water or rubbing alcohol.

3. Apply an ice pack over the sting site to reduce pain and venom absorption.

4. Seek medical attention. Small children are prime candidates for receiving antivenin. An antivenin, supplied by the Antibody Production Laboratory at Arizona State University, is available at most hospitals in Arizona. This product has been approved by the Arizona Board of Pharmacy but has never

been tested by the U.S. Food and Drug Administration. Therefore, transportation of the antivenin across state lines is illegal, and it is not available outside Arizona. Antivenin should be given only in a hospital emergency department or intensive care unit, because anaphylaxis is a potential complication.

Centipede Bites

Centipedes come in various sizes and colors and are found all over the United States and throughout the world. The giant desert centipede, which can be up to eight inches in length, is the only U.S. centipede that is dangerous to humans.

Like spiders, any centipede whose fangs can penetrate human skin can inject venom. These arthropods inject toxic substances into the skin from a pair of hollow jaws that act like fangs. Contrary to popular belief, centipedes do not inject venom with their feet. Exaggerated stories about the deadly effects of their bites and reports that the tip of each leg carries a poisonous spur have caused many people to have an unreasonable fear of centipedes. Their venom is relatively weak.

What to Look for

Generally, bite indications are burning pain and local inflammation of the wound site, with mild swelling of the lymph nodes. The bite of the giant desert centipede causes inflammation, swelling, and redness that last 4 to 12 hours. Swelling and tenderness may last as long as three weeks or may disappear and recur.

What to Do

1. Clean the wound with soap and water.
2. Apply an ice pack at the bite site.
3. Give an analgesic for pain: aspirin, acetaminophen, or ibuprofen.
4. Seek medical attention for inflamed lymph glands.

Centipedes, which have one pair of legs per body segment, are sometimes confused with millipedes, which have two pairs of legs per body segment. Millipedes cannot inject venom, but their secretions can irritate the skin. Treat by washing the area of contact with soap and water and applying a cortisone cream or ointment.

Mosquito Bites

Millions of people are bitten by mosquitoes. Mosquitoes not only are a nuisance, they also are the carriers of many diseases. In developing countries, mosquitoes transmit malaria, yellow fever, and dengue fever; in the United States, they carry encephalitis. There is no evidence that mosquitoes transmit HIV, the virus that causes AIDS.

Female mosquitoes need blood to lay their eggs. Because they breed in water, mosquitoes are most often

Preventing Mosquito Bites

To minimize being bitten by mosquitoes, follow these guidelines:

+ Wear protective clothing: pants, long-sleeved shirt, full-brimmed hat. Mosquito netting draped over a hat will protect the face and neck.

+ Use insect repellents on exposed skin. DEET-containing repellents are most effective against mosquitoes and to a lesser extent helpful in repelling ticks and black flies.

DEET is considered to have low toxicity. However, it is absorbed through the skin, and hives, skin rashes, and blisters can result when it is used for prolonged periods or in excessive amounts. The long-acting 35% solution has a polymer that prevents evaporation as well as skin absorption.

Products that contain 100% DEET are available but unnecessary, especially in children. Long-acting formulations of 35% DEET appear equally effective in protecting against mosquitoes and have far less potential for toxicity.

DEET products can be applied over other creams such as sunscreens and moisturizers. Use DEET only on exposed skin and avoid the hands of young children since children often put their hands in their mouths. Keep DEET out of the reach of small children since ingestion may be fatal. Children under five years of age should not be exposed to concentrations greater than 10%, according to the American Academy of Pediatrics. The DEET concentration should not exceed 30% for children ages five to adult.

Other, nontoxic insect repellents appear to be less effective than DEET. They may be only 25% as effective as DEET and may need to be reapplied every half hour. Mixed opinions exist about whether 100 mg of vitamin B1 (thiamine) taken daily for one week prior to being exposed is an effective preventive agent. Some experts believe that a diet high in garlic will render a person undesirable to a mosquito.

Permethrin is a pesticide, not a repellent. It should be applied to clothing and not the skin.

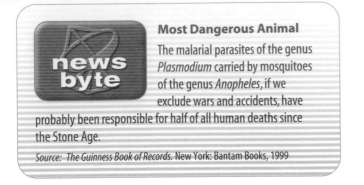
found in marshes, wetlands, and wooded areas. Mosquitoes usually can be separated into daytime and nighttime biters, but most will bite at twilight.

What to Do

1. Wash the bitten area with soap and water.
2. Apply an ice pack.
3. Apply calamine lotion to decrease redness and itching.
4. For a victim suffering a number of bites or a delayed allergic reaction, an antihistamine such as Benadryl™ every six hours or a physician-prescribed cortisone may prove useful.

Embedded Tick

Ticks are not insects but are close relatives of mites and spiders. They have eight legs and are classified as hard

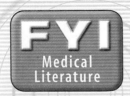
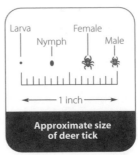

Figure 17-20 Scale of a deer tick.

ticks and soft ticks. Hard ticks are more familiar because of their wide distribution and common occurrence on domestic animals. Soft ticks are found mainly in western states. In the United States, seven kinds of hard ticks and five kinds of soft ticks carry diseases (eg, Lyme disease), are a nuisance (causing itching and swelling), or cause paralysis (toxin injected).

Ticks hatch from eggs and grow through three distinct stages: nymph (too small to see), larva (just visible), and adult (ready to lay eggs) **▲Figure 17-20**. The adult is most likely to be seen. Ticks at any stage of development can use humans for food; at each stage, they need what those who study them casually call a "blood meal" before they can grow to the next stage **▼Figure 17-21**.

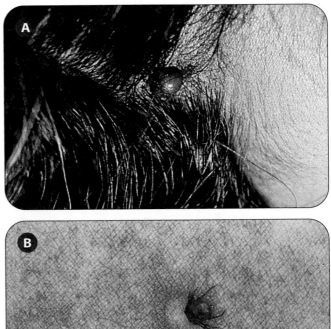

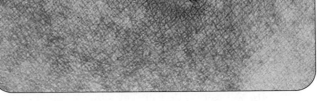

Figure 17-21, A–B **A.** Tick embedded and engorged with victim's blood. **B.** Tick embedded.

Ticks are limited in their ability to find their meals. They cannot fly, they crawl very slowly, and, without some help, they cannot travel more than a few yards from where they were hatched. When they are ready for their next meal, they may wait months, years, or even decades for the right host to come along. Bites are nearly painless, so the tick attachment is not noticed until later.

The front part of a tick consists of the head area and the mouthparts. The mouthparts have a central structure, the **hypostome,** which is shaped like a blunt harpoon. A tick makes a hole in the victim's skin with the sharp teeth (barbs) on the front of the hypostome and inserts its hypostome. The barbs anchor the tick to the skin and make it difficult to pull the tick out. Some ticks produce a substance that helps cement them to the host. As they feed, some ticks increase in size 20 to 50 times.

What To Do

Remove ticks as soon as possible (▼**Figure 17-22**). If a tick is carrying a disease, the longer it stays embedded, the greater the chance of the disease being transmitted.

Because its bite is painless, a tick can remain embedded for days before the victim realizes it. Most tick bites are harmless, although ticks can carry Lyme disease, Rocky Mountain spotted fever, and other serious diseases.

1. To pull a tick off,
   - Use tweezers or one of the specialized tick-removal tools.
   - Grasp the tick as close to the skin as possible and lift it with enough force to "tent" the skin surface. Hold it in that position until the tick lets go. This may take several seconds.
2. Wash the area with soap and water. Apply rubbing alcohol to further disinfect the area.

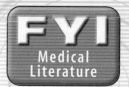

The Right Way to Remove a Tick

In one study, researchers allowed adult ticks to attach to sheep. After three to four days, they covered some ticks with petroleum jelly, some with clear nail polish, and others with rubbing alcohol. They also lit wooden kitchen matches, blew them out, and touched some ticks with the hot, smoking ends of the matches. None of these folklore methods made the ticks detach. The researchers removed other ticks by grasping them with medium-tipped, angled tweezers as closely as possible to where the mouthparts entered the skin, then steadily pulled the ticks from the skin. They found no crushed ticks or broken mouthparts. A small piece of skin may come off painlessly with the tick, which usually means that the tick was completely removed. If the tick's head or mouthparts remain in the skin, remove them as you would a splinter, with a sterilized needle. The researchers obtained the same results with ticks that had been attached for only 12 to 15 hours.

Source: G. R. Needham, "Evaluation of Five Popular Methods for Tick Removal." *Pediatrics,* 75(6):997–1002.

3. Apply an ice pack to reduce pain.
4. Apply calamine lotion to relieve any itching. Keep the area clean.
5. Continue to watch the bite site for one month for a rash. If a rash appears, see a physician. Watch for other signs such as fever, muscle aches, sensitivity to bright light, and paralysis that begins with leg weakness.

Caution:

DO NOT use the following popular methods of tick removal, which have been proved useless:
- petroleum jelly
- fingernail polish
- rubbing alcohol
- a hot match
- a petroleum product, such as gasoline

DO NOT grab a tick at the rear of its body. The internal gut may rupture and the contents may be squeezed out, causing infection.

DO NOT twist or jerk the tick, which may result in incomplete removal.

(**Figure 17-22**) Removing a tick with tweezers.

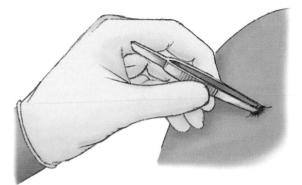

TICK REMOVAL

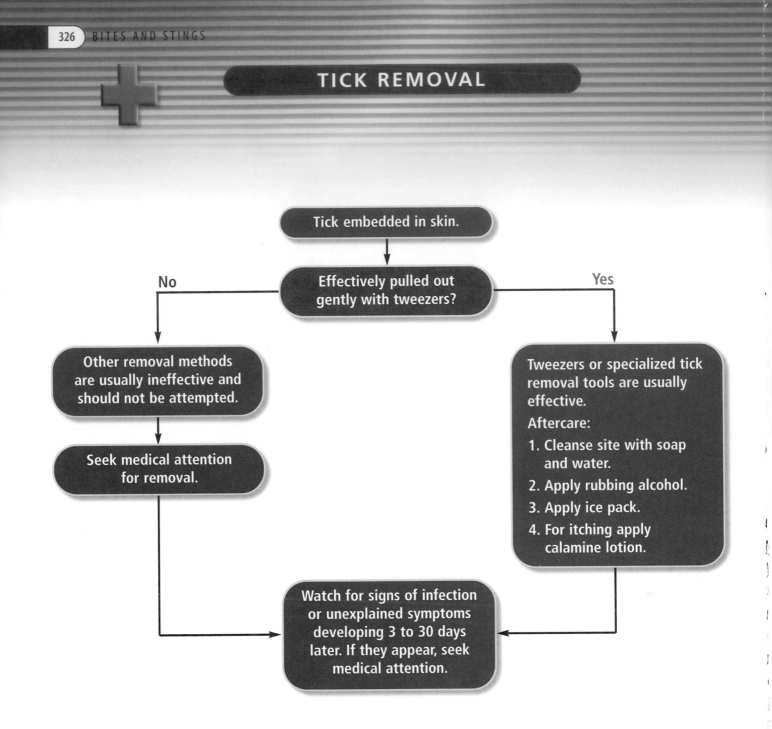

Tick embedded in skin.

Effectively pulled out gently with tweezers?

No

Yes

Other removal methods are usually ineffective and should not be attempted.

Seek medical attention for removal.

Tweezers or specialized tick removal tools are usually effective.

Aftercare:

1. Cleanse site with soap and water.
2. Apply rubbing alcohol.
3. Apply ice pack.
4. For itching apply calamine lotion.

Watch for signs of infection or unexplained symptoms developing 3 to 30 days later. If they appear, seek medical attention.

Preventing Tick Bites

+ Wear light-colored clothing so you can see any ticks on your clothes.

+ Wear a long-sleeved shirt that fits tightly at the wrists and neck and tuck the shirt into your pants.

+ Wear long pants and tuck the pant legs into your boots or socks. Or use masking tape to tape the pant legs tightly to your socks, shoes, or boots.

+ Check your clothes while you are outdoors and before entering a house. If possible, wash your clothes as soon as possible.

+ Inspect your pets for ticks before they come inside.

+ After coming indoors, shower or bathe and check your body for ticks, especially in areas that have hair or where clothing was tight. Another person could do the checking.

+ Treat your body and clothing with a repellent. The most common, EPA-approved, and effective tick repellent is DEET (N,N-diethyl-metatoluamide).

You can buy DEET under the brand names Off! or Cutters and apply it directly to your skin. Ticks crawling on the treated area are irritated by the repellent and drop off. DEET is most effective against ticks when applied to clothing from a spray can.

There have been a few reports of adverse toxic reactions to DEET, such as seizures, allergic responses, and skin irritation. To minimize reactions,

+ Apply DEET sparingly to your skin.

+ Avoid applying high-concentration products (more than 30% DEET) to the skin.

+ Do not inhale or ingest DEET-containing products or get them in your eyes.

+ Do not treat wounds or irritated skin.

+ Wash your skin after coming indoors.

+ Do not use products with more than 10% DEET on infants and small children.

You can also use 0.5% preparations of permethrin (a pesticide). Permethrin should be applied only to clothing (especially shirt sleeves, pants legs, and collars), never directly on the skin.

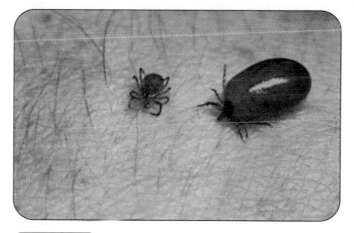

Figure 17-23 Deer ticks: not engorged and blood engorged.

Lyme Disease

In 1975, many children living near Lyme, Connecticut, developed painful swelling of the body joints. The swelling looked like arthritis but was not. Researchers finally determined that people got the sickness after being bitten by deer ticks. Infected people got rashes and flu-like symptoms about the same time. Eventually, they developed swollen joints. The sickness was named **Lyme disease,** after the town where it was first reported. (Actually, what we now call Lyme disease has been around, under other names, since the early 1900s.)

Lyme disease is caused by a bacterium that is carried by the deer tick. A deer tick is about the size of a poppy seed, except when it is swollen with blood ▲Figure 17-23 .

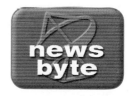

Commercial Tick Removal Tools

Original Ticked Off, Pro-Tick Remedy, and Tick Plier, also called the Tick Nipper, three commercially available tick removal tools, were compared against medium-tipped tweezers. All tools removed adults of both American dog and Lone Star species successfully. American dog ticks proved easier to remove than Lone Star ticks, whose mouthparts often remained in the skin. The researchers concluded that commercial tick removal tools can remove nymphs [too small to see with the human eye. Use a magnifying glass—the Tick Plier actually has one on it!—and adults and should be considered as good alternatives to medium-tipped tweezers.

Source: R.L. Stewart, et.al: "Evaluation of Three Commercial Tick Removal Tools," *Wilderness and Environmental Medicine,* Fall 1998; 9:137–142.

The ticks are carried into new areas by two animals, the white-tailed deer and the white-footed mouse. The ticks feed and mate on the deer, drop off, and later, as larvae, attach themselves to the mice, from which they obtain the bacteria.

In the eastern United States, the deer tick carries the bacteria; in western states, the western black-legged tick is the carrier (▶Figure 17-24). Other tick species, including the dog tick and the Lone Star tick, have been known to carry the disease. Migrating birds may carry the ticks into new areas.

FYI

Fire Ants

Fire ants are aggressive, will defensively attack anything that disturbs them, and can sting repeatedly. The fire ant bites its victim by securing itself to the skin with its mandibles, causing pain, then, using its head as a pivot, the ant swings its abdomen in an arc, repeatedly stinging the victim with an abdominal stinger. Up to 40 percent of the people who live in infested urban areas may be stung each year, and more than 30 deaths have been attributed to these insect bites.

The fire ant sting usually produces immediate pain and a red, swollen area, which disappears within 45 minutes. A blister then forms, rupturing in 30 to 70 hours, and the area often becomes infected. In some cases, a red, swollen, itchy patch develops instead of a blister. Although the stings are not usually life threatening, they are easily infected and may leave permanent scars.

Some people become sensitive to fire ant stings and should seek the advice of an allergist. Anaphylaxis (a life-threatening allergic reaction) occurs in about one to two percent of the people stung by fire ants. Therefore, if a sting leads to shortness of breath, tightness and swelling in the throat, tightness in the chest, increased pulse rate, swelling of the tongue and mouth, dizziness, or nausea, the person should be taken to a hospital emergency department immediately. Some people may lapse into a coma from even one sting.

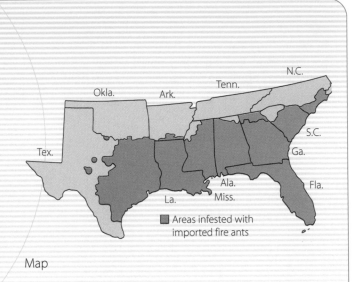

Map

First aid for fire ant stings includes placing an ice cube over the sting to reduce the pain and to slow absorption of the venom. A topical steroid cream can help combat local swelling and itching. An antihistamine may prevent some local symptoms if given early, but it works too slowly to counteract a life-threatening allergic reaction. People who are allergic to stings should always carry a kit with antihistamine tablets and a pre-loaded syringe of epinephrine.

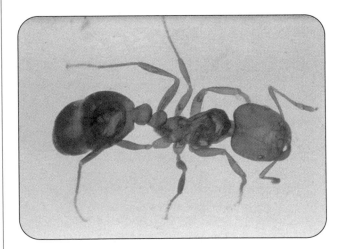

Fire ant

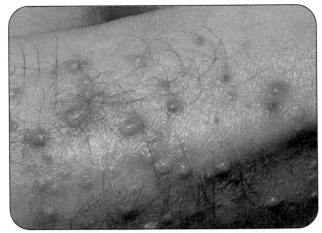

Fire ant stings

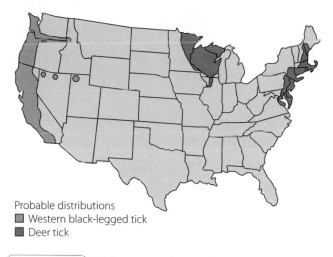

Probable distributions
■ Western black-legged tick
■ Deer tick

(**Figure 17-24**) Tick carriers of Lyme disease

Not all ticks are infected, nor do all tick bites cause Lyme disease. Other types of ticks carry other diseases including Rocky Mountain spotted fever and Colorado tick fever.

What to Look for

Signs and symptoms of Lyme disease occur any time from 3 to 30 days following a bite from an infected deer tick. The disease begins with flu-like symptoms: fever, chills, headaches, and joint stiffness.

The only visible sign of Lyme disease is the appearance of a slowly expanding, red bull's-eye rash that develops at the bite site (▼ **Figure 17-25**). The rash is common to about 70% of all Lyme disease victims. The rash may grow over a period of a few days or weeks, eventually fading in time, even without treatment. It varies in shape, but its size usually is two inches or more. The rash

(**Figure 17-25**) Lyme disease rash

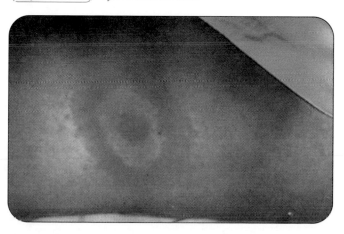

appears as a circle of white surrounded by an area of redness, thus the term "bull's eye." It is painless, but hot to the touch.

The rash alone is a good indication that a person has been exposed to Lyme disease and may be infected. Other signs and symptoms include extreme fatigue, fever as high as 104°F, and mild to severe headache.

Weeks after the initial tick bite, the victim may experience nerve and joint problems. In the later stages of Lyme disease, the most common symptom is arthritis-like swelling but little pain in a weight-bearing joint, such as the knee. In many cases, however, the diagnosis of Lyme disease comes down to a physician's judgment. The physician should always ask, "Was there ever a rash?" and "Do you live in or did you visit a tick-infested area up to a month before the symptoms appeared?"

Without proper antibiotic treatment, the disease can invade the central nervous system, resulting in meningitis, encephalitis, and Bell's palsy. Without treatment, the disease can cause stiffness in the large joints (knees and shoulders). The diagnosis of arthritis is often made by mistake. The stiffness comes and goes for periods lasting from several weeks to several years.

Medical diagnosis is difficult, because Lyme disease is often mistaken for the flu, especially if the rash is absent. Another problem is that over half the victims do not remember having been bitten by a tick. That is because the deer tick is extremely small during its infectious nymph stage of development. (The ticks do not look like the common wood or dog ticks familiar to most people.) Also, when the tick bites, it secretes a substance that acts like an anesthetic, so the human does not feel the bite.

Marine-Animal Injuries

Most marine animals bite or sting in defense, rather than attack per se. Marine venoms are similar in nature to many venoms found in reptiles and arthropods and may cause anaphylaxis or other types of reactions. The general first aid guidelines are similar to those for any disorder involving trauma, allergy, or cardiopulmonary failure. Serious allergic reactions require primary attention to keeping the airway open.

Animals That Bite, Rip, or Puncture

Sharks

Sharks are the most feared of all marine animals (▶ **Figure 17-26**), but the chance of being attacked by a shark along the North American coastline is less than

MARINE-ANIMAL INJURIES

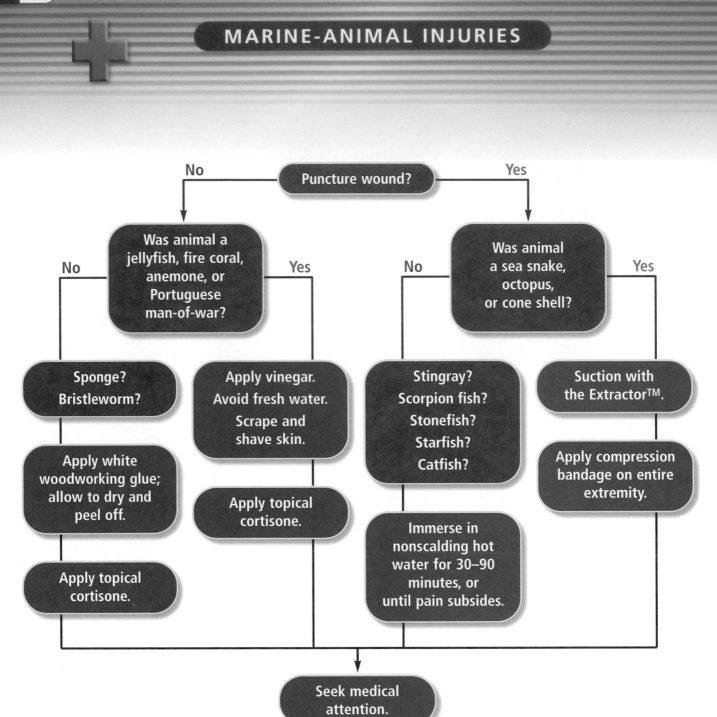

No — Puncture wound? — Yes

No ← Was animal a jellyfish, fire coral, anemone, or Portuguese man-of-war? → **Yes**

No ← Was animal a sea snake, octopus, or cone shell? → **Yes**

Sponge? Bristleworm?

Apply vinegar. Avoid fresh water. Scrape and shave skin.

Stingray? Scorpion fish? Stonefish? Starfish? Catfish?

Suction with the Extractor™.

Apply white woodworking glue; allow to dry and peel off.

Apply topical cortisone.

Apply compression bandage on entire extremity.

Apply topical cortisone.

Immerse in nonscalding hot water for 30–90 minutes, or until pain subsides.

Seek medical attention.

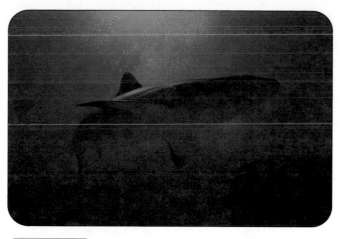

Figure 17-26 Shark.

1 in 5,000,000. Although exact figures are unavailable, it is estimated that, worldwide, no more than 50 attacks and no more than a dozen fatalities occur each year.

Most attacks occur within 100 feet of shore, and most victims are attacked by a single shark without warning. In the majority of attacks, the victim does not see the shark before the attack. The leg is the most frequently bitten part. Sharks are clearly more attracted to people on the surface than to underwater scuba divers. The greatest attraction for sharks appears to be chemicals found in fish blood—sharks can detect them in quantities as small as one part per million parts water. Shark bite wounds, among the most devastating of all animal bites, are similar to injuries caused by boat propellers or chainsaws. Immediate control of bleeding and treatment for shock are essential.

What to Do

1. Control bleeding.
2. Treat for shock.
3. Seek medical attention.

Barracudas and Eels

Barracudas are fearsome in appearance, but they have an undeserved reputation as attackers of humans. The risk of a barracuda bite is exceedingly small. First aid for a barracuda bite is identical to that for a shark bite.

Moray eels are also fierce in appearance. They are not infrequent biters of divers who handle or tease them, usually in competition for food or in pursuit of lobsters. The multiple puncture wounds created by moray eel bites have a high infection risk. Treat as you would shark bites.

Preventing Shark Attacks

No shark repellents are universally effective. Explosive and electronic devices may threaten diver safety instead of sharks. The following guidelines can help prevent shark attacks:

- Avoid swimming in areas frequented by sharks or where shark attacks have previously occurred. (In the United States, the greatest concentration of great white shark attacks is off the northern California coast.)
- Do not swim or dive alone.
- Do not swim far offshore, in murky water, or incautiously along deep dropoffs.
- People with open wounds and menstruating women should avoid swimming in areas where there is risk of shark attack.
- Avoid swimming in the vicinity of seal or sea lion colonies or turtle haulouts.
- Do not spear fish for an extended period in the same area and do not attach fish to your body.
- Avoid swimming at dawn, dusk, or night in potentially dangerous waters.

Animals That Sting

Stings from marine animals lead the list of adverse marine-animal encounters. It is important to identify the offending animal, because in many cases first aid is quite specific.

Each year, jellyfish (▶**Figure 17-27**), Portuguese man-of-wars (▶**Figure 17-28**), corals, and anemones (▶**Figure 17-29**) that lie along the shallow ocean waters of the United States sting more than one million people. Reactions to being stung by Portuguese man-of-wars and jellyfish vary from mild dermatitis to severe reactions. Most victims recover without medical attention.

Jellyfish and Portuguese man-of-wars have long tentacles equipped with stinging devices called *nematocysts*. When cast ashore or onto rocks, detached nematocysts retain their ability to sting for a long period of time, usually until they are completely dried out.

The Portuguese man-of-war sting is usually in the form of well-defined linear welts or scattered patches of welts with redness, which usually disappear within 24 hours. The jellyfish sting produces severe muscle cramping with

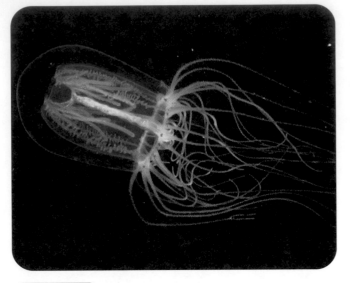

Figure 17-27 Jellyfish

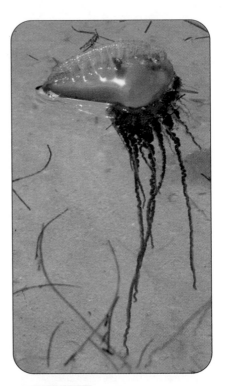

Figure 17-28 Portuguese man-of-war

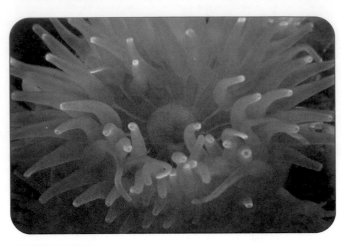

Figure 17-29 Anemones

What to Do

1. Apply vinegar to the sting area.

2. Immediately scrape off any tentacles remaining on the skin by using a credit card, stick, comb, knife blade, or similar object. Or apply shaving cream or a baking soda paste and shave the area. For large tentacles use tweezers or pliers.

3. Reapply vinegar or alcohol and soak the area for 15 minutes.

Caution:

DO NOT try to rub the tentacles off of the victim's skin—that will activate the stinging cells.

DO NOT use fresh water for rinsing because it will cause the nematocysts to fire.

DO NOT apply cold packs—they also will cause the nematocysts to fire.

DO NOT touch the tentacles with your bare hands.

multiple thin lines of welts crossing the skin in a zigzag pattern. Pain usually is a burning type that lasts 10 to 30 minutes. The welts on the skin usually disappear within an hour.

Anemones are beautiful but potentially dangerous. Many anemone stings result from the improper handling of aquarium animals.

Animals That Puncture (by Spine)

Stingrays, commonly found in tropical and subtropical waters, are peaceful, reclusive bottom feeders that generally lie buried in the sand or mud (▶Figure 17-30). Most wounds inflicted by sting rays are produced on the ankle or foot when the victim steps on a ray. The ray reacts by thrusting its barbed tail upward and forward into the victim's leg or foot. At least 2,000 stingray injuries occur each year in coastal U.S. waters. The stingray's venomous tail barb easily penetrates human skin. The sting usually is more like a laceration, since the large tail barb can do significant damage. The venom causes intense burning pain at the site.

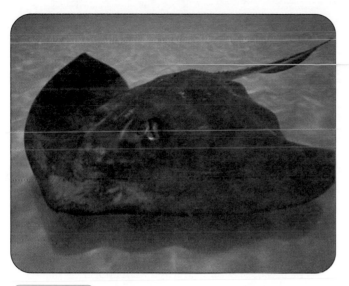

Figure 17-30 Stingray

What to Do

1. Relieve pain by immersing the injured body part in hot water (110°F) for 30 to 90 minutes. Make sure the water is not hot enough to cause a burn.

2. Wash the wound with soap and water.

3. Irrigate the area with water under pressure to wash out as much of the toxin and foreign material as possible.

4. Treat the wound like any puncture wound.

Dead Rattlesnakes Can Bite

L. M. Klauber, reported in his book, *Rattlesnakes: Their Habits, Life Histories, and Influence on Mankind,* performed experiments showing that rattlesnake heads are dangerous for 20 to 60 minutes after decapitation.

Physicians Jeffrey Suchard and Frank LoVecchio collected data on patients admitted to the Good Samaritan Regional Medical Center in Phoenix, Arizona, for rattlesnake bites. Thirty-four patients were admitted for rattlesnake bites from June 1997 to April 1998; of these, five patients (14.7%)—all men between 20 and 48 years old—were bitten by snakes that had been fatally injured and were presumed to be dead.

Patient 1 bludgeoned a rattlesnake on the head with wood, rendering it motionless, and was bitten on the right index finger when he picked up the apparently dead snake.

Patient 2 shot a rattlesnake, striking the head several times, and observed no movement for three minutes. When he lifted the snake, it bit his right index finger.

Patient 3 shot and then decapitated a rattlesnake his right index finger was bitten when he picked up the head.

Patient 4 was bitten on his left ring finger and right index finger by a decapitated rattlesnake head that had been motionless for five minutes.

Patient 5 was bitten on the left index finger by a rattlesnake he had presumed to be dead from multiple gunshot wounds, including one to the head.

Source: *New England Journal of Medicine;* 340(24):1930; June 17, 1999 .

STUDY
Questions (17)

Name_____ Course_____ Date_____

Activities

Activity 1

Mark each question as true (T) or false (F).

T F 1. An antivenin exists for black widow spider bites.

T F 2. Honeybees and wasps leave a stinger embedded in the victim's skin.

T F 3. Long and strong fangs enable black widow and brown recluse spiders to bite humans.

T F 4. No venom injection occurs in about one-fourth of all venomous snakebites.

T F 5. The same antivenin is used for all pit viper snakebites in the United States.

T F 6. Covering an embedded tick with petroleum jelly causes the tick to back out.

T F 7. Ticks can transmit disease.

T F 8. Apply ice on all animal and insect bites and stings.

Activity 2

Mark each statement as true (T) or false (F).

T F 1. Reactions to being stung by an ocean animal can be severe.

T F 2. Examples of marine animals that sting include jellyfish and Portuguese man-of-wars.

T F 3. The intense burning pain from a jellyfish sting is produced by nematocysts on the tentacles.

T F 4. Remove jellyfish tentacles on the skin by scraping them off with a credit card.

T F 5. Use rubbing alcohol or vinegar to inactivate the tentacles.

T F 6. Water can be used to inactivate the nematocysts.

Case Situations

Case 1

A 16-year-old male is stung by a swarm of bees. According to his friends, he was outside mowing the lawn when he was suddenly and repeatedly stung. He is responsive, but his face is swollen (especially around the eyes) and cyanotic about the lips. You can hear a wheezing sound when he breathes. Several large red welts appear on his back and neck. His friends report that he has asthma.

____ 1. This victim is most likely experiencing
   a. a minor allergic reaction
   b. anaphylaxis
   c. an acute asthma attack
   d. neurogenic shock

T F 2. The sooner symptoms develop after a sting, the more serious the reaction will be.

T F 3. The majority of anaphylactic deaths are caused by inability of the victim to breathe because of swollen airway passages.

____ 4. Treatment for this victim would include
   a. giving the victim prescribed epinephrine, if available
   b. giving syrup of ipecac
   c. giving activated charcoal
   d. giving CPR
   e. giving rescue breaths

Case 2

While showering after an overnight camping trip, you discover a tick embedded in your skin.

____ What should you do?
   a. Hold a heated needle or a blown-out, glowing match head to the tick.
   b. Squeeze the protruding end of the tick with your fingers and allow the blood to drain out. The body will fall out within 24 hours.
   c. Do nothing. The tick will die in 24 to 48 hours and then fall out.
   d. Use tweezers to remove as much of the tick as possible, then clean the wound with soap and water.

STUDY
Questions (17)

Case 3

While you are camping, a friend is bitten on the hand by a rattlesnake.

___ 1. How do you know it is a rattlesnake bite?
  a. The snake was brightly colored—red, yellow, and black.
  b. The snake had a triangular-shaped head.
  c. The victim's skin had two puncture marks.
  d. Both a and c.
  e. Both b and c.

___ 2. What should you do for a pit viper snakebite?
  a. Cool the bite site with an ice pack.
  b. Avoid using cold on the bite site.

___ 3. a. Do not cut through any snake bite wound.
  b. Cut through the fang marks if you are more than one hour from a medical facility.

___ 4. a. First aiders can give antivenin.
  b. Only a qualified physician should give antivenin.

___ 5. a. Apply a tourniquet.
  b. Apply suction with the Extractor™ device.

___ 6. a. If possible, identify the type of rattlesnake.
  b. Information about the snake usually is not necessary.

Case 4

A small girl is bitten by a neighbor's dog. You see an avulsed flap of skin on the girl's back.

1. How many people are bitten by dogs each year in the United States?

_____

2. Animal bites raise what two concerns?
  a. _____
  b. _____

___ 3. Which animal accounts for the most bites?
  a. dogs
  b. cats
  c. humans
  d. skunks

___ 4. Which animal accounts for the most rabies cases?
  a. dogs
  b. skunks
  c. raccoons
  d. cats

Case 5

Your three-year-old daughter runs into the house crying and holding her arms. She complains about having a black bug with a red spot on its stomach on her. You look at her arm and notice a slight redness and swelling around what is probably a spider bite.

1. A coal-black body with a red spot on its abdomen can identify which poisonous spider?

_____

_____

2. The other poisonous spider that causes severe medical problems is the

_____

3. Which of the following first aid procedures are appropriate for spider bites and scorpion stings? (Check *all* that apply.)
  ___ a. Apply a cold pack.
  ___ b. Seek medical attention immediately.
  ___ c. Capture the spider or have a definite identification.
  ___ d. Maintain open airway and restore breathing, if necessary.
  ___ e. Wash area with soap and water or rubbing alcohol.
  ___ f. Apply a constriction band 2 to 4 inches above the bite.
  ___ g. Apply calamine lotion to relieve discomfort.

Chapter Activities

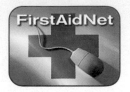

WEB Activities

Bites and Stings

Visit nsc.jbpub.com/FirstAidNet, then click on Web Activities, and select the appropriate chapter.

Dog Bites

All people, especially children, need to exercise caution when in the company of an unfamiliar dog. However, it should be remembered that a responsible owner can prevent many attacks. Suggestions for responsible dog ownership are available.

Stinging Insects

Most people, at one time or another, have been stung by an insect. For some, a single sting can be life-threatening, and immediate medical attention is necessary.

Spiders

Knowing what species of spiders live in your area will prepare you for what to expect and what to do if bitten by a spider. Being able to differentiate between the kinds of spiders, and even the gender of spiders, may save crucial minutes in treating a spider bite.

Marine-Animal Injuries

Although the beach is a wonderful place to visit, there are some potential dangers. Treatment for an injury will vary depending upon which marine animal was involved.

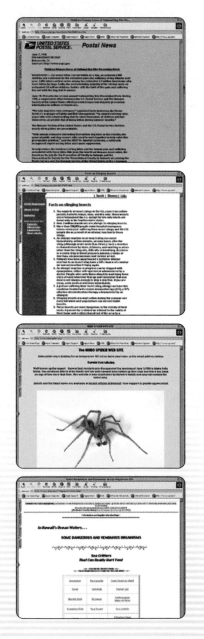

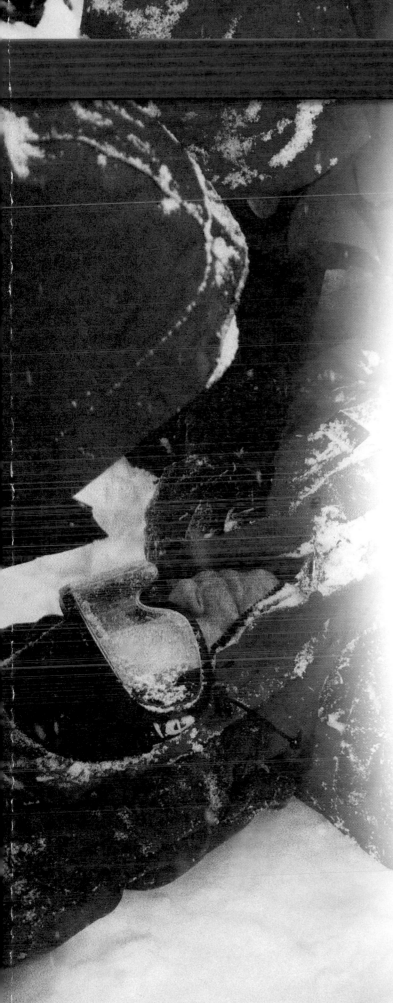

Chapter 18

Cold-Related Emergencies

Heat flows from an area with a higher temperature to an area with a lower temperature. When a person is surrounded by air or water cooler than body temperature, the body will lose heat. If heat escapes faster than the body produces heat, body temperature will fall. Normal body temperature is 98.6°F, and if the body temperature falls much below that, cold injuries can result.

How Cold Affects the Body

Humans protect themselves from cold primarily by avoiding or reducing cold exposure through the use of clothing and shelter. When that protection proves inadequate, the body has biological defense mechanisms to help maintain correct body temperature. These internal mechanisms to maintain body temperature during cold exposure include vasoconstriction and shivering. When those responses are triggered, it is a signal that clothing and shelter are inadequate.

Vasoconstriction is the tightening of blood vessels in the exposed skin. The reduced skin blood flow conserves body heat but can lead to discomfort, numbness, loss of dexterity in the hands and fingers, and eventually cold injuries.

Cold triggers shivering, which increases internal heat production and helps to offset the heat being lost. Shivering is the body's main involuntary defense against the cold. Shivering produces body heat by forcing muscles to contract and relax rapidly. About 80% of the muscle energy used in shivering is turned into body heat. When the core temperature rises, shivering is no longer needed and is shut down by the hypothalamus (in the brain). When the core temperature falls to about 86°F, the shivering reflex stops. Likewise, when there is no further fuel (glycogen) for the body, shivering stops. Several drugs suppress the shivering response, including barbiturates, beta-blocking agents, and alcohol.

Internal heat production is also increased by physical activity; the more vigorous the activity, the greater the heat production. In fact, heat production during intense exercise or strenuous work usually is sufficient to completely compensate for heat loss, even when it is extremely cold. However, high-intensity exercise and hard physical work are fatiguing, can cause sweating, and cannot be sustained indefinitely.

Susceptibility to cold injuries can be minimized by maintaining proper hydration and nutrition; avoiding alcohol, caffeine, and nicotine; and limiting periods of inactivity in cold conditions. Humans do not acclimatize to cold weather nearly as well as they acclimatize to hot weather.

The colder the surrounding temperature is, the greater the potential for body heat to escape. When the skin is exposed to cold, the brain signals the blood vessels in the skin to tighten, and blood flow to the skin decreases. This is the body's attempt to prevent heat inside the body from being carried to the skin, where it will be lost. However, due to reduced blood flow to the skin, the skin temperature falls.

When cold exposure lasts more than an hour, cooling of the skin and reduced blood flow to the hands will blunt sensation, touch, and pain and cause a loss of dexterity and agility. That can impair a person's ability to perform manual tasks and, because symptoms may go unnoticed, lead to more severe cold injuries.

Heat Loss from the Body

Normal body temperature is maintained by a balance of heat production and heat loss. Heat is produced by food metabolism and muscle activity, and shivering can increase heat production up to 500%. Shivering causes a large increase in heat production, but it rapidly consumes calories stored in the liver and muscles as glycogen. Lack of food limits the body's ability to produce heat; when glycogen stores are depleted, heat output decreases.

Heat loss occurs primarily through the skin. Blood flow to the skin varies in different parts of the body, and some areas lose more heat than others. Thermograms demonstrate high losses from the head and neck (up to 50%), axillary area (armpits), and groin area. Blood vessel constriction caused by cold conserves heat.

Body heat can be lost by four mechanisms:

- **Conduction,** or direct contact with a colder object (eg, lying on the snow), normally accounts for only a small fraction of heat loss. The exception is immersion in cold water, where heat loss can be 25 to 30 times greater than in air, and even more in moving water.

- **Convection** is the loss of heat from the body by air blowing over the skin or through porous clothing. **Windchill** is the combined effect of the ambient temperature and wind speed.

- **Evaporation,** or conversion of liquid on the skin to a vapor, normally accounts for about 20% of heat loss (two-thirds through sweating and one-third through respiration).

- **Radiation** is the primary method of heat loss, accounting for about 65% of the body's heat loss. A warm object gives off (radiates) heat to cooler air. It has been demonstrated that up to 50% of the body's total heat production can be lost by radiation through a person's unprotected head (▼**Figure 18-1**).

Susceptibility to Cold Injury

An individual's susceptibility to cold injury (nonfreezing and freezing injuries, and hypothermia) is affected by many factors. The physically unfit are more susceptible to cold injury. They tire more quickly and are unable to stay active to keep warm as long as those who are physically fit.

Dehydration reduces skin blood flow, which increases susceptibility to cold injury. Fat functions as an insulator against heat loss because it has less blood flow than muscle and loses less heat. Therefore, a very lean person may be susceptible to the effects of cold, if clothing is inadequate or wet, or if the individual is relatively inactive.

Figure 18-1 Sources of heat loss

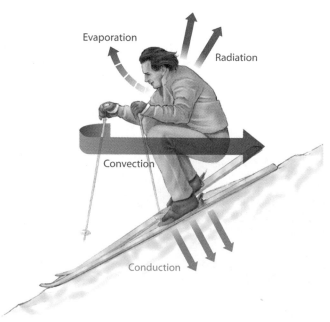

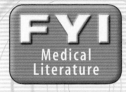

Lowest Body Temperature

A Swedish doctor who nearly drowned in an ice-covered stream thanked the medical team that revived her from what might be a record low body temperature. Anna Elisabeth Baagenholm, 29, fell into the stream while skiing in Norway. She was trapped under ice for an hour and 20 minutes. Her heart stopped beating, and she was unconscious and clinically dead. Doctors said her body temperature dipped to 56.6°F degrees from a normal of 98.6°F. Baagenholm is recovering from muscle problems, but there was no evidence of brain damage.

Source: Associated Press release.

Persons 50 years old and older may be less tolerant of the cold than younger people, due to the decline in physical fitness that often occurs with aging.

Alcohol and, to a lesser extent, caffeine cause the blood vessels in the skin to open, which can accelerate body heat loss. Also, alcohol and caffeine both increase urine formation, leading to dehydration, which can further degrade the body's defenses against cold. Most important, alcohol blunts the senses and impairs judgment, so an individual may not feel the signs and symptoms of developing cold injury.

Because nicotine decreases blood flow to the skin, smoking and chewing tobacco can increase susceptibility to frostbite. Inadequate nutrition, illness, and injury compromise the body's responses to cold and an individual's ability to recognize and react appropriately to the symptoms of developing cold injury.

People who have experienced a cold injury in the past are at greater risk of experiencing another cold injury.

Effects of Altitude

Assessing weather conditions in mountainous regions must include altitude considerations, especially if the assessment is based on weather measurements obtained at lower elevations. Temperatures, windchill, and the risk of cold injury at high altitudes can differ considerably from those at lower elevations.

In general, it can be assumed that air temperature drops 3.6°F every 1,000 feet above the original measurement site. Winds usually are more severe at high altitudes, and there is less cover above the tree line. People are more susceptible to frostbite and other cold injuries at altitudes

above 8,000 feet than at sea level, because of lower temperatures, higher winds, and lack of oxygen.

Effects of Water

Water can conduct heat away from the body much faster than air of the same temperature. When clothing becomes wet due to snow, rain, splashing water, or accumulated sweat, the body's loss of heat is accelerated, up to 25 times faster.

Swimmers and people working or wading in water can lose a great deal of body heat even when the water temperature is only mildly cool. Individuals working in cold water should be closely watched as they enter the water, since sudden plunging into cold water can produce irregular heartbeats, gasping, and hyperventilation, which can cause inhalation of water, heart failure, and drowning.

Effects of Wind

For any given air temperature, the potential for body heat loss, skin cooling, and decreased internal temperature is increased by wind. Wind increases heat loss from skin exposed to cold air, in effect lowering the temperature. The windchill index integrates wind speed and air temperature to provide an estimate of the cooling power of the environment and the associated risk of cold injury.

Windchill temperatures obtained from weather reports do not take into account artificial wind, which worsens the windchill effect of natural wind. For example, riding in an open vehicle can subject the passengers to dangerous windchill, even when natural winds are low.

Effects of Metals and Liquid Fuels

Metal objects and liquid fuels that have been left outdoors in the cold pose a serious hazard. Both can conduct heat away from the skin rapidly. Fuels and solvents remain liquid at very low temperatures. Skin contact with fuel or metal at below-freezing temperatures can result in nearly instantaneous freezing. Fuel handlers must use great care and not allow exposed skin to come into contact with spilled fuel or metals.

Minimizing Effects of Cold on the Body

When adequately protected, humans can tolerate temperatures as low as −72°F. Adequate clothing maintains the "microclimate" surrounding the body. Air is an excellent insulator, and the basis for most clothing is to trap a layer of air around the body. Layering, which has been used for centuries, allows the removal or opening of a garment to vent excess heat during times of greater activity or changes in environment and accommodates an individual's own needs and preferences. Wearing layered clothing is especially important for people who frequently change environments by going in and out of buildings or who periodically undertake vigorous physical activity.

Three important layers are recommended for most outdoor activities. The first layer (undergarments) removes perspiration from the skin, the middle layers insulate, and the outer layer or outer shell protects against wind. By understanding this principle, individuals can vary their clothing to regulate protection and stay comfortable.

For the first layer, use underwear that wicks away perspiration, that is, it stays dry by drawing moisture away from the skin to the next layer of clothing. Wet clothing transfers heat away from the body. Cotton holds moisture next to the skin so you feel cold and clammy. Silk feels warm and soft, but it also retains moisture. Fabrics such as polypropylene or one of the new types of polyesters such as Capilene™ or Thermax™ should be considered.

The middle layer can be a synthetic pile or fleece jacket that is warm and dries quickly or a wool or synthetic sweater. Synthetic insulative materials such as Thinsulate™, unlike down or wool, provide warmth without bulk or heavy weight. Insulation should be effective even when wet. In that respect, synthetics are clearly superior to natural fibers and products. Duck or goose down, for example, is virtually useless when wet, and it dries out slowly. One exception, however, is the insulating ability of wool, even when wet.

Physically active people may sweat even in extremely cold weather. Therefore, the best choice for an outside layer is a jacket that is waterproof, wind resistant, and "breathable." Materials like Gore-Tex™ allow perspiration to evaporate. A zipper is preferable, so the clothing can be opened easily to increase ventilation. Nylon and vinyl are poor choices because they produce a sauna effect by holding in perspiration.

Because the head loses more body heat than any other part (50%), heed the admonition, "If the feet are cold, cover the head." A wool or synthetic cap serves well.

Nonfreezing Cold Injuries

Nonfreezing cold injuries can occur when conditions are cold and wet (air temperatures between 32°F and 55°F) and the hands and feet cannot be kept warm and dry. The most prominent nonfreezing cold injuries are chilblain and trenchfoot.

Chilblain is a nonfreezing cold injury that, while painful, causes little or no permanent damage. It appears as red, swollen skin that is tender, hot to the touch, and possibly itchy. This can worsen to an aching, prickly ("pins and needles") sensation and then numbness. Chilblain can develop in only a few hours in skin exposed to cold.

Trenchfoot is a serious nonfreezing cold injury that develops when the skin on the feet is exposed to moisture and cold for prolonged periods (12 hours or longer). The combination of cold and moisture softens the skin, causing tissue loss and, often, infection. Untreated, trenchfoot can eventually require amputation. Often, the first sign of trenchfoot is itching, numbness, or tingling

---

If a Blizzard Traps You While You Are Driving

+ Don't panic.

+ Stay in your vehicle. Do not attempt to walk out of a blizzard. You can quickly become disoriented in blowing and drifting snow. Being lost in open country during a blizzard is almost certain death. You are more likely to be found and certainly more likely to be sheltered in your car.

+ Avoid overexertion and exposure. Exertion from attempting to push your car, shovel heavy drifts, and perform other difficult chores during the strong winds, blinding snow, and bitter cold of a blizzard may cause a heart attack—even in a person in apparently good physical condition.

+ Keep fresh air in your car. Freezing, wet snow and wind-driven snow can completely seal the passenger compartment, causing suffocation.

+ Beware the "gentle" killers: carbon monoxide and oxygen starvation. Run the motor and heater sparingly and only with the downwind window open for ventilation.

+ Keep watch. Do not permit all occupants of the car to sleep at one time.

+ Exercise by clasping hands and moving arms and legs vigorously from time to time. Do not stay in one position for long.

+ Turn on your car's dome light at night, to make the vehicle visible to work crews.

Source: National Oceanic and Atmospheric Administration.

pain. Later the feet may appear swollen and the skin mildly red, blue, or black. Commonly, trenchfoot shows a distinct waterline that coincides with the water level in the boot. Red or bluish blotches appear on the skin, sometimes with open weeping or bleeding. The risk of this potentially crippling injury is high during wet weather. People who wear rubberized or tight-fitting boots are at risk for trenchfoot regardless of weather conditions, because sweat accumulates inside the boots and keeps the feet wet.

Freezing Cold Injuries

Freezing cold injuries can occur whenever the air temperature is below freezing (32°F). Freezing limited to the skin surface is **frostnip.** Freezing that extends deeper through the skin and into the flesh is **frostbite.**

Frostbite is prevalent during military campaigns and is a known hazard for mountain climbers and explorers. As more and more recreationalists pursue cross-country skiing and snowmobiling, the number of frostbite cases probably will increase. However, it is still thought to be rare in nonmilitary situations.

Frostnip

Frostnip involves the freezing of water on the skin surface. The skin becomes reddened and possibly swollen. Although painful, there usually is no further damage after rewarming. Repeated frostnip in the same spot can dry the skin, causing it to crack and become sensitive. It is difficult to tell the difference between frostnip and frostbite. Frostnip should be taken seriously because it may be the first sign of impending frostbite.

What to Do

1. Gently warm the affected area by placing it against a warm body part (eg., bare hands, armpit, stomach) or by blowing warm air on the area. After rewarming, the affected area may be red and tingling.
2. Do not rub the affected area.

Frostbite

Frostbite occurs when temperatures drop below freezing. Tissue is not composed of water alone, so it will not freeze until it has been cooled to about 28°F. Tissue is damaged in two ways: (1) actual tissue freezing, which results in the formation of ice crystals between the tissue cells (the ice crystals enlarge by extracting water from the cells), and (2) the obstruction of the blood supply to the

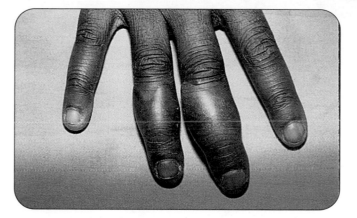

Figure 18-2 Frostbitten fingers, 6 hours after rewarming in 108°F water.

tissue, which causes "sludged" blood clots and further prevents blood from flowing to the tissues. The second type of tissue damage is more extensive than the first. In severely cold temperatures, flesh can freeze in under a minute (▲**Figure 18-2**).

Frostbite affects mainly the feet, hands, ears, and nose. Those areas do not contain large heat-producing muscles and are some distance from the body's heat-generation sources. The most severe consequences of frostbite are gangrene and amputation.

What to Look for

The severity and extent of frostbite are difficult to judge until hours after thawing, although it can be classified as *superficial* or *deep before thawing.* Even physicians have to wait until thawing has occurred before they can judge the extent of the injury.

The signs and symptoms of superficial frostbite are:

- Skin color is white, waxy, or grayish-yellow.
- The affected part feels very cold and numb. There may be tingling, stinging, or an aching sensation.
- The skin surface feels stiff or crusty and the underlying tissue soft when depressed gently and firmly.

The following signs and symptoms indicate deep frostbite:

- The affected part feels cold, hard, and solid and cannot be depressed.
- Blisters may appear after rewarming.
- The affected part is cold, with pale, waxy skin.
- A painfully cold part suddenly stops hurting.

After a part has thawed, frostbite can be categorized by degrees, similar to the classification of burns. First-degree

FROSTBITE

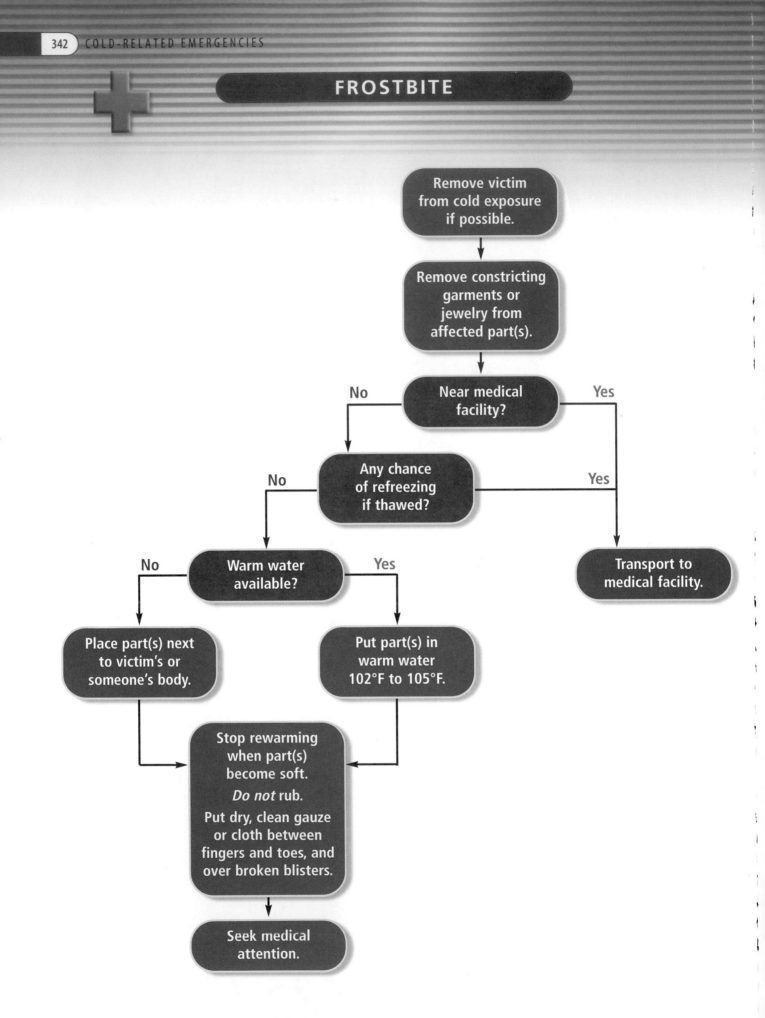

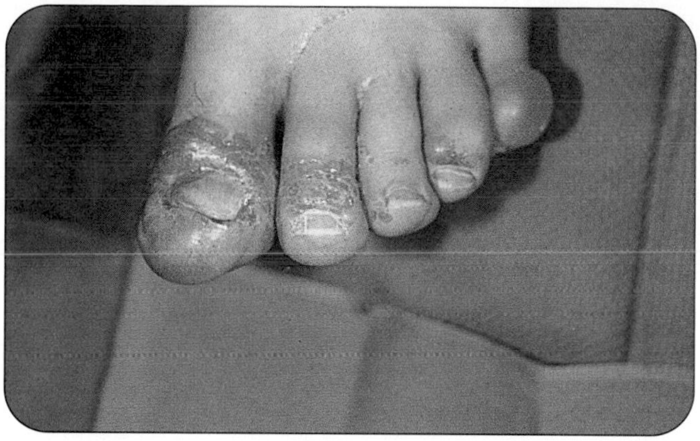

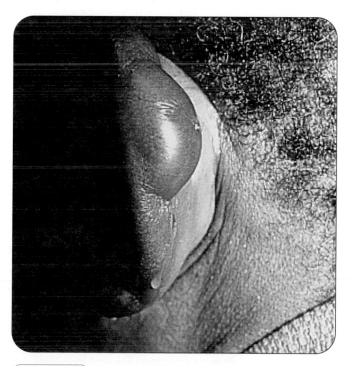

Figure 18-3 Second-degree frostbite

frostbite is superficial, while the others are degrees of deep frostbite (▲Figure 18-3) (▼Figure 18-4).

- **First-degree frostbite:** The affected part is warm, swollen, and tender.
- **Second-degree frostbite:** Blisters form minutes to hours after thawing and enlarge over several days.
- **Third-degree frostbite:** Blisters are small and contain reddish-blue or purplish fluid. The surrounding skin may have a red or blue color and may not blanch when pressure is applied.
- **Fourth-degree frostbite:** No blisters or swelling occur. The part remains numb, cold, and white to dark purple in color.

Figure 18-4 Frostbitten ear 8 hours old

Caution:

DO NOT use water hotter than 108°F—burns can result.

DO NOT use water cooler than 100°F—it will not thaw frostbite rapidly enough.

DO NOT break any blisters.

DO NOT rub or massage the part—ice crystals can be pushed into body cells, rupturing them.

DO NOT rub the affected part with ice or snow.

DO NOT rewarm the part with a heating pad, hot-water bottle, stove, sunlamp, radiator, or exhaust pipe or over a fire. Excessive temperatures cannot be controlled, resulting in burns.

DO NOT allow the victim to drink alcoholic beverages. Alcohol dilates blood vessels and causes a loss of body heat.

DO NOT allow the victim to smoke. Smoking constricts blood vessels, thus impairing circulation.

DO NOT rewarm if there is any possibility of refreezing.

DO NOT allow the thawed part to refreeze because the ice crystals formed will be larger and more damaging. If refreezing is likely or even possible, it is better to leave the part frozen.

DO NOT use the "dry" rewarming technique (putting the victim's hands in your armpits) because that takes three to four times longer than the wet, rapid method to thaw frozen tissue. Slow rewarming results in greater tissue damage than rapid rewarming.

What to Do

All frostbite injuries require the same first aid treatment. *Seek medical attention immediately.* Rewarming of frostbite seldom needs to take place outside a medical facility.

1. Get the victim out of the cold and to a warm place.
2. Remove any clothing or constricting items such as rings that could impair blood circulation.
3. Seek immediate medical attention.
4. If the affected part is partially thawed or the victim is in a remote or wilderness situation (more than one hour from a medical facility), use the following wet, rapid rewarming method.

Place the frostbitten part in warm (102°F to 105°F) water. If you do not have a thermometer, pour some of the water over the inside of your arm or put your elbow into it to test that it is warm, not hot. Maintain water temperature by adding warm water as needed. Rewarming usually takes 20 to 40 minutes or until the tissues are soft. To help control the severe pain during rewarming, give the victim aspirin or ibuprofen. For ear or facial injuries, apply warm moist cloths, changing them frequently.

5. After thawing,

- If the feet are affected, treat victim as a "stretcher" case—the feet will be impossible to use after they are rewarmed.

- Protect the affected area from rubbing against clothing and bedding.

- Place dry, sterile gauze between the toes and the fingers to absorb moisture and to keep them from sticking together.

- Slightly elevate the affected part to reduce pain and swelling.

- Apply aloe vera gel to promote skin healing.

- Give the victim aspirin or ibuprofen to limit pain and inflammation.

Hypothermia

Body temperature falls when the body cannot produce heat as fast as it is being lost. **Hypothermia** is a life-threatening condition in which the body's core temperature falls below 95°F.

Generally, the core temperature will not fall until after many hours of continuous exposure to cold air, if the individual is healthy, physically active, and reasonably dressed. However, because wet skin and wind accelerate body heat loss and the body produces less heat during inactive periods, the core body temperature can fall even when the air temperature is above freezing if conditions are windy, clothing is wet, or the individual is inactive.

Hypothermia can occur year round. Most people think of hypothermia as related only to cold outdoor exposure. It can happen indoors, in the southern states, and even on a summer day. It does not require subfreezing temperatures.

Hypothermia occurs when the body loses more heat than it produces. If the body temperature falls to 80°F, most people die. Hypothermia can occur in indoor or outdoor situations; a victim may suffer frostbite as well in an outdoor situation. Hypothermia occurs rapidly during cold-water immersion (one hour or less when the water temperature is below 45°F). Because water has a tremendous capacity to drain heat from the body, prolonged immersion (several hours) in even slightly cool water (below 70°F) can cause hypothermia. Hypothermia is a medical emergency. Untreated, it results in death.

Even though hypothermic victims may show no heartbeat, breathing, or response to touch or pain, they are not really dead. Sometimes, the heartbeat and breathing of hypothermic victims will be so faint that they can go undetected. Thus, it is important to take 30 to 45 seconds, instead of the usual 5 to 10, to check the pulse. If hypothermia has resulted from submersion in cold water, CPR should be started without delay. When a hypothermic victim is found on land, however, take a little extra time to determine whether CPR really is required. Hypothermic victims should be treated as gently as possible, because rough handling can cause life-threatening disruptions in heart rate. All hypothermic victims, even those who do not appear to be alive, must be evaluated by a physician.

In the past, the people believed to be most vulnerable to hypothermia have been hunters, hikers, and backpackers, as well as careless drinkers and accident victims. However, the condition is not limited to those groups. Disadvantaged urban dwellers exposed to the elements and elderly persons with impaired thermoregulatory mechanisms also are susceptible. Lightly clad persons almost anywhere can quickly become chilled outdoors when it is raining even though the temperatures are only cool, and persons immersed for some time in cool or cold water lose heat even more readily. Even well-conditioned athletes such as long-distance runners can be victims. Hypothermia should be considered whenever the victim's behavior and history and the weather conditions indicate abnormal heat loss. Hypothermia is an underreported cause of death in the United States. In most cases, death is attributed to other factors, with hypothermia considered a secondary cause.

The victim's history may be sufficient to determine hypothermia. Hypothermia is likely if a victim is reported by companions to be acting strangely and is shivering after exposure to cold or moisture or if he or she has been suddenly immersed in cold water. Predisposing factors are important: drinking alcoholic beverages is commonly associated with hypothermia. A typical scenario involves one or more persons in lightweight garments who drink too much, fall asleep outdoors or in a poorly heated shelter, become chilled by cold air or moisture, and remain exposed for many hours. Certain medications predispose individuals to hypothermia because they interfere with the hypothalamus, which acts as the brain's thermostat in regulating the body's heat.

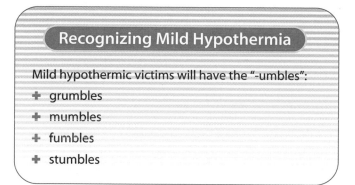

Recognizing Mild Hypothermia

Mild hypothermic victims will have the "-umbles":

+ grumbles
+ mumbles
+ fumbles
+ stumbles

Especially vulnerable to hypothermia are the very old and the very young. Infants and children have a small muscle mass, so the shivering response is poor in children and nonexistent in infants. They also have less body fat. Younger children need help to protect themselves against the cold because they cannot put on or take off clothes. The less fit are also more likely to become hypothermic.

Types of Exposure

There are three classifications of cold exposure:

* **Acute exposure** (also known as immersion) occurs when the victim loses body heat very rapidly, usually in water. Acute exposure is considered to be six hours or less in duration.

* **Subacute exposure** (also known as mountain or exhaustion exposure) occurs when exposure is 6 to 24 hours and can be either land- or water-based.

* **Chronic exposure** (also known as urban exposure) involves long-term cooling. It generally occurs on land and exceeds 24 hours.

What to Look for

Consider hypothermia in all victims who have been exposed to cold and who have an altered mental status. Suspect hypothermia in any person who has a temperature reading less than 95°F. (Keep in mind that some thermometers do not measure below that temperature.) Shivering is a good clue, but it may be suppressed when energy stores (glycogen) are depleted. Suspect hypothermia in people with frostbite and those injured in a cold environment.

Some people die of hypothermia because they or those around them do not recognize the symptoms, which are difficult to recognize in the early stages. Here are some signs to watch for:

* *Change in mental status.* This is one of the first symptoms of developing hypothermia. Examples are disorientation, apathy, and changes in personality, such as unusual aggressiveness.

* *Shivering.* Shivering is the first, and most important, body defense against a falling body temperature. Shivering starts when the body temperature drops 1°F and *can produce more heat than many rewarming methods.* As the core temperature continues to fall, shivering decreases and usually stops at about 90°F. Shivering also stops as body temperature rises. If shivering stops as responsiveness decreases, assume that the core temperature is falling. If, on the other hand, shivering stops while the victim is becoming more coordinated and feeling better, assume that the core temperature is rising.

* *Cool abdomen.* Place the back of your hand between the clothing and the victim's abdomen to assess the victim's temperature. When the victim's abdominal skin under clothing is cooler than your hand, consider the victim hypothermic until proved otherwise.

* *Low core body temperature.* The best indicator of hypothermia is a thermometer reading of the core body temperature. The ability to reliably measure core temperature depends on the availability of an appropriate thermometer and access to the victim's rectum. Normal thermometers do not register below 94°F and so do not indicate whether the hypothermia is mild or severe. Because first aid for mild hypothermia is different from that for severe hypothermia, it is helpful to have a rectal thermometer that registers below 90°F. Oral and axillary (armpit) temperatures are influenced by too many external factors to make them reliable.

* Measuring rectal temperatures in wilderness or remote locations is seldom done, mainly because low-reading rectal thermometers usually are not readily available. Also, taking a rectal temperature can be difficult, inconvenient, and embarrassing to victim and rescuer. If done outdoors, such a procedure can expose the already cold victim.

Types of Hypothermia

The difference between mild and severe hypothermia is based on the core body temperature, but taking a rectal temperature often is not possible. The other most significant difference is that with severe hypothermia the victim becomes so cold that shivering stops. That means the victim's body cannot rewarm itself internally and will require external heat for recovery.

Victims of mild hypothermia have a core body temperature above 90°F. Signs and symptoms are shivering, slurred speech, memory lapses, and fumbling hands. Victims frequently stumble and stagger, but they are usually conscious and can talk. While many people suffer cold

Table 18-1: How Cold Is It?

In addition to cold, two other factors account for body heat loss: moisture and wind. Moisture—whether from rain, snow, or perspiration—speeds the conduction of heat away from the body.

Wind causes sizable amounts of body-heat loss. If the thermometer reads 20°F and the wind speed is 20 mph, the exposure is comparable to –10°F. This is called the windchill factor. Use the following rough measures of wind speed: If you feel the wind on your face, wind speed is about 10 mph; if small branches move or if dust or snow is raised, 20 mph; if large branches are moving, 30 mph; and if a whole tree bends, about 40 mph.

To determine the windchill factor:

1. Estimate the wind speed by checking for the signs described above.
2. Look at an outdoor thermometer reading (in degrees Fahrenheit).
3. Match the estimated wind speed with the actual thermometer reading in the table below.

Windchill Factor

Estimated Wind Speed (mph)	50	40	30	20	10	0	–10	–20	–30	–40	–50	–60
	Equivalent Temperature (°F)											
Calm	50	40	30	20	10	0	–10	–20	–30	–40	–50	–60
5	48	37	27	16	6	–5	–15	–26	–36	–47	–57	–68
10	40	28	16	3	–9	–21	–33	–46	–58	–70	–83	–95
15	36	22	9	–5	–18	–32	–45	–58	–72	–85	–99	–112
20	32	18	4	–10	–25	–39	–53	–67	–82	–96	–110	–124
25	30	15	0	–15	–29	–44	–59	–74	–89	–104	–118	–133
30	25	13	–2	–18	–33	–48	–63	–79	–94	–109	–125	–140
35	27	11	–4	–20	–35	–51	–67	–82	–98	–113	–129	–145
40	26	10	–6	–21	–37	–53	–69	–85	–101	–117	–132	–148

Actual Thermometer Reading (°F) — Equivalent Temperature (°F)

(Wind speeds greater than 40 mph have little additional effect.)

Little danger (In less than 5 hours with dry skin. Greatest hazard from false sense of security.)

Increasing danger (Exposed flesh may freeze within 1 minute.)

Great danger (Flesh may freeze within 30 seconds.)

---

hands and feet, victims of mild hypothermia experience cold abdomens and backs.

Victims of severe hypothermia have a core body temperature below 90°F. Shivering has stopped. Muscles may be stiff and rigid, similar to rigor mortis. The victim's skin is ice cold and has a blue appearance. Pulse and breathing slow down, and the pupils dilate. The victim appears to be dead. In fact, 50% to 80% of all severe hypothermic victims die.

The National Association of Emergency Medical Service Physicians recommends that CPR *not* be started on a profoundly hypothermic victim if one of the following applies:

- The victim's core body temperature is less than 60°F.
- The victim's chest is frozen (cannot be compressed).
- The victim was submerged in water for more than 60 minutes.
- The victim has a lethal injury.
- Transport for controlled rewarming will be delayed.
- Rescuers are endangered.

For CPR to be effective, heart activity must be restored within a short time, which requires defibrillation, oxygen, and medications. Rescue breathing can be continued for hours when there is a pulse, but chest compressions cannot support circulation very long. CPR is also difficult to continue during a remote setting evacuation.

Also, do *not* start CPR until you have checked the victim's pulse for 30 to 45 seconds. A hypothermic victim will have an extremely slow pulse rate. CPR can cause cardiac arrest in an already beating heart.

What to Do

1. For all hypothermic victims, stop further heat loss:
   - Get the victim out of the cold.
   - Handle the victim gently. Rough handling can cause a cardiac arrest.
   - Replace wet clothing with dry clothing.
   - Add insulation (blankets, towels, pillows, newspapers) beneath and around the victim. Cover

the victim's head (50% to 80% of the body's heat loss is through the head.

- Keep the victim in a horizontal (flat) position. Do *not* raise the legs. (Elevating the legs would cause cold blood from the legs to flow into the body core and adversely affect the heart.)

- Do not let the victim walk or exercise. Do not massage the victim's body. Either activity could drive cold blood from the extremities to the torso and produce what is known as **temperature afterdrop.**

2. Call EMS for immediate medical transportation. Remember that hypothermia is more common in urban settings than in victims found in the wilderness.

3. For mild hypothermia in a remote or wilderness location, the goal is to prevent further heat loss. If protected from further heat loss, most mildly hypothermic victims are able to rewarm themselves by shivering, which generates heat.

4. For severe hypothermia in a remote or wilderness situation:

- Check ABCs (airway, breathing, circulation). Take 30 to 45 seconds to check the pulse before starting CPR.

- Evacuate the victim by helicopter. Rewarming in a remote location is difficult and rarely effective.

   Remember: *The best care can be summarized simply as: rescue, examine, insulate, and transport.*

Adding heat to a victim is extremely difficult. The longer the victim has been exposed to the cold, the longer it will take to raise the core temperature to normal. Trying to rewarm a hypothermic victim may cause cardiac arrest.

Although surface rewarming suppresses shivering, it may be the only option when the victim is far from medical care. In that case, the victim must be warmed by any available external heat source.

There are problems with the commonly recommended rewarming methods.* *Warm water immersion* requires a lot of warm water (no hotter than 106°F) and a bathtub—both rarely found in remote locations. Hot baths can produce rapid changes in the blood that can produce cardiac arrest.

---

*Bruce C. Paton, MD: "Field Treatment of Hypothermia," Second World Congress on Wilderness Medicine, Wilderness Medical Society.

Caution:

DO NOT allow the victim to physically exert (no walking, no climbing).

DO NOT try to rewarm a hypothermic victim outside a medical facility. External measures to rewarm should not be used, especially on the extremities, because surface rewarming leads to vasodilation (wider blood vessels), which can lead to a drop in blood pressure and afterdrop.

DO NOT try to rewarm a hypothermic victim outside a medical facility because rewarming the skin will stop shivering, which is the most effective way to rewarm.

DO NOT put an unconscious victim in a bathtub.

DO NOT give the victim alcohol. Alcohol interferes with shivering and accelerates heat loss by vasodilating the skin's blood vessels. The victim may feel warmer temporarily, but there is a greater risk of hypothermia.

DO NOT give the victim a warm drink. Warm drinks taste good and may give a psychological boost, but they have no warming effect and contain little energy. Warm drinks signal the brain to send more blood to the skin, which leads to some heat loss.

DO NOT give the victim a caffeine drink. Caffeine has a diuretic effect, and the victim probably is already dehydrated.

DO NOT rub or massage the victim's arms or legs. Rubbing the skin suppresses shivering, dilates the skin's blood vessels (resulting in more heat loss), and produces temperature afterdrop.

DO NOT raise the victim's legs, which allows cold blood from the legs to flow into the body core and adversely affect the heart. Keep the victim in a flat position.

Recent studies show that *body-to-body* contact in an insulated sleeping bag is ineffective for rewarming. Reasons why include the following:

- All the heat produced by the rescuer's body is not enough to rewarm a victim. For example, heat loss of adults cooled to 91°F exceeds 300 kcal (kilocalorie); heat production of a rescuer is only 100 kcal per hour.

HYPOTHERMIA

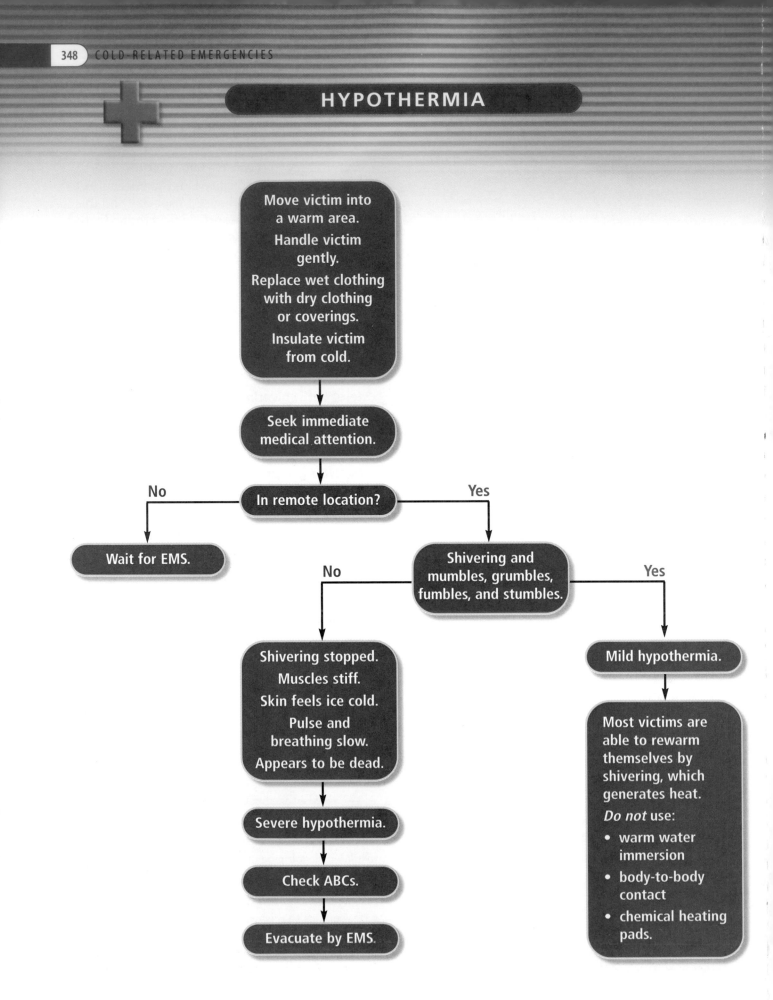

Move victim into a warm area.

Handle victim gently.

Replace wet clothing with dry clothing or coverings.

Insulate victim from cold.

Seek immediate medical attention.

In remote location?

No → Wait for EMS.

Yes → Shivering and mumbles, grumbles, fumbles, and stumbles.

No → Shivering stopped. Muscles stiff. Skin feels ice cold. Pulse and breathing slow. Appears to be dead.

Severe hypothermia.

Check ABCs.

Evacuate by EMS.

Yes → Mild hypothermia.

Most victims are able to rewarm themselves by shivering, which generates heat.

Do not use:
- warm water immersion
- body-to-body contact
- chemical heating pads.

Winter Wardrobe

	Advantages	Disadvantages	Layer
Wool	Stretches without damage; insulates well even when wet	Heavy weight; absorbs moisture; may irritate skin	1, 2, or 3
Cotton	Comfortable and lightweight	Absorbs moisture	1 (for inactive people) or 2
Silk	Extremely lightweight and durable; very good insulator; washes well	More expensive; does not transfer moisture quickly	1
Polypropylene	Lightweight; transfers moisture quickly and dries quickly	Does not insulate well; low melting point; surface may pill	1 or 2 (for active people)
Down	Durable, lightweight; most effective insulator by weight	Expensive; loses insulative quality when wet; difficult to dry	2 or 3 (especially in dry extreme cold)
Nylon	Lightweight; wind- and water-resistant; durable	May not allow perspiration to evaporate; low melting point; flammable	3
Synthetic Polyester Insulation	Does not absorb moisture, therefore insulates even when wet	Heavier than down; does not compress as well	2 or 3 (especially in wet weather)

Source: National Safety Council, *Family Safety & Health*

- There usually is only a small amount (less than 50%) of direct skin contact, which is essential for effective heat transfer, between the victim and the rescuer.
- The victim's peripheral blood vessel constriction may impair heat transfer to the body's core.
- Skin warming may slow the victim's shivering response, which effectively rewarms the body.

Because skin rewarming suppresses shivering, which slows the rate of core rewarming, body-to-body rewarming should be used only when there will be a long delay in getting the victim to medical care and when more appropriate methods of adding heat are unavailable.

Several types of *chemical heating pads* are on the market. While they may be effective for warming hands and feet, there is no evidence that they are capable of rewarming a hypothermic victim. For example, one type of heating pad is 7 inches by 9 inches and provides 14.5 kcal total heat, with a maximum temperature of about 125°F. A minimum of 20 pads would be needed to provide enough heat to rewarm a 91°F victim, even if heat transfer were 100% efficient. This method may stop the desirable effects of shivering, still leaving the victim hypothermic.

Warm drinks have no warming effect and contain little energy. Warm drinks signal the brain to send more blood to the skin. Dilation of the skin's blood vessels produces a warm feeling but causes some heat loss since the capillaries are dilated. Warm drinks taste good and provide a psy-chological boost, but it would take more than the stomach could hold and at a temperature high enough to produce burns to be effective. On the other hand, if the victim can swallow, fluids are highly recommended because dehydration is usually present.

Dehydration

Dehydration occurs because of unperceived fluid loss combined with inadequate fluid intake. In very cold weather, the humidity approaches zero, and large quantities of fluid are lost through exhaled breath.

People in a cold environment must drink even when they are not thirsty. Inactive people in comfortable climates need two quarts of water a day to prevent dehydration.

An individual's hydration status can be monitored by noting the color and the volume of the urine. The lighter the color, the better hydrated; dark yellow urine is a definite indication that fluid consumption should be increased.

Unmelted snow and ice should *not* be consumed for water. Eating snow and ice irritates the mouth, wastes body heat, and, if enough is consumed, lowers body temperature. When snow and ice are the only available sources of water, they should be melted before being consumed. Melted snow or ice should not be considered drinkable until it has been appropriately disinfected (by boiling, filtering, or using chemicals).

STUDY
Questions (18)

Name_____ Course_____ Date_____

Activities

Activity 1

Mark each question as true (T) or false (F).

T F 1. Shivering is a method the body uses to generate heat.

T F 2. You should massage frostbitten parts.

T F 3. Blisters may form as a result of frostbite.

T F 4. Smoking intensifies the harmful effects of cold.

T F 5. Frostbite is more severe if the injured area is thawed and then refrozen.

T F 6. In frostbite, the parts should be rewarmed rapidly, since rewarming reduces pain.

T F 7. Break the blisters that may develop in frostbite.

T F 8. Hypothermia can occur only in below-freezing temperatures.

Activity 2

Mark each action yes (Y) or no (N).

Which of the following actions are proper first aid for frostbite?

____ 1. Rewarm a frostbitten part by exposing it to a fire or open flame.

____ 2. Rewarm a frostbitten part by using warm water (102°F to 105°F).

____ 3. Placing frostbitten hands in another person's armpits is as effective as using warm water.

____ 4. Rub the frostbitten part to restore circulation.

____ 5. Rub the frostbitten area with snow.

____ 6. A victim with frozen lower extremities should be carried, if possible, to the nearest medical facility.

____ 7. If a victim with a severely frostbitten foot cannot be carried to medical aid, keep the part frozen and assist him in walking.

____ 8. Break any blisters that have formed.

Activity 3

Check (✓) the appropriate action(s).
Which of the following actions are proper first aid for hypothermia?

____ 1. Give hot coffee or hot chocolate to rewarm a victim.

____ 2. Treat the victim gently.

____ 3. Replace wet clothing with dry clothing.

____ 4. Get the victim out of the cold environment.

For mild hypothermia:

____ 5. Apply chemical heat pads to the head, neck, chest, and groin first.

____ 6. Place in a tub of hot water.

____ 7. Use your body heat against the victim's body while both of you are in a sleeping bag.

For severe hypothermia:

____ 8. Check the victim's breathing and pulse for at least 30 to 45 seconds.

____ 9. Quickly rewarm the victim even if you are near a medical facility.

____ 10. Arrange transportation to a medical facility.

Case Situations

Case 1

It is 5:30 P.M. on a Saturday in midwinter, and an 18-year-old female has been in the woods for most of the afternoon. She complains that her toes are numb. You find that they look grayish-blue and feel hard and frozen.

____ 1. This victim is most likely experiencing
   a. deep frostbite (also called freezing)
   b. frostnip
   c. superficial frostbite
   d. hypothermia

Check (✓) the appropriate treatment:

____ 2. Have her drink an alcoholic beverage.

____ 3. Place her feet in warm water (100°F to 105°F).

____ 4. Vigorously rub the affected area.

____ 5. Pack her feet in snow and quickly transport her to the hospital.

____ 6. Rewarm her toes by a fire.

STUDY
Questions 18

Case 2

A 50-year-old male has fallen through the ice of a local pond during his attempt to rescue a dog. Several bystanders have formed a human chain to try to reach the man, and you arrive just in time to help pull the victim from the water. He is awake and has cold, pale skin. He has intense, uncontrollable shivering.

_____ 1. While in the water, the victim lost heat through
   a. respiration
   b. convection
   c. evaporation
   d. radiation
   e. conduction

_____ 2. This victim is most likely in what stage of hypothermia?
   a. mild
   b. severe

_____ 3. Care for this victim would include
   a. having the victim walk around to generate heat
   b. wrapping the victim in blankets
   c. removing all wet clothing
   d. providing aggressive rewarming

Case 3

A middle-aged male is found beneath a railroad car on a cold night. He is semiresponsive, and you detect an alcohol smell about his body. The temperature is 10°F with a wind speed of 25 miles per hour. His hands and feet are cold and pale and feel solid. There is no evidence of other injury.

1. What injury do you suspect?

_____

_____

2. What is the first aid for this condition?

_____

_____

_____ 3. To warm frostbitten extremities, what water temperature range must be maintained?
   a. 98°F to 100°F
   b. 100°F to 102°F
   c. 102°F to 105°F
   d. above 113°F

4. How should the victim's skin feel at the conclusion of the warming process? Check all that apply.
   _____ a. Hard
   _____ b. Soft
   _____ c. Crusty

5. What precautions should you keep in mind when bandaging frostbite?
   a. _____
   b. _____
   c. _____

Case 4

A young hunter is found lying in the woods after being lost for two days. The weather has been windy and wet with occasional snow flurries. Temperatures have ranged between 20°F and 30°F. The victim is found unconscious. There are no signs of other injuries.

1. What is the initial description of this man's condition?

_____

_____

2. What is the first aid for all such cases?
   a. _____
   b. _____
   c. _____

3. What major precaution should you take with a victim who has been exposed to cold weather?

_____

_____

_____

_____

Case 5

A middle-aged male is found beneath a park bench. He is poorly clothed with no hat or coat, and overnight temperatures were around 25°F. He is conscious and tells you he is destitute with no family and was outside overnight.

1. One of the first signs of hypothermia he may be showing is

_____

_____

2. The type of exposure identified in this case is

_____

Name the other two types of exposure:
   a. _____
   b. _____

Chapter Activities

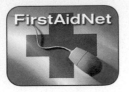

WEB Activities

Cold-Related Emergencies

Visit nsc.jbpub.com/FirstAidNet, then click on Web Activities, and select the appropriate chapter.

Cold Related Deaths

The region in which you live plays a big part on the weather you endure throughout the year. Certain altitudes and latitudes are notorious for dangerously cold weather.

Lowest Temperature Recorded

Check out your states' lowest recorded temperature ever!

Current Weather

If you haven't been outside lately, CNN brings the weather to you! Specific to your state and nearest city, this up-to-the-minute weather report can help you plan your out door activities.

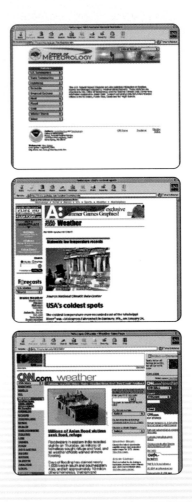

Chapter 19

Heat-Related Emergencies

When the temperature goes up, a multitude of problems can—and do—arise. Given the right (or wrong) conditions, anyone can develop heat illness. Some victims are lucky enough to suffer only from heat cramps, while less fortunate ones may be laid low by heat exhaustion or devastated by heatstroke.

How the Body Stays Cool

The human body is constantly engaged in a life-and-death struggle to disperse the heat that it produces. If allowed to accumulate, the heat would quickly increase your body temperature beyond its comfortable 98.6°F. That does not normally happen, because your body is able to lose enough heat to maintain a steady temperature. Usually, you are aware of this struggle only during hard labor or exercise in a hot environment, when your body produces heat faster than it can lose heat. In certain circumstances, your body can build up too much heat, your temperature may rise to life-threatening levels, and you can become delirious or lose consciousness. This condition is called **heatstroke** and is a serious medical emergency. If you do not rid your body of excess heat fast enough, it "cooks" the brain and other vital organs. It is often fatal, and those who do survive may have permanent damage to their vital organs. Before your temperature reaches heatstroke level, however, you may suffer **heat exhaustion** with its flu-like symptoms. By treating the symptoms of heat exhaustion, you avoid heatstroke.

How does the body dispose of excess heat? Humans lose heat largely through their skin, much as a car loses heat through its radiator. Exercising muscles warms the blood, just as the car's hot engine warms its radiator fluid. Warm blood travels through the skin's dilated blood vessels, losing heat by evaporating sweat to the surrounding air, just as the car loses engine heat through the radiator.

When blood delivers heat to the skin, the body loses heat primarily in two ways: radiation and evaporation (vaporization of sweat). When the air temperature is 70°F or less, the body releases heat into its surroundings by radiation. As the environmental temperature approaches the body's temperature, however, heat loss through radiation is greatly reduced. In fact, people working or exercising on a hot summer day actually gain heat through radiation from the sun. That leaves evaporation as the only way to effectively control body temperature.

Water Loss

Water makes up about 50% to 60% of an adult's body weight. You lose about two quarts every day through breathing, urinating, bowel movements, and sweat. That lost fluid must be replaced. Although the amount of water used each day varies from person to person, an adult requires about two quarts a day from water, beverages, and food (about 70% of most food is water). A working adult can produce two to three quarts of sweat an hour for short periods and up to 10 to 15 quarts a day. When the body's water absorption rate of 1.5 quarts per hour is pitted against a sweat loss of two quarts per hour, **dehydration** results—drinking water cannot keep up with sweat losses.

If you drink only when you are thirsty, you are already dehydrated. Thirst is not a good guide for when to drink water. In fact, in hot and humid conditions, people may be so dehydrated by the time they become thirsty that they have trouble catching up with their fluid losses. One guideline regarding water intake is to monitor urine output. You are getting enough water if you are producing clear urine at least five times a day. Cloudy or dark urine or urinating fewer than five times a day means you probably should drink more.

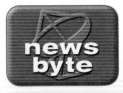

Chicago Heat Wave Was a Real Killer

A study of 58 people with classic heat stroke admitted to hospital emergency departments during the 1995 Chicago heat wave found that only one patient was cooled within 30 minutes, the generally accepted time frame. Further, nearly half of the patients admitted to intensive care units for heat stroke died within a year, 21% before discharge and another 28% after release from the hospital. Most of the survivors were left with permanent disabilities.

Source: Annals of Internal Medicine, August 1, 1998.

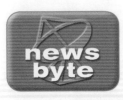

Water Loss: Do Athletes Need Sports Drinks?

An athlete who burns 4,000 to 5,000 calories per day needs to drink about four to five quarts of water or fluids. Water is best for people who work out for less than an hour. But for prolonged endurance exercise, sports drinks are better—they are absorbed slightly faster than water, and they replace carbohydrates that fuel the muscles.

Source: N. Clark: "Water: The Ultimate Nutrient." *Physician and Sportsmedicine,* 23:21

If possible while working, especially in hot weather, drink one cup (eight ounces) of water every 20 minutes. Usually, one pint (16 ounces) is the most a person can comfortably drink at once. It takes time for water to pass from the stomach into the blood, so you cannot catch up by drinking extra water later; about one quart of water per hour can pass out of the stomach.

Cool water (50°F) is easier for the stomach to absorb than warm water, and a little flavoring may make the water more tasty. The best fluids are those that leave the stomach fast and contain little sodium and less than 8% sugar. Coffee and tea should be avoided because they contain caffeine, a diuretic that increases water loss through urination. Alcoholic beverages also dehydrate by increasing urination. Soda pop contains about 10% sugar and therefore is not absorbed as well as water or commercial sports drinks (which contain about 5% to 8% sugar). Fruit juices range from 11% to 18% sugar and have an even longer absorption time.

Electrolyte Loss

Sweat and urine contain potassium and sodium, essential electrolytes that control the movement of water in and out of the body's cells. These electrolytes can be found in many everyday foods. Bananas and nuts are rich in potassium, and most American diets have up to 10 times as much sodium as the body needs. Acclimatizing to heat can also reduce sodium loss tenfold. Getting enough salt (sodium chloride) is rarely a problem in the typical American diet. In fact, most Americans consume an excessive amount of sodium, averaging 5 to 10 grams of sodium per day, although humans probably require only 1 to 3 grams. Sodium loss, therefore, is seldom a

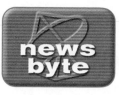

Water Intoxication in Grand Canyon Hikers

Water intoxication (hyponatremia), often seen in endurance athletes, has now been reported in recreational hikers. Water intoxication results when people replace sweat loss with plain water, instead of an enhanced product that more nearly resembles sweat. Differentiating water intoxication from heat exhaustion is difficult. Recreational wilderness hikers performing sustained exercise in the heat may require electrolyte replacement similar to endurance athletes.

Source: H. Backer et al: "Hyponatremia in Recreational Hikers in Grand Canyon National Park." *Journal of Wilderness Medicine,* 4:391–406, November 1993.

especially for those individuals who are generating heat with vigorous work.

Who Is at Risk?

Everyone is susceptible to heat illness if environmental conditions overwhelm the body's temperature-regulating mechanisms. Heat waves can set the stage for a rash of heatstroke victims. For example, in the 1995 Chicago heat wave, the death toll reached 591 in five days. Several groups are at particular risk, including the obese, the chronically ill, and alcoholics.

The elderly are at higher risk because of their impaired cardiac output and decreased ability to sweat. Infants and young children are also susceptible to heatstroke. Children (and pets) are especially vulnerable when they are left in automobiles, which can overheat in shopping center parking lots. The temperature in a parked car can soar to 150°F, even when a window is slightly open. The fluid loss and dehydration resulting from physical activity put outdoor laborers and athletes at particular risk.

Certain medications predispose individuals to heatstroke. They include drugs that alter sweat production (eg, antihistamines, antipsychotics, antidepressants) or interfere with thermoregulation.

Heat Illnesses

Heat illnesses include a range of disorders ▶Table 19-1. Some of them are common, but only heatstroke is life threatening. Untreated heatstroke victims always die.

Heat Cramps

Heat cramps are painful muscular spasms that happen suddenly. They usually involve the back of the leg muscles (calf and hamstring muscles) or the abdominal muscles. They tend to happen immediately after exertion and some experts claim they are caused by salt depletion. Victims may be drinking water without adequate salt content. However, other experts disagree because the typical American diet is heavy with salt.

Heat Exhaustion

Heat exhaustion is characterized by heavy perspiration with normal or slightly above normal body temperatures. It is caused by water or salt depletion or both. Some experts believe that a better term would be severe dehydra-

problem, unless a person is sweating profusely for long periods and drinking large amounts of water (more than one quart an hour).

Most people require only water most of the time. Commercial sports drinks can be useful if you are participating in vigorous physical activity for longer than one hour. The human body needs water more than it needs salt. Whenever extra sodium is added to your diet, drink more water. Otherwise, excessive sodium can draw water out of the body cells, accelerating dehydration.

Drinking large amounts of water (more than one quart an hour) and profuse sweating for long periods can lead to a condition called **water intoxication,** in which electrolytes are flushed from the body. Symptoms of water intoxication include frequent urination and behavior changes (irrationality, combativeness, seizures, and coma).

Effects of Humidity

Sweat can cool the body only if it evaporates (vaporizes). In dry air, you will not notice sweat evaporating. In high humidity, no sweat can evaporate. It just drips off the skin, without cooling the body. At about 75% humidity, sweating is ineffective in cooling the body.

Because humidity can significantly reduce evaporative cooling, a very humid but mildly warm day can be more stressful than a very hot, dry day. The higher the humidity, the lower the temperature at which heat risk begins,

Table 19-1: Heat Illnesses

Condition	Symptoms	What to Do
Heat cramps	Painful muscle spasms Sweaty skin Normal body temperature	1. Sit or lie down in the shade. 2. Drink cool, lightly salted water or sports drink. 3. Stretch affected muscles.
Heat exhaustion	Profuse sweating Flu-like symptoms Clammy or pale skin Dizziness Nausea, vomiting Rapid pulse Thirst Normal or slightly above normal body temperature	1. Treat mild cases the same as heat cramps (except do not stretch the muscles). 2. If persistent, gently apply wet towels and call EMS.
Heatstroke	Unresponsiveness (if responsive, victim will be confused, stagger, be agitated) Hot skin, which can be dry or wet	1. Move person to a half-sitting position in the shade. 2. Call EMS. 3. If humidity below 75%, spray victim with water and vigorously fan. If humidity above 75%, apply ice packs on neck, armpits, groin.

tion. Heat exhaustion affects workers and athletes who do not drink enough fluids while working or exercising in hot environments. Symptoms include severe thirst, fatigue, headache, nausea, vomiting, and sometimes diarrhea. The affected person often mistakenly believes he or she has the flu. Uncontrolled heat exhaustion can evolve into heatstroke.

Heatstroke

Two types of heatstroke exist: classic and exertional (►Table 19-2). **Classic heatstroke,** also known as the "slow cooker," may take days to develop. It is often seen during summer heat waves and typically affects poor, elderly, chronically ill, alcoholic, or obese persons. Because the elderly, often with medical problems, are frequently afflicted, this type of heatstroke has a 50% death rate even with medical care. It results from a combination of a hot environment and dehydration. **Exertional heatstroke** is also more common in the summer. It is frequently seen in athletes, laborers, and military personnel, all of whom often sweat profusely. This type of heatstroke is known as the "fast cooker." It affects healthy, active individuals strenuously working or playing in a warm environment. Because its rapid onset does not allow enough time for

severe dehydration to occur, 50% of exertional heatstroke victims usually are sweating. (Classic heatstroke victims are not sweating.)

There are several ways to tell the difference between heat exhaustion and heatstroke.

- If the victim's body feels extremely hot when touched, suspect heatstroke.

- Altered mental status (behavior) occurs with heatstroke, ranging from slight confusion and disorientation to coma. Between those extreme conditions,

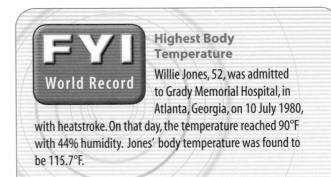

Highest Body Temperature

Willie Jones, 52, was admitted to Grady Memorial Hospital, in Atlanta, Georgia, on 10 July 1980, with heatstroke. On that day, the temperature reached 90°F with 44% humidity. Jones' body temperature was found to be 115.7°F.

Source: The Guinness Book of Records. New York: Bantam Books, 1999.

Hot-Weather Precautions

These simple preventive measures can reduce heat stress:

1. Keep as cool as possible.
   - Avoid direct sunlight.
   - Stay in the coolest available location (usually indoors).
   - Use air-conditioning, if available.
   - Use electric fans to promote cooling.
   - Place wet towels or ice bags on the body or dampen clothing.
   - Take cool baths or showers.
2. Wear lightweight, loose-fitting clothing.
3. Avoid strenuous physical activity, particularly in the sun and during the hottest part of the day.
4. Increase intake of fluids, such as water and fruit or vegetable juices. Thirst is not always a good indicator of adequate fluid intake. Fluid intake in hot weather should be $1\frac{1}{2}$ times the amount that quenches thirst. Persons who are overweight or large in build or who engage in strenuous activities, such as sports, may require more than a gallon of fluid intake daily in very hot weather. Persons for whom salt or fluid is restricted should consult their physicians for instructions on appropriate fluid and salt intake.
5. Do not take salt tablets unless instructed to do so by a physician.
6. Avoid alcoholic beverages (beer, wine, and liquor).
7. Stay in daily contact with other people.

victims usually become irrational, agitated, or even aggressive, and may have seizures.

- In severe heatstroke, the victim can go into a coma in less than an hour. The longer a coma lasts, the lower the chance for survival.
- Rectal temperature can also distinguish heatstroke from heat exhaustion, although obtaining this is usually not practical. A responsive heatstroke victim might not cooperate, taking a rectal temperature can be embarrassing to both victim and rescuer, and rectal thermometers are seldom available.

Other Heat Illnesses

Less serious heat illnesses include heat syncope, heat edema, and prickly heat:

- **Heat syncope,** in which a person becomes dizzy or faints after exposure to high temperatures, is a self-resolving condition. Victims should lie down in a cool place and, if not nauseated, drink water.
- **Heat edema,** which is also a self-resolving condition, causes the ankles and feet to swell from heat exposure. It is more common in women who are not acclimatized to a hot climate. It is related to salt and water retention and tends to disappear after acclimatization. Wearing support stockings and elevating the legs may help reduce the swelling.
- **Prickly heat,** also known as a heat rash, is an itchy rash that develops because of unevaporated moisture on skin wet from sweating. Treat by drying and cooling the skin.

What to Do

Heat Cramps

To relieve heat cramps (it may take several hours), follow these steps:

1. Rest in a cool place.
2. Drink lightly salted cool water (dissolve $\frac{1}{4}$ teaspoon salt in a quart of water) or a commercial sports

Table 19-2: Classic or Exertional Heatstroke?

Characteristics	Classic	Exertional
Age group usually affected?	Elderly	Men aged 15–45 years
Claims many victims at the same time?	During heat waves	During athletic competition
Health status of victims?	Chronically ill	Healthy and physically fit
Activity at the time of incident?	Sedentary	Strenuous exercise
Medication use?	Common	Usually none
Sweating?	Absent	Often present (50% of victims)

drink. (A commercial sports drink is easier to absorb if diluted to half strength to reduce the sugar content.)

3. Stretch the cramped calf muscle. Also, try an acupressure method: pinch the upper lip just below the nose.

Heat Exhaustion

1. Move the victim immediately out of the heat to a cool place.

2. Give cool liquids, adding electrolytes (lightly salted water or a commercial sports drink) if plain water does not improve the victim's condition in 20 minutes. Do not give salt tablets; they can irritate the stomach and cause nausea and vomiting.

3. Raise the victim's legs 8 to 12 inches (keep the legs straight).

4. Remove excess clothing.

5. Sponge with cool water and fan the victim.

6. If no improvement is seen within 30 minutes, seek medical attention.

Heatstroke

Heatstroke is a medical emergency and must be treated rapidly! Every minute delayed increases the likelihood of serious complications or death.

1. Move the victim immediately out of the heat to a cool place.

2. Remove clothing down to the victim's underwear.

3. Keep the victim's head and shoulders slightly elevated.

4. Seek immediate medical attention, even if the victim seems to be recovering.

5. The only way to prevent damage is to cool the victim quickly and by any means possible. Cooling methods include the following:

   - *Spraying* the victim with water and then *fanning*. The water droplets act as artificial sweat and cool through evaporation ▶Figure 19-1. This method is *not* effective in high-humidity (greater than 75%) conditions.

   - *Ice bags* placed against the large veins in the groin, armpits, and sides of the neck cool the body, regardless of humidity.

Preventing Heat Illness

Most heat illness occurs during the first days of working in the heat, so the main preventive measure is acclimatization (adjusting to heat). To better handle the heat, the body adjusts by decreasing the salt content in sweat and increasing the sweating rate.

Year-round exercise can help workers prepare for hot weather. Such activity raises the body's core temperature so it becomes accustomed to heat. Full acclimatization, however, requires exercise in hot weather. That can be accomplished by a minimum of 60 to 90 minutes of exercise in the heat each day for one to two weeks.

The acclimatized heart is able to pump more blood with each stroke than a heart not used to working in the heat. Sweating starts earlier, and the amount of sweat per hour doubles, from 1.5 quarts to 3 quarts or more.

Workers who live in a constantly hot climate have an advantage over those living in cooler temperatures.

Heat illnesses are avoidable. With knowledge, preparation, fluid replacement, and prompt emergency care, there is no need for heat illness to affect people working in warm weather. The following measures can help prevent heat illnesses:

+ Avoid dehydration. A good rule of thumb for fluid replacement is to drink one cup (eight ounces) every 20 minutes while working.

+ Dress in light-colored, porous, loose-fitting clothing, which reflects heat, facilitates evaporative heat loss, and allows air to circulate around your body.

+ Rest frequently, preferably in shade. This applies especially if you are not fully acclimatized, are older, are markedly overweight, or have heart disease.

+ Wipe cool water on exposed areas of the skin.

+ Dip clothing periodically in water.

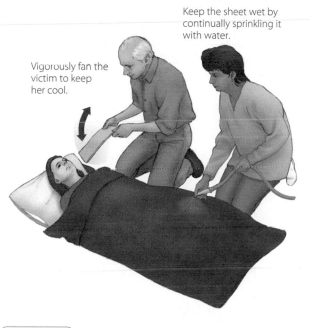

Keep the sheet wet by continually sprinkling it with water.

Vigorously fan the victim to keep her cool.

Figure 19-1 Spraying with water and fanning are effective in low humidity conditions.

Caution:

DO NOT delay initiating cooling while waiting for an ambulance. The longer the delay, the greater the risk of tissue damage and prolonged hospitalization.

DO NOT continue cooling after the victim's mental status has improved. Unnecessary cooling could lead to hypothermia.

DO NOT use rubbing alcohol to cool the skin. It can be absorbed into the blood and cause alcohol poisoning. Also, the vapors are a potential fire hazard.

DO NOT give the victim aspirin or acetaminophen. The brain's control center is not elevated, as it is with fever caused by diseases, so these products are not effective in lowering body temperature.

Table 19-3: Heat Index

Relative Humidity, %	70	75	80	85	90	95	100	105	110	115	120
	Actual Thermometer Reading (°F) / Apparent Temperature (°F)										
0	64	69	73	78	83	87	91	95	99	103	107
10	65	70	75	80	85	90	95	100	105	111	116
20	66	72	77	82	87	93	99	105	112	120	130
30	67	73	78	84	90	96	104	113	123	135	148
40	68	74	79	86	93	101	110	123	137	151	
50	69	75	81	88	96	107	120	135	150		
60	70	76	82	90	100	114	132	149			
70	70	77	85	93	106	124	144				
80	71	78	86	97	113	136					
90	71	79	88	102	122						
100	72	80	91	108							

Above 130°F = heatstroke imminent

105°F to 130°F = heat exhaustion and heat cramps likely; heatstroke with long exposure and activity

90°F to 105°F = heat exhaustion and heat cramps with long exposure and activity

80°F to 90°F = fatigue during exposure and activity

Source: National Weather Service

HEAT-RELATED EMERGENCIES

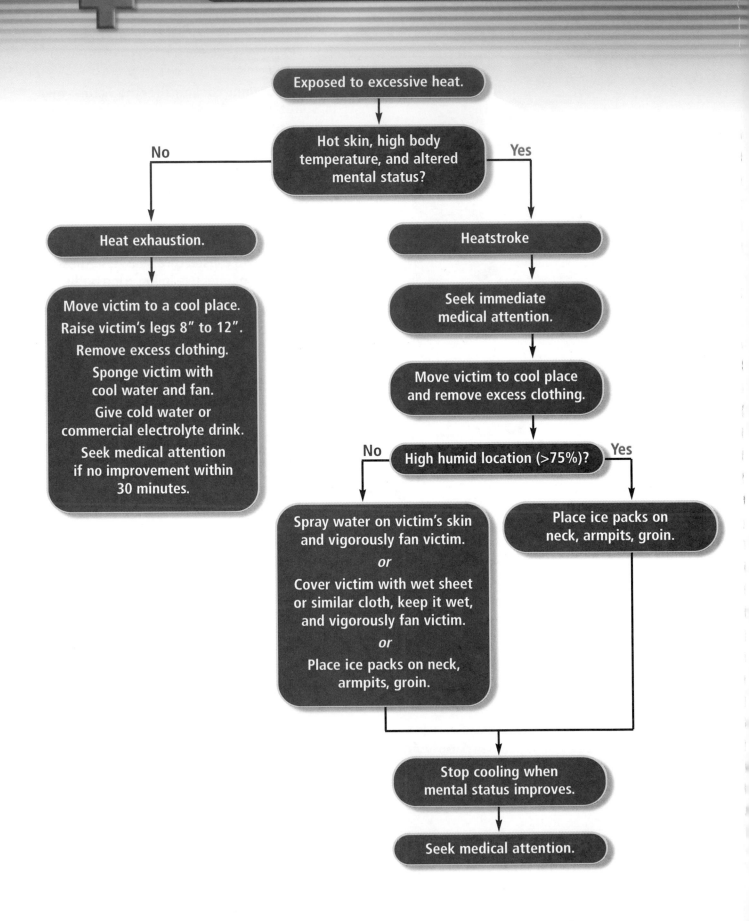

Exposed to excessive heat.

Hot skin, high body temperature, and altered mental status?

No → Heat exhaustion.

Move victim to a cool place.
Raise victim's legs 8" to 12".
Remove excess clothing.
Sponge victim with cool water and fan.
Give cold water or commercial electrolyte drink.
Seek medical attention if no improvement within 30 minutes.

Yes → Heatstroke

Seek immediate medical attention.

Move victim to cool place and remove excess clothing.

High humid location (>75%)?

No → Spray water on victim's skin and vigorously fan victim.
or
Cover victim with wet sheet or similar cloth, keep it wet, and vigorously fan victim.
or
Place ice packs on neck, armpits, groin.

Yes → Place ice packs on neck, armpits, groin.

Stop cooling when mental status improves.

Seek medical attention.

- An *ice bath* cools a victim quickly, but it requires a great deal of ice—at least 80 pounds—to be effective. The need for a big enough tub also limits this method.

- A *cool water bath* (less than 60°F) can be successful if the water is stirred to prevent a warm layer from forming around the body. This is the most effective method in high humidity (greater than 75%) conditions.

How Hot It Feels

Under normal conditions, temperature and humidity are the most important elements influencing body comfort. The Heat Index compiled by the National Weather Service lists **apparent temperatures**—how hot it feels—at various combinations of temperature and humidity (◀Table 19-3).

Heat-Related Deaths

During 1979-1996, an annual average of 381 deaths in the United States were attributable to "excessive heat exposure" (range: 148 in 1979 to 1,700 in 1980), for an average age-adjusted rate of 2 deaths per 1 million population. During this 18-year period, 6,864 deaths were attributable to excessive heat exposure: 2,914 (42%) "due to weather conditions," 343 (5%) "of man-made origin," and 3,607 (53%) "of unspecified origin." About half of all heat-related deaths occurred among persons aged greater than or equal to 65 years.

✚ Case 1

A 92-year-old man's family to conserve electricity had not been running the air conditioner in their residence. The daytime heat index recorded at the local airport during the five days preceding his death ranged form 102°F to 109°F (38.9°C to 42.8°C).

✚ Case 2

A 4-year-old girl was found in a locked car in front of a childcare center. The temperature inside the car at the time of her death was unknown; however, the estimated heat index in the area that day was 93°F (33.9°C).

✚ Case 3

A 70-year-old woman was found dead in a mobile home. When she was discovered, the air conditioner was blowing hot air, and the temperature inside the mobile home was about 115°F (46°C).

✚ Case 4

A 52-year-old man walked from the lawn he was mowing to a nearby residence and knocked on the back door. When the homeowner opened the door, the man collapsed onto the porch. He died at the hospital. His core temperature was 107.1°F (41.7°C), which, before his death was reduced to 101°F (38.3°C). The outside temperature at the time he collapsed was 109°F (42.8°C).

Source: *CDC MMWR Weekly;* 48(22):469-472 (June 11, 1999)

STUDY
Questions 19

Name_____ Course_____ Date_____

Activities

Activity 1

Mark each statement as true (T) or false (F).

T F 1. Use rubbing alcohol to cool a heatstroke victim's high body temperature.

T F 2. Use the evaporation method to cool a heatstroke victim in high-humidity conditions.

T F 3. All heatstroke victims will have hot, dry skin.

T F 4. Altered mental status is a good indication of heatstroke.

T F 5. Heat exhaustion is more serious than heatstroke.

T F 6. The underlying cause of heat cramps is depletion of blood glucose.

Activity 2

Choose the best answer.

On a hot day a man complains of pain in his legs. Choose the more appropriate treatment option.

____ 1. a. Give him a lot of cold water to drink.
     b. Give him a commercial sports drink.

____ 2. a. Massage the cramping muscle.
     b. Stretch the cramping muscle.

Mark each sign HE (heat exhaustion) or HS (heatstroke)

____ 3. Skin: hot, dry, or wet

____ 4. Skin: cool, clammy

____ 5. Sweating excessively

____ 6. Sweating usually absent

____ 7. Unresponsive

Choose the best techniques.

A woman has hot, red skin. Which *two* of the following cooling techniques could you use to quickly reduce her body temperature?

____ 8. Apply cold towels to her back.

____ 9. Place her feet and hands in buckets of cold water.

____ 10. Wrap the victim in wet sheets and fan her.

____ 11. Apply ice packs to her neck, armpits, head, and groin.

____ 12. Apply ice packs around her wrists and ankles.

Case Situations

Case 1

A middle-aged man collapses while mowing the lawn on a hot, very humid day.

____ 1. What symptoms lead you to believe that the victim is suffering from heatstroke rather than heat exhaustion?
     a. normal body temperature
     b. altered mental status
     c. high body temperature
     d. both B and C

____ 2. Which is the most serious condition?
     a. prickly heat
     b. heatstroke
     c. heat cramps
     d. heat exhaustion

____ 3. For this heatstroke victim, what should you do?
     a. Move him into the shade, remove excess clothing, cover him with damp sheets, and vigorously fan.
     b. Move him into the shade, remove excess clothing, and apply ice packs to his groin, neck, and armpits.
     c. Splash water on him to revive him.
     d. Give him a drink of water.

Case 2

A group of children summon you to a playground on a hot, humid summer day. You find a young girl sitting on the ground. She is breathing normally but is complaining of a headache and dizziness. Her skin is cool and she is sweating heavily.

____ 1. From what condition is this child suffering?
     a. heat cramps
     b. heat exhaustion
     c. heatstroke

STUDY
Questions (19)

2. What is the appropriate first aid?

   a. _____
   _____

   b. _____
   _____

Case 3

On your vacation, you spend a day at a large amusement park. It is an extremely hot and humid day. During the afternoon, you decide to rest a while and watch one of the special shows. Soon after you have been seated, an elderly man in front of you suddenly falls forward out of his seat. When you reach him, his wife reports that they have been walking around the park practically all day without stopping. His skin feels cool and clammy.

1. From what emergency condition is this man most likely suffering?

   _____
   _____

2. What first aid should you provide to this man?

   a. _____
   _____

   b. _____
   _____

   c. _____
   _____

3. The other major heat condition is heatstroke. Although not as common as heat exhaustion, heatstroke is more serious and a true medical emergency. What are the two best indicators of heatstroke?

   a. _____
   _____

   b. _____
   _____

4. What three steps constitute the emergency care for heatstroke?

   a. _____
   _____

   b. _____
   _____

   c. _____

5. How can you tell the difference between heat exhaustion and heatstroke by examining the victim's skin?

   a. Heat exhaustion_____
   _____

   b. Heatstroke_____
   _____

Chapter Activities

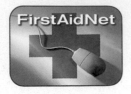

WEB Activities

Heat-Related Emergencies

Visit nsc.jbpub.com/FirstAidNet, then click on Web Activities, and select the appropriate chapter.

Heat Index

Discover how high levels of heat and humidity pose a health risk.

Heat-Related Deaths

Exposure to humidity combined with heat makes people more susceptible to heat illnesses. The region in which you live plays a big part on the weather you endure throughout the year.

Highest Temperatures Recorded

Check out your states' highest recorded temperature ever!

Current Weather

If you haven't been outside lately, CNN brings the weather to you! Specific to your state and nearest city, this up-to-the-minute weather report can help you plan your outdoor activities.

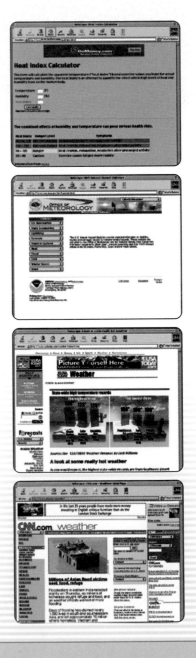

Special Situations

Part 6

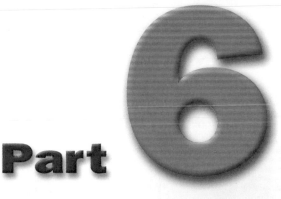

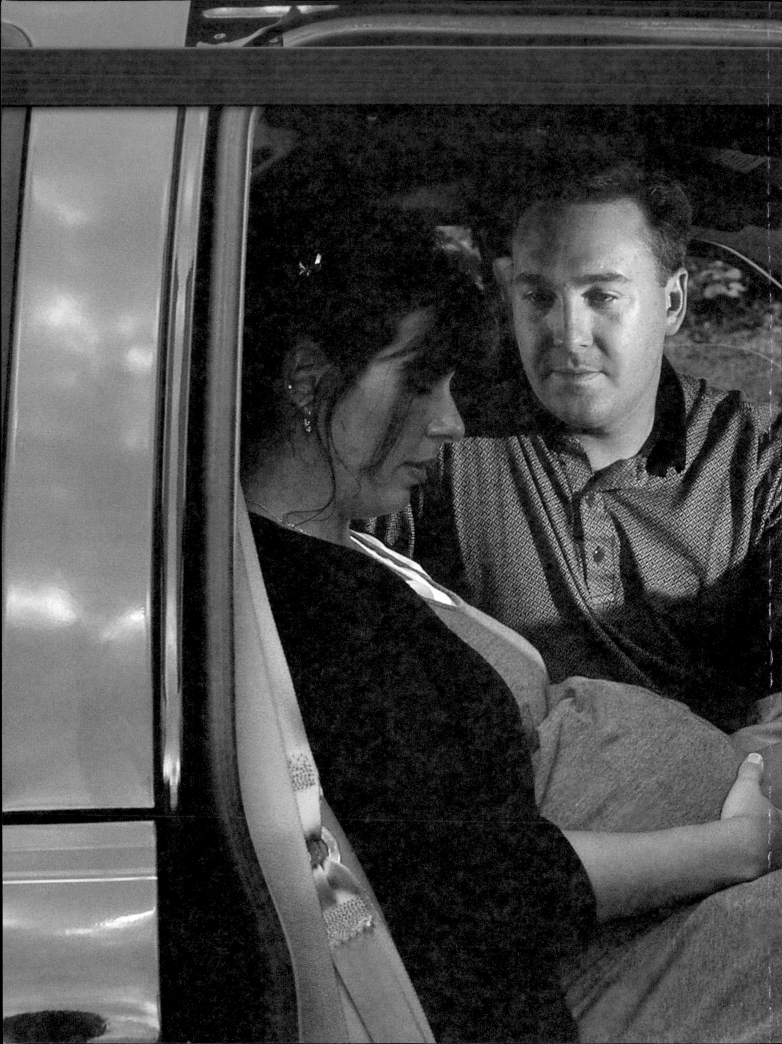

Chapter 20

Childbirth and Gynecologic Emergencies

Handling childbirth and gynecologic situations requires that a first aider be familiar with the terminology used to describe female reproductive anatomy and physiology.

- The **birth canal** includes the vagina and the lower part of the uterus.
- The **cervix** is the small opening at the lower end of the uterus through which the baby passes.
- The **placenta** (afterbirth) is the organ through which the mother and the fetus exchange nourishment and waste products during pregnancy. It is expelled after the baby's birth.
- The **umbilical cord** is the extension of the placenta through which the fetus receives nourishment while in the uterus.
- The **amniotic sac** ("bag of waters") surrounds the fetus inside the uterus. **Amniotic fluid** in the sac cushions the fetus and helps protect it from injury.
- **Crowning** occurs when the fetus's head or presenting part presses against the vagina and begins to bulge out.
- **Bloody show** is the mucus and blood that may be discharged from the vagina as labor begins.
- **Labor** is the time and the process of childbirth (defined in three stages), from the first regular uterine-muscle contractions until delivery of the placenta.
- A **miscarriage** (medical term is **spontaneous abortion**) is the delivery of a fetus before it can live independently of the mother.

Predelivery Emergencies

Miscarriage

Miscarriages usually occur during the first three months (first trimester) of pregnancy. Most happen because the fetus was not developing properly and was not able to survive. The signs and symptoms of a potential miscarriage include vaginal bleeding and pain resembling menstrual cramps. Signs of an inevitable miscarriage include heavy vaginal bleeding and cramping pain in the abdomen, and aching in the lower back.

Care for Miscarriage

1. Call EMS.
2. Have the woman place a sanitary pad over the outside of the vagina.
3. Any fetal tissue should be transported with the woman to the hospital.

Vaginal Bleeding in Late Pregnancy

If a woman has vaginal bleeding late in her pregnancy (third trimester or last three months), find out how long she has been bleeding and how many sanitary pads she has used so that you can report to medical personnel. An increase in pulse rate of more than 20 beats per minute when the victim goes from a lying-down to a sitting position suggests blood loss greater than one pint.

Care for Vaginal Bleeding in Late Pregnancy

1. Face woman on her left side to relieve pressure on the mother's circulatory system (the vena cava) from the fetus.
2. Seek medical attention.

Vaginal Bleeding Caused by Injury

External vaginal bleeding caused by trauma usually can be controlled by applying external pressure over the laceration. Internal vaginal bleeding, however, can be massive. It is both useless and dangerous to introduce packs blindly into the vagina in an attempt to control bleeding. A pack should be used *only* if bleeding is life threatening. Place the victim on her left side to help prevent vomiting, to prevent aspiration of vomitus, and to relieve pressure on the mother's circulatory system (vena cava) from the fetus. Seek medical attention.

Care for Injury-related Vaginal Bleeding

1. Use direct pressure to control external bleeding from a laceration or other injury.
2. Apply an ice pack to reduce swelling and pain.

Never place or pack dressings into the vagina unless the bleeding is life threatening. Place the woman on her left side. Seek medical attention.

Care for Noninjury-related Vaginal Bleeding

Noninjury-related vaginal bleeding can result from various causes, but treatment is similar.

1. Have the woman place a sanitary pad over the vaginal opening.
2. Seek medical attention.

Delivery

Childbirth in an out-of-hospital setting rarely occurs. Because of the infrequency, taking care of an anxious mother and her newborn infant is a stressful event for a first aider. On the other hand, assisting in the birth of a baby is one of the few situations in which first aiders have the opportunity to participate in a happy event rather than an unpleasant one.

At the scene of a woman in labor, you will need to determine if delivery is imminent or whether there is time to transport the woman to the hospital. To make that decision, answer the following questions:

- *Has the woman had a baby before?* Labor during a first pregnancy is usually longer than in subsequent pregnancies. If this is her first pregnancy, there may be more time for transport to a hospital.
- *How frequent are the contractions?* Contractions more than five minutes apart are a good indication that there will be enough time to get the mother to a nearby hospital. Contractions less than two minutes apart that last 45 to 60 seconds, especially in a woman who has had more than one pregnancy, signal imminent delivery.
- *Has the amniotic sac ruptured? If so, when?* If the sac ruptures more than 18 hours before birth occurs, the likelihood of fetal infection increases, and the hospital staff should be alerted. Delivery may be more difficult when the amniotic sac ruptures prematurely, because amniotic fluid serves as a lubricant.
- *Does the mother feel as though she has to move her bowels?* That sensation is caused by the fetal head in the vagina pressing against the rectum and indicates that delivery is imminent.

Only if the answers to those questions seem to indicate an imminent birth should you examine the mother for crowning. Look to see if there is bulging at the vaginal opening or if part of the baby is visible. Crowning indicates that the baby is about to be born and that there is no time to get to a hospital before delivery. Because this step may be embarrassing to the mother, the father, bystanders, even you, it is important that you explain fully what you are doing and why. Make every effort to protect the woman from embarrassment during such an examination by removing only enough clothing to expose the vaginal area. Use something to shield the woman from prying eyes, for example, a blanket used to make a tent, or even a human shield, with people standing with their backs toward her.

Consider transporting the woman to a hospital only if she is not straining or crowning and this is her first pregnancy. Making a hasty decision to transport the woman means that the delivery could take place under the worst possible circumstances. When there is enough time to transport the woman to a hospital, place her on her left side. That position prevents a possible drop in blood pressure caused by pressure on the inferior vena cava (large vein between the spine and the abdominal organs), which reduces venous blood returning to the heart.

If the woman is straining or crowning, has had prior pregnancies, and there is not enough time to get to the hospital, you must prepare to assist in the delivery. First, call (or have a bystander call) the EMS. Then, if the woman is in a crowded or public place, try to find a private, clean area. The mother may find it reassuring to have a companion, such as her husband, a friend, or a relative, present. Follow these guidelines:

- Wear medical exam gloves. If available, wear a mask, a gown, and eye protection.
- Do not touch the vaginal area except during delivery and, if possible, with a witness present.
- Do not let the mother use the toilet.
- Do not hold the mother's legs together.

If the baby's head is not the presenting part, the delivery may be complicated. Tell the mother not to push and attempt to calm and reassure her.

Caution:

DO NOT allow the mother to go to the toilet if delivery seems imminent.

DO NOT attempt to delay or restrain delivery in any way (eg, holding the mother's legs together).

Stages of Labor

Labor is a three-stage process that begins with the first regular uterine contractions, includes delivery of the baby, and ends with delivery of the placenta. The first stage usually lasts several hours (possibly 18 hours or more for a first baby), from the first contraction until the cervix is fully open (dilated). The cervix gradually stretches until it is large enough to let the baby pass through. (Outside a hospital setting, rescuers cannot safely check for dilation of the cervix.) The contractions usually begin as acutely aching sensations in the small of the back; in a short time, they turn into cramp-like pains recurring regularly in the lower abdomen. At first, the contractions are 10 to 15 minutes apart, are not very severe, and last less than a minute. Gradually, the intervals between contractions grow shorter, and the contractions increase in intensity. A slight, watery, bloodstained discharge from the vagina may accompany contractions or may occur before labor begins.

At the end of the first stage of labor, the amniotic sac breaks, and a pint or more of watery fluid, the amniotic fluid, discharges. Sometimes the amniotic sac breaks during the first stage of labor, but this is no cause for concern because it usually does not affect labor. If the amniotic sac breaks prematurely and labor does not begin within 12 hours, the risk of infection to mother and baby is great.

The second stage lasts from 30 minutes to 2 hours. It begins when the neck of the cervix is fully open and ends with the actual birth of the baby. The baby is normally head down; once the head gets through the pelvis, the rest of the body should follow easily.

During the third stage, which lasts about 15 minutes or more, the afterbirth (placenta) is expelled ▶Figure 20-1 .

Delivery Procedures

Ideally, you should have the following supplies for delivery:

- clean sheets, towels, and blankets to cover the mother and baby
- a plastic bag or towel to wrap the placenta for delivery to the hospital
- clean, unused, medical exam gloves to reduce the likelihood of infection
- sanitary pads
- newspapers, plastic, or a cloth sheet to place under the woman to provide for a clean delivery area

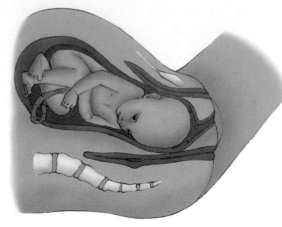

a. End of the first stage of labor

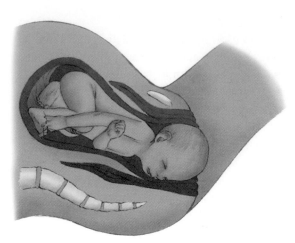

b. Head delivers face down

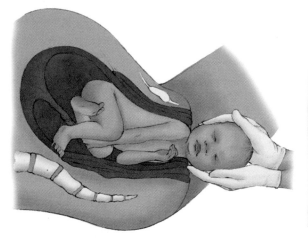

c. Support the head

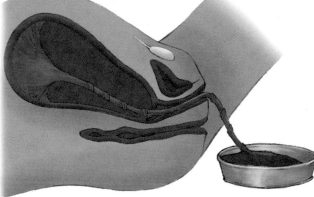

d. Placenta expelled in 5 to 20 minutes

Figure 20-1) Normal stages of childbirth.

- rubber bulb syringe for suctioning the baby's mouth and nostrils
- sterile gauze pads for wiping blood and mucus from the baby's mouth and nose
- new or clean shoelaces or similar materials to tie the cord. (Do not use thread, wire, or string because they might cut through the cord.)

What to Do

If you are faced with an imminent delivery, follow these steps:

1. Take infection-control precautions by washing your hands thoroughly and wearing medical exam gloves. If possible, wear a mask, a gown, and eye protection.

2. Have the mother lie on her back with her head slightly elevated, knees drawn up and legs spread apart. The mother might want to be in a different position. Other safe positions for childbirth include:

   - Sitting up or squatting, with someone behind supporting her. These two positions place less tension on the vaginal tissues, reducing the likelihood of a tear, and allow the force of gravity to help.

- Lying on her left side, which improves blood return to her heart and prevents aspiration should she vomit. Have someone hold the woman's right leg up out of the way.

- Kneeling in a knee-chest position, which is used in less developed countries and in cases of breech presentations.

Remind the woman to take short, quick breaths during each contraction. Between contractions, she should rest and breathe deeply through her mouth.

3. Place absorbent, clean materials (sheets, towels, etc) under the mother's buttocks.

4. Elevate her buttocks with blankets or a pillow.

5. When the baby's head appears, place the palm of your hand on top of the head and exert very gentle pressure, to prevent explosive delivery. Do not push on the fontanels (soft spots on the front and back of the infant's head).

6. If the amniotic sac does not break or has not broken, tear it with your fingers and push it away from the baby's head and mouth as they appear. The baby could suffocate if the sac is not removed.

7. As the baby's head emerges from the vagina, determine if the umbilical cord is wrapped around the baby's neck. If it is, gently slip the cord over the baby's shoulder. If you cannot do that, attempt to alleviate pressure on the cord. (See number 17 below for instructions).

8. Support the baby's head as it emerges.

9. Suction the baby's mouth and then the nostrils two or three times with the bulb syringe. Use caution to avoid contact with the back of the baby's mouth. If a bulb syringe is not available, wipe the baby's mouth and then the nose with gauze.

10. As the torso and full body emerge, support the baby with both hands—he or she will be slippery.

11. Do not pull on the baby, which could cause cervical spine damage. Do not put your fingers in the baby's armpits; pressure on the nerve centers there could cause paralysis.

12. Keep the baby level with the vagina.

13. Wipe blood and mucus from the baby's mouth and nose with sterile gauze; suction the mouth, then the nose again.

14. Dry the infant to reduce heat loss and help stimulate breathing. Rub the baby's back or flick the soles of its feet to stimulate breathing. The baby should breathe within 30 seconds, especially after the cord stops pulsing. (Do not hold the baby up by the feet and slap its buttocks—that could cause an increase in intracranial pressure.)

15. Wrap the infant in a warm blanket and place the baby on his or her side, head slightly lower than the trunk. Keep the infant level with the mother's vagina until the cord is cut. Raising the baby above the mother's abdomen (location of the placenta) while the umbilical cord is intact will allow the baby's blood to drain out and may put the baby in shock. Holding the baby below the mother's abdomen allows her blood to run into the baby, where the extra blood cells can cause serious problems such as jaundice.

16. When the umbilical cord stops pulsating, tie it with gauze between the mother and the newborn.

17. If the mother is going to the hospital soon after the birth, and it was a normal delivery, there is no need to cut the cord. Keep the infant warm and wait for the EMS personnel, who will have the proper equipment to clamp and cut the cord. If you are in a remote location, you may have to cut the cord yourself. After cord pulsations stop, tie the cord about four inches away from the baby and make a second tie 2 inches further away from the first tie. Cut the cord between the two ties.

18. Watch for delivery of the placenta, which usually takes a few minutes, but could take as long as 30 minutes. Do not pull on the end of the umbilical cord to speed the placenta's delivery.

19. When the placenta is delivered, wrap it in a towel with three-quarters of the umbilical cord and place the towel in a plastic bag. Keep the bag at the level of the infant. Take the placenta to the hospital, where it will be examined for completeness. This procedure is necessary because pieces of placenta retained in the uterus can cause persistent bleeding or infection.

20. Place a sterile pad over the vaginal opening, lower the mother's legs, and help her hold them together.

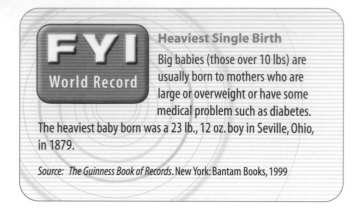

Vaginal Bleeding Following Delivery

A woman can be expected to lose from 300 to 500 ml (one to two cups) of blood after delivery. You should be aware of this amount of blood loss so it does not cause undue psychological stress to the new mother or yourself. If blood loss continues, massage the uterus. Uterine massage stimulates the uterus to contract, thus constricting blood vessels within its walls and decreasing bleeding.

1. Use your hand with your fingers fully extended.
2. Place the palm of your hand on the lower abdomen where you should be able to feel a grapefruit-sized mass.
3. Massage (knead) over the area.
4. If bleeding continues, check your massage technique.

The mother can also nurse the baby following delivery of the placenta to stimulate uterine contractions and thus help control bleeding.

Initial Care of the Newborn

Normal findings in a newborn are pulse rate greater than 100 per minute (feel the brachial artery) and a respiratory rate greater than 40 breaths per minute. The baby should be crying.

The most important care is positioning, drying, keeping warm, and stimulating the newborn to breathe. Wrap the newborn in a blanket, making sure the head is covered. Repeat suctioning if necessary and continue to stimulate the newborn if he or she is not breathing (flick soles of the feet and rub infant's back).

If the newborn does not begin to breathe within 30 seconds or continues to have difficulty breathing after one minute, you must consider the need for additional measures:

1. Ensure that the airway is open.
2. Give one rescue breath every three seconds.
3. Reassess after one minute.

Postdelivery Care of the Mother

After delivery, monitor the mother's breathing and pulse. Replace any blood-soaked sheets and blankets while awaiting transport.

Abnormal Deliveries

Most childbirths are normal and natural. Sometimes, however, complications arise. It is essential that you be calm, deliberate, and gentle in a situation that becomes even more stressful by unforeseen problems.

Prolapsed Cord

A prolapsed cord is a condition in which the umbilical cord comes through the birth canal before delivery of the head. This puts the baby in danger of suffocation (▼ **Figure 20-2**).

Figure 20-2 Prolapsed cord

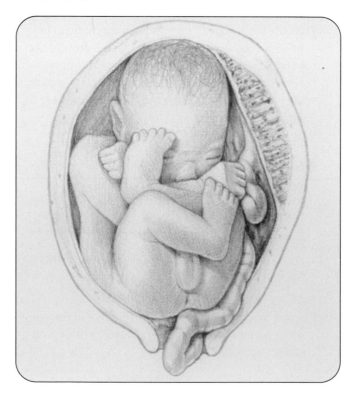

1. Position the woman with her head down or buttocks raised to use gravity to lessen pressure in the birth canal.

2. Insert your gloved hand into the vagina and gently push the presenting part of the fetus away from the pulsating cord. Again, do *not* push the cord back into the vagina.

3. Seek EMS transport *immediately*.

Breech presentation and prolapsed umbilical cord are the only two cases in which the first aider should place his or her hand in the mother's vagina.

Caution:

DO NOT attempt to push the cord back into the vagina.

Breech Birth Presentation

A breech presentation occurs when the baby's buttocks or lower extremities crown before the head or shoulders.

Figure 20-3 Breech presentation

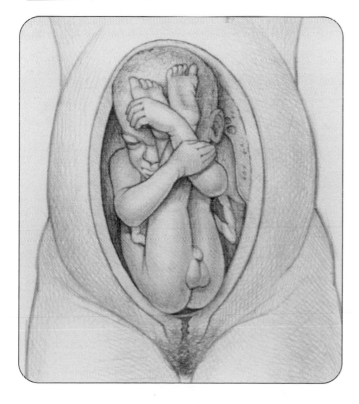

Breech presentation is the most common type of abnormal delivery, and occurs in 3% to 4% of all deliveries. Place the mother in a kneeling, head-down position, with her pelvis elevated, and seek medical care *immediately* ◄**Figure 20-3** .

If the baby's head is not delivered within three minutes of the body, you must act to prevent suffocation of the baby. Suffocation can occur when the baby's face is pressed against the vaginal wall or when the umbilical cord is compressed by the baby's head in the vagina. To establish an airway:

1. Place one hand in the vagina, positioning the palm toward the baby's face.

2. Form a V with your fingers on either side of the baby's nose.

3. Push the vaginal wall away from the baby's face until the head is delivered.

Caution:

DO NOT pull the baby's head out during a breech delivery.

Limb Presentation

Limb presentation occurs when a single arm, leg, or foot of the infant protrudes from the birth canal. A foot more commonly presents when the infant is in breech presentation ►**Figure 20-4** .

1. Place mother in head-down position with pelvis elevated. Do *not* pull on the baby or attempt to push the limb back into the vagina.

2. Call for EMS transportation *immediately*. The baby cannot be delivered in this position.

Presence of Meconium

Amniotic fluid that is greenish-yellow or brownish-yellow rather than clear means the baby has had a bowel movement, an indication of possible fetal distress during labor.

1. Suction the mouth and nostrils thoroughly, or the baby will aspirate its own waste (meconium) with its first breath. Clear amniotic fluid, however, is harmlessly absorbed through the baby's lungs.

Skill Scan **Childbirth**

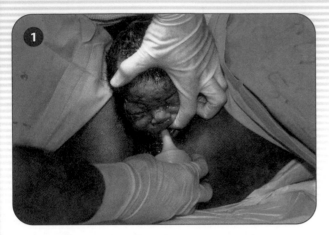

1. Support the head and suction mouth and nose.

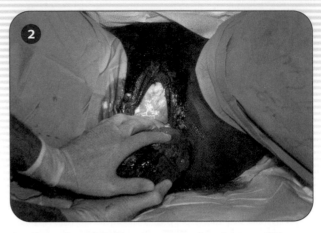

2. Once head delivers, upper shoulders will be visible.

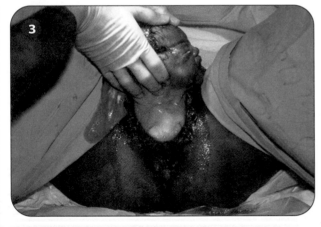

3. Support head and body as shoulders deliver.

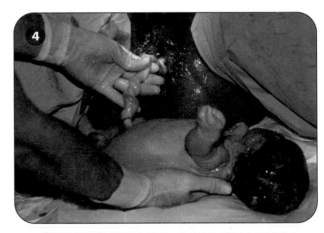

4. Clean and dry infant to reduce heat loss and stimulate breathing.

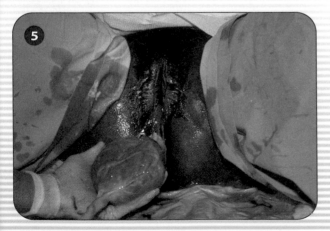

5. Allow the placenta to deliver. Do not pull on the umbilical cord.

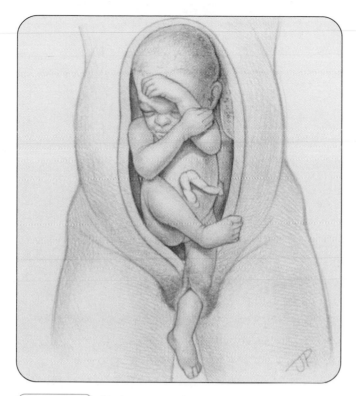

Figure 20-4 Limb presentation

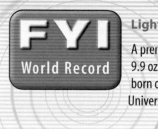
2. Maintain the baby's open airway.
3. Call for EMS transportation *immediately*.

Premature Birth

Any baby weighing less than 5.5 pounds or born before seven months of pregnancy is defined as premature and needs special care. Premature babies develop problems because they are so small and their organs are immature.

1. Keep the baby warm. Premature babies are always at risk for hypothermia.
2. Perform resuscitation, if necessary.

Gynecologic Emergencies

Gynecologic emergencies are reproductive-system problems that occur in nonpregnant females.

Vaginal Bleeding

For trauma-related soft-tissue injuries, use direct pressure to control bleeding. Apply an ice pack to reduce swelling and pain. Apply a diaper-type bandage to hold dressings in place. Never place or pack dressings into the vagina. Stabilize any foreign bodies in place. Seek medical attention.

Nontrauma vaginal bleeding can result from various causes, but treatment is the same. Have the victim place a sanitary pad over the vaginal opening and seek medical attention.

Sexual Assault and Rape

Perhaps one of the most difficult emergency situations that a first aider may have to deal with is sexual assault. Rape is the fastest-growing violent crime in the United States. Authorities suspect that only a small proportion of rape cases are reported. In most cases, the rape victim is a woman. It should be noted, however, that men, both heterosexual and homosexual, also may be raped.

There are many definitions of rape, but in general, rape involves attempted or actual forced sexual intercourse, against the will of the victim. Related physical injury is common, but the psychological trauma is more damaging. It is essential that you be calm and sympathetic when dealing with a victim of sexual assault.

Your job as a first aider is to care for the victim, not to collect evidence. Confine your questions to an assessment of the victim's injuries, not a detailed description of the events. Ask questions based on the SAMPLE survey (see Chapter 4).

Determine which injuries require immediate care. Whenever it is necessary that a female victim disrobe, have another woman present. Also whenever possible, a same-sex first aider should perform the examination.

Do not expose the genitalia unless an injury there requires immediate care (eg, severe bleeding). Examining genitalia, except when childbirth is imminent, has serious legal implications and therefore usually should not be done.

EMERGENCY CHILDBIRTH

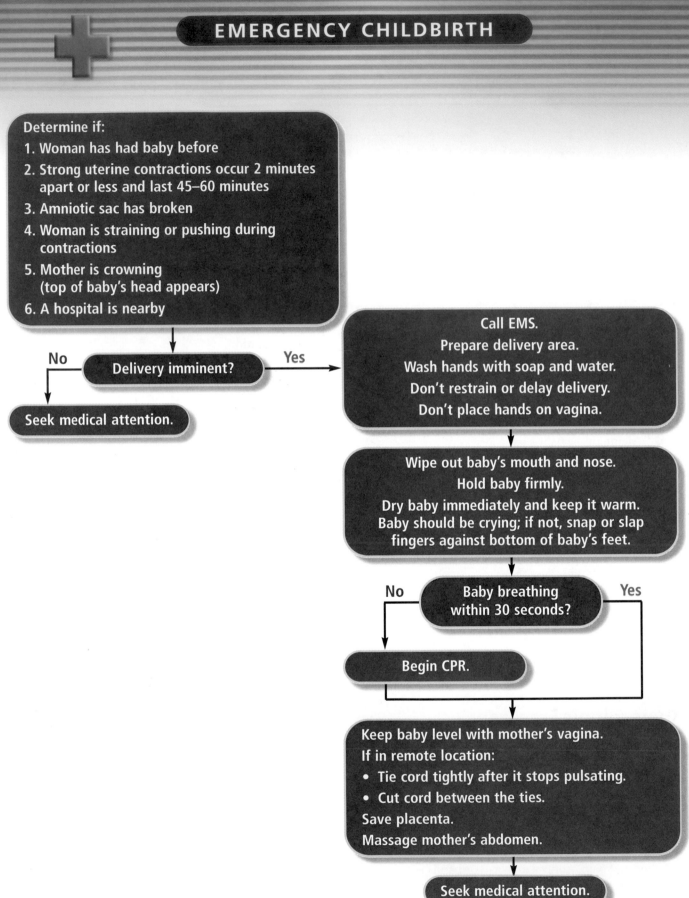

Determine if:

1. Woman has had baby before
2. Strong uterine contractions occur 2 minutes apart or less and last 45–60 minutes
3. Amniotic sac has broken
4. Woman is straining or pushing during contractions
5. Mother is crowning (top of baby's head appears)
6. A hospital is nearby

Delivery imminent?

No → Seek medical attention.

Yes →

Call EMS.
Prepare delivery area.
Wash hands with soap and water.
Don't restrain or delay delivery.
Don't place hands on vagina.

Wipe out baby's mouth and nose.
Hold baby firmly.
Dry baby immediately and keep it warm.
Baby should be crying; if not, snap or slap fingers against bottom of baby's feet.

Baby breathing within 30 seconds?

No → Begin CPR.

Yes →

Keep baby level with mother's vagina.
If in remote location:
• Tie cord tightly after it stops pulsating.
• Cut cord between the ties.
Save placenta.
Massage mother's abdomen.

Seek medical attention.

Emergencies During Pregnancy

What medical specialties take care of women?

A gynecologist specializes treating conditions related to the female reproductive cycle. An obstetrician specializes in treating pregnant women. A pediatrician specializes in treating newborn babies, toddlers, and young teens.

How is emergency care for a pregnant woman different?

There are two victims involved—mother and fetus. Even minor trauma to the abdomen can result in threatening consequences. All pregnant women with trauma to their abdomen need a medical examination in a hospital emergency department and often need fetal monitoring. Fetal viability is determined by mother viability. Position the mother on her left side to help venous blood return to the heart.

What are some indications of pregnancy problems?

+ The "big three" warning signs of a serious problem: bleeding, abdominal cramps, and weakness.

+ Morning sickness, swollen ankles, and urinary tract infections are not usually dangerous, but call the doctor anyway.

+ If a pregnant woman is "spotting," get her into bed immediately. It can signal the onset of a miscarriage.

Try, if possible, to preserve evidence but leave the actual investigation to the police. To preserve evidence, encourage the victim not to change clothes, wash, urinate, defecate, or douche. Explain to the victim in a sympathetic way that it would be best not to "clean up." Keep in mind that a rape victim, like any other victim, has the right to refuse first aid and transport to a hospital.

Even if the victim refuses aid, do not leave him or her alone. Try to have a trusted friend or relative stay with the victim. Protect the privacy of the victim. Emotional support is vital. Most large communities have rape crisis centers; furnishing the victim with the name and number of the nearest center (look in the telephone directory) is probably as important as treating any physical injuries.

Urinary Tract Infections

What should be done about urinary tract infections?

Women, especially during pregnancy, are very susceptible to urinary tract infections. Often, when one infection clears, another replaces it.

Seek advice from an obstetrician. Self-care to help relieve the burning pain include taking shallow, lukewarm sitz baths sprinkled with baking soda, urinating while standing in the shower, and practicing good personal hygiene. Wiping from front to back by a woman when going to the bathroom will help keep E-coli bacteria away from the urinary tract. Drinking more fluids helps prevent and treat urinary tract infections. Some experts report that drinking cranberry juice (tablets are also available with fewer calories) may help inhibit urinary tract infections.

A urinary tract infection can lead to the more serious bladder infection. Signs of a bladder infection include blood in urine, pain in the lower back or flank, fever, and nausea or vomiting.

STUDY
Questions (20)

Name_____ Course_____ Date_____

Case Situations

Case 1

While you are visiting your uncle and his family on their farm 20 miles from town, a blizzard blocks everyone from leaving. Your pregnant aunt starts labor. This is her first pregnancy. After about four hours of labor, you time the contractions and find they are 30 seconds in duration and about three minutes apart. You have your uncle examine his wife, and he reports no crowning.

____ **1.** Your aunt is in what stage of labor?
   a. first stage
   b. second stage
   c. third stage

____ **2.** Care of your aunt would include
   a. transport to the town's hospital
   b. calling the EMS

____ **3.** What care is considered appropriate for controlling vaginal bleeding following birth?
   a. placing a sanitary napkin into the vagina
   b. applying a warm pad over the mother's abdomen
   c. massaging the mother's lower abdomen

Case 2

A woman is expecting her first child. Her amniotic sac (bag of waters) broke an hour ago, and her contractions are now about 10 to 12 minutes apart.

1. What stage of labor is this woman experiencing?
_____
_____
_____

2. The first stage of labor typically lasts _____ hours.

3. Describe the second stage of labor and how long it typically lasts.
_____
_____
_____

Case 3

The following presents an opportunity for self-evaluation and review of situations surrounding emergency childbirth.

1. When is it necessary for a first aider to assist in or perform an emergency on-site delivery of a baby?
   a. _____
   _____
   b. _____
   _____
   c. _____
   _____

2. What factors must be considered to determine if a woman is in advanced stages of labor?
   a. _____
   _____
   b. _____
   _____
   c. _____
   _____
   d. _____
   _____

3. What should you do if you have determined that an emergency on-site delivery is necessary?
   a. _____
   _____
   b. _____
   _____
   c. _____
   _____

____ **4.** When the baby's head first appears during a normal delivery, you should
   a. gently pull on the head to ease delivery
   b. support the head gently to prevent explosive delivery

5. What should you do if the umbilical cord is wrapped around the baby's neck?
_____
_____
_____

STUDY
Questions (20)

Case 4

A pregnant woman lives in a rural setting approximately one hour from the closest medical facility. She says she is having painful contractions three to five minutes apart and feels the urge to have a bowel movement. She informs you that she has two other children. On examination you see that the woman's vagina is bulging.

1. What would be your decision regarding moving the mother-to-be? Why?

   _____

   _____

   _____

2. What is the first thing you should do once the baby's head has been successfully delivered?

   _____

   _____

   _____

___ 3. The umbilical cord is cut after the baby is delivered because the child no longer depends on it for oxygen and nourishment.
   a. True
   b. False

4. What occurs during the third stage of labor?

   _____

   _____

   _____

5. Why is it necessary to save the placenta and deliver it to the hospital with the mother and the newborn?

   _____

   _____

   _____

6. What steps should you take to care for the normal newborn child?
   a. _____

   _____

   b. _____

   _____

   c. _____

   _____

7. How does rescue breathing for a newborn differ from rescue breathing for an adult?

   a. _____

   _____

   b. _____

   _____

8. What steps are involved in caring for the umbilical cord?

   a. _____

   _____

   b. _____

   _____

___ 9. How long after the baby is born is the placenta usually delivered?
   a. 15 to 20 minutes
   b. 30 to 60 minutes
   c. one to two hours
   d. more than two hours

10. List three types of complicated deliveries.
   a. _____

   _____

   b. _____

   _____

   c. _____

   _____

11. Describe two conditions under which a first aider should have contact with the mother's vaginal area.
   a. _____

   _____

   b. _____

   _____

12. What should you do after the baby and the placenta have been delivered?

   _____

   _____

Chapter Activities

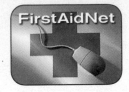

WEB Activities

Childbirth and Gynecologic Emergencies

Visit nsc.jbpub.com/FirstAidNet, then click on Web Activities, and select the appropriate chapter.

Emergency Childbirth

Emergency Medical Services help may not be available in time for some childbirths. In such cases, one must be prepared to help in the delivery.

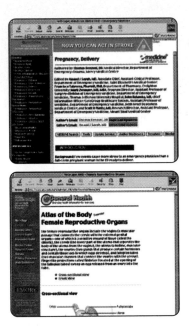

Female Reproductive Organs

Knowing the female body and the reproductive organs will help a first aider in a childbirth or gynecological emergency.

Chapter 21

Behavioral Emergencies

Behavior is how we act. Although we all act or behave differently, sometimes an individual will exhibit behavior that is unacceptable or intolerable. The abnormal behavior may be due to a psychological condition (such as a mental illness) or to a physical condition. For example, a diabetic with uncorrected low blood sugar can display aggressiveness, restlessness, or anxiety. Because the brain lacks energy in the form of blood sugar (glucose), an altered mental status results. Likewise, lack of oxygen and inadequate blood flow to the brain also cause altered mental status, resulting in similar behavior. Behavior that leads to violence or other inappropriate activities is known as a **behavioral emergency.**

Several factors can change a person's behavior, including situational stresses, medical illnesses, psychiatric problems, alcohol, or drugs. The following are common reasons for behavior changes:

- low blood sugar in a diabetic
- lack of oxygen (known as hypoxia)
- inadequate blood flow to the brain
- head trauma
- mind-altering substances, such as alcohol, depressants, stimulants, hallucinogens, and narcotics
- psychogenic or psychiatric illness that leads to psychotic thinking, depression, or panic
- excessive cold
- excessive heat

Depression

Depression can lead to suicide; in fact, 50% of all suicides involve depression. Depressed people often can be recognized by their sad appearance, crying spells, and listless or apathetic behavior. They feel worthless, guilty, and extremely pessimistic. Asserting that no one understands or cares about them and that their problems cannot be solved, they often express the desire to be left alone. Their speech may seem as if they have hardly enough energy to talk, and they may have sleeping difficulties.

Some depressed people do not feel like talking. In such cases, saying, "You look very sad," often allows the person to talk about the depressed feelings. They may burst into tears. Do not discourage their crying. Maintain a sympathetic silence and let them "cry themselves out."

A depressed person needs sympathetic attention and reassurance. He or she needs to know that the first aider is concerned. It is usually best to interview a depressed person in private, because the presence of several people may make the person uncomfortable. Tell the depressed person that many people have periods of unhappiness, but they can be helped to feel better. Mention community resources where such help can be found.

Suicide

Suicide is defined as any willful act that ends one's own life. Each year, a reported 25,000 to 30,000 Americans commit suicide; it is the tenth leading cause of death in the United States. Many experts, however, believe that suicide is vastly underreported. Suicide in the United States is increasingly a problem of adolescents, college-age students, and the very old.

The male rate for suicides is more than three times that for females. It is most common in men who are single, widowed, or divorced. Slightly more than half of all suicides—both men and women—use firearms. The next most common method is hanging. Poisoning by solids or liquids is the most common method used by people who attempt but do not complete suicide. Jumping from high places, carbon monoxide poisoning by auto exhaust, drowning, and self-inflicted wounds are less common methods.

The number of suicides peaks during spring months, rises again in the fall, and is lowest in December. Suicide rates are lowest in the Northeast and highest in the West.

Suicide attempts are eight times more common than completed suicides. In addition, although males complete suicide three times more often than females, females are reported to attempt suicide three times more often. It is not known whether males are more reluctant to seek help and therefore less likely to report their attempts. It also is not known whether the lower rate of suicide among females results from their choice of less lethal methods despite an equal desire to die.

Even though it is a major cause of death, suicide is a rare event. Except in the case of suicide clusters (three or more completed suicides closely related in time and place), no community is likely to experience many suicides.

Table 21-1: Suicide Risk Factors

The SAD PERSONS scale is a mnemonic list of known suicide high-risk characteristics. A score of 9 or greater indicates the probable need for psychiatric consultation.

Mnemonic		Characteristics	Score
S	**S**ex	Male	1
A	**A**ge	Under 19 or over 45	1
D	**D**epression or hopelessness	Admits to depression or decreased concentration, appetite, sleep, libido	2
P	**P**revious attempts or psychiatric care	Previous inpatient or outpatient psychiatric care	1
E	**E**xcessive alcohol or drug use	Chronic addiction or recent frequent use drug use	1
R	**R**ational-thinking loss	Organic brain syndrome or psychosis	2
S	**S**eparated, widowed, or divorced		1
O	**O**rganized or serious attempt	Well-thought-out plan or "life-threatening" display	2
N	**N**o social support	No close family, friends, job, or active religious affiliation	1
S	**S**tated future intent	Determined to repeat attempt	2

Determining if high-risk factors are involved will help you maintain objectivity. It is important that the first aider maintain a nonjudgmental approach. Using the SAD PERSONS mnemonic acknowledges the seriousness of the situation and reminds the first aider that ridiculing, making demeaning comments, or ignoring the person is neither helpful nor proper.

Take precautions by keeping the person under close observation, removing any potentially dangerous items (eg, glass, razors, medicines) from the immediate area, and not allowing the person to go *anywhere,* even to the bathroom, unaccompanied.

Source: R. S. Hockberger and R. J. Rothstein: "Assessment of Suicide Potential by Non-psychiatrists Using the SAD PERSONS Score." *Journal of Emergency Medicine,* 6(2):99-107, March-April 1988.

Suicide is often attempted by those who are depressed or alcoholic. At least 60% of all suicide victims previously attempted suicide, and 75% gave clear warning that they intended to kill themselves. Typically, a suicide attempt occurs when an individual's close emotional attachments are in danger or when he or she loses a significant family member or friend. Suicidal people often feel unable to manage their lives. Frequently, they lack self-esteem.

Many suicidal people make last-minute attempts to communicate their intentions. When an individual phones to threaten suicide, someone should stay on the line until the EMS reaches the scene.

Fables and Facts about Suicide

These statements are not true:

Fable: People who talk about suicide do not commit suicide.

Fable: Suicide happens without warning.

Fable: Suicidal people are fully intent on dying.

Fable: Once a person is suicidal, he or she is suicidal forever.

Fable: Improvement following a suicidal crisis means that the suicidal risk is over.

Fable: Suicide strikes more often among the rich—or, conversely, it occurs more frequently among the poor.

Fable: Suicide is inherited or "runs in a family" (ie, is genetically determined).

Fable: All suicidal individuals are mentally ill, and suicide is always the act of a psychotic person.

These statements are true:

Fact: Of every 10 people who kill themselves, 8 have given definite warnings of their suicidal intentions. Suicide threats and attempts must be taken seriously.

Fact: Studies reveal that the suicidal person gives many clues and warnings regarding suicidal intentions. Being alert to these cries for help may prevent suicidal behavior.

Fact: Most suicidal people are undecided about living or dying, and they gamble with death, leaving it to others to save them. Almost no one commits suicide without letting others know how he or she is feeling. Often this cry for help is given in code. Decoding these distress signals can save lives.

Fact: Fortunately, individuals who wish to kill themselves are suicidal only for a limited period of time. If they are saved from self-destruction, they can go on to lead useful lives.

Fact: Most suicides occur within three months after the beginning of improvement, when the individual has the energy to put morbid thoughts and feelings into effect. Relatives and physicians should be especially vigilant during this period.

Fact: Suicide is neither the rich man's disease nor the poor man's curse. Suicide is democratic and is represented proportionately at all levels of society.

Fact: Suicide does not run in families. It is an individual matter, and can be prevented.

Fact: Studies of hundreds of genuine suicide notes indicate that although a suicidal person is extremely unhappy, he or she is not necessarily mentally ill. The overpowering unhappiness may result from a temporary emotional upset, a long and painful illness, or a complete loss of hope. It is circular reasoning to say that suicide is an insane act; therefore, all suicidal people are psychotic.

Source: U.S. Department of Health and Human Resources

If you encounter a person who is attempting or threatening suicide, discreetly remove any dangerous articles. Talk quietly with the person. Encourage him or her to discuss the situation. Ask the following: *Have you attempted suicide before? Have you made any concrete plans concerning a method of suicide? Has any family member ever committed suicide?*

Individuals who have made a previous suicide attempt, who have detailed suicide plans, or who have a close relative who committed suicide are more likely to try to kill themselves. These people must be reassured and taken to medical help, usually at a hospital. Do *not* leave them alone under any circumstances.

When an individual attempts suicide, first aid care has priority. Drug overdoses must be managed. Bleeding from slashed wrists must be controlled. As you render first aid, try to encourage the person to talk about the situation. If a drug overdose is involved, collect any medication containers, pills, or other drugs found on the scene and bring the items to the hospital emergency department with the victim. In many cases, law enforcement authorities should be contacted.

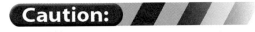

Caution:

DO NOT ignore a suicide threat. Every suicidal act or gesture should be taken seriously and the person referred to a professional counselor.

Emotional Injury

First aid for an emotional injury really means nothing more than being supportive of people with emotional injuries, whether those injuries are from physical injury or from excessive or unbearable strain on the victim's emotions.

Emotional first aid often goes hand in hand with physical first aid, because a physical injury and the circumstances surrounding it may actually cause emotional injury. On the other hand, emotional injury may occur even when there is no physical injury. Emotional injuries usually are not as obvious as physical injuries, but both can be severe and require first aid.

Although most emotional reactions are temporary, lasting only minutes, hours, or, at the most, a few days, they are seriously disabling and may upset others. It is important to know that first aid can be applied to emotional as well as physical injuries.

Typical Reactions

With few exceptions, all people experience fear in the face of an emergency. Feeling shaky, perspiring profusely, and becoming a little nauseated are common. Such reactions are normal and no cause for concern. Most people are able to collect themselves reasonably quickly.

Extensive training is not needed to recognize severe, abnormal reactions. To determine whether a person needs help, find out if he or she is doing something that makes sense and is able to take care of himself or herself.

For the most part, emotional first aid measures are simple and easy to understand. However, improvisation is often called for, just as it is in splinting a fracture. Whatever the situation, you will have your own emotional reactions toward the victim. These reactions are important—they can either enhance or hinder your ability to help the person. Especially when you are tired or worried, you may easily become impatient with the victim who seems to be "making a mountain out of a molehill." You may even feel resentful toward the victim for being a burden. Be on guard against becoming impatient, intolerant, or resentful. Victims who can see the first aider's calmness, confidence, and competence will be reassured.

On the other hand, do not be overly sympathetic or overly solicitous. Excessive sympathy for an incapacitated person can be as harmful as negative feelings. The victim needs strong help but does not need to be overwhelmed with pity.

Aggressive, Hostile, and Violent Behavior

When you are faced with aggressive, hostile, or violent behavior, size up the situation before you do anything. It may be unsafe for you and for others. The person may be standing or sitting in a threatening position. For example, does the person have clenched fists? Is he or she holding a lethal object? Is the person yelling or verbally threatening harm to anyone? If the scene appears unsafe, do not enter. If needed, contact law enforcement officers.

The angry, violent person is ready to fight with anyone who approaches and may be difficult to control. Remember that anger may be a response to illness and that aggressive behavior may be a person's way of coping with feelings of helplessness. Avoid responding with anger. Many angry or violent persons can be calmed by someone who is trained and who appears confident that the person will behave well. Encourage the person to speak directly about the cause of his or her anger. A statement like "I'm not sure I understand why you are angry" often brings results. Reassure the person that you are there to help.

A person who is violent and out of control presents a special problem. Notify the police if you are unable to communicate with a person who is dangerous to himself or herself or to others.

Calming a Person

Confronting a person who is experiencing a behavioral emergency can be a trying and frustrating experience. Use these guidelines if you must try to calm a person who is upset (▼Table 21-2):

- Acknowledge that the person seems upset and reiterate that you are there to help.

Table 21-2: Psychological First Aid for Reactions to Emergency Situations

Reaction	Symptoms	Do	Don't
Normal	Trembling Muscular tension Perspiration Nausea Mild diarrhea Urinary frequency Pounding heart Rapid breathing Anxiety	Give reassurance. Provide group identification. Motivate. Talk with victim. Observe to see that individual is gaining composure, not losing it.	Don't show resentment. Don't overdo sympathy.
Individual Panic (flight reaction)	Unreasoning attempt to flee Loss of judgment Uncontrolled weeping Wild running about	Try kindly firmness at first. Give something warm to eat or drink. Get help to isolate if necessary. Be empathetic. Encourage victim to talk. Be aware of your own limitations.	Don't use brutal restraint. Don't strike. Don't douse with water. Don't give sedatives.
Depression (underactive reactions)	Stands or sits without moving or talking Vacant expression Lack of emotional display	Make contact gently. Secure rapport. Get victim to tell you what happened. Be empathetic. Recognize feelings of resentment in victim and yourself. Give simple, routine task. Give warm food, drink.	Don't tell victim to "snap out of it." Don't overdo pity. Don't give sedatives. Don't act resentful.
Overactive	Argumentative Talks rapidly Jokes inappropriately Makes endless suggestions Jumps from one activity to another	Let victim talk about it. Find victim jobs that require physical effort. Give warm food, drink. Supervision necessary. Be aware of own feelings.	Don't suggest that victim is acting abnormally. Don't give sedatives. Don't argue with victim.
Physical (conversion reaction)	Severe nausea and vomiting Can't use some part of the body	Show interest in victim. Find small job for victim to make him/her forget. Make comfortable. Get medical help if possible. Be aware of own feelings.	Don't tell victim that there's nothing wrong with him/her. Don't blame. Don't ridicule. Don't ignore disability openly.

Source: Modified from M51-400-603-1, Department of Nonresident Instruction, Medical Field Service School, Brooke Army Medical Center, Fort Sam Houston, Texas

- Maintain a comfortable distance.
- Encourage the person to state what is troubling him or her.
- Do not make quick moves.
- Respond honestly to the person's questions.
- Do not threaten, challenge, or argue with a disturbed person.
- Tell the truth—do not lie.
- Do not "play along" with any of a disturbed person's visual or auditory disturbances.
- Involve trusted family members or friends.
- Be prepared to stay with the person for a long time. Never leave the person alone.
- Avoid unnecessary physical contact.
- Use good eye contact.

Sexual Assault and Rape

The definitions of rape and sexual assault vary widely. Rape is generally defined as forcible sexual intercourse without the consent of one participant. Categories of rape include:

- **Acquaintance rape,** which involves individuals who knew each other prior to the rape, including relatives, neighbors, or friends.
- **Date rape,** which takes place within a relationship but without the consent of one person and may involve harm or the threat of harm by the other person.
- **Marital rape,** which occurs when the victim and the offender are married to each other.
- **Stranger rape,** which occurs when the victim and the offender have no relation to each other.

The victim may hesitate to report a rape for various reasons, such as shame, guilt, fear of retaliation, or reluctance to deal with law enforcement officials or the judicial system. The victim may even begin to doubt whether a "real" rape occurred.

Rape is a traumatic crisis that disrupts the physical, psychological, social, and sexual aspects of the victim's life. The most common physical injuries are bruises, black eyes, and cuts.

As a first aider, you must be tactful and sensitive with the victim. The victim may find it extremely difficult to discuss what happened and may feel fear or hostility toward a first aider of the opposite sex. Every effort should be made to understand the victim's feelings and to respond with kindness and reassurance. The emotional trauma of rape is usually more prolonged and severe than the physical trauma. The attitude shown toward the victim during the initial care can have a serious influence, for good or ill, on future psychological and physical recovery. Convince the victim to seek counseling through community resources such as a rape crisis center and to report the crime to the police. Ask the victim not to change clothes or to bathe because doing so can alter legal evidence. For the same reason, suggest that the victim not urinate, douche, defecate, or wash before being examined by a physician. Care for any injuries incurred during the attack.

Child Abuse and Neglect

Because child abuse and neglect usually occur in the privacy of the home, no one knows exactly how many children are affected. One estimate is that 3 million children are physically abused and over 1 million are victims of sexual abuse each year. Child abuse and neglect can cause permanent damage to a child's physical, emotional, and mental development. The physical effects often include damage to the brain, vital organs, eyes, ears, arms, or legs, which, in turn, can result in mental retardation, blindness, deafness, or loss of a limb. At its most serious, abuse or neglect can result in a child's death.

Child abuse and neglect are usually divided into four major categories: physical abuse, neglect, sexual abuse, and emotional maltreatment. Each has recognizable characteristics, and all may be encountered by a first aider.

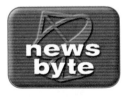

Shaken Baby Syndrome: The Shake That Can Break

Physical abuse is the main cause of serious head injury in infants. But some parents who shake a baby "to stop it from crying" or just in anger may not realize the damage they are causing. Babies have very weak neck muscles, so any shaking severely jars the head, causing blood vessels to break and causing internal bleeding. Some infant victims immediately fall into a coma and die. Others suffer mental retardation and motor disorders that become apparent years later. In short, *never* shake a baby.

Source: R. D. Krugman et al: "Shaken Baby Syndrome: Inflicted Cerebral Trauma," *Pediatrics* 92:872-875

The National Center on Child Abuse and Neglect has set forth physical and behavioral indicators of child abuse and neglect. Their list is not intended to be exhaustive; many more indicators exist than can be included. The presence of a single indicator does not necessarily prove that child abuse or neglect has occurred (►Table 21-3). However, the repeated occurrence of an indicator, the presence of several indicators in combination, or the appearance of serious injury should alert the first aider to the possibility of child abuse (►Figure 21-1, A–C). Every state has child abuse and neglect reporting laws.

First aid for an abused child's injuries is similar to the care for non-abuse injuries.

Spouse Abuse

Abuse may be the single most common source of serious injury to women. Physical domestic violence includes slapping, punching, kicking, and choking. Women also report being shot, stabbed, and bludgeoned. Injuries tend to be on the head, neck, chest, breast, abdomen, and perineum rather than the extremities.

First aid includes calling the police and the EMS and treating any injuries.

Elder Abuse

The types of physical abuse of elders vary from passive neglect to active assault. Some physically abused elderly report having had something thrown at them; some are pushed, grabbed, or shoved; others are slapped, bitten, or kicked.

First aid includes calling the police and the EMS, if warranted, and treating any injuries.

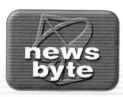

ER Staff Rarely Ask About Abuse

Although one in five women treated at U.S. emergency rooms is a victim of domestic violence, most female patients are never questioned about their experience of abuse by ER staff. Women should be routinely screened for domestic violence and history of sexual assault during primary care and routine gynecologic and prenatal visits.

Source: Obstetrics & Gynecology; 91:511-514, 1998

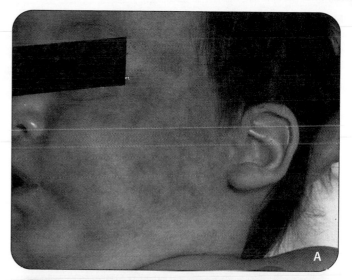

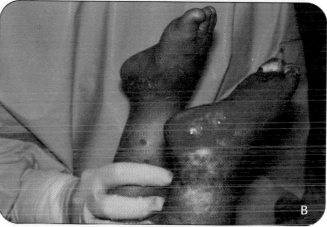

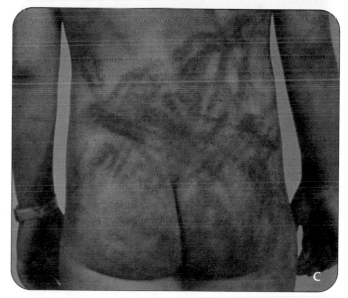

(Figure 21-1) **A.** The face is a common target for physical abuse. **B.** Stocking/glove burns of the hands and feet are almost always inflicted injuries. **C.** Rope or cord bruises are a commonly inflicted injury.

Table 21-3: Physical and Behavioral Indicators of Child Abuse and Neglect

Type of Child Abuse/Neglect	Physical Indicators	Behavioral Indicators
Physical Abuse	Unexplained bruises and welts: on face, lips, mouth, on torso, back, buttocks, thighs in various stages of healing clustered, forming regular patterns reflecting shape of articles used to inflict (electric cord, belt buckle) on several different surface areas regularly appearing after absence, weekend, or vacation especially about the trunk and buttocks Be particularly suspicious if there are old bruises in addition to fresh ones. Unexplained burns: cigar, cigarette burns, especially on soles, palms, back, or buttocks Immersion burns (socklike, glovelike, doughnut-shaped on buttocks or genitalia) Patterned like electric burner, iron, etc Rope burns on arms, legs, neck, or torso Unexplained fractures (particularly if multiple): to skull, nose, facial structure in various stages of healing, multiple or spiral fractures Unexplained lacerations or abrasions: to mouth, lips, gums, eyes to external genitalia	Wary of adult contacts Apprehensive when other children cry Behavioral extremes: aggressiveness or withdrawal Frightened of parents Afraid to go home Reports injury by parents Acts apathetic and does not cry despite injuries Has been seen by emergency personnel recently for related complaints Was injured several days before medical attention was sought
Physical Neglect	Consistent hunger, poor hygiene, inappropriate dress Consistent lack of supervision, especially in dangerous activities or for long periods Unattended physical problems or medical needs Abandonment	Begs, steals food Extended stays at school (early arrival and late departure) Constant fatigue, listlessness, or falling asleep in class Alcohol or drug abuse Delinquency (eg, thefts) States there is no caretaker
Sexual Abuse	Difficulty in walking or sitting Torn, stained, or bloody underclothing Pain or itching in genital area Bruises or bleeding in external genitalia, vaginal, or anal areas Venereal disease, especially in preteens Pregnancy	Unwillingness to change for gym or participate in physical education class Withdrawal, fantasizing, or infantile behavior Bizarre, sophisticated, or unusual sexual behavior or knowledge Poor peer relationships Delinquency or truancy Reports sexual assault by caretaker

Emotional Maltreatment	Speech disorders
	
	Lags in physical development
	
	Failure to thrive
		Habit disorders (sucking, biting, rocking, etc)
		
		Conduct disorders (antisocial, destructive, etc)
		
		Neurotic traits (sleep disorders, inhibition of play)
		
		Psychoneurotic reactions (hysteria, obsession, compulsion, phobias, hypochondria)
		
		Behavior extremes:
		  compliant, passive-aggressive, demanding
		
		Overly adaptive behavior:
		  inappropriately adult
		  inappropriately infantile
		
		Developmental lags (mental, emotional)
		
		Attempted suicide

Source: National Center on Child Abuse and Neglect

STUDY
Questions 21

Name_____ **Course**_____ **Date**_____

Activities

Activity 1

1. List eight common reasons for behavior changes:
   a. _____
   b. _____
   c. _____
   d. _____
   e. _____
   f. _____
   g. _____
   h. _____

___ 2. The term *child abuse* encompasses which of the following?
   a. physical or sexual abuse
   b. psychological or emotional abuse
   c. neglect
   d. all the above

___ 3. Who usually deliberately injures a child?
   a. a parent
   b. older siblings
   c. a teacher
   d. a stranger

___ 4. What is the speech of a depressed person like?
   a. faint, as if there is barely enough energy to speak
   b. incoherent
   c. repeats same words in conversations
   d. agitated and rambling

___ 5. Depressed persons can be recognized by their
   a. hostility and anger
   b. uncontrollable and erratic behavior
   c. energy and vivaciousness
   d. listless or apathetic behavior

___ 6. When giving psychological first aid to a depressed person, the first aider should
   a. tell the person to "snap out of it"
   b. give the person sedatives
   c. be empathetic
   d. all the above

___ 7. Which is the most common method of suicide for both men and women?
   a. hanging
   b. drug overdose
   c. firearms
   d. carbon monoxide poisoning

___ 8. Which region in the United States has the highest suicide rate?
   a. West
   b. Midwest
   c. South
   d. East

___ 9. How many attempted suicides are there for every completed suicide?
   a. 2
   b. 4
   c. 6
   d. 8

___ 10. Identify the correct statement about suicide.
   a. The majority of suicide victims gave clear warning that they intended to kill themselves.
   b. Most suicide victims had previously attempted suicide.
   c. Suicidal people frequently lack self-esteem.
   d. All the above.

___ 11. How should you react when faced with a person who is threatening suicide?
   a. Take the suicidal act or gesture seriously.
   b. Talk quietly with the individual.
   c. Encourage the person to discuss his or her situation.
   d. All the above.

___ 12. A rape victim may hesitate to report rape for which reasons?
   a. feelings of shame and guilt
   b. reluctance to deal with law enforcement officials
   c. questioning whether a "real" rape occurred
   d. all the above

STUDY
Questions (21)

____ 13. To preserve legal evidence, the rape victim should not
   a. change clothes until after medical evaluation
   b. urinate or defecate until after medical evaluation
   c. wash or douche until after medical evaluation
   d. all the above

Activity 2

1. What are the four major categories of child abuse?
   a. _____
   b. _____
   c. _____
   d. _____

2. Give several signs of possible child abuse:
   a. _____
   b. _____
   c. _____

3. How should a suspected child abuse situation be handled?
   _____
   _____

4. How should every suicide attempt be taken?
   a. _____
   b. _____
   c. _____

5. What signs indicate that a person is likely to attempt a suicide?
   a. _____
   b. _____
   c. _____
   d. _____

6. What are the four categories of rape?
   a. _____
   b. _____
   c. _____
   d. _____

7. You should try to convince a victim of rape to seek
   _____

Case Situations

Case 1

A 45-year-old male has attempted suicide by cutting both wrists. Blood is flowing from several slits across his wrists.

____ 1. This victim is experiencing _____ bleeding.
   a. arterial
   b. capillary
   c. venous

____ 2. To control the bleeding, you should apply
   a. tourniquets to both arms at the elbows
   b. direct pressure over the wounds
   c. pressure to the brachial arteries
   d. constricting bands at the wrists
   e. elastic bandages around both wrists

Case 2

A 22-year-old female has taken an overdose of aspirin. She responds to your questions about what, when, and how much was taken.

____ 1. What is the first step for this victim's care?
   a. Call the poison control center.
   b. Call the local emergency telephone number (usually 9-1-1).
   c. Call the victim's physician.
   d. Call the hospital emergency department.
   e. Call your physician.

____ 2. Which is the most likely treatment for a victim who has swallowed poison?
   a. syrup of ipecac
   b. two glasses of water
   c. epsom salts
   d. activated charcoal

STUDY
Questions (21)

Case 3

You are an elementary school teacher with a classroom full of seemingly happy and well-adjusted children. One day one of your students returns to school after a two-day absence. You notice bruises on his face and mouth. He seems wary when you get near him. He definitely has changed.

1. What do you suspect?

   _____

   _____

   _____

___ 2. What should you do?
   a. Report your suspicions to the proper authorities.
   b. Confront the parent(s).
   c. Question the child about what happened.
   d. Nothing; it is none of your business.

___ 3. How many states have child abuse and neglect reporting laws?
   a. 12
   b. 25
   c. 38
   d. all 50 states

___ 4. No one knows exactly how many children are abused.
   a. true
   b. false

___ 5. Child abuse can result in a child's death.
   a. true
   b. false

Chapter Activities

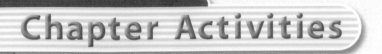

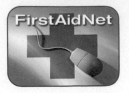

WEB Activities

Behavioral Emergencies

Visit nsc.jbpub.com/FirstAidNet, then click on Web Activities, and select the appropriate chapter.

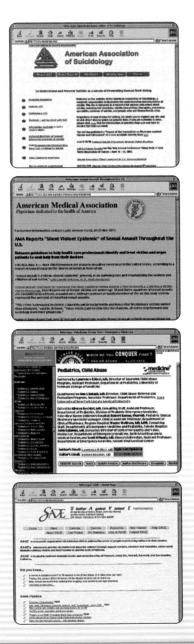

Suicide

Suicide prevention hotlines and crisis centers are excellent resources for a suicidal person. For a friend or family member, being able to recognize the early warning signs of someone threatening suicide is also crucial.

Sexual Assault

What constitutes a sexual assault? Is sexual violence a problem in the United States? Learning the difference between myths and the facts will help answer these questions and more.

Child Abuse

Child abuse can be difficult to recognize. As an outsider, you should learn to identify the signs of child abuse and know how to protect a child from future abuse.

Domestic Abuse

Victims of abuse are often fragile individuals who require special care and guidance. There are several steps you can follow to ensure the safety of an abuse victim.

Chapter 22

Wilderness First Aid

At some time, anyone living, working, traveling, or recreating in the wilderness will probably encounter dangers unfamiliar to most people. Regardless of precautions, injuries and illnesses happen.

Wilderness, as defined by the Wilderness Medical Society (WMS), is a "remote geographical location more than one hour from definitive medical care." According to that definition, "wilderness" could describe a variety of situations, including:

- recreation (eg, fishing, camping, hiking, hunting)
- occupations in remote areas (eg, farming, forestry, fishing)
- urban areas with overwhelmed emergency medical services (EMS) after a natural or manmade disaster
- residences in remote communities, farms, ranches, vacation homes
- developing countries

The millions of people in these "wildernesses" should be as medically prepared as possible to manage a problem for others and for themselves. The need for first aid with a wilderness focus appears indispensable when:

- injuries and illnesses occur in the outdoors where adverse environmental conditions such as heat, cold, altitude, rain, or snow may be a major concern
- definitive medical care is delayed for hours or days because of location, bad weather, lack of transportation, or lack of communication
- injuries and illnesses happen that are not commonly seen in urban or suburban areas (eg, altitude illness, frostbite, wild animal attacks)
- some advanced medical care (eg, reduction of some dislocations, wound cleansing) is necessary
- first aid supplies and equipment are limited
- a decision about giving unrealistic care (eg, CPR) in a remote setting must be made

Most first aid books and training courses describe situations in which the EMS response is expected within

10 to 20 minutes. In these cases the first aider usually helps for only a few minutes before an ambulance arrives. When the victim is transported, the first aider's job is finished.

Wilderness first aid is similar to that needed in urban situations, except that extra or extended skills are needed. Consideration must be given to time, distance, and availability of medical care. A first aider in the wilderness may have to remain many hours or days with a sick or injured person.

Cardiac Arrest

Because heart activity must be restored within a short time (which requires defibrillation and medications) for a cardiac arrest victim to survive, CPR has limited use in a wilderness or remote setting. That is especially true if severe trauma such as massive head or chest injury, severe blood loss, or a severed spinal cord accompanies the cardiac arrest. In addition, CPR is difficult to continue during a wilderness evacuation.

Rescue breathing can be continued for hours when there is a pulse, but chest compressions cannot support circulation for very long. The National Association of Emergency Medical Services Physicians (NAEMSP) gives the following guidelines for treating victims with normal core body temperatures or mild hypothermia (core body temperature above 90°F).

- If the victim is not breathing, give rescue breathing; if no pulse can be felt, give CPR.

- If the victim has been in cardiac arrest for more than 30 minutes without prior resuscitation efforts, do not start CPR.

- If CPR is given for more than 30 minutes without success, stop CPR (see exceptions below).

The NAEMSP recommends starting and continuing CPR for more than 30 minutes in the following situations:

- Cold-water immersion of less than one hour (hypothermia slows metabolism).
- Avalanche burial
- Hypothermia
- Lightning strike

The NAEMSP says that CPR should not be started if:

- The victim's core temperature is less than 60°F.
- The victim's chest is frozen.
- The victim has been submerged in water for more than 60 minutes.
- The procedures will place the rescuer at risk.
- An obvious lethal injury is present.

CPR for Hypothermia Victims

For the profoundly hypothermic victim, CPR should not delay evacuation to a location for rewarming and advanced cardiac life support. Rough handling of a hypothermic victim or administering CPR chest compressions when the heart is beating can cause a form of heart attack (ventricular fibrillation). Therefore, be sure there is no pulse before starting CPR. The American Heart Association recommends that a first aider take 30 to 45 seconds, instead of the usual 5 to 10, to feel for a pulse in an unresponsive hypothermic victim. Determining the existence of a pulse is difficult in cold environments because the victim will have a very slow pulse rate and the rescuer may have cold fingers. Hypothermia is one of the cases in which CPR should be continued for more than 30 minutes. See Chapter 18 for additional information on cold emergencies.

CPR for Avalanche Victims

It is suffocation and/or blunt trauma that kills avalanche victims. For pulseless victims, stabilize the cervical spine and start CPR immediately; continue for more than 30 minutes if necessary.

CPR for Lightning-Strike Victims

Start CPR on unresponsive and pulseless victims immediately. In the case of multiple victims, treat the unresponsive ones first. Continue CPR for more than 30 minutes.

Dislocations

In a wilderness situation, reducing (a technical term that means aligning) some dislocated joints is recommended. The WMS gives the following reasons for reducing a joint dislocation quickly after it happens:

- Reduction is easier immediately after the injury, before swelling develops.

- It is easier to transport a victim after reduction.

- Dramatic relief of pain results. (It is inhumane to leave a joint dislocated for several hours.)

- The joint can be stabilized and better protected.

- Reduction lessens the possibility of jeopardizing circulation in the extremity. (If the blood supply is cut off, gangrene could develop, which could result in amputation.)

- Several simple dislocations can be reduced through simple and safe techniques.

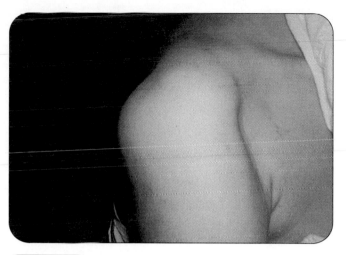

Figure 22-1 The shoulder almost always dislocates anteriorly. Note the absence of the normal rounded appearance of the shoulder.

Stop any attempts to reduce a simple dislocation if doing so increases the victim's pain or if you feel resistance in the joint.

A dislocation is considered **simple** if it involves the anterior (front) shoulder, a finger, or the patella (the kneecap, *not* the knee itself). Do *not* attempt to reduce a dislocated elbow or hip. Elbow and hip dislocations resemble fractures; reduction techniques for those joints are painful and can cause further injury.

Shoulder Dislocation

Anterior shoulder joint dislocations account for over 90% of shoulder dislocations (▲**Figure 22-1**). Because

the problem often recurs, the victim usually can readily identify the dislocation. The upper arm is held away from the body in various positions and cannot be brought next to the body into a sling-type position. The victim is unable to touch the uninjured shoulder with the hand of the injured extremity. Compare the injured shoulder to the uninjured one. Check CSM (circulation, sensation, and movement) of the hand.

There are two methods for reducing a shoulder dislocation. With either method, stop if pain increases or resistance is met. Do *not* try pulling on the victim's arm with your foot in the victim's armpit.

Traction and External Rotation

This is the easiest and most effective method for reducing an anterior shoulder dislocation (▼**Figure 22-2**).

1. Gently but steadily pull the arm out to the side while another rescuer provides countertraction against the chest wall, just below the armpit, using straps, a sleeping bag, clothing, or a flotation vest.

2. Tell the victim to relax. Massage may help.

3. As you pull, gently and slowly rotate the arm into a baseball-throwing position (take 5 to 15 minutes). Keep the arm in that position; the muscles will fatigue within 15 minutes, allowing the joint to slip back into place.

4. After successful reduction, stabilize the arm with a sling and swathe.

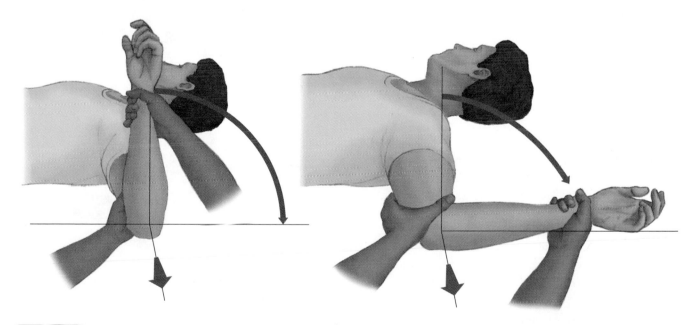

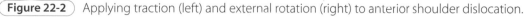

Figure 22-2 Applying traction (left) and external rotation (right) to anterior shoulder dislocation.

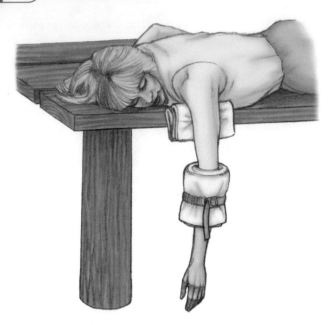

Figure 22-3 Simple hanging traction to reduce anterior shoulder dislocation.

Simple Hanging Traction

1. Lay the victim face down on a surface high enough so the injured arm can hang over the side. Place some cushioning (a folded towel or clothing) under the armpit, between the arm and the surface (▲Figure 22-3).

2. Attach a 10- to 15-pound weight to the victim's lower arm, between the elbow and the wrist. Cushion and strap the weight, being careful not to impede circulation. Keep the victim's palm facing inward.

3. It may take up to 60 minutes to stretch and tire the muscles, allowing the joint to pop back in.

4. After successful reduction, stabilize the arm with a sling and swathe.

Finger Dislocation

Deformity and loss of use identify a dislocated finger. Often, persons with this injury can reduce the finger dislocation themselves (▶Figure 22-4). In a remote location, you should try to reduce a finger dislocation only once. Do *not* attempt to reduce a dislocation at the base of the index finger or at the base of the thumb—those areas require surgery for reduction. To reduce a finger dislocation, use one of two methods (▶Figure 22-5):

1. Hold the finger in a slightly flexed position (use a cloth to prevent slipping).

2. Apply traction to the tip of the finger (pull outwards) as you push the end of the dislocated bone back into place.

3. Whether or not the reduction is successful, stabilize the joint in the **position of function** (fingers and hand in a cupping shape, as though holding a baseball).

Or

1. Hold the end of the finger with one hand and the rest of the finger in the other.

2. Pull the end of the finger first in the direction it is pointing; then, while maintaining traction, swing it back in normal anatomical position.

3. Whether or not the reduction is successful, stabilize the joint in the position of function (fingers and hand in a cupping shape, as though holding a baseball).

Patella (Kneecap) Dislocation

When dislocated, the patella displaces to the outside, with the leg bent for comfort (▶Figure 22-6). The problem

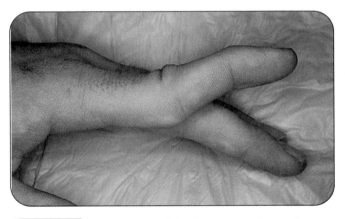

Figure 22-4 Dislocation of the finger joint. Do not be tempted to try to "pop" the joint back into place.

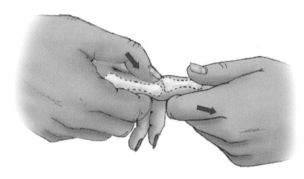

Figure 22-5 Reducing a finger dislocation

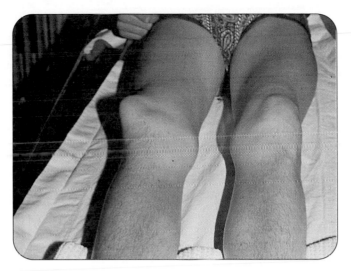

Figure 22-6 A dislocated patella will typically appear with the patella displaced lateral to the knee and with the knee moderately flexed.

often recurs, and the victim usually can identify the dislocation. For most dislocated kneecaps, you should only apply an ice pack and use a splint to stabilize the leg in place as you found it. For remote locations, however, always consider reducing a dislocated kneecap using the following method. All dislocations, whether successfully reduced in the field or not, should be seen by a physician.

1. Slowly straighten the knee as you gently push the kneecap back into its normal position. Straightening alone may replace the kneecap.

2. Stabilize the leg straight. The victim usually can walk on the injured leg.

With the knee extended (straight) and stabilized, the victim may be able to walk well enough for self-evacuation. Because of the heavy physical demands and usually higher altitudes in the backcountry, carrying a victim can take 8 to 16 rescuers rotating the task. In the wilderness, a ski pole or a tree branch makes a good walking aid. Helicopter evacuation usually is not justified for a kneecap dislocation.

Spinal Injury

The necessity of stabilizing the spine after trauma is well known. An unconscious victim with a cervical spinal injury who is moved without stabilization may become quadriplegic or die. In urban settings, spine stabilization is almost always automatically applied for survivors of violent accidents, such as automobile crashes or falls from a height.

In the wilderness, full-spine stabilization may not always be necessary—such a procedure can be difficult, impractical, impossible, or even dangerous during prolonged evacuation in severe environments. For example, an injured climber far above the timberline could wait for hours, even days, depending on the distance someone has to go for help. The injured climber would have to wait in a hostile environment and risk death from avalanche, rockfall, or hypothermia. If the victim were cleared of a spinal injury, he or she could self-evacuate.

Spinal fractures can be difficult to determine, even by physicians reading x-rays. One study found that all the spinal fractures reviewed had at least one of the following findings: midline neck tenderness, altered mental status, evidence of intoxication, or a separate painful injury away from the neck.

Assessing a Possible Spinal Injury Victim

Assessing a spinal injury can be done through a process of elimination. First, ask these four questions:

- Is the victim alert and oriented? Has the victim been drinking alcohol or using drugs?
- Does the victim have any major painful injury? Distracting injuries include fractures, deep lacerations, severe contusions, or large burns.
- Is the victim complaining of neck pain?
- Does the victim have tingling, numbness, or weakness in the extremities?

Spinal Injury

Question: Should a suspected spinal injury be stabilized as found or moved to an in-line position?

Answer: The National EMT curriculum says that the head can be placed in an in-line position unless the victim complains of pain or the head is not easily moved into that position. The anatomical (normal) position is the most stable position for all bony structures, including the spine, and movement toward that position from the position found generally is considered to be safe. Therefore, in wilderness settings, it is best to reposition suspected spinal injuries into the normal, anatomical ("eyes forward") position. If movement causes increased pain or if there is resistance to movement, it is best to splint the spine in the position found.

Next, perform these physical exams:

- Check for neck tenderness by pressing firmly on the bony part of the spine. This is a safe procedure, and there is little chance of injuring the spinal cord by feeling the bony spinal column as long as movement of the spine is prevented.
- Determine if the victim has sensation in the hands or feet and if he or she can move fingers or toes.

Here is a simple protocol for clearing a spinal injury in the wilderness: The victim does not need to be stabilized in one position if he or she is completely alert, not intoxicated, has no distracting injuries, does not complain of neck pain, can feel normal touch, and can move the fingers and toes.

Follow these guidelines to assess a suspected spinal injury:

+ Victim is responsive:
  - Determine if the mechanism of injury was a violent-impact force capable of damaging the bony spinal column. Examples are a fall from 20 feet, a high-velocity gunshot wound near the spine, and a high-velocity vehicle crash.
  - Ask questions: *Does your neck or back hurt? What happened? Can you move your hands and feet? Can you feel me touching your fingers and toes?*
  - Look and feel for D-O-T-S (deformity, open wounds, tenderness, swelling) along the bony spinal column.
  - Assess equality of strength of extremities: Have victim grip your hands; have victim push his or her feet against your hand.

+ Victim is unresponsive:
  - Determine mechanism of injury.
  - Look for deformity, open wounds, and swelling along the spinal bones.
  - Feel for deformity and swelling along the spinal bones.
  - Obtain information from others at the scene to determine information relevant to mechanism of injury and victim's mental status prior to your arrival.

Stabilizing a Spinal Injury

Providing effective spine stabilization in the wilderness often requires you to improvise methods. Initially, you can use your hands or knees to hold the victim's head in place. While kneeling at the victim's head, use your hands

Femur Fracture

Question: Do improvised traction splints work?

Answer: Although the advantages of stabilizing a broken femur by applying a traction splint are clear, there are dissenting opinions about the effectiveness of improvised traction splints. For example, Outward Bound says, "Improvised traction splints for field use employing ski poles, canoe paddles, and other pieces of equipment are usually more architecturally interesting than medically useful. The simplest, safest, and most universal splint is firm immobilization on a long board or litter without traction."

or knees to stabilize the victim's neck in relation to the long axis of the spine.

Improvised cervical collars such as a blanket, an Ensolite™ pad, or a SAM Splint™ alone are inadequate. Improvise supports by placing dirt or sand in garbage bags, stuff sacks, or roll up extra articles of clothing. Place them on both sides of the victim's head and secure them in place.

Leave the victim on the ground and avoid moving him or her. If necessary to prevent heat loss, log roll the victim, keeping the spine straight, and place insulating materials underneath.

For spinal injury procedures when EMS response time is less than one hour, see page 193.

Splinting Femur Fractures

Victims with a femur fracture can easily lose more than a quart of blood in the thigh and develop massive swelling.

Because EMS personnel have the training, the experience, and the equipment, it is best to let them apply traction splints, if possible. However, first aiders can use the methods on page 222 to stabilize a femur fracture.

Avalanche Burial

Avalanches are falling masses of snow that may also contain rocks, soil, or ice. Since the early 1970s, the number of deaths caused by avalanches has increased rapidly, as a result of the tremendous growth in backcountry winter mountain travel (skiing, mountaineering, snowmobiling). Recent statistics show that the average annual number of deaths is about 14 per year in the United States and 7 in Canada.

Avalanche Rescue

If you survive an avalanche, follow these steps to find other victims:

1. With a piece of equipment, clothing, or tree branch, mark the spot where a victim was last seen.

2. Search the area below the last-seen point for any clues of the victim. Make shallow probes into likely burial spots with a ski, ski pole, or tree limb.

3. If beacons were being used, all survivors must immediately switch their units to the receive mode and listen for a beeping sound from buried beacons.

4. If a second avalanche is possible, place one person in a safe location to shout a warning so rescuers can flee to safety.

5. Send a person to notify the ski patrol immediately if you are near a ski area and there are several rescuers. If you are the only rescuer, do a fast surface search for clues before leaving to notify the ski patrol. In remote backcountry, all survivors should remain and search until they cannot or should not continue.

Rescue transceivers or beacons are an efficient way of locating victims. Organized probe lines have found more victims than any other method, but because of the time involved, most of the victims were dead. Trained search dogs can locate buried victims quickly, but they often are brought to the scene only after long periods of burial. One trained dog can search more effectively than 30 searchers.

Avalanches kill in two ways. The first is from serious injury the victim acquires while tumbling down an avalanche path. Trees, rocks, cliffs, and the wrenching action of snow are hazards. About one-third of all deaths are related to trauma, especially trauma to the head and neck. The second way is snow burial, which causes suffocation in the other two-thirds of avalanche deaths. Inhaled snow clogs the mouth and nose, and victims can suffocate quickly if they are buried with the airway already blocked.

Snow sets up solid after an avalanche. It is almost impossible for victims to dig themselves out, even if they are buried under less than a foot of snow. The pressure of several feet of snow sometimes is so great that victims are unable to expand their chests to breathe.

A completely buried victim has a poor chance of survival. During the first 15 minutes, more people are found alive than dead. Between 16 and 30 minutes after an avalanche, an equal number are found dead and alive (50% chance of survival). After 30 minutes, more are found dead than alive.

In the absence of fatal injuries, speed of extrication from the avalanche and existence of an air pocket are the main factors that determine survival of a buried victim. There are no documented reports of anyone surviving a burial of seven feet or more.

What to Do

After you have first checked for further avalanche danger and then found a victim, follow these steps:

1. Quickly free the victim's head, chest, and stomach.
2. Send for help.
3. Clear the victim's airway and check ABCDs.
4. If a pulse is present but breathing is not, begin rescue breathing.
5. If no pulse is found, begin CPR.
6. Check for severe bleeding.
7. Examine for and stabilize a spinal injury.
8. Treat for hypothermia.

Altitude Sickness

If you live in or visit mountainous regions, you need to know about altitude sickness. Altitude sickness is not simply an exotic affliction of mountaineers but is a common environmental risk to which millions of people are exposed, often without adequate knowledge.

Altitude sickness is also called acute mountain sickness and affects about one in four people from lower elevations who visit areas 6,000 to 12,000 feet above sea level. Such elevations are common at ski resorts and on mountain hiking trails.

Altitude illnesses actually are a spectrum of a single problem, hypoxia. **Hypoxia** occurs when the body's tissues do not have enough oxygen. Altitude illnesses include **acute mountain sickness** (AMS), **high-altitude pulmonary edema** (HAPE), and **high-altitude cerebral edema** (HACE).

The actual incidence of altitude illness varies with rate of ascent and altitude attained. About 67% of climbers on Mt. Rainier in Washington suffer at least mild AMS because of rapid ascent to a moderately high altitude. The incidence of AMS in a study of Colorado skiers at lower altitudes (usually one day's ascent from Denver or lower) was only 15% to 40%.

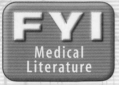

Acute Mountain Sickness

Rapid ascent from low to high altitude is often followed by headaches, fatigue, shortness of breath, sleeplessness, and loss of appetite—symptoms of acute mountain sickness. Acute mountain sickness affects climbers who ascend above 12,000 feet, but it was not thought to be common at lower altitudes. In a study of 3,158 adult visitors to Rocky Mountain elevations of 6,300 to 9,700 feet, more than 70% had at least one symptom of mountain sickness. One out of every four developed three or more symptoms, usually within 12 hours after arriving. Symptoms were most common in people age 18 to 19, people in poor physical condition or with a history of lung problems, and those whose permanent homes were at sea level. To reduce the risk of sickness, stop at an intermediate altitude for at least 36 hours and limit activities on arrival at the higher altitude.

Source: B. Honigman, et al: "Acute Mountain Sickness in a General Tourist Population at Moderate Altitudes." *Annals of Internal Medicine* 118:587–592

Although anyone can get altitude sickness, certain factors increase the risk. Under similar conditions, different people sometimes respond quite differently to altitude. For most people, at least four factors determine whether they will be sick or well after going to a higher altitude: (1) the speed of ascent (the slower the climb, the fewer the symptoms); (2) the altitude reached (the higher one goes, the more likely one will have problems); (3) one's health at the time (malnutrition, dehydration, fatigue, and any of several illnesses increase the risk); and (4) individual differences and genetic influences.

Altitude sickness occurs because oxygen levels decrease as elevation increases, and it takes a few days to adapt to the "thinner" air. At 11,500 feet, the amount of oxygen in the air is about 65% the amount at sea level, so the body has to struggle to maintain normal levels of oxygen.

What to Look for

Altitude illness typically strikes in the first 12 hours, and a headache is the most common problem. Other symptoms include loss of appetite, nausea, insomnia, fatigue, and shortness of breath with exertion. Three-fourths of all people who go from sea level to above 8,000 feet have at least one symptom (usually a headache), and the rest have three or more symptoms. Many people mistake the symptoms for a cold, the flu, or a hangover and wonder why it had to happen on their long-awaited mountain vacation.

Preventing Altitude Illness

You can take several measures to lower your risk of getting altitude sickness. First, start slowly and avoid overexerting yourself. By going easy, you allow your body to acclimatize, that is, adjust to different conditions. Simply put, your body becomes more efficient at using less oxygen. Unfortunately, it does not appear that the effects of acclimatization last after you return to your normal altitude. You must repeat the process whenever you return to higher elevations.

If you can't or won't take the time, protective medications are available by prescription. Diamox™ (acetazolamide) has been effectively used to prevent AMS (acute mountain sickness) for more than 30 years. Diamox™ also seems to prevent HAPE (high-altitude pulmonary edema) and HACE (high-altitude cerebral edema), although that is almost impossible to prove because those two conditions are rare. The simplest explanation of the benefits of Diamox™ is that it enables the body to blow off more carbon dioxide while decreasing the alkalosis (increase in blood alkalinity or reduction of acids in blood) that results.

Side effects of Diamox™ include increased urination and tingling or numbness in the fingers and toes. If you are allergic to sulfa drugs, you may be allergic to Diamox™. Also, you should wear a sunscreen with an SPF of at least 15 while taking the drug.

Diamox™ is effective for most lowlanders going to moderate altitude and perhaps for high-altitude residents returning after a short stay at low altitude. It has been called an artificial acclimatizer. Just how much Diamox™ to take and when to take it are still debated. Follow the prescribed dosage; for adults it is 125 mg twice a day starting the day of ascent.

Because dehydration can be a factor at high altitudes, drink plenty of fluids like water and juice. Mountain air is drier than air at lower elevations. You are drinking enough fluid when your urine is clear. Tea, coffee, and alcohol cause more frequent urination and may lead to dehydration. Eat lightly for a few days.

Avoid taking sleeping pills because they tend to cause shallow breathing while you sleep, which can make it harder for your body to get enough oxygen. Likewise, do not smoke because it increases carbon monoxide levels in the blood, which diminishes the body's ability to use oxygen.

What to Do

It is important to recognize the symptoms of altitude sickness and take steps to treat it. In a small number of people, simple altitude sickness can progress to pulmonary edema (HAPE), in which fluid builds up in the lungs, or cerebral edema (HACE), in which fluid collects in the brain. Although uncommon, both conditions can be fatal in less than 12 hours. Seek medical help if any of the following, more serious symptoms appear: persistent cough, shortness of breath while resting, noisy breathing, loss of balance, confusion, or vomiting.

Most people who have altitude sickness get better with rest as the body acclimatizes. But anyone who has recently ascended to above 6,000 feet, is feeling ill, and does not improve in one to two days should see a physician. If that is not possible, the victim should descend 2,000 to 3,000 feet, rest, and drink plenty of fluids. Aspirin or a similar pain reliever can be taken for a mild headache. If rest and over-the-counter medications do not provide relief, a physician may have to administer oxygen or prescribe medication.

People with mild altitude illness usually improve even at higher elevations after a few days of rest and can continue with their plans (ski, hike, hunt, etc). As long as the condition does not worsen and the victim can be carefully watched, a day or two of rest at a lower altitude may be sufficient.

All forms of altitude illness will improve when the victim simply descends a few thousand feet. If HACE is suspected, early descent is wise, because this condition is serious. The next best step after descent is to breath additional oxygen so that the inspired oxygen pressure equals that at sea level. This will also relieve the headache rapidly and completely and make breathing easier.

At 18,000 feet, humans reach their ceiling and cannot stay for more than a few weeks. Any sea-level person taken quickly to 20,000 feet will be almost incapacitated in less than half an hour, and death will occur soon thereafter.

Other Altitude-related Illnesses

- Pharyngitis and bronchitis. Because of dry air, a sore throat and coughing may develop. Care involves drinking fluids, applying an over-the-counter antibiotic ointment in the nostrils, and sucking hard candy or throat lozenges.

- Peripheral edema. The hands, ankles, and/or face (around eyes) may swell at higher altitudes. If possible, raise the affected arms and/or legs. After descending or with acclimatization to higher altitudes, the swelling diminishes. Descend if signs of the more serious altitude illness appear.

Table 22-1: Characteristics of Altitude Illnesses

	AMS	HAPE	HACE
Elevation	Above 8,000 ft.	Usually above 10,000 ft.	Above 12,000 ft.
Time after ascent	1–2 days.	3–4 days, possibly later.	4–7 days, possibly later.
Symptoms	Results from hypoxia and includes headache, sleep disturbance, fatigue, shortness of breath, dizziness, loss of appetite, vomiting.	Caused by pulmonary fluid and includes shortness of breath, dry cough, mild chest pain, weakness, insomnia, rapid pulse, cyanosis, rales (crackles), or gurgling sounds.	Caused by intracranial pressure on brain and includes severe headache (unrelieved), vomiting, Cheynes-Stokes breathing (irregular breathing pattern followed by breathing stops), ataxia (inability to walk straight line), unconsciousness.
First aid	• Stop ascending or go down. • Drink fluids. • Rest. • Take aspirin or ibuprofen. • Get prescription for Diamox™.	• Descend at least 2,000 ft. • Seek medical attention *immediately*.	• Descend 4,000 ft. • Seek medical attention *immediately*.

Notes: AMS = acute mountain sickness; HAPE = high-altitude pulmonary edema; HACE = high-altitude cerebral edema
HAPE and HACE occur when reduced oxygen causes capillary leakage and body-tissue swelling. Both conditions are life threatening.

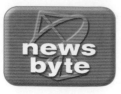

Altitude Increases Sunburn Risk

Skiers, hikers and others who enjoy outdoor activities in the mountains have long believed that it took less time to sunburn in the mountains than at lower levels. New research confirms that the higher the altitude, the quicker a person will develop sunburn. UV light energy readings were taken at solar noon in direct sunlight on cloudless days at Vail, CO, Orlando, FL, and New York, NY. The high-altitude regions in the U.S. contain areas with some of the fastest population growth and it is vital that those living or visiting these regions recognize the increase in UV exposure at higher altitudes and take extra precautions to prevent sunburn.

Source: DS Rigel, et al: "Effects of Altitude and Latitude on Ambient UVB Radiation," *American Academy of Dermatology,* 40(1):114-116, January 1999

Lightning's "Rule of 70s"

+ 70% happen in June, July, and August.
+ 70% happen between noon and 6:00 p.m.
+ 70% involve only one victim.
+ 70% of the victims survive.
+ 70% of the victims have a residual effect (hearing, vision, neurologic).

Lightning

Lightning is an awesome and frightening event (▼Figure 22-7). Lightning kills about 150 people and injures about 250 more in the United States each year (the actual numbers may be much higher). About 30% of lightning strikes to humans result in death. Lightning claims more lives in the United States than any other natural disaster, including earthquakes, blizzards, tornadoes, floods, hurricanes, and volcanic eruptions.

In the past, farmers, sailors, and other outdoor workers in isolated areas tended to be the most frequently injured. Today, a larger proportion of victims are hikers, campers, golfers, and others who are outdoors for recreational purposes.

Almost 70% of lightning deaths involve just one person; 15% involve groups of two; and groups of three or more account for another 15%. Lightning deaths happen more often during daytime hours when people are active and outdoors. Most occur in the summer months of June through September, when thunderstorms are most frequent. There are more thunderstorm days in the South than in any other region of the United States. Thunderstorms occur frequently over high mountains (▼Figure 22-8). People are better protected in urban areas where high buildings have metal frames and lightning devices.

How Lightning Injures

Lightning injures in five ways. A **direct strike** is actually being struck by lightning and is most likely to hit a

Figure 22-7 Lightning strike.

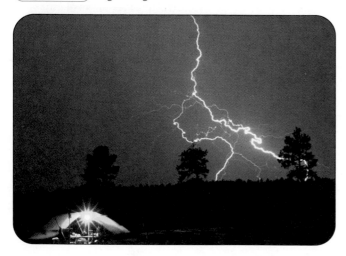

States with Highest, Lowest Death Tolls (From 1959 to 1992)

Highest		Lowest	
Fla.	333	Alaska	0
N.C.	164	Hawaii	0
Texas	156	Wash.	2
N.Y.	124	R.I.	4
Tenn.	121	D.C.	5

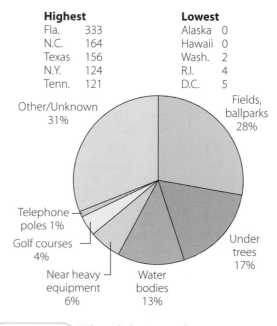

Other/Unknown 31%

Fields, ballparks 28%

Telephone poles 1%

Golf courses 4%

Near heavy equipment 6%

Water bodies 13%

Under trees 17%

Figure 22-8 Where lightning strikes

person in the open who has been unable to find shelter. Any conductor of electricity that the victim carries, especially if it is metal and carried above shoulder level (eg, umbrella, golf clubs) increases the chances of a direct hit.

A more frequent cause of injury is a **splash**, which happens when lightning strikes a tree or a building and "splashes" onto a victim seeking shelter nearby. The electrical current seeks the path of least resistance and may jump to the person because bodies have less resistance than trees or other objects. Frequently, a splash can kill groups of animals as they stand near a fence or seek shelter under trees.

Contact injury happens when a person is holding onto an object that is either directly hit or splashed by lightning.

Ground current is produced when lightning hits the ground or an object nearby. The current spreads like a wave in a pond. Although ground current is less likely to produce fatalities than direct hits or splashes, it often creates multiple victims and injuries. Large groups have been injured on baseball fields, hiking paths, and military maneuvers.

People can be injured by the explosive force of the shock wave produced as lightning hits nearby. Victims are actually thrown by this **blast effect.**

Differences Between Injuries from High-Voltage Electricity and from Lightning

Lightning contact with the body is almost instantaneous, leading to **flashover.** The current flashes over the body instead of going through it, so there are seldom burns of

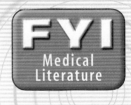

Avoid Lightning Injury

+ Be alert about weather conditions and predictions before going outdoors.

+ Do not stand underneath a natural lightning rod such as a tall, isolated tree in an open area.

+ Avoid projecting above the surrounding landscape, as you would do if you were standing on a hilltop, in an open field, or on the beach, or fishing from a small boat.

+ Get out of and away from open water.

+ Get away from tractors and other metal farm equipment.

+ Get off and away from motorcycles, scooters, golf carts, and bicycles. Put down golf clubs.

+ Stay away from wire fences, clotheslines, metal pipes, rails, and other metallic paths that could carry lightning to you from some distance away.

+ Avoid standing in small, isolated sheds or other small structures in open areas.

+ In a forest, seek shelter in a low area under a thick growth of small trees. In open areas, go to a low place such as a ravine or valley.

+ If you are hopelessly isolated in a level field or prairie and you feel your hair stand on end—indicating lightning is about to strike—drop to a baseball catcher's crotching position or stance and put your hands over both ears to help avoid an eardrum rupture. *Do not lie flat on the ground.* You want as small an area of your body as possible touching the ground to minimize the possibility of your body acting as a conductor.

+ If you are indoors during a thunderstorm, avoid open doors and windows, fireplaces, and metal objects such as pipes, sinks, and plug-in electrical appliances. Avoid using the telephone.

+ If you are in an automobile (without a cloth top), stay in it. The vehicle will diffuse the current around you to the ground. It is a myth that the rubber tires will provide insulation, but true that the metal body affords protection.

+ If a group of people is exposed, they should spread out and stay several yards apart. That way, should a strike hit, the least number will be seriously injured.

---

any magnitude. Exposure to high-voltage electricity tends to be much more prolonged, because the victim freezes to the circuit. The electrical energy surges through the tissues with little resistance to flow, causing massive internal thermal injury, with major amputations resulting.

Causes of Death and Injuries

The most common cause of death in a lightning victim is cardiopulmonary arrest. It is highly unlikely for a victim to die unless cardiac arrest is suffered as an immediate effect of the strike. Until recently, nearly 75% of those who suffered cardiac arrest from lightning injuries died, often because CPR was not attempted.

The second major cause of death and injury is central nervous system damage. When electrical current traverses the brain, brain damage can occur. Seizures, paralysis, loss of consciousness, and amnesia can result.

Most people believe that a lightning victim will be severely burned. However, due to the flashover effect, most victims suffer only minor burns. The entrance and exit burn points common with electrical burns are rare

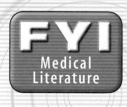

Lightning Strikes: You Are Not Immune Indoors

Most lightning strike injuries occur outdoors—at golf courses, swimming pools, lakes, and open fields. Many victims make the error of standing under a tree, which is a common target for lightning. According to one report, it is better to take refuge under a shelter or in a closed automobile. If it is not possible to go inside, it is safer to seek shelter in a thick forest or grove of several trees, rather than under an isolated tree. Also, avoid contact with metal objects such as golf clubs and carts, fishing rods, bicycles, and umbrellas. But even if you are indoors, you are not fully protected. Lightning can travel through phone lines and grounded water pipes. So during lightning storms, do not use the phone and stay out of the shower or bathtub.

Source: M. Cherington: "Lightning Injuries." *Annals of Emergency Medicine* 25:516

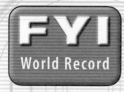

FYI
World Record

Lightning Strike Survivals

The only person in the world to be struck by lightning seven times and survive is ex–park ranger Roy C. Sullivan, of Virginia. His attraction to lightning began in 1942 (he lost his big toenail) and recurred in July 1969 (lost eyebrows), in July 1970 (left shoulder seared), in April 1972 (hair set on fire), in August 1973 (hair set on fire again and legs seared), and in June 1976 (ankle injured). He was sent to Waynesboro Hospital with chest and stomach burns on June 25, 1977, after being struck while fishing. In September 1983 he died by his own hand, reportedly rejected in love.

Source: The Guinness Book of Records (New York: Bantam Books, 1999)

with lightning. The types of burns seen with lightning strikes are punctate burns (small circular injuries resembling cigarette burns), feathering or ferning burns, linear burns, and ignited clothing and heated metal burns. On rare occasions, clothing is ignited by lightning. A victim wearing metal, such as a necklace or a belt buckle, or carrying coins in a pocket may suffer burns as the objects heat.

What to Do

1. If more than one victim has been struck by lightning at the same time, go to the quiet and motionless one first, check for ABCDs, and treat accordingly.

2. If the victim is in cardiac arrest, start CPR. Persistent care is crucial for such victims.

3. Because spinal injuries can occur with lightning strikes, precautions should be taken to stabilize the spine.

4. Raise the legs and keep the victim warm.

Wild Animal Attacks

Despite the fact that few large wild animals (bears, bison, cougars, and alligators) remain in the United States, attacks on humans still occur (▶**Figure 22-9**). Wild animal attacks outside the United States are more common. Attacks, especially fatalities, are often reported and sensationalized in the media.

The incidence of injuries from wild animal attacks is not known. Reporting is not mandatory, and many attacks are not recorded. Perhaps one or two deaths occur each year in the United States. Outside the United States, animal attacks by crocodiles, elephants, cape buffalo, lions, and tigers are a much greater cause of injury and death.

Wild animal attacks occur most often in rural or wilderness settings, a long distance from medical care.

Preventing wild animal attacks is largely common sense and awareness. An increasing number of parks and wilderness areas are posting warning signs. Recreationalists should be aware of and knowledgeable about the animal habitats through which they travel and take precautions in food handling so as not to attract animals.

Generally, if you encounter a large wild animal, try to remove yourself from the scene quietly and slowly. Running will elicit a predatory response. In most cases, a general rule is to fight back if you are attacked. Vigorous physical resistance, including striking the attacking animal with fists, a weapon, or any other object, has been effective in repelling attacks by cougars, lions, tigers, brown and black bears, and even crocodiles. Exceptions to this recommendation are the grizzly bear and a mother black bear with cubs. In these cases you should lie down and play dead.

Wilderness Evacuation

Determining the best way to evacuate a victim (helicopter evacuation versus walking the victim out versus carrying the victim on a litter) must be based on several factors:*

- the severity of the illness or injury
- the rescue and medical skills of the rescuers

---

*The recommendations presented here regarding wilderness evacuation are adapted from WMS Practice Guidelines.

(**Figure 22-9**) Large animals do not always retreat from humans and may attack rescuers.

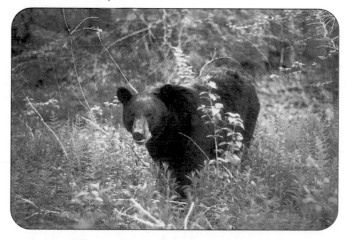

- the physical and psychological condition of the rescuers and the victims
- the availability of equipment and aid for the rescue
- the time, determined by distance, terrain, weather, and other conditions, it would take to evacuate the victim by other means
- the cost

When requesting outside assistance, you must consider the safety of incoming rescuers, their time commitment, and the cost of the rescue.

As a general rule, you should delay travel plans or start evacuating a victim from the wilderness for any of the following reasons:

- The victim is not improving.
- The victim is experiencing debilitating pain.
- The victim is unable to travel at a reasonable pace due to a medical problem.
- The victim is passing blood by the mouth or rectum (not from an obviously minor source).
- The victim has signs and symptoms of serious altitude illness.
- Infections are not improving.
- Chest pain is not from a rib cage injury.
- The victim's dysfunctional psychological status is impairing the safety of others.

When to Evacuate

Use these guidelines to decide if a victim should be evacuated.

Fractures

Rapidly evacuate the following types of fractures:

- open fractures
- extremity injuries in which circulation is absent
- spinal injuries with no sensation in the fingers or toes or inability of victim to move fingers or toes

Do not rapidly evacuate these types of injuries:

- finger or toe injuries
- minimal injuries to joints

Wounds

In the wilderness, all bleeding should be controlled and all wounds cleaned and irrigated under pressure. The standard rule is not to remove blood-soaked dressings, but to place new dressings on top. In the wilderness, you should remove blood-soaked dressings, locate the bleed-ing vessels, and reapply pressure directly over the bleeding vessels. Do not close a wound with adhesive strips, butter-fly bandages, staples, or sutures.

Evacuate a wounded victim so that a physician can suture a wound within six hours for hand or foot injuries and within 24 hours for head or trunk injuries. (If necessary, closure can be done by a physician up to about the fourth day.)

Hypothermia

Do not evacuate a victim of mild hypothermia if the victim has a normal mental status.

Evacuate victims who have severe hypothermia. It is impossible to rewarm a severely hypothermic victim in a wilderness or remote location. See Chapter 18 for more information on cold-related emergencies.

Guidelines for Ground Evacuation

If the victim is walking out, at least two people should accompany the victim. If the victim is being carried out, one or two people should be sent to notify authorities that assistance is needed and to give them specifics about the problem.

During a litter evacuation, there should be at least four, and preferably six, litter bearers at all times. Over rough terrain, eight carriers (six over smooth trail) should carry the litter 100 yards and then rest or rotate with eight other carriers. It is very demanding to carry a loaded litter for more than 15 minutes without a break.

Figure 22-10) An EMS helicopter

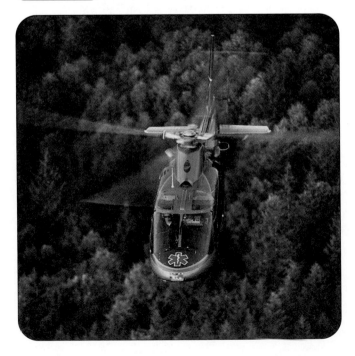

Guidelines for Helicopter Evacuation

Helicopters can reduce the time to medical care. Evacuate by helicopter only if the following conditions apply (◄Figure 22-10):

- The victim's life will be saved, or the victim will have a significantly better chance for full recovery.
- The pilot believes conditions are safe enough for helicopter evacuation.
- Ground evacuation would be unusually dangerous or excessively prolonged, or not enough rescuers are available for ground evacuation.

Caution:

DO NOT approach a helicopter until one of the aircraft personnel signals it is safe for you to approach.

DO NOT approach a helicopter from the rear, where the fast-spinning tail rotor is invisible and dangerous. Many people walk into spinning rotors each year.

DO NOT forget to protect against windchill from the rotor blades in the winter or to protect eyes against flying dirt and debris.

DO NOT approach from the uphill side. The rotor is closer to the ground on the uphill side (▼Figure 22-11).

DO NOT stand up when approaching a helicopter. Keep as low as possible in a crouched position. Because the blade is flexible, it may dip as low as four feet off the ground.

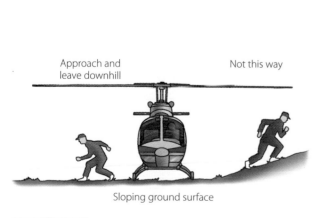

Approach and leave downhill   Not this way

Sloping ground surface

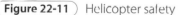

Figure 22-11   Helicopter safety

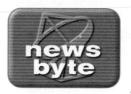
Signaling for Help

Many emergency conditions require a search for people in distress. Under such circumstances, it is always better if those being sought know how to make their presence and their location very conspicuous.

Signaling Aircraft

When creating a ground signal that an aircraft can see, remember that there are very few straight lines or right angles in nature, and that things are a lot smaller when

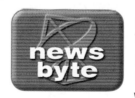

viewed from the air. Bigger is almost always better. For ground signals, make a large "V" for immediate assistance or an "X" if medical assistance is needed. Make the lines of these signals as large as you can. Construct your signal so that each line is six times as long as it is wide, such as a "V" with each side 12 feet long and two feet wide. Contrast is another key to ground signals. Examples of materials to use include: toilet paper, strips of plastic tarp, strips of tent material, tree branches, logs, and light-colored rocks. In snow, open ground, or sandy shores, signals may be tramped or dug into the surface using shadows to make the signals stand out.

Other Signals

A series of three of almost anything indicates "Help." Examples include three shouts, three shots, three blasts from a whistle, or three flashes from a light.

Use smoke by day and bright flame by night if other signaling devices are not available. Add engine oil, rags soaked in oil, or pieces of rubber to your fire to make black smoke (best against a light background). Keep plenty of spare fuel on hand. If you are tending a fire as you wait for help, keep fuel handy and throw it on the fire when you hear an aircraft —don't wait, because it takes time for smoke to form and rise.

A mirror is an effective means of sending a distress signal. On hazy days, aircraft pilots can see the flash of a mirror before survivors can see the aircraft, so it is wise to flash the mirror in the direction of a plane when you hear it, even when you cannot see it. Mirror flashes have been spotted by rescue aircraft more than 20 miles away.

To use a mirror, follow this procedure:

1. Hold the mirror up to the sun with one hand, and stretch your other hand out in front of you. Use your finger or thumb to block your view of your target.

2. Hit your extended finger or thumb with a reflection of the sun from the monitor.

3. Repeatedly flick the spot of light from the mirror across the finger or thumb and the target.

4. Try to hit the aircraft or rescuers with a flash as much as possible. Do not attempt to do series of three flashes—it's too difficult.

Survival Kit: The Bare Essentials

Minimal items	Purpose
One or two large plastic trash bags, *or* an emergency blanket ("space blanket") made of mylar	Protects against weather (wind, rain, snow). Wear one trash bag by cutting a hole in the bottom of the bag for your head; use the second bag to cover your legs.
Whistle (Mini Fox 40™ or Windstorm™)	Signal for help.
Signal mirror	Signal for help.
Metal match w/striker (magnesium)	Start a fire.
Waterproof match case containing windproof/ waterproof matches	Start a fire.
Waterproof match case or empty film canister containing several cotton balls smeared with Vaseline™ *or* commercial tinder tabs	Petroleum jelly is flammable. Make tinder using cotton balls smeared with petroleum jelly. When using, open cotton ball up to catch sparks from metal match.
Knife (multi-tool) *and/or* Wire blade survival saw	Cutting
Food (energy bars, MREs [US military surplus meals-ready-to-eat], etc.)	Provides calories and a psychological boost

STUDY Questions 22

Name_____ Course_____ Date_____

Activities

Activity 1

Mark each question as true (T) or false (F).

T F **1.** Most first aid books and training courses focus on situations in which EMS response time is quick.

T F **2.** The wilderness setting may require you to use some advanced first aid methods.

T F **3.** First aid supplies and equipment in a wilderness setting usually are limited.

T F **4.** Environmental conditions such as heat, cold, and precipitation can become major concerns.

T F **5.** CPR has limited use in remote locations.

T F **6.** Attempt to reduce all finger and thumb dislocations.

T F **7.** Straightening the leg can sometimes reduce a patella dislocation.

T F **8.** Four rescuers can easily carry a victim out of the backcountry.

T F **9.** In wilderness settings, wounds need to be closed by adhesive strips, butterfly bandages, staples, or sutures.

T F **10.** The most common cause of death from lightning is from the electrical current traveling to the brain.

T F **11.** Entrance and exit burn points are common in those struck by lightning.

T F **12.** During most animal attacks, the victim should fight back.

Activity 2

____ **1.** The Wilderness Medical Society defines *wilderness* as
   a. a remote geographical location
   b. an area or situation more than one hour from medical care
   c. both a and b

2. List five situations that would fit the WMS definition of *wilderness*:
   a. _____
   b. _____
   c. _____
   d. _____
   e. _____

3. List six reasons for wilderness first aid training:
   a. _____
   b. _____
   c. _____
   d. _____
   e. _____
   f. _____

____ **4.** In the wilderness, how long may a first aider have to remain with a sick or injured person before medical attention becomes available?
   a. many hours
   b. few minutes
   c. days
   d. both a and c

____ **5.** In a remote location, with a few exceptions, CPR can be stopped after how many minutes?
   a. 30
   b. 60
   c. 120

____ **6.** How long should you take to check an unconscious hypothermic victim's pulse?
   a. three to five seconds
   b. 5 to 10 seconds
   c. 30 to 45 seconds
   d. two minutes

STUDY Questions (22)

7. Ordinarily, first aiders should never reduce dislocations. The Wilderness Medical Society, however, gives six reasons for reducing a joint dislocation quickly after it happens.

   a. _____

   b. _____

   c. _____

   d. _____

   e. _____

   f. _____

8. In wilderness locations, what three simple dislocations can a first aider attempt to reduce?

   a. _____

   b. _____

   c. _____

___ 9. How can you identify an anterior shoulder dislocation?

   a. Upper arm is held away from the body.

   b. Arm cannot be brought next to the body.

   c. Hand of affected arm cannot touch the uninjured shoulder.

   d. All the above.

10. Name and describe the two methods of reducing an anterior shoulder dislocation:

   a. _____
   _____

   b. _____
   _____

11. What four questions should you ask to assess a suspected spinal injury in the wilderness?

   a. _____

   b. _____

   c. _____

   d. _____

12. What two physical exams should you perform to determine a spinal injury ?

   a. _____

   b. _____

13. List six factors influencing your decision to call for a helicopter evacuation.

   a. _____

   b. _____

   c. _____

   d. _____

   e. _____

   f. _____

14. What precautions should you take around a helicopter?

   a. _____

   b. _____

   c. _____

   d. _____

   e. _____

15. In what two ways do avalanches kill?

   a. _____

   b. _____

___ 16. About what percent of people from lower elevations who visit areas 6,000 to 12,000 feet above sea level experience acute mountain sickness?

   a. 25%

   b. 50%

   c. 66%

   d. 75%

___ 17. Hypoxia—the biggest factor in altitude illnesses—refers to

   a. low blood sugar

   b. anemia

   c. insufficient oxygen

   d. lactic acid

18. List the three types of altitude illness:

   a. _____

   b. _____

   c. _____

___ 19. The single best way to care for altitude illness is to

   a. carry and use oxygen

   b. descend to a lower elevation

   c. take aspirin

   d. rest and sleep

STUDY Questions 22

20. List the five ways that lightning injures people:

a. _____

b. _____

c. _____

d. _____

e. _____

21. List four large wild animals in North America that attack humans.

a. _____

b. _____

c. _____

d. _____

Case Situations

Case 1

You take a summer job at Yellowstone National Park. During your first day, you experience a headache, fatigue, and shortness of breath. You have no appetite for food.

____ **1.** What are you experiencing?

    a. heartbeat irregularity

    b. hypothermia

    c. acute mountain sickness

    d. excitement about your job and the surroundings.

2. Check the statements below that are recommended for your condition:

____ rest

____ take a short walk

____ take aspirin or ibuprofen

____ drink fluids

____ avoid drinking water

____ see a physician for medication

Case 2

During a campout at a national forest, a thunderstorm unexpectedly develops. Everyone runs for shelter from the wind and rain, but a sudden lightning strike hits two of your companions at the same time. One is motionless while the other is mumbling and asking what happened.

____ **1.** Who do you check first?

    a. responsive victim

    b. unresponsive victim

____ **2.** If needed, should you start CPR in a wilderness location?

    a. yes

    b. no

Case 3

A mountain bike slipped on gravel while descending a trail and the 19-year-old rider fell on his outstretched arm. He complains of severe pain in his shoulder and tingling in his fingers. He has no other complaints. He is holding his arm away from the body.

____ **1.** You suspect a

    a. fractured clavicle

    b. fractured scapula

    c. anterior shoulder dislocation

    d. fractured sternum

Check the other indicators of what you suspect in question 1.

____ **2.** Victim may have experienced the injury before.

____ **3.** Victim is unable to reach across and touch the opposite uninjured shoulder.

Chapter Activities

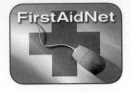

WEB Activities

Wilderness First Aid

Visit nsc.jbpub.com/FirstAidNet, then click on Web Activities, and select the appropriate chapter.

Wild Animal Attacks

You may not even have to travel into the deep woods to find a wild animal that poses a potential threat to you. Bears, fox, cougars, and raccoons can all be found in suburban areas.

Avalanches

It is a good idea to know the avalanche potential (low, moderate, high) in the area in which you live, travel, or recreate.

Lightning

Lightning storms are a big threat to persons caught without proper shelter. To see how destructive lightning can be, check out your state's report about the injuries and fatalities from this destructive natural occurrence.

Wilderness First Aid: Emergency Care for Remote Locations

This new, full-color wilderness first aid book is ideal for the outdoor enthusiast. Whether you enjoy camping, hiking, mountain biking, or fishing in remote areas, this book provides you with the information you need to treat an injured person when definitive medical care is an hour or more away. It even fits right in your backpack!

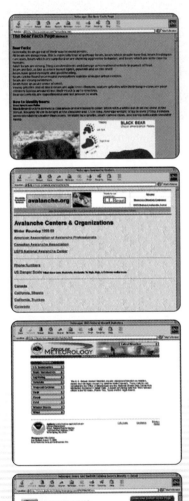

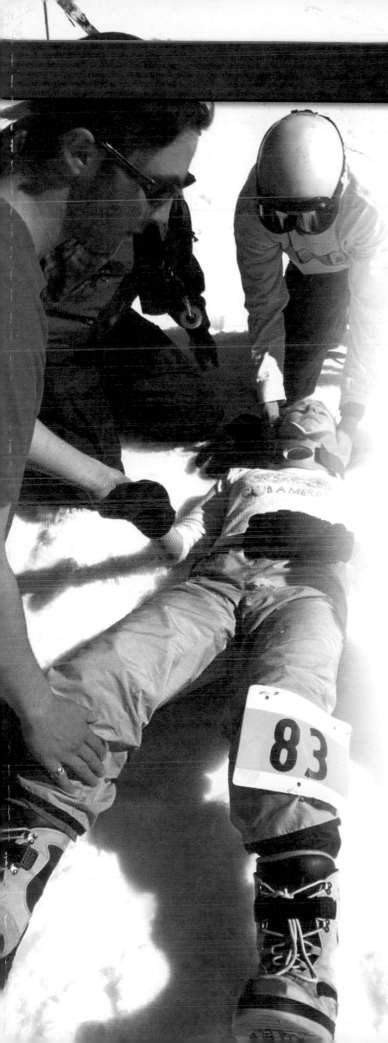

Rescuing and Moving Victims

Chapter 23

Victim Rescue

Water Rescue

Reach-throw-row-go identifies the sequence for attempting a water rescue. The first and simplest rescue technique is to **reach** for the victim. Reaching requires a lightweight pole, ladder, long stick, or any object that can be extended to the victim. Once you have your "reacher," secure your footing and have a bystander grab your belt or pants for stability. Secure yourself before reaching for the victim.

You can **throw** anything that floats—an empty picnic jug, an empty fuel or paint can, a life jacket, a floating cushion, a piece of wood, an inflated spare wheel—whatever is available (▶Table 23-1). If there is a rope handy, tie it to the object to be thrown so you can pull in the victim. Tying the object with a rope also enables you to retrieve the object and try again if you miss the first time. The average untrained rescuer has a throwing range of about 50 feet.

> *"It is chance chiefly that makes heroes."*
>
> Carlyle

If the victim is out of throwing range and there is a rowboat, canoe, motor boat, or boogie board nearby, you can try to **row** to the victim. Maneuvering these craft requires skill learned through practice. Wear a personal flotation device (PFD) for your own safety. To avoid capsizing, never pull the victim in over the side of a boat; instead, pull the victim in over the stern (rear end).

If the reach, throw, and row are impossible and you are a capable swimmer trained in water lifesaving procedures, you can **go** to the drowning victim by swimming. Entering even calm water makes a swimming rescue difficult and hazardous. All too often a would-be rescuer becomes a victim as well.

Near-Drowning

In the United States there are about 4,000 fatalities each year from drowning. In addition to the drownings, there are many cases of extreme, permanent disability that

Typical Drowning Situations

Immediate-Disappearance Syndrome

+ Victim enters water but does not return to the surface

+ Little chance of rescue

+ Caused by:

  1. diving from height and striking head

  2. hyperventilation before underwater swimming

  3. cold-induced heart attack

Distressed Nonswimmer

+ Struggles 20 to 60 seconds before sinking

+ Signs of distress: flailing arms, head tilted back, no vocalizing, appears to be playing.

Sudden-Disappearance Syndrome

+ Victim fully clothed

+ Victim apparently able to swim but is fatigued, a poor swimmer, and/or cold

+ Victim disappears after 5 to 10 minutes on surface (after clothing loses entrapped air)

Hypothermia-Induced Drowning

+ Victim seriously affected after about 15 minutes of cold-water exposure

+ Rule of 50s: Average unaware, unpracticed, and unprotected 50-year-old man would approach the 50/50 life/death point after 50 minutes of exposure to 50°F water.

Source: Adapted from David S. Smith, Ph.D.

Table 23-1: Effect of Flotation Devices on Survival Times

Situation (50° Water)	Predicted Survival Time (Hours)
No Flotation Device	
Drownproofing	1.5
Treading water	2.0
With Flotation Device	
Swimming	2.0
Holding still	2.7
HELP position	4.0
Huddle position	4.0

Drownings can be classified into three basic types. In **dry drownings** (10% to 15%), no water passes the vocal cords. Presumably, in these cases, the cords shut tightly (laryngospasm) when water touches them. Other things being equal, a near-drowning without aspiration is easier to resuscitate because water has not entered the airway.

In **wet drownings** (85% of near-drownings), water, vomitus, or foreign bodies are aspirated into the lungs. Fresh water in the lungs enters the bloodstream and has a profound destructive effect on blood cells (they swell and burst) and subsequent cardiac arrest (ventricular fibrillation). In saltwater drownings, water is taken from the bloodstream and goes into the lungs. As much as 25% of the total blood volume can be lost as fluids move into the lungs. The victims drown in their own fluids as much as in the saltwater itself.

A **secondary drowning** is one in which a victim who was resuscitated dies within 96 hours. Aspiration pneumonia is a late complication of near-drownings and occurs 48 to 72 hours after the episode. Near-drowning victims should be hospitalized or at least closely monitored.

Caution:

DO NOT swim to and grasp a drowning person unless you are trained in lifesaving.

What to Do

1. Survey the scene (see Chapter 2), then carry out a water rescue (▶**Figure 23-1**).

result from near-drowning. It is estimated that for every 10 children who drown, 36 are admitted to hospitals and 140 are treated in emergency rooms for near-drowning.

Drowning means suffocation by immersion in water or other liquid. **Near-drowning** occurs when a victim survives an immersion incident. About two-thirds of drowning victims are under 30 years old. Most of them are males.

Usually, the initial reaction to drowning is panic. Then violent struggling occurs. Frequently, as they become short of breath, victims swallow water during attempts to breathe. That water is often vomited. Further attempts to breath may then result in aspiration of water, vomitus, or foreign bodies into the lungs. Sometimes the vocal cords (larynx) close and will not allow any water to enter the lungs. A seizure may occur and then death.

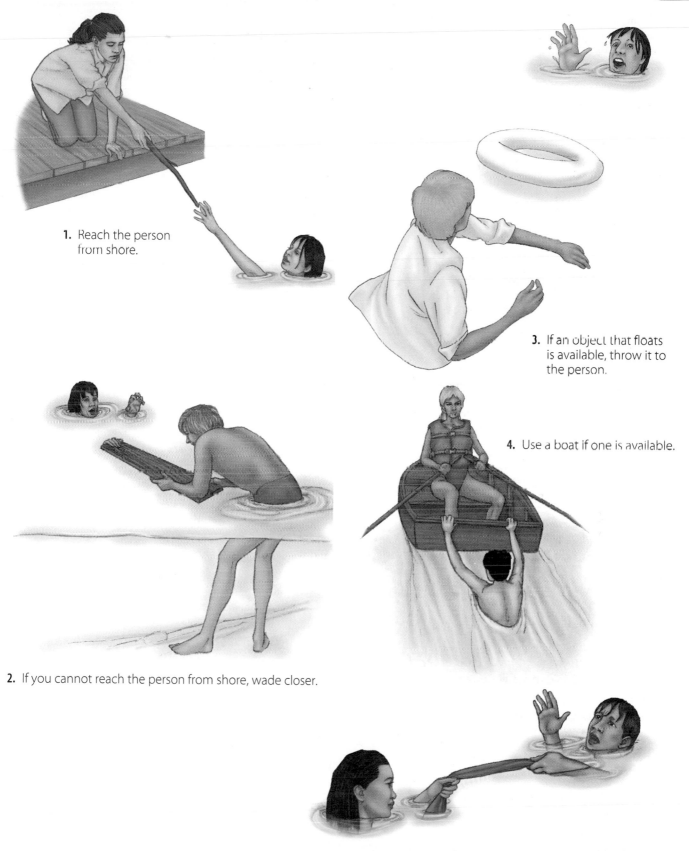

1. Reach the person from shore.

2. If you cannot reach the person from shore, wade closer.

3. If an object that floats is available, throw it to the person.

4. Use a boat if one is available.

5. If you must swim to the person, use a towel or board for him or her to hold onto. Do not let the person grab you.

Figure 23-1 Water rescue

2. If the victim was diving (or it is unknown if he or she was diving), suspect a possible spinal injury. Keep the victim in-line floating on the water surface until properly trained rescuers arrive with a backboard.

3. Check ABCDs and treat accordingly. Any pulseless, nonbreathing victim who has been submerged in cold water should be resuscitated.

4. If no spinal injury is suspected, place the victim on his or her side to allow fluids to drain from the airway.

American Academy of Pediatrics Recommendations for Preventing Childhood Drowning (by Age Group)

4 years and younger

+ Never leave them alone in bathtubs, spas, or wading pools—or near nearly filled buckets, toilets, irrigation ditches, or other standing water.

+ Recognize that swimming lessons do not "drownproof" them.

+ Fence the entire pool so that it is separated from the house. Pool covers are not a substitute for fences.

+ Learn CPR and keep a telephone and emergency equipment—such as life preservers and a shepherd's crook—poolside.

5 to 12 years

+ Provide them with swimming lessons that include safety rules.

+ Never let them swim alone or without adult supervision.

+ Make sure they wear approved flotation devices when playing in or near a body of water.

+ Teach them the dangers of jumping or diving into water and of being on thin ice.

13 to 19 years

+ In addition to relaying the safety tips above, counsel them about the dangers of substance abuse combined with swimming, diving, or boating.

+ Teach them CPR.

Source: American Academy of Pediatrics: "Drowning in Infants, Children, and Adolescents." *Pediatrics* 92(2): 292–294

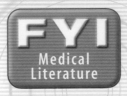

Near-Drowning: Quick Treatment Saves Lives

About 4,000 people die each year in the United States as a result of drowning. Reportedly, for every drowning, there are between 4 and 20 near-drownings. Quick action can make the difference between life and death. The outcome is usually good if the victim is submerged for less than five minutes and if CPR is started less than 10 minutes after submersion. Near-drowning victims may have spinal injuries, so care should be taken when positioning the head and neck during rescue breathing. More important, preventive measures can avoid such life-threatening events: supervise infants and toddlers, install fencing around home swimming pools, and do not use alcohol before swimming or playing water sports.

Source: M. H. Bross and J. L. Clark: *American Family Physician* 51:1545

Cold-Water Immersion

Immersion in cold water is a potential hazard for anyone who participates in activities in the oceans, lakes, and streams of all but the tropical regions of the world. The U.S. Coast Guard defines cold water as water below 70°F. However, water does not need to be that cold for a person to become hypothermic. A person can become hypothermic in water that is 77°F. Most North American lakes, rivers, and coasts are colder than that year-round. The risk of immersion hypothermia in North America is nearly universal most of the year. A person immersed in cold water loses heat about 25 times faster than someone exposed to cold air.

The U.S. Coast Guard and other rescue organizations recommend that survivors get as much of their bodies out of the water as possible to minimize cooling rate and maximize survival time. A widespread misunderstanding of the concept of windchill often causes many people to conclude that survivors have higher heat losses if they are exposed to wind, especially if they are wet, than if they are immersed in water. During recreational activities at beaches, lakes, and swimming pools, most people have experienced feeling colder after leaving the water than they do while swimming. That reinforces the misunderstanding, which has sometimes led accident victims to abandon a safe position atop a capsized vessel and reenter the water, usually with tragic results.

Cold-water immersion is associated with two potential medical emergencies: drowning and hypothermia. Numerous case histories and statistical evidence document the prominence of cold-water immersion as a cause of drowning and hypothermia. Perhaps the most famous occurrence of cold-water immersion was the sinking of the *Titanic* on April 14, 1912. After striking an iceberg, the ship sank in calm seas. Of the 2,201 people on board, only 712 were rescued, all from the ship's lifeboats. The remaining 1,489 people died in the water, despite the arrival of a rescue vehicle within two hours. Nearly all those victims were wearing life preservers, yet the cause of death was officially listed as drowning. More likely, the cause of death was immersion hypothermia.

A person's cooling depends on several factors:

- *Body fat.* The fatter a person is, the slower cooling occurs. More fat increases survival chances.

- *Body type.* Bigger people cool more slowly than smaller people. Children cool faster than adults. Women have more fat but are usually smaller, so they cool at the same rate as men.

- *Physical fitness.* Cardiovascular fitness can help meet the stress of cold-water immersion, but physically fit people usually have less subcutaneous fat for insulation.

- *Water temperature.* The colder the water, the faster a person cools.

- *Clothing.* Clothing can insulate, and some types of fabric, such as wool, are better than others.

- *Alcohol.* People who have been drinking alcohol are more likely to get into dangerous situations. Alcohol impairs judgment and coordination. Research studies have found alcohol to be implicated in 10% to 50% of all drownings. Alcohol dilates the skin's blood vessels, which allows more body heat to escape.

- *Behavior.* Swimming and treading water increase the flow of warm blood from the body's core to the muscles, thus increasing the cooling rate. Thus swimmers often die first, because they are more likely to try to tread water or swim rather than float. Likewise, so-called drownproofing, a technique of bobbing in the water (like a jellyfish), markedly increases heat loss as water circulates around the head.

A **heat escape lessening position (HELP)** has been devised, in which the victim draws the knees up close to the chest, presses the arms to the sides, and remains as quiet as possible (►**Figure 23-2 A–B**). For two or more people, huddling quietly and closely together (huddle position) will decrease heat loss from the groin and the front of the body. Both of these positions require personal flotation devices (life jackets).

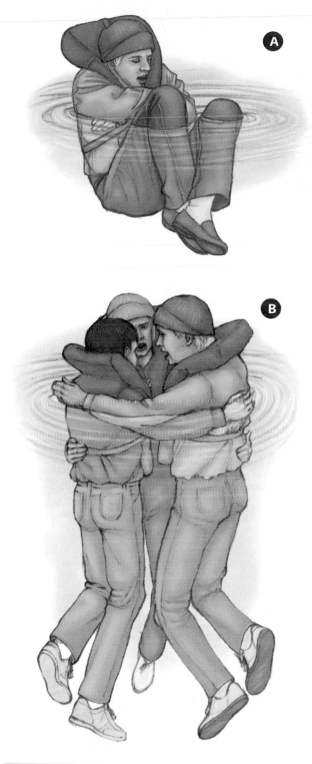

Figure 23-2 A–B **HELP or Huddle** A person wearing a flotation device can minimize heat loss and increase chances of survival by assuming the heat escape lessening position, or HELP (**A**) in which the knees are pulled up to the chest and the arms crossed. Groups of three or more can conserve heat by wrapping their arms around one another and pulling into a tight circle (**B**).

Surviving long periods of submersion has been explained by the **diving reflex** found in mammals. Some say that the diving reflex slows the heart rate, shunts blood to the brain, and closes the airway. Recent research, however, suggests that the diving reflex is present in marine mammals such as seals, porpoises, whales, and walruses but not in humans. If the diving reflex is discounted, the most likely explanation for prolonged submersion survival is that cold water produces hypothermia, which reduces the body's demand for oxygen and protects the brain.

Ice Rescue

If a person has fallen through the ice near the shore, extend a pole or throw a line with a floatable object attached to it. When the person has hold, pull him or her toward the shore or the edge of the ice.

If the person has fallen through the ice away from the shore and you cannot reach him or her with a pole or a throwing line, lie flat and push a ladder, plank, or similar object ahead of you (▼Figure 23-3). You can also tie a rope to a spare tire and the other end to an anchor point, lie flat, and push the tire ahead of you. Pull the person ashore or to the edge of the ice.

Caution:

DO NOT go near broken ice without support.

Electrical Emergency Rescue

Electrical injuries can be devastating. Just a mild shock can cause serious internal injuries. A current of 1,000 volts or more is considered high voltage, but even the 110 volts of household current can be deadly.

When a person gets an electric shock, electricity enters the body at the point of contact and travels along the path of least resistance (nerves and blood vessels). The current travels rapidly, generating heat and causing destruction.

Most indoor electrocutions are caused by faulty electrical equipment or careless use of electrical appliances. Before you touch the victim, turn off the electricity at the circuit breaker, fuse box, or outside switch box or unplug the appliance if the plug is undamaged.

If the electrocution involves high-voltage *power lines*, the power must be turned off before anyone approaches the victim. If you approach a victim and feel a tingling sensation in your legs and lower body, stop. You are on energized ground, and an electrical current is entering one foot, passing through your lower body, then leaving through the other foot. If that happens, raise one foot off the ground, turn around, and hop to a safe place. Wait for trained personnel with the proper equipment to cut the wires or disconnect them.

If a power line falls over a car, tell the driver and passengers to stay in the car. A victim should try to jump out of the car *only* if an explosion or fire threatens, and then without making contact with the car or the wire.

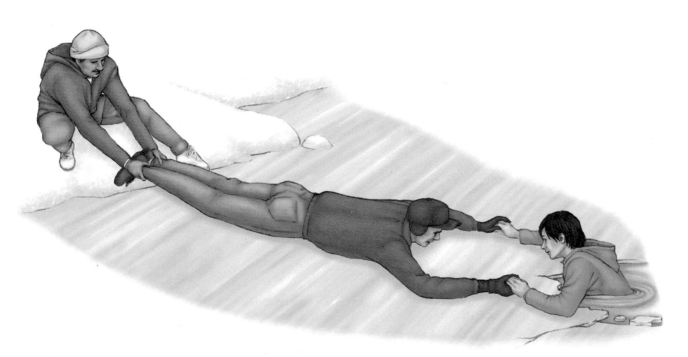

Figure 23-3 Ice rescue: Lie flat to distribute the weight.

Caution:

DO NOT touch an appliance or the victim until the current is off.

DO NOT try to move downed wires.

DO NOT use wood or metal objects, to separate the victim from the electrical source.

Hazardous Materials Incidents

At almost any highway crash scene, there is the potential danger of hazardous chemicals. Clues that indicate the presence of hazardous materials include the following:

- signs on vehicles ("explosive," "flammable," "corrosive")

- spilled liquids or solids

- strong, unusual odors

- clouds of vapor

Stay well away and upwind from the area. Only those who are specially trained in handling hazardous materials and who have the proper equipment should be in the area.

Motor Vehicle Crashes

In most states, you are legally obligated to stop and give help when you are involved in a motor vehicle crash. If you arrive at a crash shortly after it happens, the law does not require you to stop, although it might be argued that you have a moral responsibility to render any aid you can.

1. Stop and park your vehicle well off the highway or road and out of active traffic lanes. Park at least 5 car lengths from the crash. If the police have taken charge, do not stop unless you are asked to do so. If the police or other emergency vehicles have not arrived, call or send someone to call 9-1-1 or the local emergency number as soon as possible. Ways to call include:

   - finding a pay phone or roadside emergency phone

   - cellular phone or CB radio

   - ask to use a phone at a nearby house or business

2. Turn on your vehicle's emrgency hazard flashers. Raise the hood of your vehicle to draw more attention to the scene.

3. Make sure everyone on the scene is safe.

   - Ask the driver(s) to turn off the ignition or turn it off yourself.

   - Ask bystanders to stand well off the roadway.

   - Place flares or reflectors 250-500 feet behind the crash scene to warn oncoming drivers of the crash. Do not ignite flares around leaking gasoline or diesel fuel.

4. If the driver or passenger is unresponsive or might have spinal injuries, use your hands to stabilize their heads and necks.

5. Check and keep monitoring the ABCDs. Treat any life-threatening injuries.

6. Whenever possible, wait for EMS personnel to extricate the victims from vehicles, because they have training and the proper equipment. In most cases, keep the victims stabilized inside the vehicle.

7. Allow the EMS ambulance to take victims to the hospital.

Caution:

DO NOT rush to get victims out of a car that has been in a crash. Contrary to opinion, most vehicle crashes do not involve fire, and most vehicles stay in an upright position.

DO NOT move or allow victims to move unless there is an immediate danger like fire or oncoming traffic.

DO NOT transport victims in your car or any other bystander's vehicle.

Fires

Should you encounter a fire, you should

1. Get all the people out fast.

2. Call the emergency telephone number (usually 9-1-1).

Then—and *only* then—if the fire is small and if your own escape route is clear, should you fight the fire yourself with a fire extinguisher. You may be able to put out the fire or at least hold damage to a minimum. Because fire can spread so quickly, efforts to contain it within the first five minutes of a blaze can make a substantial difference in the eventual outcome.

If clothing catches fire, tear it off away from the face. Keep the victim from running, because that fans the flames. Wrap a rug or a woolen blanket around the victim's neck to keep the fire from the face or throw a blanket on the victim. In some cases, you may be able to smother the flames by throwing the victim to the floor and rolling him or her in a rug.

To use a fire extinguisher, aim directly at whatever is burning and sweep across it. Extinguishers expel their contents quickly; it takes just 8 to 25 seconds for most home models containing dry chemicals to empty.

Caution:

DO NOT let a victim run if their clothing is on fire.

DO NOT get trapped while fighting a fire. Always keep a door behind you so you can exit if the fire gets too big.

Threatening Dogs

When you enter any emergency scene, look for signs of a dog and ignore it if the animal is not threatening. Ask the owner to control a threatening dog. If you cannot be delayed, consider using a fire extinguisher, water hose, or pepper spray. For a vicious dog, call the police for assistance.

Farm Animals

Emergencies involving farm animals can be dangerous to rescuers. Horses kick and bite. Cattle kick, bite, gore, or squeeze people against a pen or barn. Pigs can deliver severe bites.

- Approach a situation involving animals with caution.
- Do not frighten an animal. Speak quietly to reassure it.
- If food is available, use it to lure the animal away from the victim.

Confined Spaces

A confined space is any area not intended for human occupancy that may contain or accumulate a dangerous atmosphere. Examples of confined spaces are tanks, vessels, vats, bins, vaults, trenches, and pits.

An accident in a confined space demands immediate action. If someone enters a confined space and then signals for help or becomes unconscious, follow these steps:

1. Call for immediate assistance, and activate the local EMS.
2. Do *not* rush in to help.
3. If you are the attendant, do *not* enter the confined space unless you are relieved by another attendant *and* you are part of the rescue team.
4. When help arrives, try to rescue the victim without entering the space.
5. If rescue from the outside cannot be done, allow trained and properly equipped (respiratory protection plus safety harnesses or lifelines) rescuers to enter the space and remove the victim.
6. Give first aid, rescue breathing, or CPR if necessary and if you are trained.

Triage: What to Do with Multiple Victims

You may encounter emergency situations in which there are two or more victims. This often occurs in multiple-car accidents or disasters. After making a quick scene survey, decide who must be cared for and transported first. This process of prioritizing or classifying injured victims is called triage. *Triage* comes from the French word trier, *to sort*. The goal is to do the greatest good for the greatest number of victims.

Finding Life-Threatened Victims

A variety of systems are used to identify care and transportation priorities. To find those needing immediate care for life-threatening conditions, first tell all victims who can get up and walk to move to a specific area. Victims who can get up and walk rarely have life-threatening injuries. These victims ("walking wounded") are classified as delayed priority (see below). Do not force a victim to move if he or she complains of pain.

Find the life-threatened victims by performing only the initial survey (ABCDs) on all remaining victims. Go to motionless victims first. You must move rapidly (spend less than 60 seconds with each victim) from one victim to the next until all have been assessed. Classify victims according to the following care and transportation priorities:

1. **Immediate care.** Victim has life-threatening injuries but can be saved.
   - airway or breathing difficulties (not breathing, breathing rate slower than eight per minute or breathing rate faster than 24 per minute)

- weak or no pulse
- uncontrolled or severe bleeding
- unresponsive or unconscious

2. **Urgent care.** Victim does not fit into either the immediate or delayed categories. Care and transportation can be delayed up to one hour.

3. **Delayed care.** Victims with minor injuries. Care and transportation can be delayed up to three hours.

4. **Dead.** Victims are obviously dead, mortally wounded, or unlikely to survive because of the extent of their injuries, age, and medical condition.

Do not become involved in treating the victims at this point, but ask knowledgeable bystanders to provide care for immediate life-threatening problems (ie, rescue breathing, bleeding control).

Reassess victims regularly for changes in their condition. Only when the immediate life-threatening conditions receive care should attention shift to those with less serious conditions.

Later, you will usually be relieved when more highly trained emergency personnel arrive on the scene. You may then be asked to provide first aid, to help move victims, or to help with ambulance or helicopter transportation.

Principles of Lifting

+ Know your capabilities. Do not try to handle a load that is too heavy or awkward—seek help.

+ Use a safe grip. Use as much of your palms as possible.

+ Keep your back straight. Tighten the muscles of your buttocks and abdomen.

+ Bend your knees to use the strong muscles of the thighs and buttocks.

+ Keep your arms close to your body and your elbows flexed.

+ Position your feet shoulder-width apart for balance, one in front of the other.

+ When lifting, keep and lift the victim close to your body.

+ While lifting, do not twist your back; pivot with the feet.

+ Lift and carry slowly, smoothly, and in unison with other helpers.

+ Before you move a victim, tell him or her what you are doing.

Moving Victims

A victim should not be moved until he or she is ready for transportation to a hospital, if required. All necessary first aid should be provided before moving a victim. A victim should be moved only if there is an immediate danger:

- There is a fire or danger of fire.
- Explosives or other hazardous materials are involved.
- It is impossible to protect the accident scene from hazards.
- It is impossible to gain access to other victims in the situation who need lifesaving care (such as in a vehicle accident).

A cardiac arrest victim is usually moved unless he or she is already on the ground or floor, because CPR must be performed on a firm, level surface.

Caution:

DO NOT move a victim unless you absolutely have to. That might happen if the victim is in immediate danger or must be moved to shelter while waiting for the EMS to arrive.

DO NOT make the injury worse by moving the victim.

DO NOT move a victim who could have a spinal injury.

DO NOT move a victim without stabilizing the injured part.

DO NOT move a victim unless you know where you are going.

DO NOT leave an unconscious victim alone unless taking a short time to call EMS.

DO NOT move a victim when you can send someone for help. Wait with the victim.

DO NOT try to move a victim by yourself if other people are available to help.

Emergency Moves

The major danger in moving a victim quickly is the possibility of aggravating a spinal injury. In an emergency, every effort should be made to pull the victim in the direction of the long axis of the body to provide as much protection to the spinal cord as possible. If victims are on the floor or ground, you can drag them away from the scene by one of various techniques.

Nonemergency Moves

All injured parts should be stabilized before and during moving. If rapid transportation is not needed, it is helpful to practice on another person about the same size as the injured victim.

Stretcher or Litter

The safest way to carry an injured victim is on some type of stretcher or litter, which can be improvised. Before using it, test an improvised stretcher by lifting a rescuer about the same size as the victim.

- **Blanket-and-pole improvised stretcher.** If the blanket is properly wrapped, the victim's weight will keep it from unwinding (▼Figure 23-4).

- **Blanket with no poles.** The blanket is rolled inward

toward the victim and grasped for carrying by four or more rescuers.

- **Board improvised stretcher.** Sturdier than a blanket-and-pole stretcher but heavier and less comfortable. Tie the victim on to prevent him or her from rolling off (▼Figure 23-5).

Commercial stretchers and litters usually are not available except through the EMS.

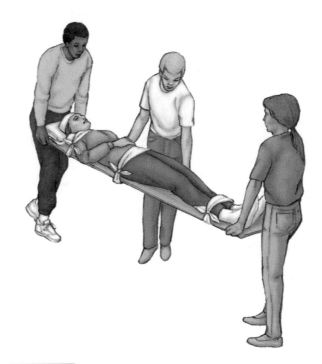

Figure 23-5) Board improvised stretcher

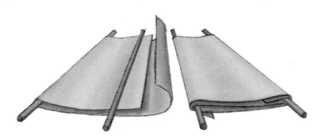

Figure 23-4) Blanket-and-pole improvised stretcher

Skill Scan Drags

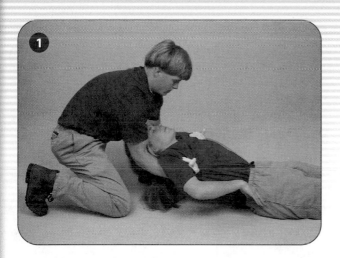

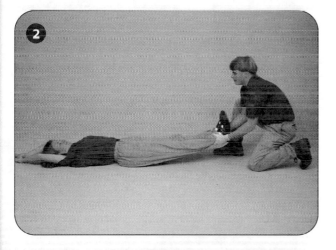

1. *Shoulder drag.* For short distances over a rough surface; stabilize victim's head with your forearms.

2. *Ankle drag.* The fastest method for a short distance on a smooth surface.

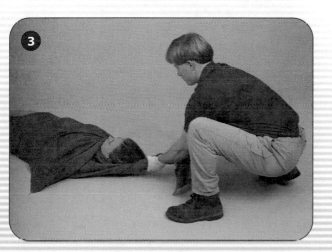

3. *Blanket pull.* Roll the victim onto a blanket and pull from behind the victim's head.

Skill Scan

One-Person Moves

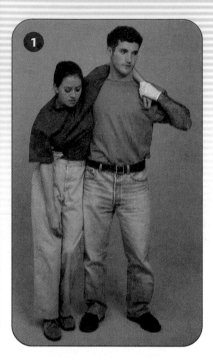

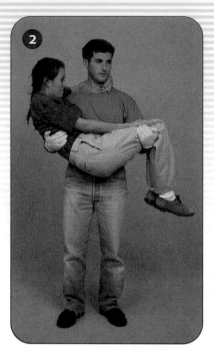

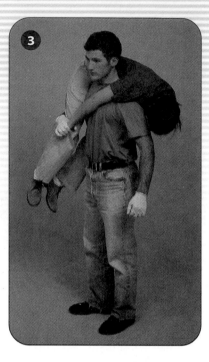

1. *Human crutch* (one person helps victim to walk). If one leg is injured, help the victim to walk on the good leg while you support the injured side.

2. *Cradle carry*. Use for children and lightweight adults who cannot walk.

3. *Firefighter's carry*. If the victim's injuries permit, you can travel longer distances if you carry the victim over your shoulder.

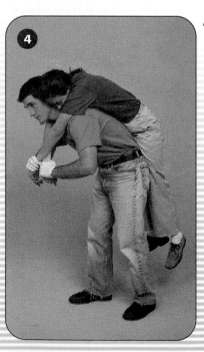

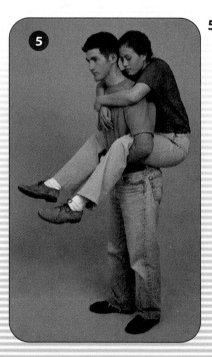

4. *Pack-strap carry*. When injuries make the fireman's carry unsafe, this method is better for longer distances.

5. *Piggyback carry*. Use this method when the victim cannot walk but can use the arms to hang onto the rescuer.

Skill Scan — Two/Three-Person Moves

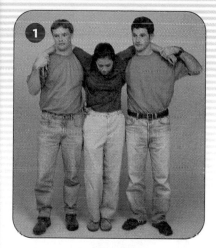

1. *Two-person assist.* Similar to human crutch.

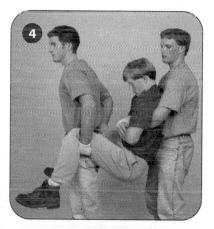

2. *Two-handed seat carry.*

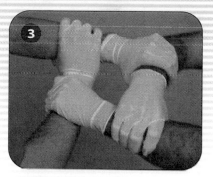

3. *Four-handed seat carry.* The easiest two-person carry when no equipment is available, and the victim cannot walk but can use the arms to hang onto the two rescuers.

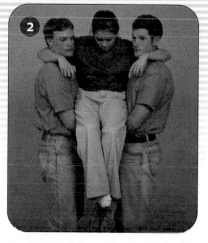

4. *Extremity carry.*

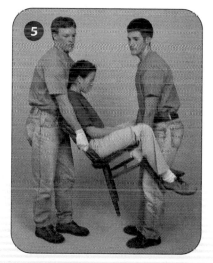

5. *Chair carry.* Useful for a narrow passage or up or down stairs. Use a sturdy chair that can take the victim's weight.

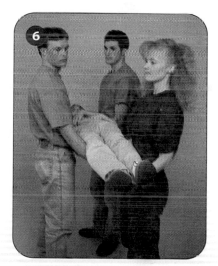

6. *Hammock carry.* Three to six people stand on alternate sides of the injured person and link hands beneath the victim.

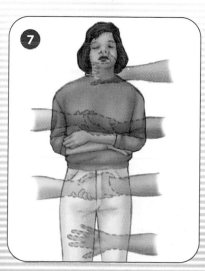

Chapter Activities

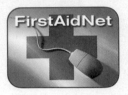

WEB Activities

Rescuing and Moving Victims

Visit **nsc.jbpub.com/FirstAidNet, then click on Web Activities, and select the appropriate chapter.**

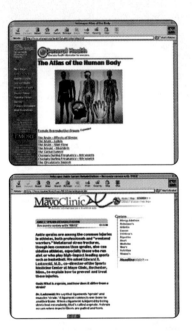

Skeletal System

This web site offers extensive visuals for a review of the body's skeletal system. Keeping up on the basics of the human anatomy can help a first aider recognize and threat an injury or illness.

Ankle Sprain

Although considered to be a common injury, ankle sprains need special attention, including knowing what types of pain reliever to take and how to prevent re-injuries.

Appendix A

First Aid Supplies

Many injuries and sudden illnesses can be cared for without medical attention. For these situations and for situations requiring medical attention later, it is a good idea to have useful supplies on hand for emergencies.

A first aid kit's supplies should be customized to include those items likely to be used on a regular basis. For example, a kit for the home will be different from one at a workplace or one found on a boat.

The list here includes nonprescriptive (over-the-counter) medications. Some drug products lose their potency over time, especially after they have been opened. Other drugs change in consistency. Buying the large "family size" of a product that you use infrequently may seem like a bargain, but it is poor economy if the product has to be thrown out before the contents are used. Note the expiration date on every medication.

Keep all medicines out of the reach of children. Read and follow all directions for properly using medications.

Keep your first aid supplies in either a fishing tackle box or a tool box. Boxes with an O-ring gasket around the cover are dustproof and waterproof.

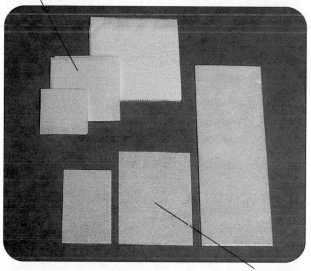

Gauze pads

Nonstick pads

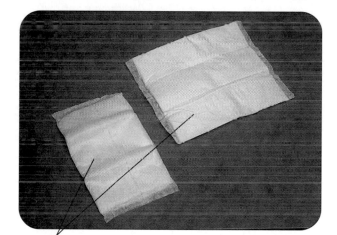

Trauma dressings

First Aid Kits

The following recommended items should be stocked inside a first aid kit in the workplace, at home, and for travel.

First aid kits should be

- Impact-resistant and made of durable material to protect against moisture, dust, and contamination

- Portable and easily carried by a handle

- Of sufficient size to store the equipment listed

- Clearly marked as being a first aid kit by words and/or symbols

- Regularly inspected and updated for completeness and content condition

Workplace First Aid Kit*

Equipment	Minimum Quantity
1. Adhesive strip bandages (1" × 3")	20
2. Triangular bandages (muslin, 36" – 40" × 36" – 40" × 52" – 56")	4

* This list does not include over-the-counter ointments, topicals, or internal medicines; consult the workplace's medical director for these.

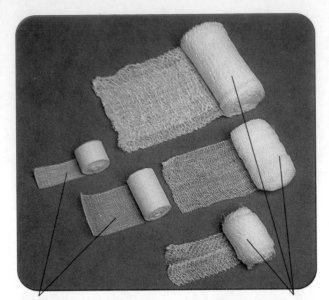

Gauze rollers   Conforming, self-adhering roller bandages

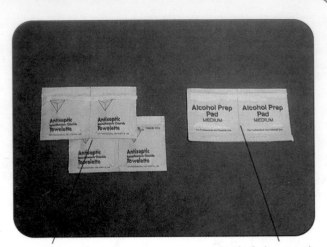

Antiseptic towelettes   Alcohol prep pads

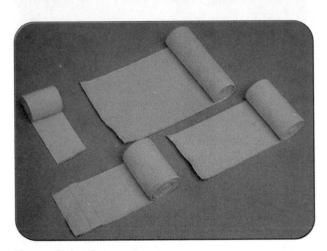

Elastic roller bandages

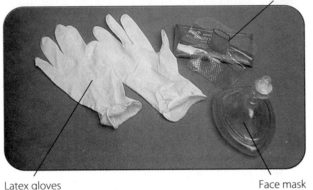

Face shield

Latex gloves   Face mask

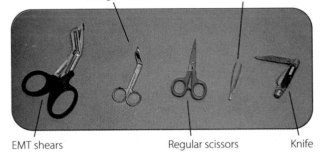

Bandage scissors   Tweezers

EMT shears   Regular scissors   Knife

3. Sterile eye pads (2 1/8" × 2 5/8")   2
4. Sterile gauze pads (4" × 4")   6
5. Sterile nonstick pads (3" × 4")   6
6. Sterile trauma pads (5" × 9")   2
7. Sterile trauma pads (8" × 10")   1
8. Sterile conforming roller gauze (2" width)   3 rolls
9. Sterile conforming roller gauze (4 1/2" width)   3 rolls
10. Waterproof tape (1" × 5 yards)   1 roll
11. Porous adhesive tape (2" × 5 yards)   1 roll
12. Elastic roller bandages (4" and 6")   1 each
13. Antiseptic skin wipes, individually wrapped   10
14. Medical-grade exam gloves (medium, large, extra large), conforming to FDA requirements   2 pairs per size
15. Mouth-to-barrier device, either a face mask with a one-way valve or a disposable face shield   1
16. Disposable instant-activating cold packs   2

17. Resealable plastic bags (quart size)   2
18. Padded malleable splint   1
     (SAM splint™, 4" × 36")
19. Emergency blanket, Mylar   1
20. Paramedic shears   1
     (with one serrated edge)
21. Splinter tweezers (about 3" long)   1
22. Biohazard waste bag   2
     (3 1/2 gallon capacity)
23. First aid and CPR manual and list   1
     of local emergency telephone numbers

Home First Aid Kit**

1. Acetaminophen, ibuprofen, and aspirin tablets: for headaches, pain, fever, and simple sprains or strains of the body. (Aspirin should not be used for relief of flu symptoms or given to children.)

2. Ipecac syrup and activated charcoal: for treatment after ingestion of certain poisons. (Use only on the advice of a poison control center or the emergency department.)

3. Elastic wraps: for wrapping wrist, ankle, knee, and elbow injuries

4. Triangular bandage: for wrapping injuries and making an arm sling

5. Scissors with rounded tips

6. Adhesive tape and 2" gauze: for dressing wounds

7. Disposable, instant-activating ice bags: for icing injuries and treating high fevers

---

**Recommended by the American College of Emergency Physicians.

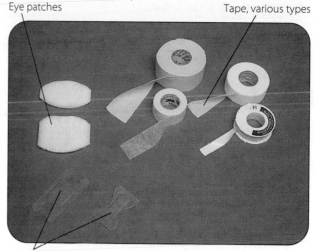

Eye patches   Tape, various types

Knuckle and fingertip bandages

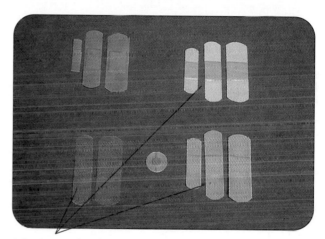

Adhesive strip bandages

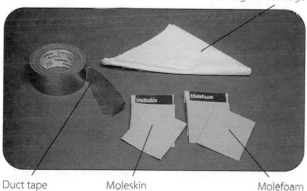

Triangular bandage

Duct tape   Moleskin   Molefoam

8. Bandages of assorted sizes: for covering minor cuts and scrapes

9. Antibiotic ointment: for burns, cuts, and scrapes

10. Gauze in rolls and in 2" and 4" pads: for dressing wounds

11. Bandage closures, $\frac{1}{4}$" and 1": for taping cut edges together

12. Tweezers: to remove small splinters and ticks

13. Safety pins: to fasten splints and bandages

14. Medical-grade exam gloves to protect your hands and reduce the risk of infection when treating open wounds

15. First aid manual

16. List of emergency phone numbers

Travel First Aid Kit**

1. Aspirin, acetaminophen, or ibuprofen: for headaches, pain, fever, and simple sprains or strains of the body. (Aspirin should not be used for relief of flu symptoms or given to children.)

2. Antihistamine/decongestant cough medicine

3. Anti-nausea/motion sickness medication

4. Bandages of assorted sizes, including adhesive bandages (e.g., Band-Aids™)

5. Adhesive tape and 2" gauze: for dressing wounds

6. Elastic wraps: for wrapping wrist, ankle, knee, and elbow injuries

7. Triangular bandage: for wrapping injuries and making an arm sling

8. Scissors with rounded tips

9. Medical-grade exam gloves: to reduce the risk of infection

10. Disposable, instant-activating ice bags: for icing injuries and treating high fevers

11. Antifungal cream (tolnaftate 1% or clotrimazole 1%): good for athlete's foot or ringworm

12. Antibacterial ointment

13. Antibiotic ointment: for burns, cuts, and scrapes

14. Thermometer with case

15. Sunscreen: SPF 15 or higher

16. Insect repellent: those that contain 35% to 55% DEET with stabilizer

17. Antidiarrheal medications (e.g., Pepto-Bismol™, Imodium AD™) tablets or liquid; follow directions carefully

18. Anti-malaria medications (if indicated)

19. Water-purifying pills or liquid (tincture of iodine or halazone tablets) or mechanical filtration devices, such as Katadyne™ water purifier

20. Steroidal cream, such as hydrocortisone cream: for insect bites

21. Tweezers: to remove small splinters and ticks

22. Safety pins: to fasten splints and bandages

**Recommended by the American College of Emergency Physicians.

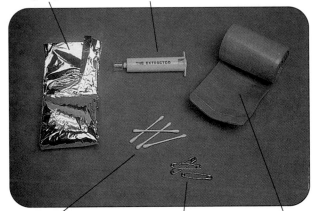

Emergency blanket   Extractor™

Cotton-tipped swabs   Safety pins   SAM Splint™

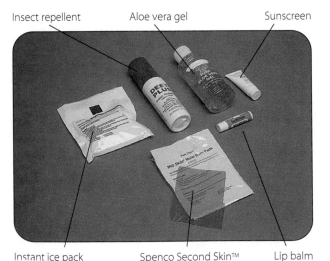

Insect repellent   Aloe vera gel   Sunscreen

Instant ice pack   Spenco Second Skin™   Lip balm

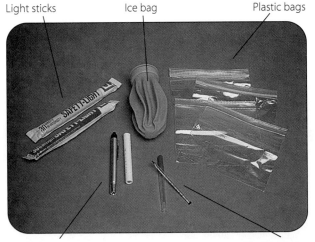

Light sticks   Ice bag   Plastic bags

Pen lights   Thermometer

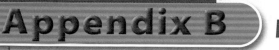

Appendix B — Medication Information

As a first aider, you may be in a situation that requires you to give a victim certain medications (or to assist a victim in taking his or her own medication). A knowledgeable first aider should be familiar with the following medications:

Over-the-counter pain relievers

- acetaminophen
- aspirin
- ibuprofen
- naproxen

Victim's physician-prescribed medications

- metered-dose inhaler
- nitroglycerin
- epinephrine

Over-the-counter medications carried in a first aid kit or available from the victim

- oral glucose
- activated charcoal

Pros and Cons of Popular Pain Relievers

Acetaminophen. Brand names: Tylenol™, Datril™
Advantages: Relieves pain and fever, does not irritate stomach
Disadvantages: Heavy or prolonged use may damage liver and kidneys

Aspirin. Brand names: Bufferin™, Anacin™
Advantages: Relieves pain, fever, inflammation; prevents heart attacks
Disadvantages: Interferes with blood clotting; may trigger stomach bleeding; may cause Reye's syndrome in children with viral infections

Ibuprofen. Brand names: Advil™, Nuprin™
Advantages: Relieves pain, fever, inflammation
Disadvantages: Interferes with clotting; may cause stomach bleeding, ulcers, irritation; heavy or prolonged use may damage liver and kidneys

Naproxen. Brand name: Aleve™
Advantages: Relieves pain and fever; one dose lasts 8 to 12 hours
Disadvantages: May cause stomach bleeding, ulcers, irritation; prolonged use may harm kidneys

Nitroglycerin

Give victim nitroglycerin (trade name Nitro-stat™) if the following conditions exist:

- Victim is an adult.
- Victim has chest pain.
- Victim has physician-prescribed sublingual tablets or spray.

Do *not* give a victim nitroglycerin if *any* of the following conditions applies:

- Victim has a head injury.
- Victim is an infant or a child.
- Victim has already taken three doses.

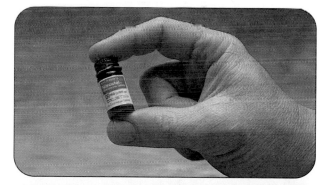

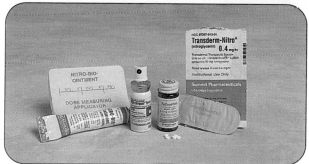

Nitroglycerin pills, spray, and patch are used for relief of chest pain.

Medication forms: tablet (about one-half the size of an aspirin); sublingual spray; and patch.

Dosage: One dose, repeated in three to five minutes. If no relief, repeat again (maximum of three doses).

Procedure

1. Check expiration date of nitroglycerin.
2. Ask victim about last dose taken.
3. Ask victim to lift tongue. Place tablet or spray dose under tongue or have victim do so. Do not touch the tablet—wear gloves because your skin will absorb nitroglycerin and it will affect your heart rate.
4. Have victim keep mouth closed, with tablet under tongue (without swallowing) until the tablet dissolves and is absorbed.

Actions

- relaxes (dilates) blood vessels
- reduces workload of heart

Side effects

- lowers blood pressure (victim should sit or lie down)
- headache
- heart rate changes

Epinephrine Auto-Injector

Give victim epinephrine (trade name Adrenaline™) if *both* of the following conditions exist:

- Victim exhibits signs of a severe allergic reaction (includes breathing distress or shock).
- Victim has physician-prescribed medication.

Medication form: liquid from automatic needle-and-syringe injection system

Dosage

- Adult: One adult auto-injector (0.3 mg)
- Child/infant: One infant/child auto-injector (0.15 mg)

Procedure

1. Obtain victim's physician-prescribed auto-injector.
2. Remove safety cap.
3. Place tip of auto-injector against victim's thigh.
4. Push injector firmly against the thigh to inject medication.
5. Hold injector in place for 10 seconds.

Actions

- dilates the bronchioles (small tubes in lungs)
- constricts blood vessels

Side effects

- increases heart rate
- dizziness
- headache
- chest pain
- nausea
- vomiting
- anxiety

Reassessment: Monitor ABCs. If victim worsens, give an additional dose; treat for shock

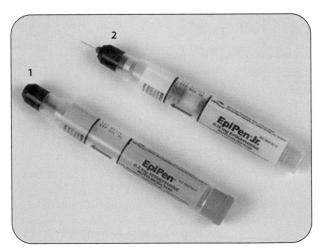

EpiPen (1-unfired, 2-fired).

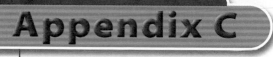

Appendix C

Automated External Defibrillators (AEDs)

Automated External Defibrillators: Jump-starting the Heart

One of the leading causes of death in the United States is sudden cardiac arrest—about 360,000 deaths each year.

What causes cardiac arrest?

Most sudden cardiac arrest victims have an electrical malfunction of the heart termed ventricular fibrillation. In ventricular fibrillation, the heart's electrical signals, which normally induce a coordinated heartbeat, suddenly become chaotic, and the heart's pumping function abruptly ceases. When the heart stops pumping blood, the victim immediately loses consciousness and is considered clinically dead. If one were to look at the heart in ventricular fibrillation, it would look like the heart is quivering like a bowl of jello. When this occurs, the heart is not pumping blood and there are only about four minutes to correct this problem before irreversible brain damage occurs. Without intervention, the victim will become biologically (irreversibly) dead within minutes.

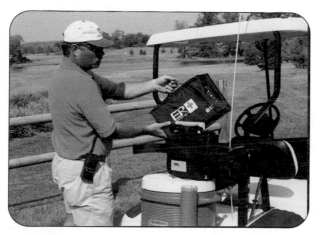

Golf staff arrive to help an apparent heart attack victim.

What is the prehospital emergency treatment for sudden cardiac arrest?

Cardiopulmonary resuscitation (CPR) alone will not reverse ventricular fibrillation. At best, CPR provides only about 30% of normal blood flow to the brain, and is simply a method to extend the time a victim may remain resuscible.

The best emergency treatment involves early access, CPR, defibrillation, and advanced care. Defibrillation is often done through the use of automated external defibrillators (AED). Television programs have acquainted the public with AEDs—the devices used to deliver controlled electrical shock to the heart via electrical pads applied to the victim's chest. These devices allow victims suffering a sudden cardiac arrest a greatly improved chance of survival.

Unfortunately, defibrillators generally reach the scene of a cardiac arrest too late or not at all. As a result of the limited distribution of defibrillators and the resulting delays in treatment, the survival rate for sudden cardiac arrest in the United States is very low.

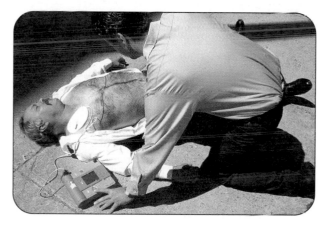

Development of defibrillators

Until recently, prehospital defibrillation was a skill reserved for personnel such as paramedics. Advances in computer technology resulted in a new generation of "smart" defibrillators. These devices, called automated external defibrillators (AEDs), are lightweight, can interpret the ECG (heart) rhythm, determine whether defibrillation is required, and deliver an electrical shock, when appropriate. The AED guides the operator through every action.

How available are AEDs?

CPR is extremely important since it buys time for the victim by allowing a defibrillator to arrive while the victim is still viable. However, it is widely recognized that early defibrillation is the single most important factor in survival from sudden cardiac arrest caused by ventricular fibrillation. Most victims suffering non-traumatic, pre-hospital cardiac arrest are in ventricular fibrillation.

The widespread deployment of AEDs increases survival rates. The strongest determinant of survival in people having an out-of-hospital cardiac arrest is the speed with which shocks are delivered.

Chances of successful resuscitation decrease by about 10% with each minute following sudden cardiac arrest. After 10 minutes, very few resuscitation attempts are successful.

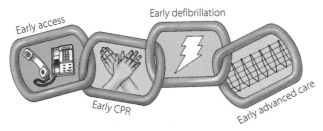

The four links in the chain of survival.

AEDs have the potential to become similar to fire extinguishers—readily available and always ready in case of an emergency. In addition to first responders such as police officers and firefighters, AEDs are appropriate in a variety of other settings. For example, companies with large facilities or high-rise buildings without easy access might keep an AED on the premises for use by physician-authorized responders. AEDs are readily available on airlines, in airports, at sporting events, in Senior Citizen Centers, and at amusement parks. Other logical locations for an AED include golf courses and households with high-risk individuals. AED use is being extended beyond healthcare profes-

sional and trained emergency personnel to trained citizens. Most states have public access defibrillation (PAD) laws that enable individuals to use AEDs and protect those who help in an emergency situation.

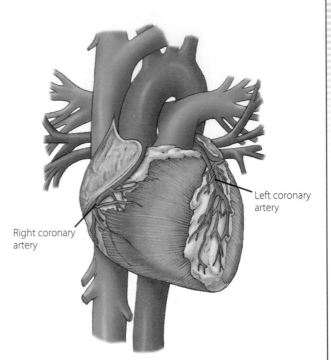

Coronary arteries of heart that supply oxygen to heart muscle.

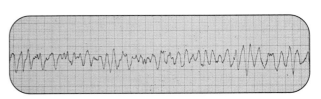

The abnormal heart rhythm ventricular fibrillation.

Are AEDs difficult to learn and use?

Because of the ease of operation, especially since ECG rhythms do not have to be taught, people can be trained in AED use in a few hours and some say the techniques are easier to learn than CPR. There are several different models of AEDs. AEDs offer voice prompts that provide operators with clear and concise instructions. AEDs have only two or three buttons: On/Off, Analyze, and Shock. Operators using defibrillators no longer need to be physicians or paramedics.

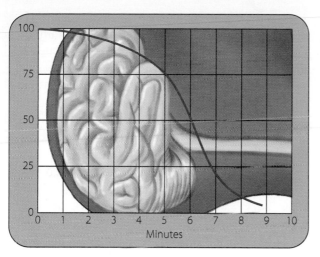

A victim's chance of survival decreases each minute without treatment.

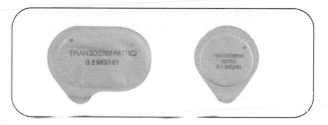

Remove medication patches prior to beginning CPR or applying an AED.

Do AEDs require a high degree of maintenance?

AEDs do not require a high degree of maintenance because the lithium-based battery system is long-lasting (over 1 year) and eliminates recharging. An AED will automatically indicate if service is needed.

What criteria determine when an AED can be used? When would one not be used?

Before AED use, a victim must be: (1) unresponsive, (2) not breathing, (3) without a pulse, and (4) over 8 years of age. Once these criteria have been established, the AED's two pads are attached to the victim to analyze the victim's heart and decide if it is in a shockable rhythm.

AEDs should not be used on victims who are: (1) under 8 years of age, (2) severely hypothermic, and (3) trauma victims. Caution must be used when the AED is being applied to a person wearing a nitroglycerin patch, or to those with implantable pacemakers or defibrillators.

While a person may complete an AED training program and have the necessary skills to apply an AED, such training does not authorize anyone to provide this treatment to victims. Defibrillation can be given only under the medical authorization of a physician who takes legal responsibility for the performance of the emergency rescuer.

How do you apply the AED?

Refer to the operating manual supplied by the manufacturer for the steps specific to the AED you will be using.

If two rescuers are present, one rescuer assesses the victim and begins CPR if necessary. The other rescuer prepares the AED and attaches it to the victim if indicated. If you are alone, assess the victim and then apply the AED prior to initiating CPR.

First, turn the unit on. Attach the defibrillation electrodes to the cables. Next, expose the victim's chest. For proper adherence and conduction the skin must be clean and dry. If necessary, dry the skin with a towel. Excessive body hair on the chest may interfere with adhesion and conduction. If this should occur, shave the area where the electrodes will be placed. Remove the backing and apply the electrodes to the victim's chest. One is placed to the right of the sternum (breastbone) just below the collarbone and above the right nipple. The other is placed to the left of the victim's left nipple with the electrode on the side of the chest, above the lower rib margin.

The AED is attached—now what?

Once the electrodes are placed, press the Analyze button. Make sure no one is touching the victim and the victim is not being moved. These actions could interfere with the analysis. If a shock is indicated, again make sure no one is touching the victim or touching any conductive material in contact with the victim (i.e., stretcher, electrode cables, oxygen tubing, resuscitator). *If anyone is in contact with the victim or these objects when the shock is delivered that person could receive a potentially life-threatening amount of energy.* It is the rescuer operating the AED who is responsible for the safety of everyone present, including him- or herself prior to delivering the shock. This can be accomplished by shouting loudly, "Everyone's clear!" Once it is safe to do so, press the shock button to deliver the electrical charge. If it is not delivered, the charge will be safely "dumped" by the machine in a few seconds. A charge is dumped when the stored energy is released by the unit's circuitry without allowing it to pass through the treatment cables or exterior of the unit. If this occurs, the analysis must be initiated again before the machine will charge for another shock. In addition, the charge can be manually dumped by turning off the power.

After delivering the first shock, you must analyze the rhythm again and repeat the previous steps. Do not check for a pulse until three shocks have been administered or a "No shock indicated" message is displayed. If there is no pulse, perform one minute of CPR. After one minute of CPR, recheck the pulse. If there is still no pulse, analyze the rhythm and deliver up to another three shocks, if indicated. Shocks are administered in sets of three unless a "No shock indicated" message is displayed. AEDs will provide voice and message prompts to guide you through this process. The energy selection for each shock is determined by the AED. If an ambulance is at the scene, your local protocols will dictate how many sets of three shocks can be administered prior to transport. If an ambulance is not at the scene, continue sets of three shocks if indicated with one minute of CPR in between until the ambulance arrives.

Glossary

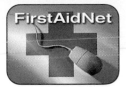 For access to the First Aid and CPR Web Enhanced Edition Interactive Glossary, please visit **nsc.jbpub.com/FirstAidNet**. Easy-to-use and state-of-the-art, this interactive glossary provides students with significant terms, definitions, pronunciations, and flash-card testing! A personal first aid and CPR resource right at your fingertips!

abandonment: A termination of a helping relationship by a first aider without consent of the victim and without replacement care to the victim by qualified medical personnel.

ABCs: Airway, Breathing, and Circulation; the first three steps in the examination of any victim; basic life support.

abdomen: The large body cavity below the diaphragm and above the pelvis.

abnormal: Not normal; malformed.

abrasion: An injury consisting of the loss of a partial thickness of skin from rubbing or scraping on a hard, rough surface; also called brush burn, friction burn.

acetone: A chemical compound found normally in small amounts in the urine; diabetic victims are said to produce a fruity odor when larger amounts are produced in blood and urine.

activated charcoal: Powdered charcoal that has been treated to increase its powers of absorption; used in a slurry to absorb ingested poison.

acute: Having rapid onset, severe symptoms, and a relatively short duration.

acute abdomen: A serious intra-abdominal condition causing irritation or inflammation of the peritoneum, attended by pain, tenderness, and muscular rigidity (boardlike abdomen).

acute myocardial infarction (AMI): The acute phase of a heart attack, in which a spasm or blockage of a coronary artery produces a spectrum of signs and symptoms, commonly including chest pain, nausea, diaphoresis, anxiety, pallor, and lassitude.

Adam's apple: The projection on the anterior surface of the neck, formed by the thyroid cartilage of the larynx.

addiction: The state of being strongly dependent on some agent, for example, drugs or tobacco.

adjunct: An accessory or auxiliary agent or measure; an oropharyngeal airway is an airway management adjunct.

Adrenalin: The proprietary name for epinephrine.

afterbirth: The placenta and membranes expelled after the birth of a child.

air: The gaseous mixture that makes up the Earth's atmosphere; composed of approximately 21 percent oxygen, 79 percent nitrogen, plus trace gases.

air embolism: The presence of air bubbles in the heart or blood vessels, causing an obstruction.

air splint: A double-walled plastic tube that immobilizes a limb when sufficient air is blown into the space between the walls of the tube to cause it to become almost rigid.

airway: An air passage.

allergic reaction: A local or general reaction to an allergen, usually characterized by hives or tissue swelling or dyspnea.

allergy: Hypersensitivity to a substance, causing an abnormal reaction.

AMI: Abbreviation for *acute myocardial infarction*.

amnesia: Loss or impairment of memory.

amniotic fluid: The fluid surrounding the fetus in the uterus, contained in the amniotic sac.

amniotic sac: A thick, transparent sac that holds the fetus suspended in the amniotic fluid.

amputation: Complete removal of an appendage.

analgesic: A pain-relieving drug; a class of drugs used to reduce pain.

anaphylaxis: An exaggerated allergic reaction, usually caused by foreign proteins.

anatomic position: The presumed body position when referring to anatomical landmarks; upright, facing the observer, with hands and arms at sides, thumbs pointing away from the body, legs and feet pointing straight ahead.

Adapted from National Highway Traffic Safety Administration, *Emergency Medical Care* (Washington, D.C.: U.S. Government Printing Office).

anesthesia: A partial or complete loss of sensation with or without loss of consciousness; can result from drug administration or from injury or disease.

aneurysm: A permanent blood-filled dilation of a blood vessel resulting from disease or injury of the blood vessel wall.

angina pectoris: A spasmodic pain in the chest, characterized by a sensation of severe constriction or pressure on the anterior chest; associated with insufficient blood supply to the heart, aggravated by exercise or tension, and relieved by rest or medication.

angulation: The formation of an angle; an abnormal angle in an extremity or organ.

anoxia: Without oxygen; a reduction of oxygen in body tissues below required physiology levels.

ante-: A prefix meaning *before* in time or place.

anterior: Situated in front of, or in the forward part of; in anatomy, used in reference to the ventral, or belly, surface of the body.

anti-: A prefix that shows a negative or reversal of the word root placed after it.

antibody: A substance produced in the body in response to an antigen that destroys or inactivates the antigen.

antidote: A substance to counteract or combat the effect of poison.

antigen: A substance that causes the formation of antibodies.

antihistamine: A substance capable of counteracting the effects of histamine.

antipyretic: A class of drugs that reduces fever.

antiseptic: Any preparation that prevents the growth of bacteria.

antivenin: An antiserum containing antibodies against reptile or insect venom.

arm: The upper extremity, specifically that segment between the shoulder and hand.

arterial blood: Oxygenated blood.

artery: A blood vessel, consisting of three layers of tissue and smooth muscle, that carries blood away from the heart.

artificial ventilation: Movement of air into and out of the lungs by artificial means.

asphyxia: Suffocation.

aspirate: To inhale foreign material into the lungs; to remove fluid or foreign material from the lungs or elsewhere by mechanical suction.

aspirin: Salicylic acid acetate; a drug known for its analgesic, fever-reducing, and anti-inflammatory properties.

asthma: A condition marked by recurrent attacks of dyspnea with wheezing, due to spasmodic constriction of the bronchi, often as a response to allergens or to mucous plugs in the bronchioles.

avulsion: An injury that leaves a piece of skin or other tissue either partially or completely torn away from the body.

axilla: The armpit.

axillary temperature: Body temperature measured by placing a thermometer in the axilla while holding the arm close to the body for a period of 10 minutes.

Babinski reflex: A reflex response of movement of the big toe; positive reflex is determined when, as the sole is stroked, the toe turns upward; negative is determined by a downward movement or no movement of the toe.

bag of waters: The amniotic sac and the fluid it contains.

ball-and-socket joint: A joint wherein the distal bone has a rounded head (ball) that fits into the proximal bone's cuplike socket; the hip and shoulder joints, for example.

bandage: A material used to hold a dressing in place.

basal skull fracture: A fraction involving the base of the cranium.

basic life support: Maintenance of the ABCs (airway, breathing, and circulation) without adjunctive equipment.

Battle's sign: A contusion on the mastoid area of either ear; sign of a basal skull fracture.

biological death: A condition present when irreversible brain damage has occurred, usually from 3 to 10 minutes after cardiac arrest.

blanch: To become white or pale.

blister: A collection of fluid under or within the epidermis.

blood: The fluid that circulates through the heart, arteries, capillaries, and veins carrying nutriment and oxygen to the body cells and removing waste products such as carbon dioxide and various metabolic products for excretion.

blood clot: A soft, coherent, jellylike mass resulting from the conversion of fibrinogen to fibrin, thereby entrapping red blood cells and other formed elements in the fibrinic web.

bone: The hard form of connective tissue that constitutes most of the skeleton in a majority of vertebrates.

bowel: See *intestine.*

brachial artery: The artery of the arm that is the continuation of the axillary artery that in turn branches at the elbow into the radial and ulnar arteries. Used to determine an infant's pulse.

brain: The soft, large mass of nerve tissue that is contained in the cranium.

breech birth (breech delivery): Delivery during which the presenting part of the fetus is the buttocks or a foot instead of the head.

bronchial asthma: The common form of asthma.

bruise: An injury that does not break the skin but causes rupture of small underlying blood vessels, with resulting tissue discoloration; a contusion.

burn: An injury caused by heat, electrical current, or a chemical of extreme acidity or alkalinity.

first-degree burn: A burn causing only reddening of the outer layer of skin; sunburn is usually a first-degree burn.

second-degree burn: A burn extending through the outer layer of skin, causing blisters and edema; a scald is usually a second-degree burn.

third-degree burn: A burn extending through all layers of skin, at times through muscle or connective tissue, having a white, leathery look and lacking sensation; grafting is more often necessary with a third-degree burn; a flame burn is usually third-degree.

burn center: A medical facility especially designed, equipped, and staffed to treat severely burned patients.

capillary: Any one of the small blood vessels that connect arteriole and venule and through whose walls various substances pass into and out of the interstitial tissues and thence on to the cells.

carbon monoxide (CO): A colorless, odorless, and dangerous gas formed by incomplete combustion of carbon; it combines four times more quickly with hemoglobin than oxygen; when in the presence of heme, replaces oxygen and reduces oxygen uptake in the lungs.

cardiac arrest: The sudden cessation of cardiac function, with no pulse, no blood pressure, unresponsiveness.

cardiopulmonary arrest: The cessation of cardiac and respiratory activity.

cardiopulmonary resuscitation (CPR): The application of artificial ventilation and external cardiac compression in victims with cardiac arrest to provide adequate circulation to support life.

carotid artery: The principal artery of the neck, palpated easily on either side of the thyroid cartilage.

carpals: The eight small bones of the wrist.

cartilage: A tough, elastic, connective tissue that covers opposite surfaces of movable joints and also forms parts of the skeleton, such as the ear and nose.

caustic: Corrosive; destructive to living tissue.

centigrade scale: The temperature scale in which the freezing point of water is 0° and the boiling point at sea level is 100°.

cerebral contusion: A bruise of the brain, causing a characteristic symptomatic response.

cerebral hemorrhage: Bleeding into the cerebrum; one form of stroke or cerebrovascular accident.

cerebrospinal fluid (CSF): The fluid contained in the four ventricles of the brain and the space around the brain and spinal cord.

cerebrovascular accident (CVA): The sudden cessation of circulation to a region of the brain due to thrombus, embolism, or hemorrhage; also a stroke or apoplexy.

cervical: Pertaining to the neck.

cervical collar: A device used to immobilize and support the neck.

chief complaint: The problem for which a person seeks help, stated in a word or short phrase.

chills: A sensation of cold, with convulsive shaking of the body.

circulatory system: The body system consisting of the heart and blood vessels.

clammy: Damp and usually cool.

clavicle: The collarbone; attached to the uppermost part of the sternum at a right angle and joined to the scapular spine to form the point of the shoulder.

clinical death: A term that refers to the lack of signs of life, when there is no pulse and no blood pressure; occurs immediately after the onset of cardiac arrest.

closed fracture: A fracture in which there is no laceration in the overlying skin.

closed wound: A wound in which there is no tear or cut in the epidermis.

clot: A semisolid mass of fibrin and cells.

coffee grounds vomitus: A vomitus having the appearance and consistency of coffee grounds; indicates slow bleeding in the stomach and represents the vomiting of partially digested blood.

coma: A state of unconsciousness from which the victim cannot be aroused even by powerful stimulation.

comminuted fracture: A fraction in which the bone ends are broken into many fragments.

communicable disease: A disease that is transmissible from one person to another.

compound fracture: An open fracture; a fracture in which there is an open wound of the skin and soft tissues leading down to the location of the fracture.

compress: A folded cloth or pad used for applying pressure to stop hemorrhage or as a wet dressing.

concussion: A violent jar or shock that injures the central nervous system.

conscious: Capable of responding to sensory stimuli and having subjective experiences.

consent: An agreement by a patient or victim to accept treatment offered as explained by medical personnel or first aiders.

implied consent: An assumed consent given by an unconscious adult when emergency lifesaving treatment is required.

informed consent: A consent given by a mentally competent adult who understands what the treatment will involve; it can also be given by the parent or guardian of a child, as defined by the state, or for a mentally incompetent adult.

constrict: To be made smaller by drawing together or squeezing.

constricting band: A band used to restrict the lymphatic flow of blood back to the heart.

contagious: A term that refers to a disease that is readily transmitted from one person to another.

contagious disease: An infectious disease transmissible by direct or indirect contact; now synonymous with *communicable disease.*

contaminated: A term used in reference to a wound or other surface that has been infected with bacteria; may also refer to polluted water, food, or drugs.

contusion: A bruise; an injury that causes a hemorrhage in or beneath the skin but does not break the skin.

convulsion: A violent involuntary contraction or series of contractions of the voluntary muscles; a fit or seizure.

core temperature: Body temperature measured centrally, from within the esophagus or rectum.

coronary: A term applied to the cardiac blood vessels that supply blood to the walls of the heart.

coronary artery: One of the two arteries arising from the aortic sinus to supply the heart muscle with blood.

CPR: Abbreviation for *cardiopulmonary resuscitation.*

cramp: A painful spasm, usually of a muscle; a gripping pain in the abdominal area; colic.

cravat: A type of bandage made from a large triangular piece of cloth and folded to form a band; used as a temporary dressing for a fracture or wound.

crepitus: A grating sound heard and the sensation felt when the fractured ends of a bone rub together.

crowning: The stage of birth when the presenting part of the baby is visible at the vaginal orifice.

CVA: Abbreviation for *cerebrovascular accident.*

cyanosis: A blueness of the skin due to insufficient oxygen in the blood.

defibrillation: Direct current electrical shock applied to stop fibrillation of the heart.

dehydration: Loss of water and electrolytes; excessive loss of body water.

depressed fracture: A skull fracture with impaction, depression, or sinking in of the fragments.

diabetes: A general term referring to disorders characterized by excessive urine excretion, excessive thirst, and excessive hunger.

diabetes mellitus: A systemic disease marked by lack of production of insulin, which causes an inability to metabolize carbohydrates, resulting in an increase in blood sugar.

diabetic coma: Loss of consciousness due to severe diabetes mellitus that has not been treated or to treatment that has not been adequately regulated.

diarrhea: The frequent passage of watery or loose stools.

digestive tract: The passages of tubes leading from the mouth and pharynx to the anus; the alimentary tract; mouth, pharynx, esophagus, stomach, small intestine, large intestine, rectum, and anus.

dilated pupil: A pupil enlarged beyond its normal size.

dilation: The process of expanding or enlarging.

dispatcher: One who transmits calls to service units and vehicles and personnel on assignments.

distal: Farthest from any point on the center or median line; in extremities, farthest from the point of junction of the trunk of the body.

drag: A general term referring to methods of moving victims without a stretcher or litter, usually employed by a single rescuer.

blanket drag: A method by which one rescuer encloses a victim in a blanket and then drags the victim to safety.

clothes drag: A method by which one rescuer can drag a victim to safety by grasping the victim's clothes and pulling him away from danger.

fireman's drag: A method by which one rescuer crawls over a victim, looping the victim's tied wrists over the rescuer's neck to support the victim's weight.

dressing: A protective covering for a wound; used to stop bleeding and to prevent contamination of the wound.

-ectomy: Suffix meaning surgical removal, as in *appendectomy.*

edema: A condition in which fluid escapes into the body tissues from the vascular or lymphatic spaces and causes local or generalized swelling.

electrocution: Death caused by passage of electrical current through the body.

embolism: The sudden blocking of an artery or vein by a clot or foreign material that has been brought to the site of lodgement by the blood current.

emesis: Vomiting.

EMS: Emergency medical services.

EMT: Emergency medical technician.

epidermis: The outermost and nonvascular layer of the skin.

epiglottis: The lidlike cartilaginous structure overhanging the superior entrance to the larynx and serving to prevent food from entering the larynx and trachea during swallowing.

epilepsy: A chronic brain disorder marked by paroxysmal attacks of brain dysfunction, usually associated with some alteration of consciousness, abnormal motor behavior, psychic or sensory disturbances; may be preceded by an aura.

epinephrine: A hormone released by the adrenal medulla that stimulates the sympathetic nervous system, producing vasoconstriction, increased heart rate, and bronchodilation.

epistaxis: Nosebleed.

esophagus: The portion of the digestive tract that lies between the pharynx and the stomach.

exhalation: The act of breathing out: expiration.

extremity: A limb; an arm or a leg.

extrication: Disentanglement; freeing from entrapment.

Fahrenheit scale: The temperature scale in which the freezing point is 32° and the boiling point at sea level is 212°.

fainting: A momentary loss of consciousness caused by insufficient blood supply to the brain; syncope.

feces: The product expelled by the bowels; semisoft waste products of digestion.

femoral artery: The principal artery of the thigh, a continuation of the iliac artery; supplies blood to the lower abdomen wall, the external genitalia, and the lower body extremities; pulse may be palpated in the groin area.

femur: The bone that extends from the pelvis to the knee; the longest and largest bone of the body, the thigh bone.

fever: An elevation of body temperature beyond normal.

fibrillation: Ineffective contractions of the heart muscles.

fibula: The smaller of the two bones of the lower leg; the most lateral bone of the lower leg.

first aid: Immediate care given to the injured or suddenly ill person. First aid does not take the place of proper medical treatment. It consists only of furnishing temporary assistance until competent medical care, *if needed,* is obtained, or until the chance for recovery without medical care is assured.

first-degree burn: A burn causing only reddening of the outer layer of skin; sunburn usually is a first-degree burn.

first responder: A person who has been trained to provide emergency care before the EMTs arrive; usually police or fire fighters.

flail chest: A condition in which several ribs are broken, each in at least two places; a sternal fracture or separation of the ribs from the sternum producing a free-floating segment of the chest wall that moves paradoxically on respiration.

forearm: The part of the upper extremity between the elbow and the wrist.

fracture: A break or rupture in a bone.

closed fracture: A fracture that does not cause a break in the skin; a simple fracture.

comminuted fracture: A fracture in which the bone is shattered.

compound fracture: A fracture in which the bone ends pierce the skin; an open fracture.

greenstick fracture: An incomplete fracture (the bone is not broken all the way through); seen most often in children.

impacted fracture: A fracture in which the ends of the bones are jammed together.

oblique fracture: A fracture in which the break crosses the bone at an angle.

open fracture: A fracture in which the skin is open; a compound fracture.

simple fracture: A fracture in which the skin is not broken; a closed fracture.

spiral fracture: A fracture in which the breakline twists around and through the bone.

transverse fracture: A fracture in which the breakline extends across the bone at a right angle to the long axis.

fracture of the hip: A fracture that occurs at the upper end of the femur, most often at the neck of the femur.

frostbite: The damage to tissues as a result of prolonged exposure to extreme cold.

frostnip: The superficial local tissue destruction caused by freezing; it is limited in scope and does not destroy the full thickness of skin.

gangrene: Local tissue death as the result of an injury or inadequate blood supply.

gastrointestinal tract: The digestive tract, including stomach, small intestine, large intestine, rectum, and anus.

glucose: Blood sugar.

glycogen: Carbohydrates stored in the liver and muscle tissue.

grand mal seizure: A type of epileptic attack; characterized by a short-term, generalized, convulsive seizure.

gullet: The esophagus; the passage from the pharynx to the stomach.

heart: The hollow muscular organ that receives blood from the veins, sends it through the lungs to be oxygenated, then pumps it to the arteries.

heart attack: Lay term for a condition resulting from blockage of a coronary artery and subsequent death of part of the heart muscle; an acute myocardial infarction; sometimes called simply a "coronary."

heat cramp: A painful muscle cramp resulting from excessive loss of salt and water through sweating.

heat exhaustion: A prostration caused by excessive loss of water and salt through sweating; characterized by clammy skin and a weak, rapid pulse.

hematoma: A localized collection of blood in an organ, tissue, or space as a result of injury or a broken blood vessel.

heme: The deep red, iron-containing group of hemoglobin.

hemiplegia: Paralysis of one side of the body.

hemoglobin: The oxygen-carrying substance of the red blood cells.

hemophilia: An inherited blood disease occurring mostly in males, characterized by the inability of the blood to clot.

hemorrhage: Abnormally large amount of bleeding.

hemorrhagic shock: A state of inadequate tissue perfusion due to blood loss.

hemothorax: Bleeding into the thoracic cavity.

hives: Red or white raised patches on the skin, often attended by severe itching; a characteristic reaction in allergic responses.

humerus: The bone of the upper arm.

hyper-: Prefix meaning *excessive* or *increased*.

hyperglycemia: An abnormally increased concentration of sugar in the blood.

hypertension: High blood pressure, usually in reference to a diastolic pressure greater than 90–95 mm Hg.

hyperthermia: An abnormally increased body temperature.

hyperventilation: An increased rate and depth of breathing resulting in an abnormal lowering of arterial carbon dioxide, causing alkalosis.

hyphema: Hemorrhage in the anterior chamber of the eye.

hypo-: A prefix meaning *less than, lack of;* a deficiency.

hypoglycemia: An abnormally diminished concentration of sugar in the blood; insulin shock.

hypothermia: Decreased body temperature.

hypovolemic shock: Shock caused by a reduction in blood volume, such as caused by hemorrhage.

hypoxia: A low oxygen content in the blood; lack of oxygen in inspired air.

immobilize: To hold a part firmly in place, as with a splint.

impaled object: An object that has caused a puncture wound and remains embedded in the wound.

incision: A wound usually made deliberately in connection with surgery; clean cut as opposed to a laceration.

infarction: The death (*necrosis*) of a localized area of tissue caused by the cutting off of its blood supply.

infection: An invasion of a body by disease-producing organisms.

inferior: Anatomically, situated below or the lower surface or part of a structure.

inflammation: A tissue reaction to disease, irritation, or infection; characterized by pain, heat, redness, and swelling.

ingestion: Intake of food or other substances through the mouth.

inhalation: The drawing of air or other substances into the lungs.

insulin: A hormone secreted in the pancreas; essential for the proper metabolism of blood sugar.

insulin shock: Not a true form of shock; hypoglycemia caused by excessive insulin dosage, characterized by sweating, tremor, anxiety, unusual behavior, and vertigo; may cause death of brain cells.

intestine: The portion of the alimentary canal extending from the stomach to the anus.

intoxicate: To poison; commonly, to cause diminished control by means of drugs or alcohol.

ipecac syrup: A medication used to induce vomiting.

-itis: A suffix meaning *inflammation.*

jaw-thrust maneuver: A procedure for opening the airway in which the jaw is lifted and pulled forward to keep the tongue from falling back into the airway.

joint: The point at which two or more bones articulate; also, commonly, a marijuana cigarette.

jugular: Pertaining to the neck; large vein on either side of the neck, draining the head via the *external jugular* or draining the brain via the *internal jugular.*

kidneys: The paired organs that filter blood and produce urine; they also act as adjuncts to keep a proper acid-base balance.

knee: The hinge joint between the femur and the tibia.

labor: The process or period of childbirth; especially, the muscular contractions of the uterus designed to expel the fetus from the mother.

laceration: A wound made by tearing or cutting of body tissues.

ladder splint: A flexible splint consisting of two stout parallel wires and finer crosswires; resembles a ladder.

laryngospasm: A severe constriction of the vocal cords, often in response to allergy or noxious stimuli.

larynx: The organ of voice production.

lateral: Of or toward the side; away from the midline of the body.

leg: The lower limb generally; specifically, that part of the lower limb extending from the knee to the ankle.

lesion: A distinct area of pathologically altered tissue; an injury or wound.

lethal: Fatal.

lethargy: A lack of activity; drowsiness; indifference.

ligament: A tough band of fibrous tissue that connects bone to bone or that supports any organ.

limb presentation: A delivery in which the presenting part of a fetus is an arm or a leg.

linear fracture: A fracture running parallel to the long axis of the bone.

linear skull fracture: A skull fracture that runs in a straight line.

litter: A stretcher.

liver: The large organ in the right upper quadrant of the abdomen that secretes bile, produces many essential proteins, detoxifies many substances, and stores glycogen.

log roll: A method for placing a person on a carrying device, usually a long spineboard or a flat litter; the person is rolled onto his or her side, then back onto the litter.

lungs: The paired organs in the thorax that effect ventilation and oxygenation.

lymph: A straw-colored fluid that circulates in the lymphatic vessels and interstitial space.

mastoid: A portion of the temporal bone that lies behind the ear and contains spongy bone tissue.

medial: Toward the midline of the body.

metacarpal bones: The five cylindrical bones of the hand extending from the wrist to the fingers.

metatarsal bones: The five cylindrical bones of the foot extending from the ankles to the toes.

morbidity: A synonym for illness; generally used to refer to an untoward effect of an illness or injury.

mortality: Refers to death from a given disease or injury; generally thought of as a statistic to state the ratio of death to recovery.

motion sickness: A sensation induced by repetitive motion, characterized by nausea and lightheadedness.

mottled: Characterized by a patchy, discolored appearance.

mouth-to-mouth ventilation: The preferred emergency method of artificial ventilation when adjuncts are not available.

mouth-to-nose ventilation: An emergency method of artificial ventilation when mouth-to-mouth cannot be used.

mucus: A viscid, slippery secretion that lubricates and protects various body structures.

muscle: A tissue composed of elongated cells that have the ability to contract where stimulated, thus causing bone and joints to move or other anatomical structures to be drawn together.

myocardial infarction: The damaging or death of an area of the heart muscle resulting from a lack of blood supplying the area; a heart attack.

nausea: An unpleasant sensation, vaguely referred to the epigastrium and abdomen, often culminating in vomiting.

necrosis: The death of an area of tissue, usually caused by the cessation of blood supply.

nerve: A cordlike structure composed of a collection of fibers that conveys impulses between a part of the central nervous system and some other region.

nervous system: The brain, spinal cord, and nerve branches from the central, peripheral, and autonomic systems.

nitroglycerin: A drug used in the treatment of angina pectoris.

noxious: Injurious.

oblique fracture: A fracture that runs diagonally to the long axis of the bone.

occipital: Pertaining to the back of the head.

ointment: A semisolid preparation for external application to the body, usually containing a medicinal substance.

open fracture or dislocation: A fracture or dislocation exposed to the exterior; an open wound lies over the fracture or dislocation.

open wound: A wound in which the affected tissues are exposed by an external opening.

oral: Pertaining to the mouth.

-otomy: A suffix meaning surgical incision into an organ, as in tracheotomy.

oxygen: A colorless, odorless, tasteless gas that is essential to life and that makes up 21 percent of the atmosphere; chemical formula: O_2.

pallor: A paleness of the skin.

palpation: The act of palpating; the act of feeling with the hands for the purpose of determining the consistency of the part beneath.

palpitation: A sensation felt under the left breast when the heart "skips a beat" because of premature ventricular contractions.

paralysis: Loss or impairment of motor function of a part due to a lesion of the neural or muscular mechanism.

paraplegia: The loss of both sensation and motion in the lower extremities, most commonly due to damage to the spinal cord.

patella: A small, flat bone that protects the knee joint; the kneecap.

pediatrics: The medical specialty devoted to the diagnosis and treatment of diseases of children.

penetrate: To pierce; to pass into the deeper tissues or into a cavity.

perfusion: The act of pouring through or into; the blood suffusing the cells in order to exchange gases, nutrients, etc., with the cells.

petit mal seizure: A type of epileptic attack characterized by a momentary loss of awareness but not accompanied by loss of motor tone.

pharynx: The portion of the airway between the nasal cavity and the larynx.

placenta: The vascular organ attached to the uterine wall that supplies oxygen and nutrients to the fetus; also called *afterbirth*.

pneumothorax: An accumulation of air in the pleural cavity usually entering after a wound or injury that causes a penetration of the chest wall or laceration of the lung.

point tenderness: An area of tenderness limited to two or three centimeters in diameter; point tenderness can be located in any area of the body; usually associated with acute inflammation, as in peritonitis (abdominal point tenderness).

posterior: Situated in the back of or behind a surface.

presenting part: The part of the baby that emerges first during delivery.

pressure dressing: A dressing with which enough pressure is applied over a wound site to stop bleeding.

pressure point: One of several places on the body where the blood flow of a given artery can be restricted by pressing the artery against an underlying bone.

pressure splints: An inflatable plastic circumferential splint that can be applied to an extremity and inflated to achieve stability after a fracture.

prognosis: The probable outcome of a disease based on assumptive knowledge.

prolapsed cord delivery: A delivery in which the umbilical cord appears at the vaginal opening before the head of the infant.

prone: A position of lying face down.

psychogenic shock: A fainting spell resulting from transient generalized cerebral ischemia; not a true shock condition.

psychosomatic: An indication of an illness in which some part of the cause is related to emotional factors.

pulse rate: The heart rate determined by counting the number of pulsations occurring in any superficial artery.

pump failure: A partial or total failure of the heart to pump blood effectively.

pupil: The small opening in the center of the iris.

quadrant: One of the four quarters of the abdomen.

quadriplegia: Paralysis of both the arms and the legs.

radial artery: One of the major arteries of the forearm; the pulse is palpable at the base of the thumb.

radiation sickness: The condition that follows excessive irradiation from any source.

radius: The bone on the thumb side of the forearm.

rape: Sexual intercourse by force.

rash: An eruption of the skin, either localized or generalized.

rectal temperature: The core body temperature obtained by inserting a thermometer into the rectum and retaining it for a minute; normally 1°F higher than oral temperature.

regurgitation: A backward flowing, as the casting up of undigested food from the stomach to the mouth.

respiration: The act of breathing; the exchange of oxygen and carbon dioxide in the tissues and lungs.

respiratory arrest: The cessation of breathing.

respiratory system: The system of organs that controls the inspiration of oxygen and the expiration of carbon dioxide.

resuscitation: The act of reviving an unconscious victim.

rib: One of the 24 bones forming the thoracic cavity wall.

rigid splint: A splint made of a firm material that can be applied to an injured extremity to prevent motion at the site of a fracture or dislocation.

roller dressing: A strip of rolled-up material used for dressings.

Rothberg position: Heart attack victim placed in sitting position with legs up and bent at the knees.

saliva: The clear, alkaline fluid secreted by the salivary glands.

scab: A crust formed by the coagulation of blood, pus, serum, or any combination of these on the surface of an ulcer, erosion, abrasion, or any other type of wound.

scapula: The shoulder blade.

sclera: The white, opaque, outer layer of the eyeball.

second-degree burn: A burn penetrating beneath the superficial skin layers, producing edema and blisters.

seizure: A sudden attack or recurrence of a disease; a convulsion; an attack of epilepsy.

semiconscious: Stuporous; partially conscious.

shell temperature: The temperature of the extremities and surface of the body.

shivering: A trembling from cold or fear; it produces heat by muscular contractions.

shock: A state of inadequate tissue perfusion that may be a result of pump failure (cardiogenic shock), volume loss or sequestration (hypovolemic shock), vasodilation (neurogenic shock), or any combination of these.

anaphylactic shock: A rapidly occurring state of collapse caused by hypersensitivity to drugs or other foreign materials (insect venom, certain foods, inhaled allergens); symptoms may include hives, wheezing, tissue edema, bronchospasm, and vascular collapse.

septic shock: A shock developing in the presence of, and as a result of, severe infection.

sign: Any objective evidence or physical manifestation of a disease

simple fracture: A fracture that is not compound; the skin is not broken over the break in the bone.

skeleton: The hard, bony structure that forms the main support of the body.

skin: The outer integument or covering of the body, consisting of the dermis and the epidermis; the largest organ of the body, it contains various sensory and regulatory mechanisms.

skull: The bony structure surrounding the brain; it consists of the cranial bones, the facial bones, and the teeth.

sling: A triangular bandage applied around the neck to support an injured upper extremity; any material long enough to suspend an upper extremity by passing the material around the neck; used to support and protect an injury of the arm, shoulder, or clavicle.

sling and swathe: A bandage in which the arm is placed in a sling and is bound to the body by another bandage placed around the chest and arm to hold the arm close to the body.

small intestine: The portion of the intestine between the stomach and the colon.

snowblindness: Obscured vision caused by sunlight reflected off snow.

spasm: A sudden, violent, involuntary contraction of a muscle or group of muscles attended by pain and interference with function; a sudden but transitory constriction of a passage, canal, or orifice.

spineboard: A wooden or metal device primarily used for extrication and transportation of victims with actual or suspected spinal injuries.

spiral fracture: A fracture in which the line of break runs diagonally around the long axis of the bone.

spleen: The largest lymphatic organ of the body; located in the left upper quadrant of the abdomen.

splint: Any support used to immobilize a fracture or to restrict movement of a part.

sprain: A trauma to a joint that injures the ligaments.

sputum: Expectorated matter, especially mucus or matter resulting from diseases of the air passages.

status asthmaticus: A severe, prolonged asthmatic attack that cannot be broken with epinephrine.

status epilepticus: The occurrence of two or more seizures with a period of complete consciousness between them.

sterile: Free from living organisms, such as bacteria.

sterilize: To render sterile or free from bacterial contamination; to make an organism unable to reproduce.

sternum: The long, flat bone located in the midline in the anterior part of the thoracic cage; articulates above with the clavicles and along the sides with the cartilages of the first seven ribs.

stomach: A hollow digestive organ in the epigastrium that receives food from the esophagus.

stool: Feces; the matter discharged at defecation.

stove-in chest: See *flail chest*.

strain: An injury to a muscle caused by a violent contraction or an excessive, forcible stretching.

stretcher: A carrying device that enables two or more persons to lift and carry a person who is lying down.

stroke: A cerebrovascular accident of sudden onset.

sublingual: Under the tongue.

sucking chest wound: An open pneumothorax.

suffocate: To impede breathing; to asphyxiate.

suicide: The act of deliberately taking one's own life.

sunstroke: A form of heatstroke due to prolonged sun exposure.

superior: In anatomy, used to refer to an organ or part that is located above another organ or part.

supine: Lying in a face-upward position.

suture: The material used to close a surgical wound or to repair a gaping wound.

swathe: A cravat tied around the body to decrease movement of a part.

symptom: A subjective sensation or awareness of disturbance of bodily function.

syncope: Fainting; a brief period of unconsciousness.

syndrome: A complex of symptoms and signs characteristic of a condition.

synovial fluid: A clear fluid that lubricates joints; it is secreted by the synovial membrane.

tachycardia: Abnormally rapid heart rate, over 100 beats per minute.

tarsal: Pertaining to the tarsus (the ankle).

temperature: The degree of heat of a living body; varies in cold-blooded animals with environmental temperature and is constant, within a narrow range for warm-blooded animals; 98.6°F oral temperature and 99.6°F rectal are considered normal for humans.

tendon: A tough band of dense, fibrous, connective tissue that attaches muscles to bone and other parts.

tetanus: An infectious disease caused by the bacteria *Clostridium tetani* that is usually introduced through a wound, characterized by extreme body rigidity and spasms of voluntary body muscles.

thermal: Pertaining to heat.

thigh: The portion of the lower extremity between the hip and the knee.

third-degree burn: A full-thickness burn destroying all skin layers and underlying tissue; has a charred or white, leathery appearance and is insensitive.

thoracic: Pertaining to the chest.

thrombosis: Formation of a blood clot, or *thrombus*.

tibia: The larger of the two bones in the leg; the shinbone.

tissue: An aggregation of similarly specialized cells and their intercellular substance, united in the performance of a particular function.

tourniquet: A constrictive device used on the extremities to impede venous blood return to the heart or obstruct arterial blood flow to the extremities.

toxin: Any poison manufactured by plant or animal life.

trachea: The cartilaginous tube extending from the larynx to its division into the primary bronchi; the windpipe.

traction: The act of exerting a pulling force.

transient ischemic attack (TIA): Symptoms of a stroke lasting from several minutes to several hours, with a return to normal neurological function.

triage: A system used for sorting victims to determine the order in which they will receive medical attention.

triangular bandage: A piece of cloth cut in the shape of a right-angle triangle; used as a sling or folded for a cravat bandage.

trunk: The body excluding the head and limbs; the torso.

ulcer: An open lesion of the skin or mucous membrane.

ulna: The larger bone of the forearm, on the side opposite that of the thumb.

umbilical cord: The flexible structure that connects the fetus to the placenta.

umbilicus: The navel.

unconscious: Without awareness; comatose.

universal access number: A telephone number that can be called in emergency situations and that ties in with the police, fire, and emergency medical services; in most areas the number is 9-1-1.

universal dressing: A large (9-in. by 36-in.) dressing of multilayered material that can be used open, folded, or rolled to cover most wounds, to pad splints, or to form a cervical collar.

uterus: The muscular organ that holds and nourishes the fetus, opening into the vagina through the cervix; the womb.

vagina: The canal in the female extending from the uterus to the vulva; the birth canal.

vasoconstriction: The narrowing of the diameter of a blood vessel.

vein: Any blood vessel that carries blood from the tissues to the heart.

venom: A poison, usually derived from reptiles or insects.

venous blood: Unoxygenated blood, containing hemoglobin in the carboxyhemoglobin state.

ventilation: Breathing; supplying of fresh air to the lungs.

ventricular fibrillation: A rapid, tremulous, and ineffectual contraction of the cardiac myofibrils, producing no cardiac output; cardiac arrest.

vertebrae: The 33 bones of the spinal column.

vertigo: Dizziness; a hallucination of movement; a sensation that the external world is spinning; it may be right or left, upward or downward.

vital signs: The indication of life through values that reflect mental status, blood pressure, pulse rate, and respiration rate.

vitreous fluid: A jellylike, transparent substance filling the inside of the eyeball.

voice box: The larynx.

vomiting: The forceful, active expulsion of stomach contents through the mouth, as opposed to regurgitation, which is passive.

vomitus: The matter ejected from the stomach by vomiting.

wheal: A swelling on the skin, produced by a sting, an injection, external force, or internal reaction.

wheeze: A high-pitched, whistling sound characterizing an obstruction or spasm of the lower airways.

windchill factor: The relationship of wind velocity and temperature in determining the effect of cold on a living organism.

windpipe: The trachea.

womb: The uterus.

wrist: The joint or the region of the joint between the forearm and the hand.

xiphoid process: The sword-shaped cartilaginous process at the lowest portion of the sternum that ossifies in the aged and has no ribs attached to it.

Photo and Illustration Credits

Part 1
Opener   © Kenneth Murray, Photo Researchers, Inc.

Chapter 1
Opener   © Mark E. Gibson

Chapter 2
Opener   © Brian Peters, Masterfile

Part II
Opener   © Howard M. Paul

Chapter 3
Opener   Digital Imagery © 2000 PhotoDisc, Inc.; **Figures 3-3B, 3-4, 3-5, 3-6, 3-8, 3-9, 3-10, 3-11, 3-12, 3-13, 3-15** courtesy of American Academy of Orthopaedic Surgeons (AAOS)

Chapter 4
Opener   © 1998 Bob Winsett/Index Stock Imagery/Picture-Quest; **Figure 4-2**, D-O-T-S Skill Scan Steps 1 and 4 courtesy of AAOS

Part III
Opener   Digital Imagery © 2000 PhotoDisc, Inc.

Chapter 5
Opener   © Bruce Ayres, Tony Stone

Chapter 6
Opener   © 1988 Peter Menzel/Stock, Boston/PictureQuest; **Figure 6-8A** courtesy of AAOS

Part IV
Opener   © Audrey Gibson

Chapter 7
Opener   © Christopher Morris/Black Star Publishing/PictureQuest; **Figures 7-2, 7-12, 7-15A & B** courtesy of AAOS; **Figure 7-8B** courtesy of Dr. Lawrence B. Slack; **Figures 7-7, 7-10** © Howard Backer

Chapter 8
Opener   © Frank Pedrick/Index Stock Imagery/PictureQuest

Chapter 9
Opener   © Owen Franken/Stock, Boston/PictureQuest; **Figure 9-2** courtesy of AAOS; **9-6** © Howard Backer

Chapter 10
Opener   © 1992 Tim Lynch/Stock, Boston/PictureQuest; **Figures 10-1, 10-2** courtesy of AAOS

Chapter 11
Opener   © Custom Medical Stock Photo; **Figure 11-3** courtesy of North Carolina EMSC Prehospital

Chapter 12
Opener   © 1999 Jim Pickerell/Stock Connection/PictureQuest

Chapter 13
Opener   Steve Ferry, P & F Communications; **Figure 13-3** courtesy of AAOS

Chapter 14
Opener   © Custom Medical Stock Photo

Part V
Opener   Mike Bucy, Fireshots.com © Emergency Media Services

Chapter 15
Opener   © Wedgworth, Custom Medical Stock Photo; **Figure 15-11** courtesy of AAOS

Chapter 16
Opener   © 1991, Stephen Agricola/Stock, Boston/Picture-Quest; **Figure 16-3** courtesy of AAOS; **Figure 16-4** © Bachmann/Photo Researchers; **Figure 16- 5** © Richard Sobol/Stock, Boston/PNI; **Figure 16-6** © CNRI/Phototake/PNI; **Figure 16-7** © Michael Newman/Photoedit/PNI

Chapter 17
Opener   © David Dennis, Animals Animals; **Figure 17-2** reproduced with permission from the Journal of the AVMA; **Figure 17-12** courtesy of Bruce Paton; **Figure 17-13B** © Kim Taylor, 1989; **Figure 17-13D** © Ron Sanford; **Figure 17-26** © Eric Popp, 1994; **Figure 17-27** © Chris Seaborn, Tony Stone Images; **Figure 17-28** © Doug Perrine, Innerspace Visions; **Figure 17-29** © Kevin McDonnell, 1995; **Figure 17-30** © M. Mesgleski, 1989

Chapter 18
Opener   © Howard Backer

Part VI
Opener   © 1995 Patrick Ward/Stock, Boston/PictureQuest

Chapter 19
Opener   © Bob Daemmrich/Stock, Boston/PictureQuest

Chapter 20
Opener   Peter Baker Studios; **Figures 20-2, 20-3, 20-4** reproduced with permission from Mayo Clinic *Complete Book of Pregnancy and Baby's First Year*; William Morrow and Co., New York, NY. © 1994 Mayo Foundation of Education and Research; Childbirth Skill Scan images courtesy of AAOS

Chapter 21
Opener   © Linda Gheen; **Figures 21-1A–C**, courtesy of Ron Dieckmann, MD

Chapter 22
Opener   © Rob Matheson/The Stock Market; **Figures 22-1, 22-4, 22-6, 22-10, 22-11** courtesy of AAOS; **22-7** © Ray Nelson, 1994; **Figure 22.9** © Daniel E. Marks

Chapter 23
Opener   © Mark E. Gibson

Appendix B
Figure B-1 courtesy of AAOS; **Figure B-2** © Andrea Randolph

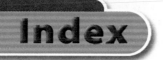

Reference Guide